Encyclopedia of Pestilence,
Pandemics, and Plagues

ADVISORY BOARD

Ann G. Carmichael, Co-Director of the Center for the Study of the History of Medicine, Indiana University

Katharine Donahue, Head of History and Special Collections, Louise M. Darling Biomedical Library, UCLA

John Parascandola, President of the American Association for the History of Medicine (2006), former Chief of the History of Medicine Division (HMD) of the National Library of Medicine, and Public Health Services Historian in the U.S. Department of Health and Human Services

Christopher Ryland, Assistant Director for Special Collections at Vanderbilt University's Annette and Irwin Eskind Biomedical Library

William C. Summers, Professor of Molecular Biophysics and Biochemistry and Professor of History of Science and Medicine at Yale University

Encyclopedia of Pestilence, Pandemics, and Plagues

Volume 1, A–M

Edited by
JOSEPH P. BYRNE

Foreword by
Anthony S. Fauci, M.D.

GREENWOOD PRESS
Westport, Connecticut • London

Library of Congress Cataloging-in-Publication Data

Encyclopedia of pestilence, pandemics, and plagues / edited by Joseph P. Byrne ; foreword by Anthony S. Fauci.
     p. cm.
  Includes bibliographical references and index.
  ISBN: 978-0-313-34101-4 (set : alk. paper)
  ISBN: 978-0-313-34102-1 (v. 1 : alk. paper)
  ISBN: 978-0-313-34103-8 (v. 2 : alk. paper)
  1. Epidemics—Encyclopedias.   2. Communicable diseases—Encyclopedias.   I. Byrne, Joseph Patrick.
  [DNLM: 1. Disease Outbreaks—Encyclopedias—English. 2. Communicable Diseases—Encyclopedias—English. WA 13 E564 2008]
RA652.E535   2008
614.4003—dc2   2008019487

British Library Cataloguing in Publication Data is available.

Library of Congress Catalog Card Number: 2008019487
ISBN: 978–0–313–34101–4 (set)
       978–0–313–34102–1 (vol. 1)
       978–0–313–34103–8 (vol. 2)

First published in 2008

Greenwood Press, 88 Post Road West, Westport, CT 06881
An imprint of Greenwood Publishing Group, Inc.
www.greenwood.com

Printed in the United States of America

The paper used in this book complies with the Permanent Paper Standard issued by the National Information Standards Organization (Z39.48-1984).

10 9 8 7 6 5 4 3 2 1

Contents

List of Entries

Guide to Related Topics

Epidemiology

Factors in Disease Outbreaks

Institutions

Medical Personnel

Foreword

Pandemics, epidemics, and infectious diseases have long been the deadliest challenges to human existence, greatly outstripping wars, accidents, and chronic diseases as a cause of mortality. They have filled history books and have been woven into the fabric of popular and religious culture: examples include the Pharaonic "plagues" of the Old Testament and the many later "plagues" of ancient Greece and Rome; the writings of Boccaccio, Machaut, and Petrarch about the Black Death; Daniel Defoe's long-running 1722 best seller memorializing London's 1665 plague epidemic, *A Journal of the Plague Year*; and the dying consumptive heroines of Dumas and Murger, widely read and then reimagined operatically in *La Traviata* and *La Bohème*.

Much about infectious diseases has changed in the modern era, with the availability of vaccines, antimicrobial therapy and other interventions; however, much remains eerily familiar. We still face the unpredictable appearance of new diseases such as SARS, H5N1 avian influenza, and HIV/AIDS. We still read and see and listen to the plague artistry of earlier times, with the same morbid fascination, but we also find and cherish contemporary "plague art." Popular histories about epidemics continue to become best sellers, such as John Barry's *The Great Influenza*, about the 1918–1919 pandemic. *Outbreak*, a film about a deadly viral pandemic threat, has been seen by millions of people and remains popular more than a decade after its 1995 release. "Andromeda strain," taken from the title of a 1969 book about a potentially world-ending pandemic, has even entered the standard English vocabulary.

Although a deep-seated public fascination with plagues, pestilences, and pandemics is obvious, many encyclopedic works on the subject already sit on library shelves. Is there anything new to say in 2008 that has not already been said countless times before? I think the answer is a resounding *Yes*. Our understanding of infectious diseases has grown steadily in the past two decades, thanks in large part to the new tools of molecular biology. Much of this new knowledge is incorporated into the entries in this encyclopedia.

Let us put this new knowledge into perspective. More than a century ago, Robert Koch's 1876 publication on anthrax, the first fully characterized infectious disease, was followed by an explosion of microbiological knowledge. A new "microbial era" quickly produced passive immunotherapies, vaccines, and antimicrobials. Long before 1900, scientists began to predict the eventual eradication of infectious diseases. Unfortunately, optimism was premature: old epidemic diseases such as tuberculosis and dengue fever simply refused to go away, and more than 30 new ones have been recognized in the past four decades alone.

The U.S. Institute of Medicine's influential 1992 report—*Emerging Infections: Microbial Threats to Health in the United States*—took a new approach, one that profoundly impacted our thinking about "newly emerging" and "reemerging" infectious diseases. Since that report, it has become more widely recognized that men and microbes exist in complex dynamic ecosystems that are continually perturbed and unsettled not only by interactions between the microbes and humans themselves, but also by human movement, crowding, climate, environmental damage, and many other interrelated factors. With their superior ability to adapt to new ecologic opportunities by rapid replication and genetic change (e.g., by mutation), microbes always threaten to gain the upper hand over their slowly evolving human counterparts. Such microbial genetic advantages must be offset by human ingenuity and by a broader understanding of infections in their total context. This includes not only variables of the microbial agent, the human host, and the environment, but also the impact of societal choices, behaviors, and policies on disease emergence, spread, and control. Addressing the problem in this way requires not only the efforts of basic scientists, epidemiologists, and physicians, but also entomologists, environmental specialists, policy makers, bioinformatics experts, and many others, working together in interdisciplinary partnership.

Pestilence, pandemics, and plagues have always been among the greatest challenges to continued human existence. In learning about them we learn about who we are and about our human history, and we make connections across millennia that reinforce our identity, our heritage, and our shared human experience. The more we learn about emerging infectious diseases, the more we understand how deadly and persistent the challenge is and will remain, and the better able we will be to respond to future challenges that the microbial world is certain to present to us.

Readers should find this encyclopedia stimulating and informative. There are many lessons to be learned, but among the most important is this: the next pandemic waits in the wings for some convergence of critical determinants not yet imagined by any of us. How we respond may make a difference not only for ourselves, but for the rest of the world as well.

Anthony S. Fauci, M.D., Director of the National Institute of Allergy
and Infectious Diseases of the National Institutes of Health

Preface

This encyclopedia of infectious diseases in history grew out of a proposal for an encyclopedia of the Black Death that followed two volumes I wrote for Greenwood Press on the second plague pandemic. Greenwood's editors were correct to suggest a much broader, interdisciplinary work, given that existing works on the history of epidemic disease tended to be either chronological or topical by disease, or topical by place. Given the opportunity, I engaged a truly first-rate editorial board of medical historians, M.D.s, a microbiologist, and medical history librarians.

With their indispensable help, I crafted a list of entries that would take the nonspecialist advanced high school or college student from the basics of bacteria and viruses, through the intricacies of the human body and immunity to disease, to the major infectious diseases (and some others of growing relevance). Historical outbreaks constituted a second category of entries. We chose the major pandemics of plague, influenza, and cholera, of course, but we also included more tightly focused outbreaks that allowed for a closer analysis of the phenomena, their impacts, and the ways people dealt with them. A third major group of articles, we felt, needed to discuss the range of care-giving and treatments that developed independently of or in response to the great disease outbreaks. Physicians, nurses, pharmacists, hospitals, leprosaria, sanatoria, as well as sulfa drugs and antibiotics found their places in these pages. Related to these entries are those outlining major theories of disease and medicine that dictated cultural responses to epidemic disease. Desiring to be synthetic as well as specific in coverage, we decided to commission a series of longer entries on historical (and contemporary) factors that have affected the emergence and spread of epidemic diseases. Some of these are natural (air, water, the environment) but many are social, economic, and political: colonialism, war, poverty, urbanization, and the sexual revolution, for example. A final broad category covers effects or responses to disease, including media and artistic responses, international health organizations, and effects on personal liberties. We chose these categories and topics with a view to both the basics and to geographical and chronological diversity. We make no claims of completeness or comprehensiveness but do hope that we have provided a variety of materials that will stimulate and aid research, both informing and leading the reader to other fruitful sources.

To aid internal searching, we have provided an alphabetical list of all entries in the front matter, as well as an index at the end of Volume 2. Each entry includes a list of related entries under "See also," while terms with their own entries that appear in the text are boldfaced for easy identification.

Arcing across the nearly 300 articles are certain themes that should serve a student well: colonialism, war, the development of Western medicine, the roles of migration and modern globalization, and the continuing plight and challenges of much of the underdeveloped world in the face of established and emerging diseases. We have chosen some of these themes and grouped relevant entries in the Guide to Related Topics that follows the List of Entries in the front matter. Entries have been written and edited for use by students with minimal backgrounds in biology, and a glossary of predominantly biomedical terms has been appended. Each entry has a list of suggested readings, and many have useful Websites. A broad bibliography of Websites, books, and articles appears at the end of Volume 2.

In acknowledging my own debts to those who made this work possible, I would like to begin with the 101 authors from around the world who lent this project their time and expertise. The outstanding credentials of our editorial board members—Ann Carmichael, Katharine Donahue, John Parascandola, Christopher Ryland, and William Summers—are listed elsewhere, but let me assure the reader that without their contributions from conception to final editing, these volumes would have but a fraction of their merit. Each has gone well beyond any contractual obligations, each in his or her own ways, and any and all flaws are mine alone. Greenwood Press has provided me with a very helpful and supportive editor in Mariah Gumpert who has overseen this work from start to finish. I also wish to acknowledge the local efforts of Sarah Bennett, who developed the illustration program for the encyclopedia, Rebecca and Elizabeth Repasky who compiled the glossary and edited portions of the text, and Elizabeth Schriner who gathered many of the Website citations scattered about these pages. Finally, I wish to thank Belmont University, my home institution, for providing me with the academic leave and many of the means necessary to pull this project together.

Introduction

In *War of the Worlds*, English novelist H. G. Wells presented the gravest of imaginable threats to human life on earth: bellicose extraterrestrial invaders. Humanity laid prostrate, our weapons useless, our future bleak. The final outcome reflected Wells's genius as well as his time: simple terrestrial germs killed off the mighty aliens, and the war was won. What caused humans mere mild discomfort proved fatal to the beings whose bodies were not prepared for the microbial onslaught. Of course, this has long been part of the human condition on our own planet. Epidemiologists call this phenomenon a "virgin-soil epidemic," and throughout history human populations have lost their battles with "simple terrestrial germs." Plague killed perhaps 40 percent of the Western world in the late 1340s; Mayas and Aztecs fell by the tens of thousands to the measles and smallpox brought by European colonists; and in the nineteenth century, Africa's pathogen-rich environment earned it the fitting nickname "white man's graveyard."

We literally swim in a sea of germs, and our bodies are coated inside and out with a wide range of bacteria, viruses, mites, fungi, and other tiny hitchhikers. Most are benign, many helpful, and some potentially harmful. But add the wrong microbe into the mix, and the mighty human organism, like Wells's Martians, shudders and halts—and may shut down altogether.

When these microbes can be transmitted to other people, we call the resulting illnesses infectious disease. When the same disease extends across a broad population, we call it an epidemic. Anthropologists generally agree that humans became susceptible to epidemics when we settled in large villages and early cities in the later Neolithic period of human prehistory. Our own "war of the worlds"—the human organism vs. deadly microorganisms—has thus been going on for thousands of years, and until recently we have unvaryingly lost. And although modern science has reduced many former scourges to minor threats, we remain locked in mortal combat with many—both old and new—and in apprehension of the next wave of pathogenic assault. The founders of the scientific method noted that we have to understand nature and its processes before we can control them, but knowledge about microbes came very recently and still does not ensure victory.

Thirty years before this writing, scientists, policy-makers, doctors, volunteers, nurses, donors, and civil servants finally eliminated deadly smallpox from nature. But though it was the first, it is still the only human disease to be eradicated, despite the best intentions and efforts of experts, technicians, officials, and men and women of good will. Each year the World Health Organization and the U.S. Centers for Disease Control and Prevention monitor the fluctuating incidence of a long list of diseases and the lives they take. Old standards such as malaria, tuberculosis, and polio beef up the statistics, as do recent arrivals such as AIDS, Lyme disease, and West Nile Fever, and reemerging conditions such as cholera and Hansen's disease (leprosy). Footnotes account for the patterns of flux: wars, changing economic and social conditions, new encroachments on virgin natural areas, human migration, and natural processes such as genetic mutation and environmental change. Through jet travel, a minor, local outbreak of an exotic disease can find its way into dozens or hundreds of human communities within days. The "war" is far from over.

There is an ongoing flow of books that tell the story of "man vs. microbe," or narrow parts of it, and many of these are listed at the end of entries or in the bibliography at the end of these two volumes. These serve the general reading public as well as the historian and student of medical history. The present work cannot replace a ripping good medical yarn, and its editor and his collaborators have no intention of trying to do so. Instead we seek to place in the hands of the interested lay reader or student a collection of thought-stimulating and question-answering essays that will complement deeper research or merely provide accurate, condensed information to the curious. The fact that sites on the Internet seem capable of doing just this may seem to make a work like ours, or any reference book, rather quaint and clumsy by comparison. In fact, each of our contributors has taken the Web, as well as other publications, into account in preparing the present articles. The result is a sound, authoritative source covering a very wide and interdisciplinary range of topics connected to the history and science of infectious disease.

As I edited each entry and added the bolding to cross-listed terms, and compiled the "see also" lists, I was struck by and increasingly satisfied with the rich texture of interrelationships among the entries. Each reader, each student preparing to write on a relevant topic, should make use of the several tools that we have provided to help one profit from this texture. Each entry mentions related entries and provides recent or classic books and/or articles on its topic. The List of Entries—and, even better, the Guide to Related Topics—goes further in suggesting relationships between subjects. The index gives a quick overview of topics that go beyond the entry titles, and provides a clear gauge of the depth of coverage in these two volumes.

The types of discussion that fall under the broad heading of infectious disease are far more varied than may first seem evident. If I consider my senior year in high school, I can imagine using this volume in English Lit (seventeenth-century plague literature); U.S. History II (Spanish Flu in 1918 to 1919); Advanced Biology (any given disease); fourth-year German (Thomas Mann and his tuberculosis); and Religion (comparative religious theories of disease). At the other end, our essays on topics such as "News Media and Epidemic Disease," "War, the Military, and Epidemic Disease," "Colonialism and Epidemic Disease," or "Urbanization and Epidemic Disease" could spawn and help shape senior or even masters-level university theses. Teachers preparing units or professors preparing courses on medical history or disease in history will find our content stimulating and relevant, and, we believe, written at a level appropriate to our students. As I stated in the Preface, this work is by no means comprehensive or definitive, nor is it meant to be. If the reader is patient and systematic, however, I firmly believe it will prove to be very useful indeed.

A

ACQUIRED IMMUNE DEFICIENCY SYNDROME. *See* Human Immunodeficiency Virus/Acquired Immune Deficiency Syndrome (HIV/AIDS).

AIDS. *See* Human Immunodeficiency Virus/Acquired Immune Deficiency Syndrome (HIV/AIDS).

AIDS IN AFRICA. Over 25 years have gone by since the onset of the **Human Immunodeficiency Virus/Acquired Immune Deficiency Syndrome**, or HIV/AIDS, **pandemic** in the world, and yet the syndrome continues to take lives throughout the developing world, particularly in Sub-Saharan Africa. In the 10 worst affected countries, all of them in eastern and southern Africa, rates of HIV infection range from 16 percent to over 40 percent. Estimates by United Nations AIDS (UNAIDS) indicate that at the end of the year 2007, 22.5 million people were living with HIV in Africa, and that approximately 1.7 million additional people were infected with HIV during that year. During the same year, over 1.6 million people were estimated to have died from this syndrome. Since its onset in the 1980s, well over 11 million **children** on the continent have been orphaned by AIDS.

Initial Response to the Epidemic. Given these staggering statistics, many have observed that the human and social ramifications of AIDS are complex and wide-ranging. They threaten stability, exacerbate inequalities within and between countries, undermine previous gains in development, and harm children. At the onset of the **epidemic** in the early 1980s, initial responses were often guided by fear and ignorance. At that time, AIDS evoked intense fear in the United States, where many began a clarion call for **quarantine**—which historically has been the usual method of dealing with epidemics. The call for quarantine was made in spite of the fact that previous efforts to control epidemics such as **leprosy, cholera, tuberculosis,** and drug addiction through quarantine of large numbers of people were never successful. Association of the disease with homosexuality and Afro-Caribbeans from Haiti added layers of stigma to both victims and the disease itself.

By the mid-1980s, the disease was reported in Rakai District in Uganda, as well as other central African countries. Although the geographic origins of AIDS may never be known, at that time many Western scholars, including prominent geographers in the United States, began to point a finger at Africa as the origin of the **virus**. Indeed, the complex but hypothetical map drawn by Gary Shannon, Gerald Pyle, and Rashid Bashshur in 1991, showing the routes that the epidemic took to diffuse from Central Africa via Europe and Haiti to America, became accepted as the truth rather than as mere speculation on the part of these authors. This unleashed hysteria throughout the developed world. Specifically, Belgium began testing African students for the virus, arguing that it was useless to invest scholarships in students who were ill and were soon going to die. Similarly, the U.S. government under President Ronald Reagan (1911–2004) advocated the quarantining, deportation, or denial of entry visas to those with the virus.

As the pandemic began to spread rapidly in the late 1980s in Sub-Saharan Africa among men and women (i.e., heterosexual as opposed to homosexual transmission), some scholars began to offer prejudiced explanations as to why it was spreading so rapidly. They stated that the virus had jumped from monkeys to humans because Africans were having sex with monkeys. Others stated that it had jumped to humans through the peculiarities of African culture in which Africans applied monkey blood to their genitals as an aphrodisiac. Since the disease in the United States was initially found among homosexual men, some scholars set out to uncover homosexuality in Africa, even when the facts failed to support their paradigm. Indeed, on the assumption that homosexuality is a universal phenomenon, scholars looked across the continent to find homosexual populations, gay bathhouses, and other elements of a homosexual cultural landscape. Failing to find this evidence, they concluded that African homosexuality must be carefully concealed.

These ethnocentric and racist explanations from the developed countries, combined with the fear of stigmatization, denial of entry visas by Western countries, and the possible loss of the lucrative tourist **trade**, resulted in vehement denials by many African leaders about the existence of the epidemic in their countries. Some counteracted the accusations by claiming that AIDS was a disease of white people. For example, President Daniel arap Moi of Kenya (b. 1924) spent the first four years of the growing pandemic denying that there was any HIV in his country and ascribing reports of it to a deliberate hate campaign against his country. He threatened to remove the visas and deport any foreign journalist reporting AIDS and waited until 1986 before allowing even the most innocuous "AIDS guidelines" to be published. Meanwhile, he instructed the Ministry of Health to under-report the known cases, on the grounds that many of those with AIDS were "not Kenyans." While this was going on, the seropositivity rate of commercial sex workers in Nairobi rose from 17 percent to almost 100 percent by 1990. A similar story of denial was repeated in other countries such as Malawi, Tanzania, Zambia, and South Africa. It was not until 1990 that African governments reluctantly started to acknowledge that the disease was spreading widely throughout their countries. This acknowledgment came too late to launch an effective AIDS control program. The damage was already done.

Even in the early 2000s, many African leaders continued to be in denial and questioned the existence, cause, and treatment of AIDS. For example President Thabo Mbeki (b. 1942) of South Africa stunned the AIDS industry and its critics in February of 2000 when he announced that he would host an international panel of experts to examine the science of AIDS, its treatment, and the role of the **pharmaceutical** companies. The panel that met in Pretoria in May 2000 included both supporters and critics of the "HIV-causes-AIDS model." At this panel "HIV-causes-AIDS" critics embraced the opportunity to participate in an open exchange of scientific ideas, whereas proponents of the notion that HIV causes AIDS expressed indignation, not-so-veiled threats, and insults. Thabo Mbeki, the first head of state to rethink the HIV-causes-AIDS issue, was and remained suspicious of the idea of a single virus causing AIDS. Although Mbeki was ridiculed in the media as being out of touch with reality, his call for a reconsideration of the epidemic was soon being taken seriously. Mbeki's debate received great attention, and a number of issues emerged from the debate, including the recognition of **poverty** as an issue in HIV/AIDS infection. Other African leaders have propagated the story that HIV/AIDS was created in U.S. labs and exported to Africa to kill Africans. Rumors are rife in many African settings that even the condoms touted to stop the **transmission** of AIDS are already tainted with the virus at manufacturing plants in Western countries and then exported to Africa to infect Africans. It is within this context that the lukewarm response of African leaders to tackling the disease needs to be understood. Without this context, it is difficult to understand why African governments and peoples are often skeptical of receiving or implementing HIV prevention programs from developed countries.

Geographic Spread.   Regarding the geographic spread of the epidemic in Africa, John Iliffe, in his book *The African AIDS Epidemic* (2006), masterfully synthesizes the plethora of studies that have been conducted from the 1980s to the present, tracing the geographic beginnings and spread of AIDS throughout the continent. Iliffe weaves together a story that attempts to explain the origins, nature, and spread of the virus from its detection in the early 1980s to its current progression throughout the continent. He places the origins of the disease somewhere in central Africa, where it spread slowly to East Africa. In the 1990s, the disease moved to southern Africa, where it has wreaked havoc and where the pandemic remains the most intense. Using sentinel surveillance data that began to be collected in the mid-1980s, along with advanced mapping techniques, Ezekiel Kalipeni and Leo Zulu traced the geographic trajectory of the disease. Their findings, as shown in the accompanying maps, support Iliffe's picture and clearly delineate the progression of the disease from somewhere in central Africa, to eastern Africa, and finally to southern Africa.

The maps show interpolated HIV prevalence rates and the spatial-temporal progression of HIV/AIDS across Sub-Saharan Africa for the years 1986, 1990, 1994, 1999, and 2003. These maps show that southern Africa has consistently had HIV prevalence rates in excess of 5 percent since 1986, and parts of North and West Africa have generally had the lowest prevalence, below 5 percent. However, over time the epicenter of HIV/AIDS (10 to 20 percent prevalence) located in the Great Lakes region of East Africa (Burundi, Rwanda, Tanzania, and Uganda) and an isolated pocket in West Africa (Guinea-Bissau) in 1986 had by 1990 expanded in both prevalence level and spatial extent within the Great Lakes region and had developed a second nucleus in the southern Africa region (Zimbabwe, Zambia, Mozambique, and Malawi). By 1994 a more intense (15 to over 30 percent) southern Africa epicenter had expanded to include Botswana and parts of South Africa, whereas the Great Lakes nucleus had broken down into isolated pockets, and a new nucleus had developed over Ethiopia/Eritrea. The years 1999 and 2003 saw an even more intense southern Africa expansion to include Namibia, South Africa, Swaziland, and Lesotho, with isolated, less intense pockets in the East Africa region (Kenya, Uganda, Tanzania, and Ethiopia) and in Cameroon and Côte d'Ivoire in West Africa. The spatial-temporal trends

so vividly brought out by these maps largely conform with UNAIDS estimates of an escalating epidemic in southern Africa and with signs of stabilization or decline in the East
African region. In the early 2000s, southern Africa remained the worst-affected subregion
in the world, with HIV prevalence rates in excess of 25 percent, a sharp rise from around
5 percent in 1986. In short, these maps lend credence to the saying that "there is not just
one epidemic in Africa, but many." West Africa and North Africa have consistently experienced lower rates than the other regions, although in some countries in West Africa, the
epidemic is creeping up. Even within the other high-risk regions, some areas have lower
rates than others.

Causes and Consequences.   Once the disease was established in Africa in the early
1980s, it found fertile ground and began to spread like wildfire. The causes of the rapid
spread are many and complex. There are both macro- and micro-level dimensions that put
African peoples at very high levels of vulnerability to this disease. These dimensions are
rooted in the history of the continent, especially its colonial interlude. The historical
context of **colonialism** and its economy based on labor migration, contemporary gender
issues, **poverty** and disease burden, global forces, government commitment, and the
cultural context have all intertwined in complex ways to put peoples of Sub-Saharan
Africa at risk of contracting HIV. It must be understood that while people's behavior and
actions are inherently important factors in determining vulnerability to HIV, the context
is even more critical. Thus, any assessment of HIV vulnerability has to include global,
national, regional, and community factors that influence or exacerbate personal
vulnerability. Thus the political, cultural, social, and economic contexts—and particularly
the colonial economy based on labor migration—made Sub-Saharan Africa susceptible to
the rapid spread of the epidemic. These factors result in situations of powerlessness of
individuals and communities at large.

The impacts of HIV/AIDS on the critical infrastructures that sustain the security, stability, and viability of modern nation-states are manifold. For the African peoples, the consequences have been tragic. In Africa, HIV/AIDS continues to undermine education and
health systems, economic growth, micro-enterprises, policing and **military** capabilities,
political legitimacy, family structures, and overall social cohesion. The initial impact of
AIDS is the suffering of individuals and their immediate families. But a more insidious
impact is its threat to the development gains of communities and nations. African countries are hard-pressed to provide health care, treatment, and support to a growing population of people with HIV-related illnesses. In times of ongoing economic and political
turbulence, African governments are finding it difficult to launch costly aggressive campaigns to reduce the increasing annual toll of new HIV infections by enabling individuals
to protect themselves and others. It is further estimated that, so far, over 20 million people
in Africa have died from this epidemic, leaving behind millions of orphans and other survivors. This has put further strain on communities and on national development. In the
worst-hit countries, life expectancy has declined significantly. Average life expectancy in
Sub-Saharan Africa is now 47 years, when it could have been 62 without AIDS.

The Way Forward.   Yet in spite of the tragic consequences that have been brought
upon the peoples of Africa by this epidemic, there is light at the end of the tunnel.
Belatedly, the international community has been begun to galvanize itself in providing
life-saving antiretroviral medications. Although the number of people receiving these
vital medications is minuscule in comparison with the need, the efforts at providing such
medications at subsidized rates or for free are commendable. Governments in the West, in

cooperation with international pharmaceutical corporations, are also in the process of supporting the ongoing research on vaccine development. Other positive trends are the growth of grassroots political activism in Africa and the emergence of compassionate organizations such as The AIDS Support Organization (TASO) in Uganda, and Treatment AIDS Campaign (TAC) in South Africa. These are all signs of the local and international cooperation necessary to at least stabilize but possibly even reverse the patterns of the pandemic disease.

Indeed, there is growing evidence that in some countries the epidemic has leveled off. In others it is actually on the decline (e.g., Uganda), and in still others, where government commitment was strong immediately after the epidemic was recognized, the prevalence rates have been kept at very low levels (e.g., Senegal). Although the epidemic continues to ravage the continent, Uganda and Senegal appear to have implemented successful and sustainable efforts to combat the HIV/AIDS crisis. In Uganda, HIV prevalence and incidence rates that were on the increase in the 1980s began to decline significantly during the 1990s. In Uganda's capital city, Kampala, the prevalence rate in 1992 was as high as 20 percent among pregnant women visiting prenatal clinics; today it is about 7 percent. In other sites in Uganda, mostly rural, this rate was 9 percent, whereas today it is about 4 percent. Seroprevalence among 15- to 19-year-old pregnant women, which is believed to be reflective of HIV incidence, fell sharply from the early 1990s until 1996, and since then has remained low. In the case of Uganda, success stems from the fact that although most African governments buried their heads in the sand, the government of Uganda acknowledged the AIDS crisis as early as 1986 and began mobilizing both domestic and international support to combat it. In addition to high-level political support with multi-sectoral response, Uganda's prevention efforts included a range of social strategies. These included raising the legal age for sexual intercourse; social mobilization that reduced stigmatization and discrimination; decentralized planning and implementation for behavior change communication (BCC), which reached the general population and key target groups; confidential voluntary counseling; social marketing and use of condoms; increased emphasis on control and prevention of sexually transmitted infections; and a decrease in multiple sexual partnerships.

The second success story is Senegal, which acted early enough to tackle the disease before it had spread widely in the general population. Whereas politicians in some other countries ignored the threat of AIDS for fear of alienating conservative supporters by initiating a discussion about safe sex, politicians in Senegal vigorously supported efforts to confront the epidemic. The government of Senegal mobilized its meager resources to set up an ambitious program to stop HIV in its tracks. Senegal's program hinged on strong political leadership that was willing to work hand in hand with religious and community leadership, and on mobilization of the young, including sex workers and their partners, to practice safe sex. Whereas it is true that Sub-Saharan Africa remains by far the worst affected region in the world, these two examples of success offer a sign that it is possible to stem the tide of the epidemic if governments and concerned communities work together. *See also* AIDS in the United States; Animal Diseases (Zoonoses) and Epidemic Disease; Hemorrhagic Fevers in Modern Africa; Hospitals since 1900; International Health Agencies and Conventions; Non-Governmental Organizations (NGOs) and Epidemic Disease; Personal Liberties and Epidemic Disease; Poison Libels and Epidemic Disease; Popular Media and Epidemic Disease: Recent Trends; Race, Ethnicity, and Epidemic Disease; Sexuality, Gender, and Epidemic Disease; Vaccination and Inoculation.

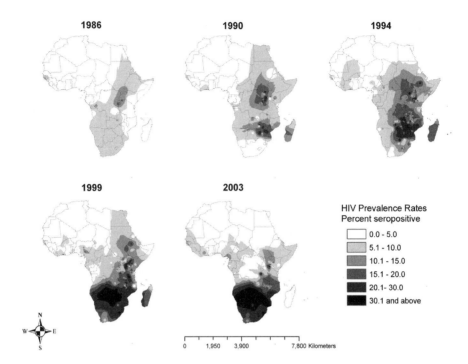

HIV/AIDS Prevalence Rates for Selected Years. Courtesy Ezekiel Kalipeni and Leo Zulu. Adapted from Kalipeni, E. and Zulu, L. 2008. "Using GIS to Model and Forecast HIV/AIDS Rates in Africa, 1986–2010." *Professional Geographer* 60(1).

Further Reading

Barnett, Tony, and Alan Whiteside. *AIDS in the 21st Century: Disease and Globalization*. New York: Palgrave Macmillan, 2002.

D'Adesky, Anne-Christine. *Moving Mountains: The Race to Treat Global AIDS*. New York: Verso, 2004.

Feldman, Douglas A., and Julia Wang Miller. *The AIDS Crisis: A Documentary History*. Westport, CT: Greenwood Press, 1998.

Global AIDS Alliance. http://www.globalaidsalliance.org/

Gould, Peter. *The Slow Plague: A Geography of the AIDS Pandemic*. Cambridge, MA: Blackwell Press, 1993.

Hunter, Susan. *Black Death: AIDS in Africa*. New York: Palgrave Macmillan, 2003.

Iliffe, John. *The African AIDS Epidemic: A History*. Oxford: James Currey, 2006.

Kalipeni, Ezekiel, and Leo Zulu. "Using GIS to Model and Forecast HIV/AIDS Rates in Africa, 1986–2010." *Professional Geographer* 60.1 (2008); forthcoming.

Kalipeni, Ezekiel, Susan Craddock, Joseph Oppong, and Jayati Ghosh, eds. *HIV/AIDS in Africa: Beyond Epidemiology*. New York: Blackwell Publishers, 2004.

Kanabus, A., and J. Fredriksson-Bass. 2007. *HIV and AIDS in Africa*. http://www.avert.org/aafrica.htm.

Mari, Christopher. *Global Epidemics*. New York: H. W. Wilson Co., 2007.

National Institutes of Health. *AIDS History*. http://aidshistory.nih.gov/

Shannon, Gary William, Gerald F. Pyle, and Rashid Bashshur. *The Geography of AIDS: Origins and Course of an Epidemic*. New York: Guilford Press, 1991.

UNAIDS. *AIDS Epidemic Update 2007*. Geneva: UNAIDS, 2007.
UNAIDS. http://www.unaids.org/en/

EZEKIEL KALIPENI

AIDS IN THE UNITED STATES.   Acquired immunodeficiency syndrome (AIDS) was first recognized in American medical literature in mid-1981. It was named just over a year later to describe the multiple symptoms seen in patients that were the result of an underlying immune deficiency caused by infection with the **human immunodeficiency virus (HIV)**. In the United States, AIDS was discovered in major homosexual communities of large cities and often initially called "gay-related immune deficiency (GRID)" or "gay cancer." By 1983 medical practitioners and the public came to realize that AIDS could and did affect many others, especially intravenous drug users who shared needles and those who received tainted blood products during medical procedures. The U.S. Food and Drug Administration approved the first successful drug therapy, AZT, in 1987. While AIDS activist groups protested the supposed lack of government interest in AIDS and AIDS-related research, laboratories developed multidrug "cocktails" with varying levels of effectiveness, releasing the first in 1993. In recent years, AIDS has become entrenched in marginalized communities where preventive and therapeutic interventions have been unavailable or have not been adopted.

Recognition of AIDS as a New Disease.   Medical research studies indicate that the first, unrecognized cases of AIDS probably occurred in West Africa, where the causative virus mutated from a form that infected monkeys to one that could infect humans. Why, then, was AIDS first recognized as a new disease in the United States? The answer lies in the differences between the ways in which medicine is practiced by **physicians** and experienced by patients in Africa and in the United States. Individuals in Africa who succumbed to AIDS in the decades before 1981 were most often poor, rural people who rarely consulted physicians practicing Western medicine. Conversely, such physicians, upon seeing an African with a fever and wasting, would likely attribute the symptoms to any of a host of diseases present in tropical countries. The earliest AIDS patients in the United States, in contrast, were largely Caucasian, upper-middle-class people with health insurance who regularly consulted physicians when they fell ill. Their physicians recognized a disruption in the medical history of their patient populations that led them to question idiosyncratic diagnoses and wonder about the possibility of a novel disease process.

Specifically, in the late 1970s, U.S. dermatologists began seeing young men with rare cancerous lesions (Kaposi's sarcoma) normally found on elderly Mediterranean men. In early 1981, infectious disease physicians encountered patients with infections, especially *Pneumocystis carinii* pneumonia (PCP), associated normally with patients whose immune systems had been compromised because of cancer treatments. In June 1981, the cases seen in Los Angeles were described in a short paper in the *Morbidity and Mortality Weekly Reports*, a weekly publication issued by the U.S. **Centers for Disease Control and Prevention** (CDC) in Atlanta. Additional papers followed in July and August, all of which observed that the affected patients were previously healthy homosexual men living in gay communities in large cities.

By June 1982, cases of AIDS outside gay communities had been observed, including cases in newborn babies, heterosexual patients who had undergone surgery, Haitian immigrants, and persons who regularly received blood products to treat their hemophilia (a genetic disease characterized by the inability to clot blood). AIDS became known at this time as the "4-H" disease because it had been observed in homosexuals, heroin addicts, Haitians, and hemophiliacs. Epidemiologists understood, however, that these categories of patients also suggested a blood-borne cause. If AIDS were transmitted by blood, the nation's supply of whole blood and blood products was at risk, a finding that many people, including those who managed blood banks, did not want to believe. Hemophiliacs previously tolerated the possibility of infection with **hepatitis** B virus because the value of the clotting factor produced from pooling serum outweighed that risk. Hemophiliacs and their families were horrified, however, by the prospect that the lifesaving blood product might harbor a lethal disease agent. After 1983, when the virus was first isolated in the Paris laboratory of Dr. Luc Montagnier, HIV was demonstrated to be the cause of AIDS. By mid-1984 transfusion-transmitted viruses were no longer considered acceptable risks in reaping the benefits of blood products. An enzyme-linked, immunosorbant assay (ELISA) for antibodies to HIV, developed for use in laboratory research on the etiology of AIDS, was adapted in 1985 as a screening test for blood and blood products. In 1987 the U.S. Food and Drug Administration (FDA) issued regulations requiring such screening, and in 1988 the FDA began inspecting 100 percent of FDA-regulated blood and plasma donor facilities to enforce screening regulations.

Another consequence of the development of sensitive **diagnostic** tests for HIV was the transformation of the definition of AIDS. Between 1981 and 1986, the CDC issued successive statements about which opportunistic infections and cancers could be used as the basis for a diagnosis of AIDS. Diseases such as *Pneumocystis carinii* pneumonia, candidiasis (a yeast-like infection) of the esophagus or lungs, toxoplasmosis of the brain, and Kaposi's sarcoma were included early. General wasting symptoms, such as ongoing diarrhea and severe pelvic inflammatory disease in women, were less clearly a part of the "syndrome" caused by the acquired immunodeficiency. Details about the various diagnoses mattered because health insurers and the U.S. federal government based reimbursement payments and access to clinical trials on such information. In August 1987, the CDC revised its definition of AIDS from a list of particular illnesses to any illness that resulted from a long-term infection with HIV. Since that time, the name used for the disease has been "HIV/AIDS."

Social, Religious, and Political Reactions to AIDS.   The social stigma carried by AIDS as a sexually transmitted disease resulted in what some public health leaders called "a second **epidemic** of fear." From 1983 to 1987, when public fear and panic were at their most destructive, some religious groups proclaimed that AIDS was God's vengeance on the gay community for violating what they viewed as **biblical** prohibitions against homosexuality. Injecting drug abusers were also viewed as people who made wrong "lifestyle" choices that led to disease. Hemophiliacs, surgery patients who received infected blood, and women who were infected by their spouses, in contrast, were viewed as "innocent" victims of AIDS. This division of people with AIDS into guilty and innocent categories led advocates of conservative views to support research on drugs to treat AIDS but to oppose any public expenditure for condom distribution or needle exchange programs for drug addicts. Teaching personal responsibility—through sexual abstinence and "just say no" to drugs campaigns—was their preferred approach to AIDS prevention efforts. Social and religious reluctance to discuss **sexuality** in any public setting exacerbated the obstacles to effective public education about AIDS.

Individuals diagnosed with AIDS or as having antibodies to HIV were sometimes fired from their jobs. Police officers, firefighters, ambulance personnel, and other health-care workers occasionally refused to take care of AIDS patients. Young Ryan White (1971–1990) in Indiana and three brothers—Ricky (1977–1992), Robert (1978–2000), and Randy (b. 1979) Ray—in Florida, all hemophiliacs who contracted AIDS from contaminated blood products, were denied entrance to schools. Even as medical research demonstrated that AIDS was not transmissible through casual contact, the epidemic of fear moved an arsonist in Arcadia, Florida, to set fire to the Ray brothers' house and the school board in Kokomo, Indiana, to insist that Ryan White take classes over the telephone to avoid accidentally touching his classmates.

The most important tool used by public health leaders to counter this fear was accurate communication about AIDS. Sharing new information as soon as it became available often made the difference between keeping and losing staff at hospitals, firehouses, police departments, and other public service agencies. A concerted education program about AIDS and how it was transmitted helped to diffuse fear in school systems. On the national level, U.S. Surgeon General C. Everett Koop (b. 1916) issued an informational report on AIDS in 1986 and two years later mailed a flier titled "Understanding AIDS" to every household in the United States.

October 2, 1985, marked a turning point in the history of AIDS in America. On that date, Hollywood actor Rock Hudson (1925–1985) died of AIDS. Hudson's death seemed to bring home the point to a broad public that anyone, even a movie star, could contract AIDS. The publicity surrounding Hudson's death motivated the U.S. Congress to appropriate significantly more money for AIDS research than it had been willing to commit previously. During the 1990s, other celebrities with AIDS—including the tennis player Arthur Ashe (1943–1993) and Elizabeth Glaser (1947–1994), wife of actor Paul Michael Glaser—as well as others without AIDS, such as Elizabeth Taylor (b. 1932), became public spokespersons for raising money to combat AIDS and raising awareness that people with AIDS should be treated fairly and with compassion.

Throughout the 1980s within the gay community, AIDS activists worked from the earliest years of the epidemic to provide care for sick individuals, to raise money for foundations, to lobby the federal government to increase research, and to make possible therapies available more quickly than the traditional drug approval process would allow. To draw attention to their cause, some of the activists staged public demonstrations, or "street theatre," designed to attract national media attention. In 1987 the organization AIDS Coalition To Unleash Power (ACT UP) was formed by activists in New York City with the initial goal of gaining the release of experimental drugs. Soon ACT UP expanded to advocate for other AIDS issues as well. ACT UP's numerous protests were so successful that they became a model for advocates for other diseases.

A more politically vexed public health policy was the decision about whether to close bathhouses in the gay communities of San Francisco, Los Angeles, and New York. The bathhouses represented for many in the gay community a civil rights triumph. After years "in the closet" for fear of losing jobs or being physically attacked, they could openly declare their gay identities and socialize in public at gay bathhouses and bars. They argued that bathhouse clients were intelligent enough to begin protecting themselves once informed of the need for safe **sex**, and that because they were the principal population at risk for AIDS, conducting AIDS prevention education at the bathhouses would lower the rate of **transmission** of the virus in the entire community. Others in the gay community, bolstered by some public health

"BATHHOUSES REFLECT AIDS CONCERNS,"
NEW YORK TIMES, OCTOBER 14, 1985

Attendance has declined at the 10 homosexual bathhouses in New York since the onset of the AIDS epidemic, according to the city's Department of Health. But some of the owners report that business remains profitable despite mounting public pressure that the baths be closed.

"I've gone through my own particular moral crisis with this," said Bruce Mailman, a homosexual and a Lower East Side real-estate entrepreneur who owns the St. Marks Baths, as well as the Saint, a homosexual discotheque. "Am I profiting from other people's misery? I don't think so. I think I'm running an establishment that handles itself as well as it can under the circumstances."

Mr. Mailman reports a 50 percent decline in attendance since 1982, while Jim Schwartz, who describes himself as a minority stockholder at the East Side Sauna, one of the city's smaller bathhouses, said business had declined 25 percent, from nearly 2,000 customers a week to about 1,500.

Neither of the owners was willing to describe his profits in detail, but both said that if they were not making money they would close their doors, as five other local bathhouses have done in recent years.

FORUMS FOR EDUCATION
With nearly 14,000 cases of AIDS reported nationwide, 6,700 in New York, homosexual men are increasingly calling for the closing of the baths, and many are criticizing homosexuals who profit from their operation.

Both Governor Cuomo and Mayor Koch are reconsidering their positions that such places, licensed by the city's Health Department, are useful forums for educating homosexuals about the sexual practices that spread acquired immune deficiency syndrome, which is usually fatal.

"Because the circumstances have changed, because political opinion makes us bad guys, that doesn't mean I'm doing something morally incorrect," said Mr. Mailman.

leaders, believed that since multiple unprotected sex acts took place in bathhouses, classic public health practice dictated that closing the bathhouses would help stop transmission. In 1984 the argument was settled in San Francisco when political and public health leaders agreed that the bathhouses should be closed. The following year Los Angeles and New York City also moved to close bathhouses.

Public education programs in the United States about AIDS were strongly split in content according to which group produced them. Those funded by the U.S. government emphasized "getting the facts" about AIDS. There was virtually no emphasis in government-funded educational campaigns on communicating specifically to the gay community or on discussing safe sex through the campaign's posters. AIDS community action groups and other private-sector groups took the lead in producing stark, graphic messages that communicated the urgent need for condom use and clean needles.

One segment of American society that proved particularly difficult to reach with AIDS prevention messages was the African American community. Traditionally, the black church had been the most effective vehicle for communicating health messages within the African American community, but strong sentiments against homosexuality within the black church made safe gay sex extremely difficult to address. The African American community also had scant trust of health messages from the federal government because of the infamous Tuskegee **syphilis** study, in which African American men in Alabama had been left untreated for the disease without their knowledge or consent in order for the effects of syphilis in untreated patients to be observed.

AIDS Doubters and AIDS Quackery. In 1987 Peter Duesberg (b. 1936), a distinguished molecular biologist, authority on retroviruses, and member of the U.S. National Academy of Sciences, published a paper asserting that HIV was merely a benign passenger virus and not the cause of AIDS. Leading scientists refuted Duesburg's theory, but his arguments drew adherents from people who wished to believe that AIDS had no link to viral causation and could be cured by living a "healthy" lifestyle. Questioning the cause of AIDS also fueled the industry of unorthodox treatments for AIDS. From the earliest days of the epidemic, desperate patients had been willing to try almost anything advertised as a cure. Early in the epidemic, promoters of questionable cancer treatments expanded their claims to encompass AIDS because of its link to Kaposi's sarcoma. As the underlying immune deficiency in AIDS became common knowledge, remedies purporting to boost the immune system flowered. The growth of the World Wide Web in the late 1990s allowed the AIDS doubters to spread their message widely and opened the door to multiple **quack** therapies and urban legends relating to AIDS.

AIDS in the New Millennium.   In 2001 the world marked 25 years since the earliest recognition of AIDS. By this date AIDS in America had been transformed from a disease identified almost exclusively with affluent homosexual men into a disease of marginalized groups—injecting drug abusers and poor minority populations. Between 2001 and 2004, 50 percent of HIV diagnoses were among African Americans and 20 percent were among Hispanics, even though those groups constituted only 12 percent and 14 percent of the U.S. population respectively. Men who had sex with other men still accounted for more than 70 percent of AIDS cases in the United States. This was also true in Canada and in Latin America as a whole. Among Caribbean island populations, however, AIDS now strikes men and women equally.

Americans have played a leading role in efforts to halt AIDS in the rest of the world. In poorer regions of the world, AIDS patients cannot afford the cost of antiviral drugs, even those whose prices have been greatly reduced. In 2007 the U.S. government committed $30 billion over five years to fight AIDS in developing countries. Major philanthropic organizations, such as the Bill and Melinda Gates Foundation, have also invested heavily in research on ways to prevent AIDS as well as in helping those already infected.

For the United States, AIDS has become essentially a chronic disease. In 2005, the CDC reported just over 433,000 people living with AIDS in the United States and 17,000 deaths from AIDS during the year. Between 1993 and 2003, highly active antiretroviral therapy (HAART) produced an 80 percent drop in the death rate from AIDS. Since the 1986 release of Azidothymidine, or AZT, new AIDS drugs have been developed that target different points in the life cycle of HIV. In 1995 a new class of drugs called protease inhibitors was approved, and in 2007 integrase inhibitors were introduced. Even more antiviral drugs are in research and development. None of these drugs, however, can eliminate HIV from an infected person, and the disease requires drug treatment with toxic side effects for the rest of an infected person's life. Because of the rapid mutation of HIV, moreover, a conventional vaccine against AIDS has proved impossible to make, and it may take decades before novel approaches to the vaccine concept produce positive results.

The very success in managing AIDS in the United States has produced worry among public health officials that young people will not understand the serious side effects that accompany antiviral regimens and be lulled into thinking that AIDS is no longer a danger. Among affluent homosexual men—the initial group struck so hard by AIDS—some risky behaviors have reemerged. Many gay bathhouses in major cities, closed in the mid-1980s, reopened quickly with regulations restricting unsafe sexual practices in public areas. Sexual activity in the bathhouses' privately rented rooms was and still is

The first thing
that should go on between
two consenting adults.

The sexual revolution may be over,
but the casualties are still mounting.
Don't be counted among them. Use condoms.

Milwaukee AIDS Project
273-AIDS

"The sexual revolution may be over, but the casualties are still mounting. Don't be counted among them. Use condoms." Milwaukee AIDS Project (1980s). Courtesy of the National Library of Medicine.

unregulated, illustrating the ongoing tension between **personal liberty** and the community's right to coerce healthful behavior. Exacerbating the problem has been the widespread use of the drug methamphetamine, which in the twenty-first century has fueled a return to unsafe sex with multiple partners in bathhouses.

It has been a hard-won truth that AIDS in America is best prevented in the twenty-first century with traditional, twentieth-century public health techniques. Educational campaigns about how HIV is transmitted help individuals protect themselves by abstaining from sex or engaging in safe sex practices. Efforts to expand testing for HIV and reduce the stigma of a positive diagnosis likewise help individuals to know their personal status and protect their sexual partners. Before 2005 public health efforts to exchange clean needles for used ones to protect injecting drug users from AIDS had been illegal under most state drug laws, but volunteer programs were often tolerated by law enforcement. In that year, however, needle exchange won official support in California, and since then, other states and municipalities have endorsed this effort. *See also* AIDS in Africa; AIDS, Literature, and the Arts in the United States; Cinema and Epidemic Disease; Disease, Social Construction of; Drug Resistance in Microorganisms; Human Immunity and Resistance to Disease; Literature, Disease in Modern; Medical Ethics and Epidemic Disease; Popular Media and Epidemic Disease: Recent Trends; Poverty, Wealth, and Epidemic Disease; Public Health Agencies, U.S. Federal; Race, Ethnicity, and Epidemic Disease; Religion and Epidemic Disease; Scapegoats and Epidemic Disease; Sexual Revolution; Trade, Travel, and Epidemic Disease.

Further Reading

The AIDS Reader. http://www.medscape.com/viewpublication/93

Baldwin, Peter. *Disease and Democracy: The Industrialized World Faces AIDS.* Berkeley: University of California Press, 2005.

Davis, Julia. *Evolution of an Epidemic: 25 Years of HIV/AIDS Media Campaigns in the U.S.* Menlo Park, CA: Henry J. Kaiser Family Foundation, 2006.

Engel, Jonathan. *The Epidemic: A Global History of AIDS.* Washington, DC: Smithsonian Books, 2006.

Feldman, Eric, and Ronald Bayer, eds. *Blood Feuds: AIDS, Blood, and the Politics of Medical Disaster.* New York: Oxford University Press, 1999.

National Institutes of Health. *History of AIDS.* http://aidshistory.nih.gov/

Public Broadcasting Service. http://www.pbs.org/wgbh/nova/aids/

Shilts, Randy. *And the Band Played On: Politics, People, and the AIDS Epidemic.* New York: St. Martin's Press, 1987.

Treichler, Paula. *How to Have Theory in an Epidemic.* Durham, NC: Duke University Press, 1999.

UNAIDS. *AIDS Epidemic Update.* Geneva, Switzerland: World Health Organization/UNAIDS, 2007.

Watney, Simon. *Policing Desire: Pornography, AIDS, and the Media,* 2nd edition. Minneapolis: University of Minnesota Press, 1989.

VICTORIA A. HARDEN

AIDS, LITERATURE, AND THE ARTS IN THE UNITED STATES.   AIDS has been variously called an "**epidemic** of signification" and the first postmodern epidemic. In the early years after its discovery, the syndrome was diagnostically defined only by its second-hand disease manifestations (its "signifiers") rather than by the infectious agent itself.

(Only later was the viral cause identified, and a test for its antibodies developed.) Perhaps more than any other infectious epidemic, **HIV/AIDS** has resulted in an excess of public discourse attempting to define what it means, over and above its status as a public health issue.

Because the first observed vectors of transmission, namely intravenous (IV) drug use and homosexual sex, and the first populations in which it was observed, namely poor, IV drug users, and gay men, were socially stigmatized behaviors and socially stigmatized groups, AIDS has absorbed more than its share of metaphorical significance: God's wrath, a CIA experiment gone awry, a punishment for violating Nature, and so forth. The struggle to comprehend the epidemic, therefore, became a struggle to control its representations in public discourse, literature, and the arts. That gay men are disproportionately represented in the worlds of fine arts, performing arts, and literature meant that many culture workers in the 1980s and 1990s would undertake the task of remembering lives lost, encouraging survivors, and calling citizens to action on behalf of the infected. That the world of cultural production tends to be progressive in its politics meant that some artists became activists in opposition to America's swerve toward conservatism in the 1980s.

Literature. AIDS emerged in 1981 as a text, first in published reports in mainstream journalism, then in sensationalized accounts in tabloid media, then in Christian fundamentalist apocalyptically tinged accounts. In their quest to take control of the tendencies to demonize or to sentimentalize the infected, writers were among the first artists to contend with the epidemic.

Some of the earliest fiction attempting to represent AIDS came from gay writers publishing in marginal small presses rather than mainstream venues. Paul Reed's 1984 *Facing It: A Novel of A.I.D.S.* (arguably one of the first, if not the first, AIDS-themed novel) was published by Gay Sunshine Press, and Samuel R. Delany's 1985 "The Tale of Plagues and Carnivals; or, Some Informal Remarks toward the Modular Calculus, Part Five" appeared as an appendix to his science-fiction book, *Flight from Nevèrÿon.* Toby Johnson's futuristic and dystopian 1987 *Plague: A Novel about Healing* was published by the gay publisher Alyson Publications. Knights Press published several novels, including *The World Can Break Your Heart* (1984) by Daniel Curzon, *The Wrong Apple* (1988) by David Rees, *Genocide: The Anthology* (1989) by Tim Barrus, and *Gardy and Erin* (1989) by Jeff Black, among others.

By the late 1980s, more mainstream writers and publishing houses brought out AIDS-themed fiction. Christopher Bram's *In Memory of Angel Clare* (1989) recounted the lives of a circle of friends after losing another friend to AIDS. Sarah Schulman's unflinching *People in Trouble* (1990) and *Rat Bohemia* (1995) resisted sentimentality, explored political engagement, and represented the responses to AIDS of straight and queer women. Alice Hoffman's *At Risk* (1988) explored a middle-class child's infection with HIV (by a blood transfusion), her development of AIDS, and the social stigma associated with her diagnosis. James McCourt's *Time Remaining* (1993) was by turns brilliantly witty and poignantly elegiac.

Love lost and mortality are not unusual themes in poetry, and AIDS certainly provoked an outpouring of elegiac verse, collected in anthologies such as *Poets for Life: Seventy-Six Poets Respond to AIDS* (edited in 1989 by Michael Klein) and *Brother to Brother: New Writings by Black Gay Men* (edited in 1991 by Essex Hemphill). Some poets produced sustained lyric sequences thematically dealing with AIDS, including Robert Boucheron's *Epitaphs for the Plague Dead* (1985), Paul Monette's *Love Alone: 18 Elegies for*

Rog (1988), Thom Gunn's *The Man with Night Sweats* (1992), Walter Holland's *A Journal of the Plague Years* (1992), Mark Doty's *Atlantis* (1995), and Essex Hemphill's collection of prose and poetry *Ceremonies* (1992).

Performing Arts. The arts of stage and screen were profoundly affected by the AIDS epidemic, which was reflected in a new cultural phenomenon, the benefit performance to raise funds for AIDS service organizations, and in a variety of new artistic creations. The deaths from AIDS of ballet dancer Rudolf Nureyev, Broadway director Michael Bennett, musician Liberace, and actors Brad Davis and Rock Hudson, among others, gave AIDS a high public profile and allowed mainstream America to identify with the epidemic.

Dramatists engaged the epidemic in its first years. Larry Kramer's *The Normal Heart* (1985) chronicled early AIDS activism (eventually supplemented with his plays *Just Say No* [1989] and *The Destiny of Me* [1993]), whereas William Hoffman's *As Is* (1985) situated the epidemic within human relationships. Comic playwright Harvey Fierstein created a trilogy of one-acts titled *Safe Sex* (1987). Terrence McNally's *Love! Valour! Compassion!* (1994) was a humorous and poignant reflection on mortality and friendship. Perhaps the most ambitious stage treatment was Tony Kushner's 1991 *Angels in America: A Gay Fantasia on National Themes*, an epic drama in two parts over two performances totaling about seven hours (directed by Mike Nichols for HBO in 2003).

The 1980s and 1990s also saw the emergence of solo-performance art as a politically engaged agitprop medium designed to catalyze audiences to action in the face of growing political, religious, and economic conservatism. Usually in the form of monologues, frequently engaging the audience directly and physically, sometimes featuring a naked performer, solo-performance art was confrontational in its politics and sexuality, dismantling the notion of sex as a "private" (and therefore apolitical and invisible) matter. So successfully did performers like Tim Miller, Karen Finley, John Fleck, and Holly Hughes test the limits of what constitutes theatrical performance, that grants from the National Endowment for the Arts that they had been awarded were withdrawn after political pressure from the first Bush administration. A tamer version of this phenomenon was David Drake's *The Night Larry Kramer Kissed Me* (1993, made into a film in 2000), a memoir of his coming out and a fantasy of a world after AIDS.

Musical composers contributed to this creative outpouring. John Corigliano's Symphony No. 1 was precipitated by his seeing the traveling AIDS Memorial Quilt. Jazz composer and pianist Fred Hersch composed "Tango Bittersweet," pianist and composer Kevin Oldham, a "Concerto for Piano," composer Lee Gannon a "Triad-O-Rama" for wind quintet, and Calvin Hampton a set of variations on "Amazing Grace" (collected in a 1994 CD entitled *Memento Bittersweet*). Vocal performer Diamanda Galas created a series of searing vocal performance pieces, including *The Divine Punishment* and *Saint of the Pit* (1986, 1989), *Masque of the Red Death* (1988), *Plague Mass* (1990), and *Vena Cava* (1992).

The Broadway musical would seem an unlikely genre for a reflection on the AIDS epidemic, but two stand out. William Finn's *Falsettos* (1992) depicted gay men dealing with AIDS with the support of family and friends (and won Tony Awards for Best Book and Best Score). Jonathan Larson, an aspiring Broadway composer, achieved posthumous fame when his rock musical *Rent*, set in Manhattan's East Village and based on Puccini's opera *La Bohème*, opened in 1996 shortly after his death (from an undiagnosed congenital heart defect). The musical, which substitutes AIDS for the opera's tuberculosis, generated some controversy after novelist Sarah Schulman pointed out its parallels to her novel *People in Trouble*, published six years before.

Major Hollywood filmmakers were slow to bring AIDS to the big screen. That role was ably performed by independent filmmakers such as Bill Sherwood's *Parting Glances* (1986), Craig Lucas's *Longtime Companion* (1990), Todd Haynes's *Poison* (1991), and Gregg Araki's *The Living End* (1992). Television surprisingly brought some of the earliest popular representations of people with AIDS, including Daniel Lipman and Ron Cowen's *An Early Frost* (NBC, 1985), playwright Harvey Fierstein's *Tidy Endings* (HBO, 1988) and Terrence McNally's *Andre's Mother* (PBS, 1990). *Tongues Untied* (1991), directed for PBS by black filmmaker Marlon Riggs, explored the lives of African American gay men and homophobia in black communities, creating a larger public controversy about funding for public television because of its frankness about sexuality. The Hollywood release *Philadelphia* (1993), starring one of America's most beloved and affable actors, Tom Hanks, as a lawyer with AIDS who is fired by his firm, finally brought a mainstream cinematic treatment, though in a nonthreatening and sexually chaste mode.

Visual Arts.   Graphic and visual arts can either be among the most public (mechanically reproduced and circulated) or among the most cloistered (the sole copy existing in a private collection) of the arts. The arts scene during the 1980s witnessed an economic boom for some artists as new wealth sought out (and paid ever higher prices for) new art as an "investment" or status marker. Many of these artworks were the detached, ironic, and apolitical grandchildren of Andy Warhol.

However, the AIDS epidemic decimated the art world (including its creators, critics, and brokers) to the point that, beginning in 1989, December 1 of each year has been declared a Day Without Art in order to engage art communities in the struggle against AIDS. During the 1980s and 1990s, some politically engaged visual artists employed graphics, photography, collage, and installations in order to represent the lives of HIV-infected people and to advocate action to end the epidemic.

Art collectives like Gran Fury working with the AIDS Coalition to Unleash Power (ACT UP) created striking postmodern graphics (e.g., posters, signs, crack-and-peel stickers) for direct-action demonstrations. ACT UP also created at New York's Museum of Contemporary Art an installation entitled *Let the Record Show*, which drew parallels between the actively hostile or merely complacent religious and political authorities in power at the time with Nazi war criminals on trial at Nuremberg after World War II.

By late in the twentieth century, photography had emerged as an art form, not just a journalistic tool, which, when focused on AIDS, documented the lives of HIV-infected people and their caregivers, as well as the activists working on their behalf. Photographers like Nicholas Nixon, Gypsy Ray, Jane Rosett, Brian Weil, and Sal Lopes counteracted the prevailing sensationalism of many media images and the invisibility of the poor and ethnic or racial minorities living with AIDS.

Two photographers drew special notoriety for the frankness of their depictions of the body and their hostility to mainstream sensibilities. Robert Mapplethorpe, who died of HIV-related illness in 1989, produced a body of work that contrasted its cool formalism with its candid sexuality. A posthumous retrospective of his work was canceled by the Corcoran Gallery of Art in Washington, D.C., (prompting the arts community to boycott the museum) and when the director of Contemporary Arts Center of Cincinnati, Dennis Barrie, presented the exhibition, he was charged with a violation of obscenity laws (but later acquitted by a jury). An activist artist and a person with AIDS, David Wojnarowicz, became embroiled in a larger controversy about public funding for the arts through the National Endowment for the Arts, involving conservative Republican Senator Jesse Helms and Christian fundamentalist minister Donald Wildmon of the American Family Association.

Equally libidinal but somehow tamer, more accessible, and less confrontational were the graphics of Keith Haring, who died of AIDS in 1990. A "guerilla" artist whose cartoon graffiti drawings appeared on subways and urban wallscapes before his work became commercialized, Haring contributed graphic designs to AIDS education publications and activist materials. His life and career were celebrated in a musical, *Radiant Baby*, in 2003.

A classic American folk art genre was revived in the AIDS epidemic: the quilt. The AIDS Memorial Quilt began as an effort simply to document the names of those who had died (the NAMES Project), but grew as a grassroots effort to provide a more personal memorial for those who had died by using an artifact of material culture that often comforts the ill or afflicted, a quilted blanket. Consisting of 3-foot by 6-foot panels (the approximate size of a funeral plot) now numbering over 40,000, with each panel stitched and embroidered by family or friends to represent the unique quality of an individual lost, the AIDS Memorial Quilt has been exhibited (in parts, because it is too large for one public space) throughout the world.

During the first two decades of the AIDS epidemic, literature and the arts were media to express grief and rage, to celebrate sexuality at a time when the erotic was represented as dangerous, and to engage those affected by AIDS in solidarity and productive action. *See also* AIDS in Africa; AIDS in the United States; Black Death: Literature and Art; Cinema and Epidemic Disease; Literature, Disease in Modern; Plague Literature and Art, Early Modern European; Popular Media and Epidemic Disease: Recent Trends; Poison Libels and Epidemic Disease; Religion and Epidemic Disease; Scapegoats and Epidemic Disease; Sexuality, Gender, and Epidemic Disease; Trade, Travel, and Epidemic Disease.

Further Reading

Atkins, Robert, and Thomas W. Sokolowski. *From Media to Metaphor: Art About AIDS*. New York: Independent Curators, 1991.

Baker, Rob. *The Art of AIDS: From Stigma to Conscience*. New York: Continuum International, 1994.

Bordowitz, Gregg. *The AIDS Crisis is Ridiculous and Other Writings, 1986–2003*. Cambridge, MA: MIT Press, 2006.

Clark, Charles F. *AIDS and the Arrows of Pestilence*. Golden, CO: Fulcrum, 1994.

Crimp, Douglas, ed. *AIDS: Cultural Analysis, Cultural Activism*. Cambridge, MA: MIT Press, 1988.

Crimp, Douglas, with Adam Rolston. *AIDS Demo Graphics*. Seattle: Bay Press, 1990.

Foertsch, Jacqueline. *Enemies Within: The Cold War and the AIDS Crisis in Literature, Film, and Culture*. Urbana: University of Illinois Press, 2001.

Long, Thomas L. *AIDS and American Apocalypticism: The Cultural Semiotics of an Epidemic*. Albany: State University of New York Press, 2005.

Miller, James, ed. *Fluid Exchanges: Artists and Critics in the AIDS Crisis*. Toronto: University of Toronto Press, 1992.

Murphy, Timothy F., and Suzanne Poirier, eds. *Writing AIDS: Gay Literature, Language, and Analysis*. New York: Columbia University Press, 1993.

Nelson, Emmanuel S. *AIDS: The Literary Response*. Boston: Twayne, 1992.

Pastore, Judith Laurence. *Confronting AIDS through Literature: The Responsibilities of Representation.* Urbana: University of Illinois Press, 1993.

Sontag, Susan. *AIDS and Its Metaphors.* New York: Farrar, Straus, Giroux, 1989.

Treichler, Paula. *How to Have Theory in an Epidemic.* Durham, NC: Duke University Press, 1999.

THOMAS LAWRENCE LONG

AIR AND EPIDEMIC DISEASES. Historically, the conception that imbalances between the **human body** and the environment create illness frequently gave air a primary role in both natural and transcendental explanations of communally experienced illness.

Early considerations of air and disease occur in several texts of the **Hippocratic Corpus** (e.g., *On the Nature of Man* 9, *Breaths* 6, *Regimen in Acute Diseases* 2, *Epidemics* 2.1 and 3, *Airs, Waters, Places*), and a co-mingling of natural and transcendental etiologies appears around the term *miasma* ("pollution"). Miasmas resulting in **epidemic** plagues could be brought on by "polluted" actions (such as in Sophocles's [495–406 BCE] *Oedipus the King*) or by air rendered unhealthy by natural processes. Over time, prevailing medical theory held that plagues were caused by air fouled by wet organic materials decomposing and entering the air through heat (Diodorus Siculus [c. 90–30 BCE] 12.58.3; **Galen** *De febrium differentiis* 1.6). However, other related theories, such as a concentration of unhealthy atoms in the air (Lucretius [99–55 BCE] 6.1093–97), minute airborne creatures (Varro [116– 27 BCE] *On Rural Farming* 1), or noxious materials brought up by earthquakes (Seneca [4 BCE–65 CE] *Naturales quaestiones* 6.27) also occur.

In general, it was broadly accepted well into the nineteenth century that miasmas resulted from decaying organic material and that they were the cause of epidemic diseases that we would now recognize as disparate (e.g., **cholera, smallpox, influenza,** and

---

THE CAUSE OF CHOLERA: NOT CONTAGION BUT MIASMA (1831)

It is chiefly for the purpose of quieting these unnecessary alarms, that this essay is published; in which it is intended to prove, (notwithstanding all the assertions to the contrary) that the mild Cholera of this country [England], is essentially the same disease, and proceeds from the same cause, as the malignant Indio-Russian Cholera; modified, however, by the state of the bodies of the individuals attacked. Besides this, the cause, symptoms, mode of prevention, and the plan of treatment, which has been successfully employed, is laid down.

If the disease had been viewed in the light afforded by the celebrated **Sydenham** [1624–1689], whose accurate observation of the operation of morbific causes upon the body have justly entitled him to the appellation of the English **Hippocrates**, many of the evils, which have resulted from the unqualified and groundless statements of the contagious nature of Cholera, would have been prevented. In the chapter on Epidemic Diseases he says, "There are various constitutions of years, which owe their origin neither to heat nor cold, dryness nor moisture, but which depend upon some secret and inexplicable action in the bowels of the earth, whence the air is contaminated with certain effluvia, which subject the body to particular diseases, so long as that constitution predominates."

In this short sentence, we have a rational explanation of the origin of spasmodic Cholera, which has traveled from Asia, through Europe to England, not by contagion above ground, but by underground alterations and consequent emanations of certain effluvia from the earth, by which the atmosphere is contaminated.

From Isaac Pidduck, M.D., *The Identity of the Asiatic, Russian, and English Cholera: Its Cause, Symptoms, Prevention and Cure* (London, 1831), pp. 3–4.

diphtheria). As urban centers grew, thanks in part to **colonization** and the **Industrial Revolution**, miasmatic theory influenced advancements in Western public health that were aimed to curb epidemic outbreaks through better civil engineering and health reforms. These advancements often went hand-in-hand with convictions that people, especially the poor and the uncivilized, needed both moral and hygienic regulation and education.

From the Renaissance through the nineteenth century, however, competing theories of **transmission** and disease generation, influenced by developments in the natural sciences, challenged miasmatic theory. These theories contended that specific contaminants entered or contacted the body through the air or **water** and caused specific diseases to grow rather than to occur spontaneously from miasmatic air. One of the earliest was **Girolamo Fracastoro's** suggestion (1546) that seed-like particles caused infectious disease. However, these theories did not gain the upper hand until the nineteenth century through the work of pioneers such as **John Snow, Louis Pasteur**, Joseph Lister (1827–1912), **Robert Koch**, and Theodor Klebs (1834–1913). Some physicians and health reformers, such as Florence Nightingale (1820–1910), vigorously opposed the new theories. However, the rapidly spreading **influenza pandemic of 1889–1890** hastened worldwide acceptance of the new theories and turned attention toward air contamination by specific aerosolized agents as a cause of many epidemic illnesses. The subsequent identification of these various agents and their methods of transmission led to modern medical and public health approaches toward airborne illness and air pollution, as well as to weaponization of some airborne agents such as anthrax for **biological warfare** or **bioterrorism**. *See also* Astrology and Medicine; Avicenna (Ibn Sina); Contagion and Transmission; Contagion Theory of Disease, Premodern; Corpses and Epidemic Disease; Disinfection and Fumigation; Environment, Ecology, and Epidemic Disease; Flight; Germ Theory of Disease; Greco-Roman Medical Theory and Practice; Islamic Disease Theory and Medicine; Pneumonic and Septicemic Plague; Sanitation Movement of the Nineteenth Century; Urbanization and Epidemic Disease.

Further Reading

Porter, Roy. *The Greatest Benefit to Mankind.* New York: Norton, 1997.

Rosenberg, Charles. *Explaining Epidemics and Other Studies in the History of Medicine.* New York: Cambridge University Press, 1992.

Watts, Sheldon. *Epidemics and History.* New Haven: Yale University Press, 1997.

ERIC D. NELSON

ANIMAL DISEASES (ZOONOSES) AND EPIDEMIC DISEASE. Animal **epidemics**, or epizootics, also affect humans. Epizootics mean less food for people, making them more susceptible to disease. Zoonotic diseases—those transmissible between humans and animals—usually begin with birds, reptiles, amphibians, or mammals, and end up in human populations (although the reverse occurs as well). Contemporary biologists Fuller Torrey and Robert Yolken estimate that microbes originating with nonhuman animals in the past and those currently transmissible to humans from nonhuman animals cause approximately three-quarters of all human infections. Humans and cattle both suffer from **tuberculosis, smallpox** and cowpox are closely related, and human **measles** is a cousin to rinderpest in cattle and canine distemper. True zoonoses, those diseases currently transmissible between animals and humans, include **bubonic plague**, rabies, and anthrax. These infections have caused both devastating epidemics and less dramatic endemic diseases (such as tuberculosis and **dysentery**) that have caused even more deaths over time.

Transmission of zoonoses can occur in numerous ways that depend on genetic and ecological changes in populations of humans, animals, and microorganisms. Historical outbreaks of disease have pointed to the importance of understanding the ecology and evolution of zoonotic diseases. For example, in 2006 scientists determined that a mutated bird **virus** caused the **influenza pandemic of 1918–1919**, which killed between 20 and 100 million people. This was announced in the midst of an Asian outbreak of avian (bird) **influenza**. Some epidemiologists feared that the bird infection would jump to humans, creating a deadly **pandemic**, like that of 1918–1919. A long history of biological relationships between humans and animals has given the pathogens and their hosts plenty of opportunities to develop new ecological and evolutionary strategies. People, animals, and pathogens may trigger epidemics by finding a new species to infect, traveling on a ship or plane, or undergoing a genetic mutation, for example.

This article focuses on bubonic plague and influenza to demonstrate how ecological and evolutionary changes have helped cause epidemics (or, in a global context, pandemics). The same questions could be asked about any zoonotic disease. Bubonic plague depends on ecological interactions between wild reservoirs (Asian and North American rodents) and the movements of people along **trade** routes. The example of influenza draws attention to the importance of the biological mechanisms used by pathogens to adapt to new ecological circumstances. The influenza virus undergoes genetic alteration rapidly and easily jumps between species—sometimes initiating epidemics or pandemics. The two case studies that follow provide a model for understanding and writing about the ecology and evolution of zoonotic diseases.

The Ecology of Bubonic Plague.   Bubonic plague is caused by *Yersinia pestis*, a **bacterium** that diverged evolutionarily from its nearest relatives only a few thousand years ago. This organism infects native rodents on the Asian steppes. It hitched a ride to Europe with rats, which first arrived in the Mediterranean basin on ships from central Asia around 500 CE. The **Plague of Justinian** of the sixth century followed, killing around 40 percent of the population of Constantinople and up to a quarter of the human population of the entire eastern Mediterranean. Smaller outbreaks occurred for the next 200 years or so, until bubonic plague disappeared in European populations. *Y. pestis's* major European reservoir, the black rat (*Rattus rattus*), continued to spread and expand in numbers, however, and local wild populations of rodents also became infected. As human population densities and trading activities recovered over the years, the ecological conditions were right for plague to appear again.

In 1338, plague broke out among people living on the Asian steppes in what is now Kyrgyzstan; it spread along trade routes to India, China, and the Middle East where it killed an estimated 35 million in China alone. Ten years later, it arrived with rats on ships coming to the ports of Genoa, Messina, and Sicily. By this time, black rats had adapted very successfully to living in close contact with European people, and as plague spread among the rats, it spread to people also. Historians have estimated that between 1348 and 1352 up to one-third of Europe's entire population died of the **Black Death** and the chaos that accompanied the epidemic. Although rats had been suspected as a reservoir of plague, the disease's causative organism was found much later, in the 1890s, by **Alexandre Yersin** and **Shibasaburo Kitasato**. *Y. pestis* was transmitted between animals and to humans by another animal: a vector, the flea.

The **third plague pandemic** originated in China in the 1860s and spread quickly. An estimated 12 million people died, mainly in India and China. This pandemic affected every continent on the globe except Antarctica. Infected rats carried plague from Hong Kong to Honolulu to San Francisco in 1900, where it hit Chinese neighborhoods near the docks hardest. *Y. pestis* had just been given its greatest ecological break in centuries—a vast land mass with new populations of animals and people to colonize. Rapidly infecting prairie dogs and ground squirrels in the North American West, the microbe has crossed the Rocky Mountains and is moving eastward. Although rare in people and domesticated animals in wealthier countries, plague still kills people in the developing world and in areas suffering from natural or human-made disasters.

Scientists now understand that *Y. pestis* has evolved to what researchers Sharon Collinge and Chris Ray call "spectacular generalism": it occurs naturally in more than 200 species of mammals and over 260 species of fleas worldwide. This makes it easy for plague to spread from wild animals to domesticated animals, such as cats, and thence to humans who otherwise would have little direct exposure to wild rodents. *Y. pestis* has now established itself so firmly around the world that its eradication is all but impossible, and future outbreaks will occur.

As long as people and the wild reservoirs avoided each other, plague did not cause human pandemics. From its limited range in wild central Asian rodents, *Y. pestis* tagged along as rats spread along human trade routes, both over land and by sea. Rats adapted very successfully to cohabitation with populations of humans, especially in crowded cities. Once established in these rats, *Y. pestis* spread to people, thus ensuring positive conditions for its continued survival. In this framework, humans are only one species of many that provide a substrate for the microbe's evolutionary success; but for us, bubonic plague remains one of history's most devastating and terrifying zoonotic diseases.

The Evolution of Influenza.   Influenza is a disease caused by a family of viruses (although this idea was not agreed upon by scientists until the 1930s). Influenza viruses have caused disease in humans for quite some time; major outbreaks have occurred approximately every 40 years since 1800. Influenza was responsible for the third most devastating pandemic in history (following the Justinian plague and the Black Death). In 1918–1919, 20 to 100 million people around the world died from influenza and its complications. Scientists and historians have estimated that about one-third of the world's population was infected and sickened by influenza. Influenza flourished in the chaos of World War I: in the trenches, bomb shelters and basements, railway cars, and encampments of people weakened by malnutrition. It also spread rapidly across the United States, a nation not as directly impacted by the **war**. The influenza pandemic of 1918–1919 remains an historical puzzle that involves not just human but also animal populations.

The disease seemed to "explode" simultaneously in Asia, Europe, and the United States, and it came in three waves that spanned over a year. The human pandemic coincided with outbreaks of similar respiratory diseases in pigs (swine) and horses. Both human and swine populations seemed immunologically naïve to the pandemic virus (a piece of information noted by witnesses at the time), which made it unlikely that the virus had "incubated" in pigs before jumping to human populations. Within a few years of the 1918–1919 pandemic, moreover, influenza seemed to have become an ordinary (far less fatal) disease. After the horrors of 1918, as modern historian Alfred Crosby has argued, most people wished to forget about influenza (Crosby, 1989).

Following World War II, **World Health Organization** researchers surveyed animals and people around the world, looking for influenza. They took blood samples from human, swine, horse, and bird (avian) populations, compared them serologically, and banked them. This research began the process of understanding what had happened in 1918 because the researchers found virus strains in all of the human and animal populations. Scientists recognized that animal populations served as reservoirs and mixing vessels for human influenza. In the 1990s, geneticists began to apply newly available scientific tools to old questions about the influenza pandemic of 1918–1919. Where had the virus come from? Why had it emerged so quickly, only to disappear just as quickly?

In terms of mutation and ability to infect new species, influenza has evolved for speed. It exists on the edge of what geneticists call "error catastrophe": it mutates so promiscuously and rapidly that its genome teeters on the brink of dysfunctionality. These potential problems are, however, outweighed by the advantages of being able to mutate and adapt to new hosts very quickly. These genetic characteristics help to explain how influenza (and other infections) can transcend species barriers so efficiently. Indeed, the strain of the virus that caused the 1918–1919 pandemic, "H1N1," has been called "the mother of all pandemics." H1N1 was the origin of all known strains circulating in populations of people and pigs circa 2000. Descendents of the 1918 virus are responsible for all recorded pandemics since that time; moreover, swine have served as the major reservoir for H1N1 strains (which have now recently reemerged in humans as the result of a laboratory accident).

Using preserved autopsy material from people who died of influenza in 1918, scientists have concluded that the deadly virus from that pandemic was an avian-like strain that had mutated dramatically. In contrast, it was determined that subsequent pandemics (with lower mortality) in 1957 and 1968 had been caused by the reassortment of genetic segments from wild bird viruses. Scientists believe that the 1918 virus appeared so rapidly and was so deadly because it had undergone dramatic mutations with which humans' and pigs' immune systems were unfamiliar. Although the virus seemed to have disappeared just as quickly as it came, it had only moved out of the human population; it continued to live and evolve in swine. In both pigs and people, herd immunity provided the most likely explanation for the virus' decrease in virulence in the 1920s. In the early 2000s, an outbreak of H5N1 influenza in Asian birds caught the attention of scientists when about 200 people became infected, and several died. All of the infected people had had close contact with infected birds, but fears of the virus mutating so that it could be spread directly between people conjured up visions of the 1918–1919 pandemic. No historical data exist to support the idea of avian outbreaks preceding the 1918 pandemic. However, it has become clear that we must understand the circulation of viruses in human *and* animal populations, through time and across space, in order to predict and prepare for future outbreaks. *See also* Bubonic Plague and related articles; Human Immunity and Resistance to Disease; Influenza Pandemic, 1889–1890; Plague: End of the Second Pandemic; Plague in San Francisco, 1900–1908; Plague in China; Simond, Paul-Louis.

Further Reading

Barnes, Ethne. *Diseases and Human Evolution*. Albuquerque: University of New Mexico Press, 2005.

Collinge, Sharon, and Chris Ray. *Disease Ecology: Community Structure and Pathogen Dynamics*. Oxford: Oxford University Press, 2006.

Crosby, Alfred W. *America's Forgotten Pandemic: The Influenza of 1918*. New York: Cambridge University Press, 1989.

National Library of Medicine Exhibition. http://www.nlm.nih.gov/exhibition/animals/index.html

Taubenberger, J. K., and David Morens. "1918 Influenza: The Mother of All Pandemics." *Emerging Infectious Diseases* [serial on the Internet]. January 2006. http://www.cdc.gov/ncidod/EID/vol12no01/05-0979.htm

Torrey, E. Fuller, and Robert H. Yolken. *Beasts of the Earth: Animals, Humans and Disease*. New Brunswick, NJ: Rutgers University Press, 2005.

SUSAN D. JONES

ANIMAL RESEARCH.   Although animals were occasionally used for scientific experimentation at least since the days of ancient Greece, animal experimentation did not become significant until the **Scientific Revolution**, when discoveries such as the circulation of the blood clearly demonstrated that such experiments could lead to useful scientific knowledge. Even then, some raised objections to animal experimentation on both moral and scientific grounds.

With the emergence of physiology as a scientific discipline in the early nineteenth century, the use of animals in experimentation became much more widespread. As other biomedical sciences, such as pharmacology and bacteriology, were established later in the century, animal experimentation also became central to their focus. This increased use of animals in experimentation also led to the first organized efforts promoting animal welfare, such as the founding of societies for the protection of animals, in the nineteenth century. In England and America a vigorous anti-vivisection movement emerged. Although the term "vivisection" originally referred to dissection of living animals, by this time it had come to be applied to animal experimentation in general.

As animal experimentation led to the introduction of important medical advances around the turn of the twentieth century, such as the development of an antitoxin for the treatment of **diphtheria**, an infectious disease that especially affected children, the popularity of the anti-vivisection movement waned. Animals were also utilized in the production and testing of the antitoxin, as well as in the research leading to its discovery. Animal research was involved in the development of many other preventive and treatment methods for infectious disease, among other illnesses, such as the **polio** vaccine and **antibiotics**. Animals also became increasingly important in the twentieth century in the testing and standardization of the new **pharmaceuticals** and other therapies developed as a result of biomedical research.

The use of animals in the life sciences has undergone further expansion since the Second World War. Increases in funding for medical research, the number of chemicals in the marketplace, and the regulations governing drugs and other products have all contributed to the growing use of animals in research and testing. Under U.S. law, for example, new drugs for infectious and other diseases must be tested first in animals for efficacy and safety before they can be approved for clinical trials involving **human subjects**. Tens of millions of animals are used annually in the United States today for research, testing, and education.

The postwar period has also witnessed a revival of the animal protection movement, especially since the publication of ethicist Peter Singer's *Animal Liberation* in 1975. Animal rights activists and the scientific community have frequently clashed over the necessity and ethics of using animals in medical research. The efforts of the animal rights movement have helped to increase sensitivity about the treatment of animals and to enact animal welfare legislation, such as the Animal Welfare Act of 1966 and subsequent amendments. There has also been an increased emphasis on the development of alternatives to animals, for example, greater use of nonsensitive organisms (such as bacteria) and computer modeling, but it does not seem likely that the need for animals in research will be eliminated any time soon. Thus animal research is likely to remain an important tool of biomedical science and an area of controversy for the foreseeable future.

Further Reading

French, Richard D. *Antivivisection and Medical Science in Victorian Society*. Princeton: Princeton University Press, 1975.
Guerrini, Anita. *Experimenting with Humans and Animals: From Galen to Animal Rights*. Baltimore: Johns Hopkins University Press, 2003.
Rudacille, Deborah. *The Scalpel and the Butterfly: The War Between Animal Research and Animal Protection*. New York: Farrar, Straus, and Giroux, 2000.
Rupke, Nicolaas A., ed. *Vivisection in Historical Perspective*. London: Routledge, 1987.

JOHN PARASCANDOLA

ANTIBIOTICS. Antibiotics are the class of drugs used to treat infections caused by **bacteria**. When the term was coined in 1941, it referred specifically to substances produced by one microorganism that inhibit or kill another form of microorganism. More recently, the term has been generalized to include drugs synthesized in the laboratory or **pharmaceutical** factory.

Antibiotics work by inhibiting a variety of metabolic processes of bacteria. **Penicillin** and similar drugs destroy the cell walls of some bacteria. Other antibiotics inhibit the ability of bacteria to make DNA, RNA, or proteins essential for metabolism and replication. Many of the mechanisms that bacteria use to construct proteins are different from the processes that higher animals use, so it is possible for antibiotics to target specific bacteria without harming the patient.

The first uses of substances to fight infections are likely lost in prehistory. Many ancient peoples used honey as a wound dressing without recognizing that it possesses hydrogen peroxide and other antibacterial compounds and that its high sugar content makes bacterial growth impossible. They also plastered wounds with moldy bread, foreshadowing the eventual development of penicillin. These primitive efforts were effective in treating superficial wounds and skin infections, but were worthless in treating internal infections.

The ability to treat internal infections effectively began in the early twentieth century. Salts of mercury, arsenic, and other metals were used to treat syphilis, but were highly toxic. Later, organic aniline dyes led to the use of **sulfa drugs**, which were much safer antibacterial treatments. In 1928 penicillin, the first true antibiotic, was discovered, but its commercial production lagged until the Second World War. The use of sulfa drugs and penicillin on the battlefield dramatically decreased combat mortality and led to rapid growth of antibiotic production for the civilian population.

The initial enthusiasm for these new "miracle drugs" was followed by disappointment because relatively few types of bacteria were affected by them. Gram-positive bacteria, such as streptococcus and staphylococcus, have a cell wall and are susceptible to the effects of penicillin. Gram-negative bacteria lack a cell wall and include a host of disease-causing organisms that are unaffected by penicillin. The promise of treatment for infections caused by these organisms led to the rapid development of new antibiotics.

Streptomycin was the first major antibiotic to be developed after penicillin. It is a member of the aminoglycoside family, and its initial role was in the treatment of **tuberculosis**, but it also is effective against some Gram-negative bacteria. Streptomycin was derived from *Streptomyces*, a species of soil bacterium, by Ukrainian American biochemist Selman Waksman (1888–1973). He and others postulated that sites of high bacterial population would be likely to have a variety of bacteria that produce antibiotics as a matter of survival, decreasing the competition from other species in the same area. This hypothesis led to the productive pursuit of other antibiotics from soil and even sewage samples.

The development of the tetracycline family of antibiotics soon followed. This group of drugs is important because they were the first "broad spectrum" antibiotics, effective against a wide variety of both Gram-negative and Gram-positive bacteria. This ability of the tetracyclines to treat many types of infection was balanced by a disadvantage. Penicillin, streptomycin, and similar drugs are bactericidal—they kill bacteria outright. Tetracyclines and many other antibiotics are bacteristatic—they inhibit the ability of bacteria to reproduce and rely on the ability of the immune system to clear the infection by destroying the still-living bacteria.

The class of bactericidal antibiotics with the greatest number of drugs is the cephalosporins. The first of the cephalosporins were isolated from bacteria growing in a sewer in 1948. There are now well over 50 drugs in the cephalosporin class, and its members have widely varying properties. They have different patterns of absorption and penetration into different internal organs. Most important, the members of the group have great variation in the spectrum of bacteria that are susceptible to them. The number and variation of the cephalosporins demonstrate the ability to manipulate the molecular structure of antibiotics to alter their effects.

Once the ability to manipulate the structure, and therefore the function, of the cephalosporins had been harnessed, the ability to totally synthesize antibiotics without a biological source followed. This led to the development of the fluoroquinolones, the best known of which is ciprofloxacin. Cipro is a very broad-spectrum antibiotic that became an everyday word during the anthrax scares of 2001.

Another problem of antibiotic use is that bacteria have a tremendous ability to develop resistance to nearly any antibiotic. It was initially thought that this happened only after bacteria were exposed to a drug, but not for a long enough time to kill them all. It was believed that the survivors would then transmit their ability to resist the antibiotic to future generations of the bacteria. It is now apparent that even before some antibiotics are made commercially available, bacteria can develop a resistance to the drugs, possibly through exposure to the natural antibiotics produced by other bacteria in the natural environment.

There are a number of practices that increase the likelihood that bacteria in a host will develop resistance. One is failure to complete a full course of antibiotics, instead stopping before all the bacteria have been killed. Another is using an overly broad spectrum of treatment, which kills both the disease-causing organism and the human host's normal "friendly" bacteria, thus allowing the overgrowth of more resistant species. Perhaps one of the greatest causes of resistance is the widespread use of broad-spectrum antibiotics as nutritional supplements in animal feed. This practice encourages the emergence of resistant forms that contaminate the meat and make their way into the food chain, thus infecting us.

Some "superbugs" appear to be able to develop resistance faster than new antibiotics can be developed. This pattern of rapid mutation of bacteria along with the decreasing rate of production of new antibiotics has led to concern that we may again enter an era of bacterial diseases that are untreatable by any safe drugs—that we may witness a chilling return to the fearsome pre-antibiotic era. *See also* Capitalism and Epidemic Disease; Drug Resistance in Microorganisms; Human Body; Human Immunity and Resistance to Disease.

Further Reading

Amyes, Sebastian G. B. *Magic Bullets, Lost Horizons: The Rise and Fall of Antibiotics*. London: Taylor and Francis, 2001.

Gould, Ian M., and J. W. van der Meer. *Antibiotic Policies: Theory and Practice*. New York: Springer, 2004.

Walsh, Christopher. *Antibiotics: Actions, Origins, Resistance*. Washington, DC: ASM Press, 2003.

Charles V. Bender

ANTONINE PLAGUE.   *See* Plagues of the Roman Empire.

APOTHECARY/PHARMACIST.   Medicines are among humanity's oldest tools, and the making of medicines is the central concern of the modern field of pharmacy. Despite pharmacy's prehistoric origins, a specialized occupation dedicated to the production and distribution of medicines—the pharmacist—did not arise until the Middle Ages. Before that time, healers of all sorts, including domestic healers and religious leaders, usually mixed together their own remedies and administered them to their patients.

The ancestors of today's pharmacists arose in the flowering of Islamic culture in Baghdad in the late eighth century CE. This new city quickly became a center of scholarship and of trade, including exotic spices and drugs. A specialized shopkeeper appeared, the *sayādilah*, who concentrated his business in the making and selling of medicines. In the decades that followed, governmental authorities initiated a system of licenses and inspections, and the idea of regulated medicine makers spread across the cities of the Arab world. During the eleventh century, the concept of specialized medicine sellers emerged in southern Europe where Islamic culture had its greatest influence. By the middle of the thirteenth century, public medicine shops were so common that Frederick II (1194–1250), as King of Sicily, issued edicts that called for the separation of medicine and pharmacy and the regulation of apothecary shops. As their shops spread through Europe, apothecaries became incorporated into the guild system that regulated trade and political life in the late medieval and Renaissance cities, usually joining spice merchants, grocers, or physicians. Not all guildsmen, however, were actively involved in the trade: the Italian poet Dante Alighieri (1265–1321), for example, became a member of the guild of apothecaries and physicians of Florence for political reasons.

Some European medicine dealers took on a version of the name "apothecary," which was derived from the Latin *apotheca* or storehouse. These shopkeepers were identified directly with the goods they sold. In other parts of Europe, the specialist's name was derived from the Greek *pharmakon* meaning medicine, the source of the modern term "pharmacist." In this case, the occupational name was derived from the work done, as was the case with other trades such as smith or cooper.

Guilds and Pharmacopeias.   A primary activity of apothecary and physician guilds was to promote the compiling and publication of pharmacopeias. These books of drug standards and medicine formulas served to guide apothecaries as they filled the prescriptions written by physicians. The guilds also set standards for the training of apprentices and the quality of medicines in shops. Eventually, apothecaries grew in power and prestige to the point at which they split off to form their own associations such as the Worshipful Society of Apothecaries of London (1617).

In the 1500s, changes swept through the fields of medicine and pharmacy. Followers of **Paracelsus** applied the emerging technologies of chemistry to the making of medicines, greatly expanding the drug armamentarium of physicians. Moreover, European explorers to the New World brought back other new plant drugs, such as cinchona bark and tobacco, which increased the stock of apothecary shops. Apothecaries became versed in chemistry and botany to serve their clientele. By the 1600s, French pharmacists like Nicaise LeFebvre (c. 1610–1669) and Nicolas Lemery (1645–1715) were writing the leading chemistry texts of the era. In the eighteenth and nineteenth centuries, pharmacists such as Carl Wilhelm Scheele (1742–1786), Antoine Baumé (1728–1804), Martin Klaproth (1743–1817), and Carl Freidrich Mohr (1806–1879) produced some of the greatest achievements in early modern chemistry. By combining their chemical expertise with their knowledge of plant drugs, pharmacists Friedrich Wilhelm Sertürner (1783–1841), Joseph Bienaimé Caventou (1795–1877), and Pierre Joseph Pelletier (1788–1842) isolated pure crystalline alkaloids including morphine and quinine in the early 1800s. These drugs revolutionized both medical practice and research by granting precision to the prescriptions of physicians and the experiments of scientists.

Modern Europe.   Most apothecaries, of course, were not explorers or scientists. They were owners of small shops specializing in the making and selling of medicines. Their status in society, however, did benefit from the fame of their profession's achievements and the highly regulated nature of their practice. In northern Europe, especially, governmental units tightly controlled pharmacy, limiting competition and setting up price schedules for medicines. Apothecaries operated as solid members of the middle class, and across most of Europe they had a status similar to physicians well into the twentieth century. Since the end of World War II, restrictive regulations on the number pharmacists and pharmacies have gradually disappeared across most of Europe. Pharmacists have maintained their standing as middle-class heath professionals through the general adoption of college diplomas as a requirement for licensure.

Anglo-American Differences.   In the Anglo-American context, however, the occupation of pharmacist developed differently. Beginning in the late seventeenth century, English apothecaries shifted more closely toward the role of general practitioners of medicine. Because university-trained physicians were rare and expensive, most ailing people consulted apothecaries, who charged only for the medicine they sold, not for advice. Moreover, the apothecaries had benefited from stories that they stayed behind their counters even during plague times, when physicians abandoned London and other cities. As more and more apothecaries moved into medical practice, a new class of shopkeepers—the chemists and druggists—appeared to take over the routine making and selling of medicines. In sharp contrast with the Continent, government authorities in England did not choose to regulate pharmacy until well into the 1800s.

During this period of change and turmoil within the English health scene, the North American colonies were settled. Until towns and villages reached a critical size to support specialized shops like those of apothecaries, most medicines in the English colonies were sold in general stores or by wholesale druggists in the largest coastal ports, who serviced the needs of ships or plantations. According to *Kremers and Urdang's History of Pharmacy*, American community pharmacy arose from four distinct roots: the apothecary shop, the general store, the wholesale druggist, and the doctor's shop. The last type of establishment was run by a physician who diagnosed, prescribed, and dispensed all out of a small shop. The practices of medicine and pharmacy in the United States did not clearly begin to separate until the middle of the 1800s.

Two events of the early 1800s marked the beginnings of professional pharmacy in the young United States. In 1820, nine physicians gathered at the Capitol in Washington, D.C., and founded the *United States Pharmacopoeia*. This book of drug standards was meant to guide apothecaries and wholesalers as they prepared the basic ingredients that went into medicines. The book was needed because physicians had come to rely on druggists and apothecaries. The second event was the establishment of the Philadelphia College of Pharmacy in 1821. This local association of apothecaries organized to foster professional development through publications and a school for apprentices. During the middle third of the 1800s, other local societies sprung up following the Philadelphia example. In 1852, the American Pharmaceutical Association was formed and has fostered professional development to the present day.

In the late nineteenth century, large-scale manufacturing methods were applied to the making of prescription ingredients as well as proprietary remedies. In the face of industrialization, pharmacists organized state associations, which worked to pass state pharmacy laws that regulate practice. At the same time, Schools of Pharmacy also began to appear alongside medical schools at large state universities.

The early days of the twentieth century witnessed reforms that included the expansion of the pharmacy education system and the introduction of a requirement for pharmacy school diplomas (begun in New York in 1910). By the 1930s, pharmacy school expanded to a uniform four-year Bachelor of Science degree requirement. Because most American pharmacists continued to practice in a drugstore setting, however, their professional status suffered. It was only in the post–World War II era, when the modern pharmaceutical industry began to mass-produce medicines effective against a wide spectrum of diseases, that the prestige of American pharmacists rose. By 1970 the proportion of prescriptions requiring compounding expertise dropped significantly. Pharmacists gained stature within the health-care system by providing drug information and counseling to their patients. In the early 1990s, American pharmacy embraced the practice model of "pharmaceutical care," which called for pharmacists to assume responsibility for proper drug outcomes. In addition, pharmaceutical education began the shift to a single Doctor of Pharmacy (Pharm. D.) degree.

In the early years of the twenty-first century, the roles of pharmacists continue to evolve. Still in charge of the distribution of medicines, pharmacists seek more authority

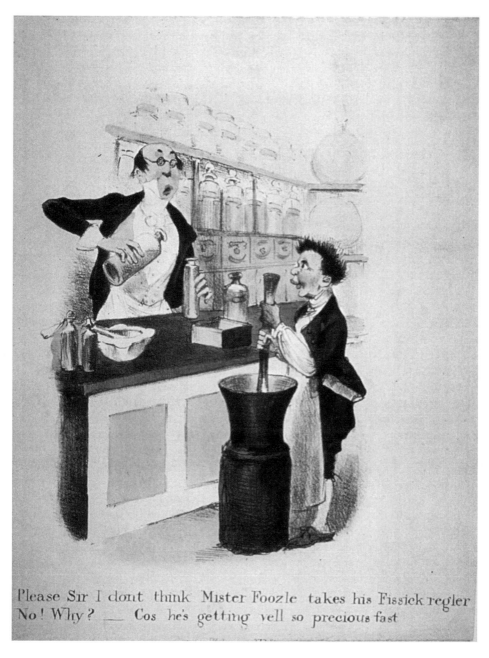

Please Sir I dont think Mister Foozle takes his Fissick regler No! Why? — Cos he's getting vell so precious fast

Interior of pharmacy in 1800s. Pharmacist behind the counter is pouring mixture into a jar while the assistant, in the foreground, prepares mixture in a butter churn. A pestle and mortar and other containers are shown on the counter; apothecary jars can be seen on shelves in the background. Caption: "Please Sir I dont think Mister Foozle takes his Fissick regler No! Why?—Cos he's getting vell so precious fast." Courtesy of the National Library of Medicine.

over proper drug use and a larger role in matters pertaining to public health. *See also* Antibiotics; Bimaristan/Maristan; Capitalism and Epidemic Disease; Empiric; Folk Medicine; Islamic Disease Theory and Medicine; London, Great Plague of (1665–1666); Pest Houses and Lazarettos; Pharmaceutical Industry; Plague and Developments in Public Health, 1348–1600; Poison Libels and Epidemic Disease; Public Health Agencies in the West before 1900; Public Health in the Islamic World, 1000–1600; Quacks, Charlatans, and Their Remedies; Sulfa Drugs.

Further Reading

Anderson, Stuart. *Making Medicines: A Brief History of Pharmacy and Pharmaceuticals.* London: Pharmaceutical Press, 2005.

Bender, George. *Great Moments in Pharmacy.* Detroit: Northwood Institute Press, 1966.

Cowen, David L., and William H. Helfand. *Pharmacy: An Illustrated History.* New York: Abrams, 1990.

Higby, Gregory J. and Elaine C. Stroud, eds. *American Pharmacy: A Collection of Historical Essays.* Madison, WI: American Institute of the History of Pharmacy, 2005.

Kremers and Urdang's History of Pharmacy. Revised by Glenn Sonnedecker. Philadelphia: Lippincott, 1976.

University of Arizona. http://www.pharmacy.arizona.edu/museum/tour.php

GREGORY J. HIGBY

ARMSTRONG, RICHARD (1805–1860). Although not a medical practitioner, Richard Armstrong was deeply involved in fighting the **smallpox epidemic** that swept the Hawaiian Islands in 1853. A member of King Kamehameha III's (1813–1854) privy council, he led the **vaccination** program during the epidemic and afterward conducted a census to determine the disease's toll. In the aftermath of the disaster, he and another cabinet member, Dr. Gerritt Judd (1803–1873), were accused of having mishandled the government response to the epidemic. He defended his actions in public hearings and managed to retain his government position, whereas Judd, who had led the Royal Commissioners of Health, was forced to resign.

A teacher and Princeton Theological Seminary–trained minister, Armstrong and his family moved to Hawaii in 1832 to serve as missionaries. Armstrong served at several churches in the Hawaiian Islands before becoming Minister of Public Instruction in 1848, a position he would hold until his death in a riding accident in 1860.

The smallpox epidemic began in February, 1853, when the *Charles Mallory,* a merchant ship from San Francisco, appeared in Honolulu's harbor flying the yellow flag that signaled disease aboard. The single afflicted sailor, who eventually recovered, was isolated on a reef in the harbor while the rest of the crew was vaccinated and **quarantined** at Waikiki. This quick action seemed to have kept the **contagion** from spreading, but in May, more cases began to appear, probably unrelated to the *Mallory's* sailor. After the *Mallory* incident, Armstrong had been charged with directing an intensive vaccination program as part of a comprehensive plan developed by the Royal Commissioners of Health and had secured a supply of vaccine by the end of March.

The vaccination program was plagued with problems, including difficulty in securing good quality vaccine supply. Whereas most whites complied with government orders to be immunized, many native Hawaiians avoided the vaccinations, preferring the **folk medicine** of native healers called *kahuna.* Lacking sufficient medical personnel to handle the workload, Armstrong trained laymen to give immunizations and vaccinated a number of people himself.

Rev. Armstrong drew upon his connections to the missionary community to spread smallpox information through churches. He set up vaccination stations at both Protestant and Catholic churches. He also persuaded the king to designate June 14 as a national day of prayer and fasting.

The epidemic peaked in October 1853 and had run its course by the middle of January 1854. The islands had a population of over 73,000 just prior to the epidemic, and official statistics generated by Armstrong's 1854 census set the toll of the epidemic at 6,405 cases of smallpox resulting in 2,485 deaths. These figures are generally agreed to be inaccurately low. Convinced that at least two-thirds of all cases went unreported, Armstrong himself contended that the actual death toll was over 6,000. This catastrophe prompted Hawaiian lawmakers in 1854 to make vaccination of natives and visitors compulsory. *See also* Measles Epidemic in Fiji (1875) and Eugenics; Smallpox in Canada and the United States since 1783; Smallpox in Colonial Latin America; Smallpox in Colonial North America; Smallpox in European Non-American Colonies; Trade, Travel, and Epidemic Disease.

Further Reading

Daws, Gavan. *Shoal of Time: A History of the Hawaiian Islands.* Honolulu: University of Hawaii Press, 1974.

Greer, Richard. "Oahu's Ordeal: The Smallpox Epidemic of 1853." *Hawaii Historical Review* 1 (1965): 221–242.

TERESA LESLIE

ARTHROPODS.   *See* Insects, Other Arthropods, and Epidemic Disease.

ASTROLOGY AND MEDICINE.   From ancient Sumerians and Egyptians to modern Chinese who use traditional medicine, medical practitioners of many cultures have assumed and sought to account for the influence of planets and stars on the human body and on **epidemic** diseases. Islamic scholars significantly developed Greek astrology during the ninth and tenth centuries CE, creating its central place in Western medicine. **Physicians** relied on astrology to understand and treat epidemic disease into the eighteenth century. An ancient art, astrology differed from astronomy in its emphasis on the supposed effects of stars and planets on earthly life. Practitioners of both disciplines observed celestial bodies—their magnitude, motions, phases, and so forth. Astrologers, however, searched for causal relationships between earthly events and celestial motion. Though generally not astrologers themselves, physicians used astrology as a tool to understand the physical constitution and temper of their patients and to determine the best courses of treatment.

There were two varieties of astrology practiced in the premodern West: prognosticative (or "natural") astrology, which physicians and the Catholic Church accepted, and unapproved judicial astrology, which used celestial events to foretell the future. Many **quacks** regularly practiced the latter, and cash-strapped professional astrologers sometimes attempted it as well. Prognosticative astrologers confidently utilized complex quantitative methods as they tried to interpret celestial phenomena they completely misunderstood. Medical students in medieval and early modern Europe learned this form of astrology to

AN ASTROLOGICAL EXPLANATION OF THE BLACK DEATH'S CELESTIAL ORIGINS IN 1345

Because Saturn was dominant, he brings cold (greater than the sun could counter) to each country under his rule, and because of the sign in which the conjunction occurred men will experience the onset of lingering illnesses such as tuberculosis, catarrh, paralysis, and gout; passions of the heart arising from unhappiness; and the deaths of those who have endured long weakness. And since the conjunction was in the air sign of Aquarius it signified great cold, heavy frosts, and thick clouds corrupting the air; and since this is a sign that represents the pouring out of water, the configuration signifies that rivers will burst their banks and the sea flood. And because of the persistently cold atmosphere bitter humors cannot be expelled from the sea as usual, and because of the persistent cold there will be few fish in the sea and those that are there will rot because of the cold, which traps vapors and humors in their bodies. For his part, Mars in that sign denotes strife among men, and sudden death that comes among all sorts of men, especially among children and adolescents, and illnesses entailing fevers and the spitting of blood, and also violent death and ulcers.

From astrologer Geoffrey de Meaux, astrological treatise in Bodleian Library, Oxford, MS Digby 176; translated by Rosemary Horrox in her *The Black Death* (New York: Manchester University Press, 1994), p. 172.

help them understand health and disease. Curricula included both cosmology and planetary astrodynamics, though many physicians learned how to chart horoscopes without understanding the underlying astronomical theory. The primary focus was on the correlation between astrological influences and disease and on the practical application of this understanding.

Astrologers used astronomers' observational data recorded in complex tables to track the positions of planets in the 12 divisions of the heavens, denoted by the familiar "signs" of the zodiac. They constructed a chart (geniture) to map effects of the thousands of planetary (and other celestial) movements on a specific individual. This did not predict particular events but presented many probable outcomes based on trends. The primary factors believed to influence an individual's "nature" shaped genitures vastly more complex than modern popular horoscopes. One zodiacal sign or "house" dominated a person, but the relative and changing positions of the five known planets, the moon, and the sun also mattered. So did the relative positions of all of these bodies at the time of the individual's birth, the "aspects." Together these gave the astrologer a complete portrait of a client's natural "dispositions."

Physicians considered two kinds of astrological influence when diagnosing diseases. One was specific to an individual, as a result of the sum of celestial forces acting on him or her from conception beyond birth; this component described a person's predispositions, chronic conditions, or disabilities. The second was the celestial influence on the terrestrial environment: weather, waters, crops, and so forth. Physicians held certain astrological events or moments responsible for the rise and spread of diseases now known to be infectious; a "malign" planet like Saturn in the right position caused plague outbreaks by "putrefying" air. The outbreak of the **Black Death** in 1347, for instance, was interpreted as the result of the 1345 "Great Conjunction" of Jupiter and Saturn, which prominent astrologers considered the harbinger of most of that decade's mishaps, including serious economic problems. Later plagues were also attributed to conjunctions and sometimes to comets. Geographical locations influenced by malign celestial bodies were considered breeding grounds for pestilence. For treatment, physicians, following **humoral theory**, considered appropriate plant and mineral substances by correlating the astrological influence on the medicine and the disease or provided purgative or bloodletting treatments only when astrologically appropriate. Medicinal astrology in the West disappeared with the successes of the **Scientific Revolution**. *See also* Chinese Disease Theory and Medicine; Islamic Disease Theory and Medicine; Medical Education in the West, 1100–1500; Medical Education in the West, 1500–1900; Plague in Europe, 1500–1770s; Plague in Medieval Europe, 1360–1500.

Further Reading

French, Roger. "Astrology in Medical Practice." In *Practical Medicine from Salerno to Black Death*, edited by Luis Garcia-Ballester, et al., pp. 30–59. New York: Cambridge University Press, 1994.

Grafton, Anthony. *Cardano's Cosmos: The Worlds and Works of a Renaissance Astrologer*. Cambridge, MA: Harvard University Press, 1999.

Hare, E. H. "Medical Astrology and its Relation to Modern Psychiatry." *Proceedings of the Royal Society of Medicine* 70 (1977): 105–110.

National Library of Medicine. http://www.nlm.nih.gov/hmd/arabic/magical_tb.html

Saliba, G. "The Role of the Astrologer in Medieval Islamic Society." In *Magic and Divination in Early Islam*, edited by Emilie Savage-Smith, pp. 341–370. Burlington, VT: Ashgate, 2004.

DENNIS GREGORY CARAMENICO

AVICENNA (ABU ALI AL-HUSAYN IBN ABDULLAH IBN SINA; 980–1037). The medieval Persian philosopher and **physician**, known in the West as Avicenna, had an enormous influence on the interpretation and treatment of plague **epidemics** in the Middle East and in Europe. Born in Bukhara, southern Uzbekistan, he mastered all the Greek sciences by the age of 18. Physician and political administrator at an early age, he became the envy of many and fled from place to place, writing by night on horseback, his memory serving as reference. Avicenna finally settled in the capital, Isfahan, in central Iran, and after a protracted bout of colic, died and was buried in Hamadan, northwest of Isfahan.

Though his mother tongue was Persian, Avicenna wrote mainly in Arabic, not only on medicine and the sciences, but also on philosophy, music, and poetry. His most famous work, al-Qanun fi al-tibb (*The Canon of Medicine*) is a record of all the medical knowledge of his time, including translations of Greek writings that would otherwise have been lost, supplemented with his own observations. Clear and well ordered, *The Canon*, more accessible than **Hippocrates** or **Galen**, was translated into Latin in the twelfth century and remained an essential medical textbook until the nineteenth century. Avicenna recognized the presence of infectious diseases such as **leprosy**, scabies, **smallpox, measles**, and pestilential fevers (plague) and adopted, from the Greeks, the theory that epidemics are caused by pollution in the **air** (miasma). In Volume III of *The Canon*, in the chapter "Epidemics [Plague] and similar fevers," Avicenna wrote that impure air is like boggy, stagnant **water**; pollution is caused by smoky winds that cover the land with dust, by contact with swamps, by rotting carcasses, and by contaminated bodies. When air is polluted, his advice was to stay indoors. Plague epidemics, he wrote, thrive on hot, damp air, usually occurring at the end of summer and in the autumn. Avicenna described the symptoms of plague infection as the appearance of swellings (buboes) on armpits, groin, or behind the ears. Pestilence, he said, contaminates plants, the animals that feed on them, and the people who consume these animals. He saw an increase in the number of frogs, insects, and rats that surfaced as a sure sign of an impending epidemic, but only as a forewarning; he did not recognize the causal relationship between rats and plague.

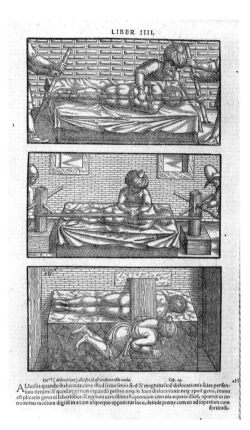

Illustrations showing dislocation and massage. From *Liber canonis, de medicinis cordialibus, et cantica* [canon of medicine] by Avicenna, published by J. Hervagius, Basle in 1556. Courtesy Wellcome Library, London.

The uncertainty that dominated Islamic, as well as European, opinion about the cause of an epidemic made it very difficult for physicians to find a cure for plague. Treatment centered on ways to improve air quality or advice to flee to uncontaminated areas. Avicenna recommended bloodletting; applying Armenian clay to buboes; improving the air with aromatic fruits and herbs; cooling the patient's surroundings by spraying water and vinegar; fumigating with camphor, pomegranate peel, myrtle, and sandalwood; and, in line with previous Islamic and Greek recommendations, giving the patient a daily potion of aloes, saffron, and myrtle. *See also* Contagion Theory of Disease, Premodern; Greco-Roman Medical Theory and Practice; Islamic Disease Theory and Medicine; Rhazes.

Further Reading

Avicenna. *Canon of Medicine.* Translated by Laleh Bakhtiar. Chicago: Abjad Book Designers, 1999. Contains only Book I.

Gohlman, W. *The Life of Ibn Sina: A Critical Edition and Annotated Translation.* Albany: State University of New York Press, 1974.

Grmek, Mirko D., ed. *Western Medical Thought from Antiquity to the Middle Ages.* Cambridge, MA: Harvard University Press, 1999.

Khan, Aisha. *Avicenna: Muslim Physician and Philosopher of the Eleventh Century.* New York: Rosen Central, 2006.

National Library of Medicine. http://www.nlm.nih.gov/hmd/arabic/authors.html#ibnsina

Pormann, Peter E., and Emilie Savage-Smith. *Medieval Islamic Medicine.* Edinburgh: Edinburgh University Press, 2007.

SELMA TIBI-HARB

AYURVEDIC DISEASE THEORY AND MEDICINE.   Long before there were written languages, the peoples of the regions now called Pakistan and India, following patterns established further back than memory could reach, set broken bones, treated wounds, and tended the disease-stricken. Some of these practices included strong doses of religious belief in disease-causing demons and healing deities, others were based on astrological cults, and still others on the observations of **empirics**. Elements of some of these manifold traditions may remain in contemporary **folk medicine**, but only one major strain has survived, having been recorded first in Sanskrit during the fifth century BCE, about the time of the Greek **Hippocrates**, and over centuries after. These texts served medical students in schools that taught the "knowledge for longevity," one translation of the Indian term Ayurvedic, an elite and learned tradition. Ayurvedic medicine remains actively studied and practiced today alongside Western medicine in India, and the Indian government even supports its teaching and practice. In the West, Ayurveda is often treated as a trendy "alternative" medicine.

Distinctively nonreligious, Ayurveda does share with Buddhism a concern for moderation or "the middle way" in all things, especially diet, mood, and morality. Practitioners believe that the human body consists of tissues, the three humor-like *doṣas* or *tridoṣa,* and wastes awaiting removal. To these are added the body's seven "constituents": chyle, blood, fat, flesh, bone, marrow, and (the highest) semen. The *tridoṣa*—wind, bile, and phlegm— are byproducts of food that move through the body's tubes, and blockages in these cause many of the conditions labeled disease. Regulation of these through a regimen of **diet,** exercise, and bathing is the key to good health.

But the body is also acted on by the **environment,** which is what brings on **epidemics,** or *janapada-uddhvamsa.* When a single disease afflicts many in a given area, the cause clearly must be in the place: its **air, water,** vegetation, pests, and even earthquakes and ghosts. Time (seasons, conjunctions of events) also plays a role, and Ayurvedic texts reflect this concern with their inclusion of astrological material. The earliest surviving text, *Caraka's Compendium* from northwest India, equates epidemic preconditions with "corruption" of the air, water, locale, and time. Essentially, each is unusual or abnormal in one or more distinctive, negative ways: the air is too humid or smoky, the water is sour or cloudy. These four corruptions are rooted in "bad judgments" made recently or in the past by the social leaders in the area, which resulted in bad acts or unrighteousness. In a kind of cascading effect, the unrighteousness grows, virtue is overwhelmed, the gods abandon the area, and the abnormalities of corruption set in. These affect the inhabitants in roughly the same fashion, and an epidemic arises, the specifics of the disease being dependent on the specifics of the corruption. Bad karma corrupts. The role in epidemic disease of **contagion,** or spread of disease by personal contact, is hinted at but never fully developed in Ayurvedic texts

In Caraka's account, the appropriate medicines must be gathered before conditions deteriorate, or their potency will likewise drain away. Ayurvedic doctors used long lists of both animal and plant materials as medications, and Caraka's text asserts boldly "when people are treated [prophylactically] with medicine they will not become sick." The use of emetics, purgatives, enemas, sinus clearing, and later bloodletting, douches, sweating, massage, and other therapeutic procedures meant to affect the *tridoṣa* took their place as well, both as prophylaxes for and treatments of disease. Though highly traditional, Ayurvedic medicine changed and evolved over time: minerals appear in the pharmacopoeia around 1000 CE; **syphilis** (French/*phiranga* disease) appeared among treated diseases around 1500; and more effective means of diagnosis replaced less reliable ones over time. Though practiced in India by at least 1700, **inoculation** is never mentioned in Ayurvedic texts. *See also* Astrology and Medicine; Chinese Disease Theory and Medicine; Galen; Greco-Roman Medical Theory and Practice; Humoral Theory; Islamic Disease Theory and Medicine.

Further Reading

Conrad, Lawrence I., and Dominik Wujastyk, eds. *Contagion: Perspectives from Pre-Modern Societies.* Burlington, VT: Ashgate, 2000.

Majumdar, Ashok. *Ayurveda: The Ancient Indian Science of Healing.* Allahabad, New Delhi: Wheeler Publishing, 1998.

Wujastyk, Dominik. "New Age Ayurveda or What Happens to Indian Medicine When it Comes to America." *Traditional South Asian Medicine* 6 (2001): 10–26.

———. *The Roots of Ayurveda.* New York: Penguin Books, 2003. Includes material quoted above.

JOSEPH P. BYRNE

B

BABESIOSIS. While treating patients for the **bacteria** that cause **Lyme disease**, medical practitioners eventually realized that tick bites, such as painless bites from period-sized deer ticks, were "dirty" and carried a wide range of infections. One of the most important of these deer tick infections is the tiny parasitic infection caused by protozoa of the genus *Babesia*, which is named for Romanian biologist Victor Babes (1854–1926). This is an infection that affects the interior of red blood cells, with effects similar to **malaria**. Babesiosis and other conditions caused by *Babesia* are considered emergent. The two main reasons it has escaped detection in so many countries for so many decades are the lack of advanced testing to detect its presence and the fact that little attention has been given to this type of disease by the modern world medical community. The veterinary medicine community has done much more study and treatment of *Babesia* infection in **animals**—for example, cattle—than have **physicians** treating humans.

Babesia diseases are not rare. In one study, 36 percent of Mexican citizens tested were infected with the species *Babesia canis*. This infection is not supposed to be common in humans and is typically understood to be an infection that affects dogs. In another study, 3 to 8 percent of U.S. blood donors had *Babesia microti*. Researchers have found that *Babesia* is a common coinfection and is present in 66 percent of patients with Lyme. This coinfection causes the patient to commonly suffer from nearly 50 different symptoms, which include fever, waves of warmth, sweating, chills, and fatigue. *Babesia* can also cause red blood cells to become deformed inside tiny organ capillaries and cause dozens of debilitating symptoms. It may also possibly increase the probability of strokes and heart attacks as the result of blood clots.

Because of the tiny size of the *Babesia* protozoa, testing for this infection is challenging. For example, bloodstains of infected people can require hours of manual searching with a **microscope** at high, 1000x magnification. This tedious searching is rarely performed. The severe diagnostic limitations of blood smear testing are similar to those experienced in the process of malaria testing. Under the microscope, malaria appears very similar to *Babesia* when present within the red blood cell. In one Baylor Texas Medical Center study of 59 patients with clear, clinical malaria, 80 percent were given the wrong initial diagnosis based on blood, and some patients died as a result.

Babesia Signs and Symptoms.   Babesiosis can cause many different signs and symptoms, including a period of high fever or persistent low fever, listlessness, chills, sweats, headaches, excessive sleep, fatigue, and muscle or joint aches. *Babesia, Bartonella, Mycoplasma,* and mold spore surface mycotoxin exposure should always be considered in patients who do not respond well to indicated Lyme treatment. The research is universally clear that *Babesia* with Lyme is much more disabling for patients, and the treatment requires more aggressive and diverse options.

Treatment.   Most *Babesia* research suggests the best treatment for adult patients is Mepron (atovaquone) 750 mg at least twice a day combined with Zithromax (azithromycin) 250 mg twice daily. The research on all treatments is very limited, and each treatment is usually based on as few as one to nine studies, most of which were not performed at an advanced academic level. Much of the current research represents only small groups of patients or animals receiving clinical care utilizing various treatment options. Further, most of the treatments suggested are applications of malaria research because malaria has some similarities with *Babesia*.

Another treatment option for *Babesia* involves the use of Artemisia plant derivatives. This approach is taken from Chinese medicine and is now recommended as a leading treatment against malaria according to the **World Health Organization** (WHO) and the United Nations Children's Fund (UNICEF). For example, many drugs are derived from the Artemisia plant; some are potentially damaging to hearing and are toxic to the brain, whereas others are well tolerated. Some Artemisia advertisements falsely call this herb "Wormwood," because it is popularly called "Sweet" or "Annual Wormwood," but it does not have Wormwood's toxic chemicals. Effective forms of Artemisia preparations kill *Babesia* by methods that include free radical formation, so multiple antioxidant supplements are recommended to catch free radicals and help the red blood cells regain their smooth surface. These also help to prevent Artemisia medications or nutrients from causing free radical damage to other organs.

Babesia is an emerging pathogen, which means in part that new species are being discovered, and medical science is far from mastering the infections it causes. *See also Bartonella* Diseases.

Further Reading

Centers for Disease Control and Prevention. *Babesiosis.* http://www.dpd.cdc.gov/dpdx/HTML/Babesiosis.htm

Hildebrandt, A., et al. "Human Babesiosis in Germany: Just Overlooked or Truly New?" *International Journal of Medical Microbiology* (September 2007): 336–346.

Kjemtrup, A. M., and P. A. Conrad. "Human Babesiosis: An Emerging Tick-borne Disease." *International Journal of Parasitology* 30 (2000): 1323–1237.

Schaller, James. *The Diagnosis and Treatment of Babesia.* Self-published by Hope Academic Press, 2007.

Schaller, James, M.D. http://www.personalconsult.com/pubindex.html#babesia

JAMES SCHALLER

BACTERIUM/BACTERIA.   Bacteria are small, free-living, single-cell organisms without a true nucleus and bounded by a rigid cell wall composed of protein and carbohydrate components. These organisms reproduce asexually by binary fission (splitting). As a group they are among the most numerous and diverse organisms in the world. Individual bacteria, however, are only visible with the aid of the **microscope**. Bacteria are distinguished from other single-cell organisms such as yeasts, molds, and **protozoa** by the lack of an organized nucleus as well as by more subtle biochemical properties.

The study of the unseen world of these organisms was first revealed through the use of the microscope, invented in the early decades of the 1600s. These early microscopes were simply single lenses of high curvature, such as small spherical glass beads of very short focal length. The best of these "simple" microscopes had a magnification of about 200x.

The acknowledged pioneer in both microscope construction and careful observation was the Delft cloth merchant **Athony van Leeuwenhoek**. Leeuwenhoek produced a series of landmark communications to the Royal Society of London which extended from 1673 until his death in 1723. Leeuwenhoek described what appeared to be little animals ("animalcules") in many seemingly "pure" substances, from melted snow and vinegar to extracts of spices from the Far East. These are the first reports on the organisms we now take to be the subject of the field of microbiology. Not only did Leeuwenhoek note that these little animals had regular structures, which he arranged in a simple classification scheme, but he also reported that some were motile (able to move themselves) and that they seemed to increase in number, that is, to grow and multiply over time.

Although many objects that Leeuwenhoek described are now recognized as amoeba, paramecia, diatoms, and small multicellular organisms such as rotifers, some of the smallest objects appear to have been true bacteria. Leeuwenhoek's classification scheme is the distant precursor of that in use today. He described four types of these tiny organisms based on shape and size: round cocci, rod-shaped bacteria (two sizes), and helical spirillia.

In 1773 Otto Friedrich Müller (1730–1784) published a treatise on "infusoria," the name for the collection of organisms that were found in various teas and other water extracts of plant and animal materials. Müller, using the improved microscopes of the eighteenth century, including the "compound" microscope with multiple lenses, recognized two main groups of infusoria, Monas and Vibrio, which contain bacterial forms.

Müller's scheme was used in the late eighteenth century and was extended in 1838 with the famous study by Carl Gustave von Ehrenberg (1795–1876), who published *Die Infusionthierchen als vollkemmene Organismen*, a large folio atlas with extensive hand–colored, engraved plates. Ehrenberg, like his predecessors, did not make a distinction between protozoa and bacteria. They were all classified as Infusoria, and all were believed to have tiny stomachs and other parts analogous to those of larger animals. His classification scheme was detailed, complex, and extensive. Of relevant interest are his descriptions of the family Vibrionia, which was comprised of five genera: *Bacterium*, *Vibrio*, *Spirochaeta*, *Spirillum*, and *Spirodiscus*. In spite of Ehrenberg's detailed descriptions, we cannot unequivocally identify many of his organisms with current microbial classifications.

Throughout the nineteenth century, the classification of microorganisms evolved and developed, but all attempts were limited by the fact that they were superficially descriptive, not physiologic, morphologic but without the aid of chemical stains, and mixtures rather than homogeneous samples of the organisms.

As soon as bacterial culture became routine, following the work of the nineteenth-century bacteriologists, it was noted that growth requirements and culture conditions were properties that were useful in characterizing the various bacterial types. These physiological studies paralleled the study of metabolism in both plants and animals and showed that bacteria were similar in many ways to higher forms of life.

Although bacteria share basic metabolic pathways with all other organisms, they are in general much more adaptable and exhibit a great diversity of special physiological and metabolic processes. As free-living, single-cell organisms, functional and biochemical specialization that is a hallmark of multicellular organisms is not usually available to them as a survival strategy.

The relationship of bacteria to disease, fermentation, and putrefaction was elucidated toward the end of the nineteenth century initially through the work of **Louis Pasteur, Robert Koch,** and their colleagues. So-called **germ theories of disease** provided an explanation for the specificity of various diseases while also explaining mechanisms of **contagion**, pathogenesis as a result of bacterial toxins, and subsequently, **immunity** to infectious diseases.

Bacteria living in diverse environments have many special structures, chemicals, and metabolic pathways to exploit their particular ecological niches. Thus, the membrane lipids of bacteria living at low temperature differ significantly from those of bacteria adapted to warm temperatures. The differing lipid compositions allow maintenance of membrane fluidity at different temperatures. The adaptive utilization of a wide variety of carbon compounds for energy, the presence or absence of the requirement for oxygen for energy production, and the production of secondary metabolites that are toxic to environmental competitors are all examples of this biological diversity. This diversity of bacterial metabolism has been exploited for many useful purposes, including such age-old processes as production of vinegar by *Acetobacter* and such recent discoveries as **antibiotic** production from *Streptomyces*.

Many bacteria have evolved special, mutually beneficial relationships with other organisms. The bacteria that inhabit the intestines of animals are supported by the food that the animal eats, but at the same time, the bacteria produce certain essential nutrients as byproducts, which are absorbed by the animal host. One such example is the vitamin, biotin. The intestinal bacteria *Escherichia coli* produce all the biotin needed by humans. In the case of certain animals that subsist on a diet of grass, such as cattle, special bacteria in their stomachs can digest cellulose to produce sugars which are absorbed by the cattle as their main source of nutrition. These animals, called ruminants, are absolutely dependent on being colonized by these cellulose-digesting bacteria. A similar situation exists in some plants (legumes) which harbor bacteria in small root nodules. These bacteria are able to absorb atmospheric nitrogen and convert it (by a process called nitrogen fixation) into ammonia and related compounds, the most important of which are the amino acids. These amino acids are then provided to the plant for protein synthesis and growth. The process of nitrogen fixation is crucial to the existence of life on earth. An extreme case of this type of mutual benefit is represented by the subcellular organelles called mitochondria which exist in most eucaryotic cells. There is strong evidence that mitochondria evolved from bacteria which long ago invaded the cytoplasm of some cells, became a useful source of oxidative energy production for the cell, and along the way lost the ability to live independently.

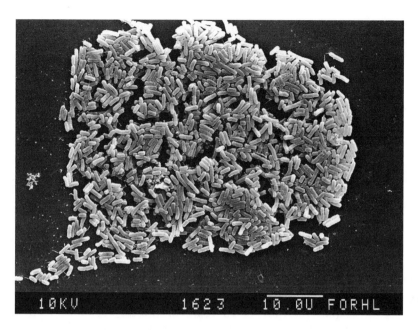

Scanning Electron Micrograph (SEM) of *Escherichia coli.* Courtesy of David Gregory and Debbie Marshall, Welcome Library, London.

One type of growth process distinguishes bacteria from many higher organisms: the ability, when placed in unfavorable environments, to develop into a dormant state known as a spore form. Spores are living cells which are metabolically quiescent, surrounded by a durable wall, and relatively dehydrated in comparison with normal cells. Under normal growth conditions, spores germinate to produce normal vegetatively growing bacteria again. The spore forms of bacteria are highly resistant to drying, to temperature (they are not killed by boiling water temperature, but require high pressure steam above 120°C to be killed), and to ultraviolet light. Sporulation is a survival strategy that is common to bacteria that live in diverse environments and is less common in bacteria that inhabit more constant ecological niches such as the mammalian intestine, for example.

The widespread presence of bacteria and their adaptability to many ecological niches provide them with the ability to move about in nature with speed and efficiency. Humans perceive such survival strategies as contagion and the basis for **epidemic** disease. Bacteria can often be spread by simple physical contact, which transfers a few organisms to a new location. Often, however, **water** or **air** currents serve to carry bacteria to new environments. Some bacteria have evolved to be carried by other organisms (called vectors) such as insects or other animals. One important example is the transmission of human plague bacteria by the bite of the rat flea.

Although bacteria do not have a membrane-bounded organelle, the nucleus in which the genetic apparatus of the cell resides, their genetic organization is similar to that of all other cellular life. Genes are encoded in DNA, and the genetic code of bacteria is identical to that of higher organisms (with a few interesting variations in the evolutionarily ancient Archea). Most bacteria reproduce by binary fission so they form clonal populations, all descended from a founder organism. However, some bacteria have evolved mechanisms for mating and genetic exchange as a way to increase genetic diversity and, presumably, evolutionary fitness. So-called bacterial sex has been a very useful tool for analysis of genetic mechanisms at the molecular level.

Further Reading

Dubos, René J., with an addendum by C. F. Robinow. *The Bacterial Cell in its Relation to Problems of Virulence, Immunity and Chemotherapy*. Cambridge, MA: Harvard University Press, 1955.

Dyer, Betsey Dexter. *A Field Guide to the Bacteria*. Ithaca: Cornell University Press, 2003.

Tomes, Nancy. *The Gospel of Germs: Men, Women, and the Microbe in American Life*. Cambridge, MA: Harvard University Press, 1999.

WILLIAM C. SUMMERS

BARTONELLA DISEASES.   *Bartonella* is the cause of one of the most serious emerging bacterial infections in the world. It has the potential to infect tens of millions of people because it is found throughout the entire world, with the exception of the polar ice caps, and can easily infect patients in cities, suburbs, or rural areas. Further, in contrast to many vector-borne infections, *Bartonella* can be spread by many vectors and by many means: flea bites, flea feces, dust mites, cats, and dogs can carry this infection in their paws and saliva, and can infect a person by a scratch, lick, or playful bite.

Bartonella is so common that laboratory findings show that 40 percent of California cats have contact with the illness. Since one-third of all homes in the United States have a cat, this means that many of the 70 million cats in the United States can playfully bite, lick, or scratch a human and infect him or her. But it is very probable that the 40 percent figure seriously understates the case. Researchers have discovered that blood samples with *Bartonella* infection sent to labs have routinely been falsely declared negative, meaning that labs routinely miss the presence of the pathogen in both humans and animals. A new blood cell stain by Dr. Stephen Fry and new genus-level DNA testing (PCR testing) both hold hope for better diagnosis in the future.

Amazingly, however, *Bartonella* has still other agents to spread its infection: lice, ticks, and certain flies. Finally, examination of fetus pregnancy tissue shows that *Bartonella* clearly infects the placenta, and infected baby mice are born smaller than normal.

Bartonella typically hides in the human and animal body, literally infecting red blood cells and the cells lining the blood vessels, and it can suppress the immune system and remain undetected. If other **bacteria** were floating in blood or lining the red blood cell endothelial cells, they would likely cause death within hours or days; yet Bartonella escapes detection.

It was formerly thought that most types of *Bartonella* were harmless to cats and humans, but emerging research has found that close examination under the **microscope** shows tissue damage to cats from *Bartonella*. In the same manner **Lyme disease** was initially seen as merely an arthritis disease and ***Babesia*** as a pathogen that simply caused fevers, fatigue, and sweats. With each passing year it becomes clearer that both of these infections have hundreds of symptoms. *Bartonella* is similar in the number of new strains being found and the increasing evidence for diverse human body damage.

Bartonella was initially discovered and named after Alberto L. Barton (1874–1950), a Peruvian **physician**. In 1909 he published an article on elements found in the red blood cells of patients with dangerous Oroya fever. In this article he identified the blood parasite (*Bartonella bacilliformis*) that is the causative agent of Oroya fever and verruga peruana. The organism is now placed in the genus *Bartonella*, which was named after him in 1915. It was first considered a **virus**, and then a bacterium having only three species. Now it is known to have approximately 10 species, including a newly discovered species that infects humans, *Bartonella rochalimae*. Most experts expect to find additional species. In 2005 French researchers found *Bartonella* DNA in the tooth pulp of French soldiers buried in 1813 in Vilnius, Lithuania, indicating that Napoleon's troops suffered from *Bartonella* diseases as well as typhus and others well known to historians.

As research on the effects of *Bartonella* has proceeded, it has become clear that it causes over 200 signs and symptoms in humans. These include numbness or loss of sensation; dizziness; headaches; oxygen deprivation; abscesses; gingivitis; muscle spasms and/or weakness; joint pain; liver disease; intestinal disorders; and kidney, bladder, and genital disorders. Also common are fatigue, sleep and memory problems, and drowsiness. Because it is a red blood cell infection and blood enters all tissues, the illnesses *Bartonella* causes in humans can involve any organ. For years this infection was naïvely felt to be only as serious as a cold, with a few transient enlarged lymph nodes, skin tag-like papules, and maybe an occasional small painless rash. Now, however, we know that a percentage of patients die from heart rhythm damage caused by *Bartonella* fat spots made in the heart. Others experience weakening blood vessel walls that can lead to a stroke. Still others with *Bartonella* struggle with agitated depression, bipolar disorder, panic disorder, addiction, or aggressive rage, all of which makes them prone to suicide. The psychiatric treatment of a patient with *Bartonella* is highly specialized, and most family physicians and psychiatrists do not know how to treat a patient suffering from *Bartonella*-induced psychiatric disorders.

Yet despite advances in understanding and agreement on the seriousness of *Bartonella* infection, lab testing and health-care worker training in the diagnosis of this infection are poor, and so the vast majority of infected and ill patients go undiagnosed, misdiagnosed, and untreated.

Treatment.   Currently, no standard of medical care exists for *Bartonella*. Many treatments tested in the laboratory do not seem to work in live animals or humans. Research shows that routinely prescribed **antibiotics** fail in individuals ill with *Bartonella*, particularly if only given for a few weeks, and that even after the blood is cleared some infection remains in the walls of the blood vessels, and repeat pulsed treatment is needed for a cure. This is the probable cause for so many "relapses" in past studies—short treatment and a lack of appreciation that the antibiotic was not killing the *Bartonella* hiding in the blood vessel walls. However, longer-term treatment with breaks, followed by restarted pulsed treatment, is not yet routine. Because no treatment is universally agreed upon at this time, and no book in English exists on advanced clinical *Bartonella* medicine, no standard has currently clearly been shown to be effective in the eyes of the broad medical community. As traditional medicine looks for new effective antibiotics, researchers have found that some modern Chinese medicine antibiotic herbal treatments are effective; however, they are under-prescribed, and patients still require pulsed treatment once their blood has been initially cleared of infection.

Further Reading

Centers for Disease Control and Prevention. *Cat Scratch Disease.* http://www.cdc.gov/healthy-pets/diseases/catscratch.htm

Raoult, Didier, et al. "Evidence for Louse-transmitted Diseases in Soldiers of Napoleon's Grand Army in Vilnius." *Journal of Infectious Disease* 193 (2006): 112–120.

Schaller, James. *The Diagnosis and Treatment of Bartonella.* Self-published by Hope Academic Press, 2008.

Schaller, James, M.D. http://www.personalconsult.com/pubindex.html#bartonella http://www.pubmedcentral.nih.gov/articlerender.fcgi?artid=172916

Wormser, G. P. "Discovery of New Infectious Diseases: Bartonella Species." *New England Journal of Medicine* 356 (2007): 2381–2387.

JAMES SCHALLER

BEHRING, EMIL VON (1854–1917).   Emil von Behring is one of the founders of the science of **immunology**. Prior to his work, the prevailing concept was that the body's ability to fight infection could be attributed to the cellular response, the ability of phagocytes and other cells to engulf and destroy **bacteria**. He was one of the first proponents of the humoral aspects of immunology that led to using antitoxins and antibodies to fight infection.

Von Behring was born in East Prussia on March 15, 1854. While in high school he developed an interest in medicine and later attended Friedrich Wilhelm University in Berlin where he received his medical degree in 1878. His early medical career occurred during a time of great progress in medicine's ability to deal with infectious diseases. **Louis Pasteur** developed **germ theory, Robert Koch** refined the ability to grow and identify bacteria, **Paul Ehrlich** introduced the use of specific chemical agents to treat infections, and Elie Metchnikoff (1845–1916) formulated the concepts of the cellular immune response.

During his work as a military physician, von Behring recognized the importance of infected wounds as a cause of deaths. In the 1860s, British surgeon Joseph Lister (1827–1912) instituted the use of carbolic acid sprays during surgery as a method of preventing contamination of surgical incisions and subsequent infection. Following on this idea, von Behring attempted using the antiseptic iodine compound iodoform internally as a means of fighting the effects of infection by neutralizing toxins produced by bacteria, but the side effects of the iodoform were themselves too severe to allow its use. Nonetheless, he persisted in his attempts to reduce the effects of infections not by killing the bacteria causing the infection, but by destroying the toxins produced by the bacteria.

Diphtheria was an ideal disease for von Behring to study. Many of the deaths from diphtheria are not the result of the local infection itself, but rather the effects of toxins produced by the bacteria. Von Behring and his associates, primarily **Shibasaburo Kitasato**, first confirmed that bacteria-free filtrates contained toxins that, when injected into animals, caused the systemic signs of these diseases. When very minute doses of the toxins were injected, an adequate amount did not exist to cause disease. However, repeated minute doses did protect the animals from ill effects of subsequent larger doses. They postulated that the animals had developed an ability to neutralize the toxins with an antitoxin that the animals themselves had produced. They next injected the serum of an animal that had the ability to neutralize the toxin into animals that were infected. Those infected animals developed no signs of disease, thus demonstrating that the ability to neutralize the toxin could be passed on with injection of the antitoxin. In 1891 von

Behring administered an injection of antitoxin obtained from a sheep into a girl dying of diphtheria, saving her life and establishing the value of antitoxin therapy.

Emil von Behring received the first Nobel Prize in Physiology or Medicine in 1901 in recognition of his work on the antitoxin serum therapy of diphtheria. He died of pneumonia in 1917. *See also* Animal Research; Disinfection and Fumigation; Human Immunity and Resistance to Disease.

Further Reading

Linton, Derek S. *Emil von Behring: Infectious Disease, Immunology, Serum Therapy.* Philadelphia: American Philosophical Society, 2005.

Simmons, John Galbraith. *Doctors and Discoveries: Lives that Created Today's Medicine from Hippocrates to the Present.* Boston: Houghton Mifflin Company, 2002.

CHARLES V. BENDER

BIBLICAL PLAGUES.   The scriptures of ancient **religions** contain many accounts of pestilence, often reported in catastrophic language. This is not surprising because these episodes were often dramatic events that swept through populations, killing many and frequently occurring at times of social disorder, population displacement, or **environmental** adversity. It must therefore have always seemed probable that these scourges were a form of divine punishment for moral or devotional failure. The ancient apocalypticism, which characterized the thinking of early Christianity, readily interpreted the social disaster and institutional collapse associated with these pestilential events as a battle that had been duly lost against the Power of the Lord. A similar subtext of divine displeasure underlies the ancient accounts of pestilence in the Sumerian epic of Gilgamesh, in the Indian Mahabharata, and in Oedpius's Greek city-state of Thebes.

There are many overt references to epidemic outbreaks of infectious disease in the Hebrew Scriptures, also known as the Old Testament of the Christian Bible. There were the plagues of Egypt during Israel's bondage in that powerful land, occurring late in the Middle Kingdom. One plague entailed "sores that break into pustules on man and beast." Another plague, more notorious, killed the first-born Egyptian children on the night of the original Jewish Passover: "and there was a great cry in Egypt, for there was not a house where there was not one dead." The Book of Deuteronomy records that after the Israelites escaped from Egypt, braving the parted waters of the Red Sea, Moses received subsequent divine instruction on Mount Sinai to exact a ransom to God from each of the newly liberated Israelites in order "to avert plague."

During the two immediate pre-Christian millennia, as city-states and civilizations came increasingly into commercial and military contact, infectious agents were often exchanged. The initial contact of a virgin population with a novel microbe would have often caused violent **epidemics**. For example, in Deuteronomy it is recorded that the Hittites suffered in great anguish from the 20 years of pestilence that followed their capture, importation, and enslavement of Egyptians as prisoners-of-war. The enslaved Egyptians would almost certainly have inadvertently carried with them a range of infectious agents from the microbial repertoire of their more ancient civilization (to which the Egyptians would have developed some low-level immune resistance). Once loosed among the less cosmopolitan and immunologically defenseless Hittites, however, these alien microbes wreaked havoc, despite the anguished and wailing pleadings of the prostrated Hittite priests.

THE BIBLICAL PLAGUES OF THE APOCALYPSE

And the seven angels came out of the temple, having the seven plagues, clothed in pure and white linen, and having their breasts girded with golden girdles. And one of the four beasts gave unto the seven angels seven golden vials full of the wrath of God, who liveth for ever and ever. And the temple was filled with smoke from the glory of God, and from his power; and no man was able to enter into the temple, till the seven plagues of the seven angels were fulfilled.

And I heard a great voice out of the temple saying to the seven angels, Go your ways, and pour out the vials of the wrath of God upon the earth. And the first went, and poured out his vial upon the earth; and there fell a noisome and grievous sore upon the men which had the mark of the beast, and upon them which worshipped his image. And the second angel poured out his vial upon the sea; and it became as the blood of a dead man: and every living soul died in the sea. And the third angel poured out his vial upon the rivers and fountains of waters; and they became blood. And the angel said: For they have shed the blood of saints and prophets, and thou hast given them blood to drink; for they are worthy.

And the fourth angel poured out his vial upon the sun; and power was given unto him to scorch men with fire. And men were scorched with great heat, and blasphemed the name of God, which hath power over these plagues: and they repented not to give him glory.

And the fifth angel poured out his vial upon the seat of the beast; and his kingdom was full of darkness; and they gnawed their tongues for pain, and blasphemed the God of heaven because of their pains and their sores, and repented not of their deeds.

And the sixth angel poured out his vial upon the great river Euphrates; and the water thereof was dried up, that the way of the kings of the east might be prepared. And I saw three unclean spirits like frogs come out of the mouth of the dragon, and out of the mouth of the beast, and out of the mouth of the false prophet. For they are the spirits of devils, working miracles, which go forth unto the kings of the earth and of the whole world, to gather them to the battle of that great day of God Almighty. And he gathered them together into a place called in the Hebrew tongue Armageddon.

And the seventh angel poured out his vial into the air; and there came a great voice out of the temple of heaven, from the throne, saying, It is done. And there were voices, and thunders, and lightnings; and there was a great earthquake, such as was not since men were upon the earth, so mighty an earthquake, and so great.

From Revelations 15:6–16:18 (KJV)

The Hebrew First Book of Samuel recounts how, in the seventh century BCE, the Lord smote the neighboring Philistines for their seizure of the Israelites' Ark of the Covenant. The text records that "after they [the Philistines] had carried it about, the hand of the Lord was against the city with a very great destruction. And He smote the men of the city, both small and great, and they had emerods in their secret parts." Over 5,000 men were smitten "with a great slaughter." Historians have long been tantalized by these embarrassingly located emerods. The word refers to tumors—so were these emerods swollen lymph nodes in the groin, the telltale swellings of the **bubonic plague**? Even more tantalizing, indeed remarkable, the Bible records that the penitent Philistines offered up "golden mice." Was this an inspired allusion—and, if so, an extraordinarily prescient one—to the rodents whose infected fleas spread the bubonic plague **bacterium**?

In Leviticus, the Hebrew priests are made the judges of ritual uncleanness, including "**leprosy**," and are instructed to banish the impure from the bounds of the camp. The term "leper," translated by medieval Europe's scholars from the original Hebrew, was taken to refer to the specific condition then recognized as leprosy. Most probably, the word was actually generic, referring to conditions of gross and menacing disfigurement of face and limbs, and deemed in biblical times to be the mark of divine rejection or displeasure. For this reason, or because of folk wisdom about the possibility of some type of **contagion**, those afflicted were often required to identify themselves by ringing a hand-bell. A description of lepromatous leprosy—the most severe, systemic, form—appears in Hindu Sanskrit texts from around 600 BCE. Although there is no corroboration from skeletal remains in the Indian subcontinent, the writings seem to indicate that the disease was familiar within that part of the world.

The vicissitudes of pestilence were not confined to the Biblical Lands. By around 2,500 years ago, agrarian-based civilizations had begun to form in many fertile regions around the world. Each region duly acquired its own distinctive new infections, and local exchanges of these diseases between populations then occurred, sometimes with devastating consequences. Over time, however, coevolutionary pressures tended to render these endemic infections less virulent—a change that benefited both parties, in terms of survival probabilities. Various ancient texts, including the Sumerian *Epic of Gilgamesh* from 4,000 years ago, the ancient court texts from Egypt and China, and the Hebrew Scriptures, indicate that by the second millennium BCE epidemic outbreaks of these pestilences were no longer dire enough to enfeeble the civilized societies in the Middle East and constrain their imperial ambitions. This apparent virulence-lessening evolution of infectious agents in order to enhance accommodation with their human hosts was, however, less evident elsewhere. In the less consolidated and often later-developing civilizations of the Yellow River (China) and the Ganges Valley (India), and in the Aegean-Mediterranean coastal region, the ecological balance between microbes and humans was less settled.

Later, there came from the early Christian era the extraordinary text of the biblical Book of Revelation. The purported author, St. John (who had been exiled by the Romans to the Greek island of Patmos), gives a lurid account of pestilential diseases as a fearsome instrument of God. He describes the Four Horsemen of the Apocalypse, the fourth (pestilence, riding on a white horse) being the harbinger of near-certain death. These four horsemen are instructive in reminding us that, around two millennia ago in the eastern Mediterranean region, warfare, enslavement, famine, and pestilence were the four main recurring scourges of human happiness, health, and survival. *See also* Diagnosis of Historical Diseases; Leprosy in the Premodern World; Plagues of the Roman Republic; Religion and Epidemic Disease.

Further Reading

Freemon, F. R. "Bubonic Plague in the Book of Samuel." *Journal of the Royal Society of Medicine* 98 (2005): 436.

Karlen, Arno. *Plague's Progress: A Social History of Disease*. London: Gollancz, 1995.

Kohler W, and M. Kohler. "Plague and Rats, the 'Plague of the Philistines'", and "What Did Our Ancestors Know about the Role of Rats in Plague." *International Journal of Medical Microbiology* (November 2003): 333–340.

Mars, J. S., and C. D. Malloy. "An Epidemiologic Analysis of the Ten Plagues of Egypt." *Caduceus* 12 (1996): 7–24.

McMichael, Anthony. *Human Frontiers, Environments and Disease: Past Patterns, Uncertain Futures.* New York: Cambridge University Press, 2001.

McNeill, William. *Plagues and Peoples.* New York: Penguin, 1994.

Trevisanato, S. I. "The Biblical Plague of the Philistines Now Has a Name, Tularemia." *Medical Hypotheses* 69 (2007): 1144–1146.

Weiss, Robin. The Leeuwenhoek Lecture 2001. "Animal Origins of Human Infectious Disease." *Philosophical Translations of the Royal Society London B: Biological Sciences* 356 (2001): 957–977.

ANTHONY MCMICHAEL

BIMARISTAN/MARISTAN.   *Bimaristan* is the Arabic form of the Persian word designating the hospital in the Arabo-Islamic tradition. The question of the origin of hospitals in the Arabo-Islamic world has been long debated. The bimaristan is most probably a continuation of the hospital in the Byzantine world (*xenodocheion*), the origin of which has probably to be sought in Egyptian Christian monasticism rather than in fourth-century Christian charitable foundations in Asia Minor, as some historians believe. The fifteenth-century historian Al-Maqrizi asserted that Caliph Al-Walid established the first bimaristan in Damascus in 707. Hospitals clearly flourished in Baghdad from the early tenth century and spread across the Islamic world. The exception is Al-Andalus (Spain), where hospitals seem to have been built only from the very end of the fourteenth century. They were generally endowed with a *waqf*, a grant of productive agricultural land with the peasants tied to it, though some were directly funded by the state.

Bimaristan were large architectural structures with many wards for the patients. Some wards were devoted to such specialties as gynecology (but not obstetrics), psychiatry, and surgery. Bimaristan also included several peripheral units such as a kitchen(s), pharmacy, school, library, shops, and even in some cases an entire caravanserai. Some scholars believe that many had **leprosaria** located adjacent to them, as at Dimnah Hospital, in al-Qayrawan, established around 830. **Physicians** with different specialties, working in collaboration with different corps of assistants and nurses, visited the patients daily, performed surgical interventions, and prescribed appropriate medications. Hospitals provided the populace with a wide range of services not strictly limited to the treatment and cure of illness. These included some forms of public hygiene and prevention of diseases, as well as other social functions such as a retirement place for the elderly. They were directed by a chief physician and managed by a civil administrator. Among the most important bimaristan were the 'Adudi hospital in Baghdad, the hospital in Rayy, and the Mansuri hospital in Cairo. Over time, hospitals became important scientific and teaching institutions, as physicians did not limit their activity to the care of the sick but also conducted theoretical investigations, the results of which they communicated to audiences of students. Some of the historic hospitals of the Islamic world remained active well into the nineteenth century.

It is difficult to assess the role that the bimaristan might have actually played in the management of **epidemics** in the Islamic world because of the etiology attributed to epidemics in Muslim theology and **Islamic disease theory and medicine**. Since physicians in the Islamic world subscribed to both **miasma theory** and **humoral theory**, prevention relied on such methods as **fumigating** by burning perfumes and odoriferous substances, practicing a quiet lifestyle, and embracing a **diet** consisting of such foods as raw onions, lentils, pomegranates, grapes, vinegar, and lemon juice. As for the treatment, it consisted first of bleeding the patients in order to eliminate the supposed excess of corrupted humor out of the blood and body. Caregivers also administered topical remedies of differing natures according to the disease. Although bimaristan certainly helped in educating the population by promoting supposedly preventive methods and dispensing such treatments, they probably did not have a specific impact on the prevention, diffusion, and eradication of epidemics. *See also* Apothecary/Pharmacist; Astrology and Medicine; Avicenna (Ibn Sina); Black Death (1347–1352); Hospitals in the West to 1900; Plague in the Islamic World, 1360–1500; Plague in the Islamic World, 1500–1850; Public Health in the Islamic World, 1000–1600.

Further Reading

Dols, Michael D. "The Origins of the Islamic Hospital: Myth and Reality." *Bulletin of the History of Medicine* 61 (1987): 367–390.

Horden, Peregrine. "The Earliest Hospitals in Byzantium, Western Europe and Islam." *Journal of Interdisciplinary History* 35 (2005): 361–389.

Muslim Heritage. http://www.muslimheritage.com/uploads/The_Origin_of_Bimaristans_in_Islamic_Medical_History.pdf

Pormann, Peter E., and Emily Savage-Smith. *Medieval Islamic Medicine.* Washington, DC: Georgetown University Press, 2007.

Rahman, Fazlur. *Health and Medicine in the Islamic Tradition: Change and Identity.* Chicago: Kazi, 1998.

Risse, Guenter B. *Mending Bodies, Saving Souls: A History of Hospitals.* New York: Oxford University Press, 1999.

Tabbaa, Y. "The Functional Aspects of Medieval Islamic Hospitals." In *Poverty and Charity in Middle Eastern Contexts*, edited by M. Bonner, et al., pp. 95–119. Albany: State University of New York Press, 2003.

ALAIN TOUWAIDE

BIOLOGICAL WARFARE.   **Warfare** and disease have always gone together, and in all wars prior to World War II (1939–1945), deaths from disease surpassed deaths from combat, for both soldiers and civilians. It is no wonder, then, that there have been attempts to harness disease as a weapon. The term for such a practice is biological warfare (BW): the use by countries of microbes or toxins as a weapon to cause disease. This is distinct from **bioterrorism** or biocriminality, which is the use of disease as a weapon by individuals or groups.

Biological Warfare before the Twentieth Century.   Diseases are complex phenomena, and controlling them sufficiently for use as weapons was not truly possible in a rational fashion until the twentieth century, after the microbial causes of infectious diseases had begun to be understood. Nevertheless, there were sporadic cases of biological warfare in prescientific times. Several incidents of the use of plant toxins as weapons are recorded in ancient times. And in Europe in the fourteenth century, there were several alleged instances of attempts to transmit disease into besieged cities by hurling biological material over the walls. In one such report, at the beginning of the **Black Death**, Mongol armies besieging the Crimean city of Kaffa in 1346 hurled corpses of their plague dead, apparently starting a plague **epidemic** within the city.

Probably more common was the use of disease as a weapon by European settlers in the New World. Several deliberate attempts to transmit **smallpox** to Native Americans have been recorded, usually by giving them contaminated material from a smallpox victim. However, only one has been documented beyond any reasonable doubt: a 1763 incident at Fort Pitt (now the site of Pittsburgh, PA), in which civilian and military leaders of the Fort gave besieging Indians two blankets and two handkerchiefs from smallpox patients. No results were recorded. There were probably additional such incidents that went unrecorded. But even accounting for these, the practice appears to have been rare. However, given the ravages of smallpox on indigenous peoples in the New World, it is likely that some of these attempts caused outbreaks and possibly many deaths.

There have also been suggestions that the British might have used smallpox as a weapon during the American Revolution, although the evidence is scanty. In both the siege of Boston in 1775 and the siege of Quebec in 1775–1776 there were suspicions that civilians with smallpox were sent out of the cities to infect Continental Army troops. Similar actions may have been taken in the South, using escaped slaves infected with smallpox. The British planned to return them to their owners, as many slave-holders were supporters of the revolution. Whether the plan was executed is not known.

World War I (1914–1918).   By the time of World War I, infectious diseases were beginning to be understood, and the scientific basis for using them as weapons was being laid. One of the belligerents, Germany, established a systematic program of secret agents in neutral countries that were trading partners of France and Britain—mainly in the United States (neutral until 1917) and Argentina, with smaller programs in Spain, Norway, and Romania. These secret agents tried to infect animals, mainly horses and mules being shipped to the Allies, by pouring cultures of the causative agents of glanders or anthrax in the animals' feed or by jabbing them with contaminated needles. It is unclear whether this program had any success in infecting animals—it appears likely that it did not, but the reasons are unclear. It is notable that the German government explicitly ruled out attack on humans with biological weapons: that was considered to be immoral.

After the war, the nations of the world negotiated a treaty banning both biological warfare and chemical warfare (chemical weapons such as mustard gas had been extensively used in the war). Called the Geneva Protocol of 1925, it has become one of the pillars of the international arms control regime.

World War II (1939–1945).   Despite the Geneva Protocol, Japan made extensive use of crude biological weapons during World War II, against the Chinese. **Bubonic plague** was transmitted by dropping infected fleas from airplanes, or by releasing infected rats in cities. Intestinal diseases like **typhoid fever** and **cholera** were spread by infecting wells and food left behind during a Japanese retreat. The results are unclear, but it is estimated that these events left hundreds of thousands of Chinese dead. Another 10,000 are thought to have been killed during Japanese experimentation on prisoners.

Although the atrocities of Japanese biological warfare became known after the war, and most of the officers in charge were captured by U.S. forces, none was tried for war crimes. They were all given immunity in exchange for their cooperation with U.S. military. This deal was probably motivated largely by fear that the information would fall into Soviet hands (because the Soviet Union was a co-prosecutor in the Tokyo War Crimes Tribunal). However, a desire to see the results of human experiments and of actual use of biological weapons may also have played a role, as the U.S. biological warfare program could not use **human subjects**, and the United States had never actually used the weapons.

Although Japan was the only country to use biological weapons during World War II, several were attempting to develop them. The British developed and stockpiled a low-tech weapon—cattle biscuits laced with anthrax spores—to be used against German live-stock as retaliation if Germany used unconventional weapons. These were never used and were destroyed after the war.

A number of countries, including the United States, the United Kingdom, and the Soviet Union, also had programs to develop traditional military munitions—bombs, artillery shells, mortar rounds, and so forth—to deliver live biological agents. Although much progress was made, no country had a militarily useful weapon by the end of the war. Quite notably, Germany did not have a biological weapons program of any significance; Hitler was adamantly opposed to them, for unknown reasons. France had a biological weapons program before the war, but it was ended by France's defeat by the Germans. It was restarted, however, after the war ended.

The Cold War Era.   Most countries' BW programs petered out in the 1950s or 1960s, leaving the United States and USSR as the only nations with major programs. The United States developed a number of pathogens (for both humans and animals) as weapons and made stockpiles of these in bombs, shells, and spray tanks. The Soviet Union appears to have lagged far behind the United States in its capabilities and probably had no usable weapons in this time period.

Although the U.S. military had developed biological weapons for battlefield use, it rec-ognized that their utility was quite limited: they could be easily protected against with a respirator, their effects would be delayed by one to several days, they would be very sensi-tive to the weather conditions, and their effects would be unpredictable. However, they offered great potential to attack civilians covertly. A single plane, equipped with a spray device and several tens of kilograms of a concentrated preparation of a biological agent, could blanket hundreds of square kilometers, causing very large numbers of deaths.

Nevertheless, in 1969 Richard Nixon (1913–1994) announced that the United States would unilaterally destroy its biological weapons and would in the future only develop defensive capabilities. This followed the advice of an expert panel that considered the weapons essentially useless, as the United States had alternatives to biological weapons, most importantly nuclear weapons. It also recognized that possessing biological weapons sent a message to the world that these were useful weapons, and encouraged other nations to follow suit, whereas disarming suggested the weapons had limited utility.

This disavowal prepared the way for a second major treaty limiting biological weapons: the Biological Weapons Convention (BWC) of 1975. This treaty banned the develop-ment, production, and stockpiling of biological weapons, plugging the gaps in the Geneva Protocol (which only banned their use).

Despite the treaty, the Soviet Union secretly maintained, and even expanded, its pro-gram. It was not until 1992 that Russia (which had inherited most of the Soviet Union's weapons programs) admitted that it had been violating the BWC and decreed an end to the bioweapons program. After its weak start in the 1950s and 1960s, this program had matured in the 1970s and 1980s with major successes in developing plague, anthrax, and smallpox, among others, as weapons. Soviet developers designed them to be delivered on intercontinental ballistic missiles, as second-strike weapons to follow an initial nuclear attack.

The Contemporary World.   Other countries are also known to have violated the BWC since it came into force. South Africa's minority white government had a modest program to develop biological and chemical agents for nonbattlefield use, such as assassination and special forces use. This was voluntarily ended when the black majority government came to power in 1994.

Iraq under Saddam Hussein (1937–2003), too, had a program, and actually developed several agents to the point of accumulating modest stockpiles of (militarily insignificant) filled munitions. Iraq devoted a great deal of effort to preventing UN inspection teams (UNSCOM, and its successor UNMOVIC) from learning of the program, but eventually the basic outlines became clear. UNSCOM was then able to destroy the production facilities. After the second Iraq war, the U.S.'s Iraq Survey Group confirmed that the biological weapons program had been effectively terminated, although Iraq appears to have been maintaining the ability to restart the program quickly after UN inspectors left the country.

Several other countries are suspected by Western intelligence agencies of trying to develop biological weapons, but the available evidence is quite weak, and it remains to be seen if any of these suspicions are true.

In addition to suspicions that some countries may be trying to develop biological weapons, there have been periodic accusations that some countries have actually used them. The most prominent of the allegations includes charges that the United States used them against China and North Korea during the Korean War; that the United States used them repeatedly against Cuba; that the Burmese (Myanmar) government used them against insurgent indigenous tribes; and that the Rhodesian government used them against blacks during the Zimbabwean war of independence. Some of these allegations are almost certainly false (evidence suggests that the United States did not use biological agents in Korea or Cuba), and the others are generally thought to be unlikely.

For the moment, the total ban on biological weapons, one of the major triumphs of arms control in the twentieth century, seems to be robust, and it is unlikely that the world will see biological weapons used in warfare. Use by terrorists is another matter, and there is concern that this could be a serious problem in the near future. *See also* Bioterrorism; Poison Libels and Epidemic Disease; Smallpox and the American Revolution; Smallpox in Colonial North America; War, the Military, and Epidemic Disease.

Further Reading

Dando, Malcolm. *Bioterror and Biowarfare: A Beginner's Guide*. Oxford: Oneworld, 2006.

Geissler, Erhard, and Moon, John Ellis van Courtland, eds. *Biological and Toxin Weapons: Research, Development, and Use from the Middle Ages to 1945*. New York: Oxford University Press, 1999.

Harris, Sheldon. *Factories of Death: Japanese Biological Warfare 1932–45*. New York: Routledge, 1994.

Koenig, Robert. *The Fourth Horseman: One Man's Mission to Wage the Great War in America*. New York: Public Affairs, 2006.

Leitenberg, Milton. *The Problem of Biological Weapons*. Stockholm: Swedish National Defense College, 2004.

Mayor, Adrienne. *Greek Fire, Poison Arrows and Scorpion Bombs: Biological and Chemical Warfare in the Ancient World*. Woodstock, NY: Overlook Duckworth, 2004.

Wheelis, Mark, Lajos Rózsa, and Malcolm Dando, eds. *Deadly Cultures: Biological Weapons since 1945*. Cambridge, MA: Harvard University Press, 2006.

MARK WHEELIS

BIOTERRORISM.   Bioterrorism is (a) the use, or the threat of use, of biological agents as weapons, (b) by individuals or groups (but not by nations), (c) for political, ideological, or religious motives. By biological agent we usually mean any microorganism that causes diseases in plants, animals, or humans, or any toxic compound produced by a living organism (termed toxins). This is not an official definition; in fact there is no generally agreed upon definition of terrorism, much less of bioterrorism. But this definition distinguishes bioterrorism from two other closely related activities: biological warfare and biocriminality. Biological warfare is the use of biological agents as weapons by nations; biocriminality is the use of such agents for personal motives, such as financial gain or revenge.

The 2001 U.S. Anthrax Letter Attacks.   Bioterrorism has a rather short history, and there have been very few actual attempts. Most prominent, at least for Americans, is the 2001 anthrax letter attacks. In this incident, letters containing spores of the causative agent of anthrax, *Bacillus anthracis*, were sent to several U.S. media outlets (print and TV) and to two U.S. senators. A total of five letters were sent, infecting 22 people, 11 with the pulmonary form of the disease, and 11 with the cutaneous form. Five of the victims with pulmonary anthrax died.

Ironically, it appears that the perpetrator did not intend to kill anyone. All of the envelopes contained warnings that they contained anthrax spores and advised taking **antibiotics** (which would prevent the disease). Most victims were postal workers exposed unintentionally when spores leaked out of the envelopes during sorting or recipients who did not take the warning seriously and discarded the letters and contents without notifying authorities or taking protective steps. Dozens or hundreds of deaths probably would have resulted if the perpetrator had had a serious intent to harm.

At least two of the letters contained high-purity spores, and this led investigators to conclude that the perpetrator was an insider in the U.S. military-scientific community with experience in preparing anthrax spores (the U.S. has, for many years, produced anthrax spores for defensive testing). This conclusion has since been softened, and the FBI now appears to think that a wider range of people might have had the expertise necessary to carry out the crime. Nevertheless, most investigators and scientists believe that the perpetrator must have been a Ph.D.-level microbiologist, with experience in working with dangerous microbes, and possibly with access to classified biodefense information.

In another irony, this case may not even be an example of bioterrorism. Because we do not know the motive, we cannot be sure whether this was an incident of bioterrorism or biocriminality.

Although the anthrax letters were not intended to cause casualties, there have been two attacks that were intended to do so: a 1984 bioterrorist attack in The Dalles, Oregon, by the Rajneesh sect, and attempted bioterrorist attacks in Japan by the Aum Shinrikyo sect from 1990 to 1995.

The 1984 Rajneesh Attacks.   In 1981 an East Indian sect, including many American, Western European, and Australian members, relocated from India to the Big Muddy ranch in rural Oregon south of the county seat, The Dalles, on the Columbia River. The sect's guru was the Bhagwan ("enlightened one") Shree Rajneesh (1931–1990). They incorporated a town (named Rajneeshpuram) on the ranch and built accommodations for several thousand people. However, by 1984 things were going poorly; many lawsuits had been brought against the group, its incorporation of Rajneeshpuram as a town was being challenged, and the outlook for the group's remaining in Oregon was bleak. The Rajneesh responded with a plan to take over the county government by electing their members to office in the election scheduled for November 1984.

The number of sect members is unclear, but was probably around 2,000, whereas there were about 15,000 registered voters. The Rajneesh intended to import thousands of homeless people from urban areas all over the country to overcome the numerical disadvantage. In anticipation that even with the influx of homeless people the election might be very close, a few senior sect leaders (including the nurse who ran the sect's infirmary, who provided the technical expertise) hatched a plot to make townspeople sick on election day. Their strategy was to pour suspension of the bacterium *Salmonella enteritica* (obtained by the nurse) on foods in salad bars in restaurants in The Dalles. To test the method, they attacked two restaurants around September 8 and many more (10 to 20) around September 20. The result was a major outbreak of salmonellosis (diarrhea, vomiting, fever). The **Centers for Disease Control and Prevention** (CDC) eventually identified 751 cases, 45 of whom were hospitalized. However, salmonellosis is typically under-diagnosed by as much as an order of magnitude, so it is virtually certain that there were at least several thousand cases. The successful trial was not followed by an election-day attack, however, as recruiting of the homeless fell far short of its goals, and it was clear that the Rajneesh had no hope of winning the election.

Interestingly, this outbreak was never suspected to be a bioterrorist attack, despite having a number of suspicious features that should have alerted public health personnel, and despite widespread public suspicion that the Rajneesh were involved. This was before there were serious concerns about bioterrorism (which began in the early 1990s); a similar outbreak today would certainly be recognized as a deliberate attack.

The attack was recognized as bioterrorism about a year later, when an independent police investigation of the sect turned up evidence that the Rajneesh were responsible for the outbreak. Two of the instigators of the attack were tried and convicted of first- and second-degree assault and product tampering, as well as unrelated crimes, and were sentenced to 20 years imprisonment. However, both were released after two and a half years and deported.

The 1990–1995 Aum Shinrikyo Attacks.   The only other major attempt at bioterrorism was also perpetrated by a religious sect, this one the Japanese group known as Aum Shinrikyo. It was led by Shoko Asahara (b. 1955), who had developed a large following after a magazine published a photo showing him apparently levitating. At its peak, the sect had more than 15,000 members in Japan, and many thousands more abroad. Many members were young professionals, with good incomes, so the sect was also very wealthy.

To further its goals, Aum plotted to take over the government by running candidates for the Diet (Japan's parliament). When none of their candidates won, the cult's leadership decided to use violence and instituted an ambitious, $20 million program to acquire a wide variety of weapons, from assault rifles to attack helicopters, as well as nonconventional weapons like chemical and biological weapons. Their biological attacks on Japanese cities spanned the years from 1990 to 1995. Most were attempts to disseminate botulinum toxin in an aerosol, using sprayers mounted in vehicles or in briefcases. Botulinum toxin is a protein that causes the disease botulism; it is one of the most toxic substances known. However, Aum seems not to have succeeded in producing it, and the material they disseminated appears not to have contained any toxin.

Aum also tried to disseminate anthrax spores but again failed. The group's most ambitious attack, in the summer of 1993, was from the roof of one of its buildings in Tokyo and involved spraying thousands of liters of *Bacillus anthracis* culture into the air over several days. The failure to cause any cases of disease was the result of several factors: the group had an avirulent strain of B. *anthracis* (one used as a veterinary vaccine); its dissemination device produced large droplets, rather than the tiny ones needed to cause pulmonary disease; and the concentration of spores in the cultures was very low.

Because these attempts were uniformly unsuccessful in causing disease, they were not detected by the authorities. However, Aum had more success with chemical weapons, and its attack on the Tokyo subway with sarin led to rapid police action. Aum's leaders were arrested and tried for various crimes. About a dozen senior leaders, including Asahara, have been convicted of murder (for the sarin attacks) and sentenced to death.

Hoaxes.   Although actual bioterrorist attacks have been extremely infrequent, hoaxes have been very common, particularly in the United States, which has seen well over a thousand. Hoaxes commonly involve an envelope containing a white powder (talcum powder, baking soda, or some other innocuous material) and a letter claiming that the powder is anthrax spores or some other hazardous biological material. Each one of these hoaxes has to be taken seriously by authorities, who need to counsel potentially exposed people, test the powder, and open a criminal investigation. The cumulative costs of responding have probably been more than $100 million in the United States alone.

In most cases the perpetrators have not been caught, and many of the incidents may be criminal rather than terrorist in nature. Some are clearly terrorist acts, however; for instance, motivated by religious and ideological fervor, many hoaxers target abortion clinics in an effort to harass and intimidate them. This is clearly bioterrorism.

The record of serious bioterrorist attempts to cause mass casualties is clearly very sparse, suggesting that the threat of bioterrorism may not be as serious as many have estimated. For 15 years senior American policy makers have been making very public claims that America's greatest vulnerability is to bioterrorism; nevertheless, no international terrorist group has yet taken up biological arms. Although there are periodic reports that Al Qaeda has some interest in chemical and biological weapons, there is no evidence that such interest has gone beyond some very rudimentary exploratory steps. The success of the perpetrator of the U.S. anthrax letter attacks in making highly purified anthrax spore preparations serves as a caution, however. If the expertise of the anthrax letter attacker were combined with the desire of organizations such as Al Qaeda to cause mass casualties, the result could be very serious. Furthermore, the failure of the FBI to arrest and convict the perpetrator may lead terrorists to believe that this kind of attack is safer than traditional ones, and that by escaping detection they may be able to mount multiple attacks.

Thus, the threat of bioterrorism needs to be taken seriously, and the danger is probably increasing steadily as time goes by. Yet even in the United States funds are not unlimited, and bioterrorism prevention and response funding should be viewed in the context of other priorities, such as the death toll from natural infectious diseases. For instance, ordinary influenza causes approximately 35,000 deaths per year in the United States, almost all of them preventable by immunization; this dwarfs anything that a terrorist attack could reasonably be expected to cause. This does not mean that bioterrorism funding should be diverted to flu **vaccination** programs, but it does suggest the need for a mechanism to balance competing needs in public health. *See also* Biological Warfare; Bubonic Plague; Smallpox.

Further Reading

Cole, Leonard A. *The Anthrax Letters: A Medical Detective Story.* Washington, DC: Joseph Henry Press, 2003.

Dando, Malcolm. *Bioterror and Biowarfare: A Beginner's Guide.* Oxford: Oneworld, 2006.

Greysmith, Robert. *Amerithrax: The Hunt for the Anthrax Killer.* New York: Berkeley Books, 2003.

The History of Bioterrorism [film]. http://www.bt.cdc.gov/training/historyofbt/

Leitenberg, Milton. *The Problem of Biological Weapons.* Stockholm: Swedish National Defense College, 2004.

Tucker, Jonathan, ed. *Toxic Terror: Assessing Terrorist Use of Chemical and Biological Weapons.* Cambridge, MA: MIT Press, 2000.

Wheelis, Mark, and Masaaki Sugishima. "Terrorist Use of Biological Weapons." In *Deadly Cultures: Biological Weapons since 1945*, edited by Mark Wheelis, Lajos Rózsa, and Malcolm Dando, pp. 284–303. Cambridge, MA: Harvard University Press, 2006.

MARK WHEELIS

BLACK DEATH (1347–1352).   The Black Death is the term most often applied to the initial outbreak of **bubonic plague** that began the second **pandemic** of plague. This outbreak, which spread across Europe, the Levant, and North Africa between 1347 and 1352, brought bubonic plague into Europe from the Asiatic steppes where it had long been endemic. Following this **epidemic**, Europeans experienced recurrent outbreaks of plague over the next four centuries. As a result of the many effects of the plague on society and culture, many historians consider this half-decade a turning point in European history.

Although the term "Black Death" came into common use only in the nineteenth century, it has remained a popular descriptive term for this epidemic. Many accounts of the Black Death offer an explanation for the term based on physical symptoms, but it actually comes from a misunderstanding or mistranslation of the Latin *atra mors*, which can mean either "terrible death" or "black death." Those living through this epidemic did not give it a specific name, but used general terms including pest, pestilence, plague, and mortality.

The Black Death was one of the most significant events of the late medieval world and spawned numerous changes, most visibly in the drastic reduction of population in those areas affected. Estimates of the overall mortality from the Black Death are difficult to obtain, as none of these areas kept accurate or consistent census or burial records. Historians working with a variety of local studies, however, continue efforts to approximate overall mortality. Those estimates currently range between 45 and 60 percent across the affected areas.

Historical Record.   The historical record of the Black Death is extensive, as there are numerous first-hand accounts of the epidemic from Europe, North Africa, and the Near East. Best known are the accounts of Italian chroniclers, such as Gabriele de' Mussis (c. 1280–?) who described the transfer of disease from besieging Mongol troops to besieged residents of the Black Sea port of Caffa (Kaffa; modern Feodosiya) via dead bodies catapulted over the city's walls. Another Italian writer, Giovanni Boccaccio

(1313–1375), included a vivid description of the plague in the introduction to his collection of short stories *The Decameron*, the frame story of which is set during the pestilence in Florence in 1348. These and many other accounts and descriptions have been translated and are increasingly accessible, often in abridged form, in studies on the Black Death.

In addition to individual chronicles detailing events, evidence of the reaction to and impact of the Black Death may be found across all areas of society that generated any type of records. These include municipal, ecclesiastical, medical, and scientific authorities. Scholars have made use of diverse records such as city council meeting minutes, municipal statutes, sermons, tax rolls, court records, medical and scientific treatises, and personal letters to uncover information about the Black Death.

Nature of the Disease. That some disease swept through Europe in the mid-fourteenth century, causing death rates unlike anything previously experienced, is clear. What is less clear is the exact cause of those deaths. Although bubonic plague is generally assumed to be the infectious agent, it is important to note that a number of scholars have raised questions about whether plague—in its three forms of bubonic, **pneumonic**, and **septicemic**—truly fits the symptoms, spread, seasonality, and mortality rates described by chroniclers in the early modern era. Few satisfactory alternatives have been proposed, however, and in the absence of conclusive evidence otherwise, most historians continue to attribute the Black Death to bubonic plague. In addition, recent work in paleomicrobiology has confirmed the existence of DNA from *Yersinia pestis* (the causative bacteria of bubonic plague) in tooth samples from plague-era graves in France, lending credence to the argument for the existence of plague there. Nonetheless, the Black Death remains a case study in the difficulties of **diagnosis of historical disease** and **historical epidemiology**.

Accounts and descriptions of the Black Death exist in such numbers that only a general summary of the symptoms given in them is possible. All of the accounts describe a horrible and painful disease that struck suddenly and killed rapidly. It was the rapid course of the disease that most contemporaries commented on, recording accounts of acquaintances healthy in the morning but dead by nightfall. Descriptions of symptoms most often include some sort of swellings (also referred to as tumors, boils, or apostemes) in the groin or armpit, which were exquisitely painful and the contents of which (when lanced open) were foul smelling. Others describe pustules, blisters, or black spots, the coughing or spitting of blood, and a high fever followed by great thirst and delirium or prostration. Because the disease spread quickly among family members or households, many blamed the contaminated breath of the sick for spreading the disease.

Origins and Spread. Bubonic plague, endemic to certain mammal populations but not to humans, has natural reservoirs scattered across the Asian steppes region. The epidemic of 1347–1352 likely began from one of these, spreading as a result of Mongol traders opening new trade routes. Chroniclers describe outbreaks of disease among the Mongols or "Tatars" in the early 1340s. By 1346 outbreaks had occurred in the region between the Caspian and Black Seas. According to contemporary accounts, Genoese traders helped spread the pestilence outward after visiting the city of Caffa, a Genoese colony located on the Black Sea. While there, traders became trapped by a Mongol siege of the city. Plague broke out among the Mongols, who responded by catapulting the bodies of the dead over the city walls. Some ships managed to leave Caffa in the fall of 1347, passing through Constantinople (Istanbul) and stopping briefly in Messina

(Sicily) before returning to Genoa. Although the movements of these **trade** ships may well have helped the outward spread of the Black Death, evidence from the Near East and Africa show that it was quickly spreading in several directions by the late 1340s. In 1347 it appeared in Constantinople, Greece, Venice, and most of the Mediterranean islands (Crete, Sicily, Sardinia, Mallorca) as well as Alexandria in Egypt. Once in the Mediterranean, the epidemic spread both northward across Western Europe and westward across North Africa in 1348. In Europe it spread across Spain, southern France, and most of Italy in 1348, then passed to Germany, England, and Norway in 1349. Continuing northeastward, plague infected Eastern Europe and the Low Countries in the next year, and then finally arrived in Russia in 1351–1352.

 Religious Responses. By far, the strongest reaction in Christian lands was a religious interpretation of the plague as a punishment from God. This belief, held across all levels of society, led to conflicting responses. As Boccaccio eloquently describes, some, believing there was little that mankind could do in the face of such a scourge, abandoned morality in favor of pleasures. Others turned to extreme piety and prayer in an effort to appease an angry God. In parts of Europe, the **flagellant** movement (named for the *flagellum* or whip) flourished for a time. These groups of **pilgrims** moved about from town to town holding displays of public piety in which they offered bodily penance in the form of whippings as a supplement to traditional prayers. The movement initially gained many converts and strong popular approval, but within a year had lost official support and was forbidden by Pope Clement VI (1291–1352) in October 1349. Less drastically, communities across Europe organized a variety of public processions, pilgrimages to shrines, and other forms of communal piety. Responding in part to a surge in pilgrimages to sacred sites in Europe, including Canterbury and Santiago de Compostela, the papacy declared 1350 a jubilee year, offering plenary indulgences (remission from the obligation to carry out penance for confessed sins) to all those who visited the principle churches of Rome that year.

 Alongside prayers to the Virgin Mary, Mother of Mercy, came prayers to St. Sebastian, a third-century martyr who became increasingly associated with plague. Sebastian, a member of the imperial guard under Roman Emperor Diocletian (r. 284–305), was sentenced to death for his Christian beliefs. Shot with arrows and left for dead, he was found while still alive and nursed back to health. His subsequent execution by bludgeoning made him a true martyr, but his survival of the arrows created the association with plague. Fourteenth-century thinkers often described the sudden onset of the disease as akin to being shot by an arrow (and the communal onset as a sort of rain of arrows from heaven). Thus, Sebastian's success in surviving *his* (real) arrows made him an empathetic patron saint who would likewise work to protect people from *their* (metaphorical) arrows.

 A tragic religious response to the Black Death, encouraged in part by the anti-semitism preached by the flagellants, was the persecution and massacre of Jews. As the epidemic spread and the death toll mounted, many searched for **scapegoats** to blame for the disease. Accusations were leveled against various groups of outsiders, most notably Jews who came under suspicion of deliberately spreading disease. Despite the efforts of many civil and ecclesiastical authorities (including the papacy) to protect Jewish residents, thousands were rounded up and executed in Spain, in southern France, and across central Europe.

 Social Response. One of the most striking features of accounts of the Black Death is the overwhelming fear expressed by most authors. Accounts of the epidemic are rife with stories of **flight** and abandonment, though whether these stories are objective records of fact or simply literary expressions is unclear. But regardless of how commonly "brothers abandoned brothers . . . fathers and mothers refused to nurse and assist their own children" as Boccaccio describes, it is clear from the records of this epidemic that there was a notable shift in society. The most common prescription of the era, reproduced into a variety of languages, was to "flee far, fast, and for a long time," and flight (from cities to countryside, from one town to another) was a common reaction during this and later epidemics. The observed patterns of illness led to popular beliefs that it spread from person to person, which would have been the case with pneumonic plague. Whereas medical theories held on to the miasmatic concept of disease (caused by "corruption" in the air), the popular belief in **contagion** led to a noticeable fear not just of disease, or even just of the sick themselves, but also of the potentially sick. Public venues such as markets, churches, or public squares were increasingly avoided, and care for the

> **AN IRISH FRANCISCAN FRIAR DESCRIBES THE HORRORS OF THE BLACK DEATH (1349)**
>
> Since the beginning of the world it has been unheard of for so many people to die of pestilence, famine or any other infirmity in such a short time. Earthquakes, which extended for many miles, threw down cities, towns and castles and swallowed them up. Plague stripped villages, cities, castles, and towns of their inhabitants so thoroughly that there was scarcely anyone left alive in them. This pestilence was so contagious that those who touched the dead or the sick were immediately infected themselves and died, so that the penitent and confessor were carried together to the grave. Because of their fear and horror men could hardly bring themselves to perform the pious and charitable acts of visiting the sick and burying the dead. Many died of boils, abscesses and pustules that erupted on the legs and in the armpits. Others died in frenzy, brought on by an affliction of the head, or vomiting blood . . . . Among the Franciscans at Drogheda 25 brothers died before Christmas, and 23 died at Dublin . . . . At Kilkenny the pestilence was strong during Lent, and eight Dominicans died between Christmas and 6 March. It was very rare for just one to die in a house; usually husband, wife, children and servants went the same way, the way of death.
>
> From John Clynn, OFM, in *Annalium Hibernae Chronicon* (edited by R. Butler); translated by Rosemary Horrox in her *The Black Death* (New York: Manchester University Press, 1994), p. 84.

sick often fell to either the very pious—those willing to place themselves in danger—or the very poor, who may have sought to profit however they could. Burials, which could no longer be carried out individually as a result of the excessive number of **corpses** accumulating, were likewise left in the hands of the charitable or the desperate. The accumulation of bodies faster than they could be buried led to a variety of psychological reactions—guilt, fear, anger, sorrow—none of which is directly measurable but all of which are indirectly evident in the sources.

Medical Response.   Although medical theory lagged behind popular conceptions in formulating a theory of contagion, medical personnel developed a variety of theories on how plague spread and how it could be prevented. In some areas, especially Italy, efforts were made to understand better the disease by conducting autopsies on victims. These principally discovered problems in the lungs, which helped reinforce the **humoral theory** of corrupted air causing disease. The disease was viewed as being so virulent that it was believed to be spread by the very breath of the infected (which it may have been, in the case of pneumonic plague). Prescriptions for prevention of plague included the burning of aromatic herbs (often carried out in public squares) to cleanse the air as well as the regulation of **diet** to maintain humoral balance. Other plague treatises advocated keeping one's mouth covered with a handkerchief or the use of a posy of sweet-smelling herbs while in public. One author advocated ensuring a patient's eyes had been covered before entering the room, believing that the disease could be passed along via direct eye contact.

A notable disparity existed in reactions to plague between Christian and Muslim populations, both within Spain and in the Middle East. Though plague took a high toll on both groups, and though both believed plague to be sent from God, their reactions were distinct. Whereas Christians blamed human sin as the cause of God's anger and punishment, Muslims viewed plague as a disaster to be endured, one which offered a martyr's death to its victims. Muslim submission to the will of God meant a strong focus on prayer rather than the flight and self-preservation seen among Christians, though observers noted many cases of Muslim flight. There was no scapegoating or placing of blame among Muslims, and likewise little tolerance for theories of contagion, which challenged God's supreme power over all events. Ibn al-Khatib, a Spanish Muslim medical writer in Spanish Granada, offered a treatise in which he argued for the contagious nature of plague, an argument that likely led to his subsequent persecution for heresy and his ultimate exile.

Historical Effects.   The Black Death is acknowledged as a momentous event in European history, one that affected all aspects of society. Alongside the more obvious demographic and economic effects, scholars have also argued for indirect psychological effects, manifested in art, intellectual development, and social changes. Part of the difficulty in assessing these changes, however, is the fact that the Black Death was just the first (though the most widespread and the most lethal) epidemic of many during the second pandemic that would continue to haunt Europe until its gradual disappearance in the eighteenth and nineteenth centuries.

The overall mortality of the Black Death has fascinated historians for generations, but reliable figures remain elusive. Accurate census numbers from the era prior to the Black Death simply do not exist, nor do reliable death or burial records for more than scattered territories. Thus, calculating the overall impact on Europe as a whole is extremely difficult, if not impossible. Nevertheless, estimates have steadily risen in recent generations from roughly a third of Europe to nearly two-thirds. It is considered safe to assume at least half of Europe died in the Black Death, and possibly more than half. These deaths occurred in all levels of society, from the very poorest to royalty, including King Alfonso XI of Castile (1312–1350) who fell sick and died in 1350 while besieging Gibraltar. Those who tended to the sick suffered the highest losses, including **physicians, surgeons**, clergy, and notaries (who recorded last wills). These losses had their own ripple effects, as medical and clerical positions stood empty or were filled with less qualified (or less dedicated) applicants. Throughout Europe the drastic population decline had repercussions on several generations that, coupled with recurrent epidemics, meant that population levels did not recover in most regions until the late fifteenth century.

One significant result of Black Death was an overall shift in rural population away from marginal agricultural lands and onto more fertile ones. The evidence of a large number of deserted villages in Europe, once taken to be a result of massive mortality, is now recognized as resulting from both deaths and relocation as survivors moved in search of better economic opportunities.

Economic Impacts.   The most obvious economic impact of the Black Death was a rise in the standard of living for survivors. For both free and enserfed farmers, the loss of so much population meant that lands stood open awaiting workers. This provided greater opportunities for them to gain mobility and to negotiate favorable terms of employment. For landowners, finding and retaining workers now meant paying higher wages or offering

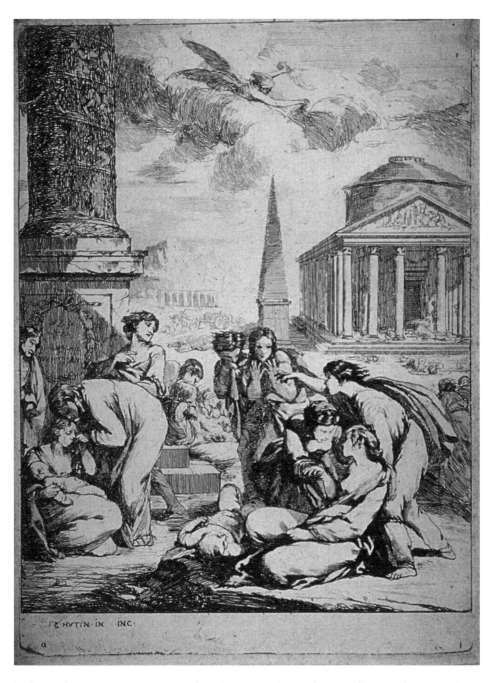

Eighteenth-century street scene showing several people attending to plague victims. Etching by Huttin. Courtesy of the National Library of Medicine.

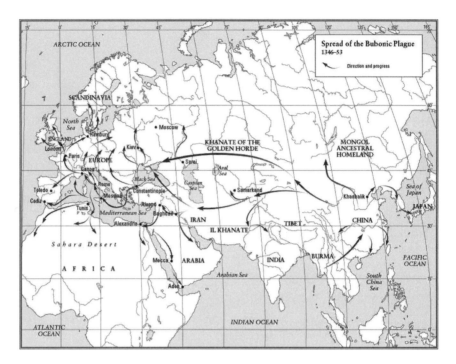

Map of the spread of the Black Death across Asia, the Middle East, Europe, and Africa.

better terms of living. Across many trades, wages and prices rose dramatically in the immediate aftermath of the Black Death, as there were simply fewer skilled workers to provide goods and services.

As early as 1349 authorities across Europe (at both the local and national levels) began to respond to these economic shifts by regulating wages, prices, and the mobility of workers. Wages were held to pre-plague levels and attempts were made to prevent secret agreements offering bribes or bonuses. These statutes led to further political and economic tensions as workers sought to capitalize on gains while employers sought to rescind them.

Cultural Changes.   Alongside the written records that reflect people's experiences with the Black Death are artistic depictions. A wealth of art, created both in direct response to the Black Death and in response to subsequent epidemics in later generations, reflects themes of death and the transitory nature of life, wealth, and power. Images increasingly showed "King Death," personified as a skeleton, stalking or attacking victims, often now armed with a scythe. The *Danse Macabre* ("The Dance of Death") became a common theme, illustrating how quickly and easily death could interrupt life and "dance" the unsuspecting victim into the grave. In addition, new cults devoted to plague saints Sebastian and Roch (Roche) sprang up, and both are depicted with greater frequency after the Black Death.

The intellectual impact of the Black Death is the hardest to quantify, but there is evidence that the massive population loss created new intellectual space for upcoming generations to fill. The loss of intellectual continuity, which allowed older ideas and traditions to slip slightly seems to have provided opportunities for new approaches, such as the increased use of the vernacular in a variety of writings, and for new ideas, such as the Renaissance humanists' new interest in reviving ancient models. Though there is no consensus on the issue, many scholars have argued that the Renaissance, which emerged on the heels of the Black Death, owes its birth to the intellectual upheavals and questions raised by the epidemic and its successive waves. Although historians do not agree on the extent to which the Black Death represented a "turning point" in history, it clearly had long-lasting repercussions and must be taken into account as a contributing factor for long-term social, economic, and intellectual shifts. *See also* Astrology and Medicine; Black Death and Late Medieval Christianity; Black Death, Economic and Demographic Effects of; Black Death, Flagellants, and Jews; Black Death: Literature and Art; Black Death: Modern Medical Debate; Environment, Ecology, and Epidemic Disease; Islamic Disease Theory and Medicine; Medical Education in the West, 1100–1500; Plague and Developments in Public Health, 1348–1600; Plague in Medieval Europe, 1360–1500; Plague in China; Plague in the Islamic World, 1360–1500; Plague of Justinian, First Pandemic; Public Health in the Islamic World, 1000–1600; Quarantine; Religion and Epidemic Disease.

Further Reading

Ancient Mysteries: The Black Death [film]. A&E, 1997.

Benedictow, Ole J. *The Black Death 1346–1353: The Complete History*. New York: The Boydell Press, 2004.

Brown University Department of Italian Studies. http://www.brown.edu/Departments/Italian_Studies/dweb/plague/index.shtml

Byrne, Joseph P. *The Black Death*. Westport, CT: Greenwood Press, 2004.

Christakos, George, et al. *Interdisciplinary Public Health Reasoning and Epistemic Modeling: The Case of the Black Death*. New York: Springer, 2005.

Cohn Jr., Samuel K. *The Black Death Transformed: Disease and Culture in Early Renaissance Europe*. New York: Arnold and Oxford University Press, 2002.

Dols, Michael. *The Black Death in the Middle East*. Princeton, NJ: Princeton University Press, 1977.

Herlihy, David. *The Black Death and the Transformation of the West*, edited by Samuel K. Cohn Jr. Cambridge, MA: Harvard University Press, 1997.

Horrox, Rosemary, ed. *The Black Death*. Manchester: Manchester University Press, 1994.

The Plague [film]. History Channel, 2006.

Platt, Colin. *King Death: The Black Death and Its Aftermath in Late-Medieval England*. Toronto: University of Toronto Press, 1996.

Scholiast. http://www.scholiast.org/history/blackdeath/index.html *In Search of History: Scourge of the Black Death* [film]. History Channel, 2005.

University of Virginia History Department. http://www3.iath.virginia.edu/osheim/intro.html

Williman, Daniel, ed. *The Black Death: The Impact of the Fourteenth-Century Plague*. Binghamton, NY: Center for Medieval and Early Renaissance Studies, 1982.

Ziegler, Philip. *The Black Death*. New York: Harper and Row, 1969.

KRISTY WILSON BOWERS

BLACK DEATH AND LATE MEDIEVAL CHRISTIANITY.   When the **Black Death** swept across Asia, North Africa, and Europe in the mid-fourteenth century, it killed between one-third and one-half of the population. In Christian areas, the Church mobilized immediately, as it had with natural disasters in centuries past. In doing so it drew from two distinct but related sources: the Bible and Catholic tradition. The Bible made it clear that plagues, regardless of the type, were a sign of God's judgment. In sermons, priests counseled against sin and encouraged penitent behavior by reciting the stories of Noah, Sodom and Gomorrah, and Nineveh. The story of Nineveh illustrates the clearest parallel to a plague visitation and the power of faith, as it tells of a king willing to join his people in a public penance that ultimately appeases God and spares the nation from obliteration. Specific forms of penance included fast days, communal prayer, processions, pilgrimage, monetary offerings, and devotion to saints. Equally important were public displays of thanksgiving, with church communities joining together to praise and thank God when deaths declined. These rituals were standard for all natural disasters, lending a degree of the ordinary to that which was otherwise unimaginable.

The devotion to saints at this time took on a unique form, with the recognition of saints who were considered particularly potent against the plague. Many prayed to the Virgin Mary, mother of Jesus, and artists depicted her as shielding her clients (devotees), and sometimes entire towns, from an angry God. The late third-century Saint Sebastian is the most recognizable of the plague saints, with his naked, arrow-strewn body clad only in a loincloth. In late medieval paintings and statues, his arrows are metaphorical "arrows of the pestilence," and the story of his recovery from these wounds stands as an account of escape from the plague. St. Michael the Archangel also figures in the late medieval Christian plague-time paintings that once adorned churches and covered processional placards. As the Christian tradition tells of Michael driving a dragon-like Satan from Heaven, so did late medieval Christians consider him able to drive away the Black Death. The only plague-specific saint of international repute was the purported fourteenth-century Saint Roche (known in various countries as San Rocco, Saint Rock, and San Roque). Few of the details of his biography are verifiable, but by the early fifteenth century, believers knew him as a healer of plague victims who had become ill and recovered from the disease. One can identify him in paintings by his dog, his pilgrim's staff, and his unusual gesture: he points under his tunic to suggest that he has a bubo on his upper thigh.

In spite of these church-sponsored efforts, it was clear that the Black Death was a more menacing threat than other scourges. It could kill an entire household within a matter of days and often reduced town populations by a quarter in a single season—all while its victims suffered enormous pain. Naturally, those who witnessed the horrors feared that they were living in the end times, as told in the book of Revelation. Late medieval writers embraced apocalyptic thinking, imagining that the end result of God's plague-time wrath might be a nation of animals only, with the entire human population extinguished.

Some of the faithful became more zealous in their determination to avert damnation. Among this small portion of the faithful were the **flagellants**, a group known more for their oddity than for the number of their followers. The flagellant movement did not last, as its adherents' extreme behavior and directives threatened church authority. Other zealous Christians used the plague as an opportunity to clear their cities of Jews. They spread rumors that the Jews worldwide had joined together to poison wells, staging a medieval terrorist attack. Still others saw the conversion or murder of Jews as essential to the cleansing of the world in anticipation of the coming of Christ at the apocalypse. In 1349 citizens of several European cities attacked Jewish communities in spite of Pope Clement's (1291–1352) efforts to prevent such killing. These activities were short-lived, however, as people soon saw that the Black Death appeared to kill entirely at random, making it impossible to identify a particular community of people, let alone a specific water source, as its origin. More troubling was that the disease killed saints as well as sinners and the very young as well as the very old. Late medieval Christians expressed again and again their difficulty in thinking about the infants, virgins, monks, and nuns struck down by plague. Surely, they reasoned, these people were not all sinners. This led some to conclude that God chose to end the lives of such devout individuals because he was sparing them from life in a corrupt world.

Many late medieval Christians sought urgently for answers and finally found the church ineffective. It is not surprising that some began to turn to other sources of spiritual and physical aid. Scholars debate the degree to which the Black Death was the primary cause of the anti-clerical movement in Europe, but all agree that it contributed to it. With bodies in pain, social structures in disarray, and the church unable to provide safety—even for its most devout or innocent members—late medieval Christian communities struggled to manage plague-time chaos on all levels and to make sense of their lives in the aftermath. *See also* Biblical Plagues; Black Death, Economic and Demographic Effects of; Black Death, Flagellants, and Jews; Black Death: Literature and Art; Bubonic Plague; Pilgrimage and Epidemic Disease; Plague in Medieval Europe, 1360–1500; Plague Memorials; Plague of Justinian, First Pandemic; Poison Libels and Epidemic Disease; Religion and Epidemic Disease; Scapegoats and Epidemic Disease.

Further Reading

Byrne, Joseph P. *Daily Life during the Black Death*. Westport, CT: Greenwood Press, 2006.

Dohar, William J. *The Black Death and Pastoral Leadership: The Diocese of Hereford in the Fourteenth Century*. Philadelphia: University of Pennsylvania Press, 1995.

Horrox, Rosemary, ed. *The Black Death*. New York: Manchester University Press, 1994.

Zeigler, Philip. *The Black Death*. New York: Harper and Row, 1969.

REBECCA TOTARO

BLACK DEATH, ECONOMIC AND DEMOGRAPHIC EFFECTS OF. The **Black Death pandemic** of 1347 to 1352 had devastating results for the population of Europe, and it led to many dramatic changes within European societies and economies. Though scholars disagree over matters of degree, the general trends are broadly accepted: one-third to one-half of Europeans died; a good deal of wealth and property changed hands through inheritance; most of those who died in major cities were replaced rather quickly by migration from the countryside; wages dropped and prices rose; and both local and national laws sought to dampen what authorities saw as negative effects of the population disaster.

One problem with establishing exact figures for medieval population loss is that there are few reliable demographic statistics. One of the best-documented regions is England. A poll tax was collected in 1377, which was essentially a census of English citizens in order to establish and collect a head tax. A previous census had been taken in 1086, and this census allows historians to estimate the toll that the plague took on at least the English population. Another source for population figures is church burial records, but these were neither universally maintained nor accurate throughout Europe, nor have they survived in large numbers. Even so, most historians agree that the population of Europe fell by at least one-third in the initial outbreaks of 1347–1352; perhaps as many as 70 to 80 percent of some regions (particularly cities and towns in Italy and England) were lost in that and subsequent outbreaks in the late fourteenth century. Contemporary poets and chroniclers, some of whom did not survive the plague, describe losses of 90 percent of their towns' populations, although many of these accounts may be exaggerations. Italy may have had the highest losses, because of high population density and because it was the first region in Europe to be hit; Eastern Europe, the most sparsely populated and the last to be struck, may have had the lowest.

Some populations were devastated more thoroughly than others. Populations of cities, which were densely packed and thus more susceptible to contagion, seem to have had higher mortality rates than rural areas, but even this was not consistent: villagers, too, died in appalling numbers. Clergy had higher mortality rates than lay people because they had more contact with plague victims when they delivered last rites and other sacraments. Because priests had such a high mortality rate, the Church was particularly devastated. New priests were quickly ordained in the decades following 1347; as a result, most were not fully trained and entered their new profession unprepared. This led to a gradual decrease in respect for clergy.

The plague seemed to strike the young most of all, especially during later outbreaks, an impression noted by many contemporaries. Those who survived the initial outbreak were apparently more likely to survive subsequent outbreaks and grow older (though exposure to plague is not known to confer immunity). This meant that the demographic state of Europe was drastically altered by the Black Death; by the early 1400s, many towns had more elderly than young; adults in their twenties and thirties were rather few in number. The sheer number of people who died meant that the economics of Europe also changed. Craftsmen and skilled laborers died of plague, and, in order to replace them, craft guilds began to recruit and approve underage members. Guilds, like society as a whole, had to replace deceased members and train new ones quickly. Plague losses also meant that guilds, and towns in general, were willing to accept strangers and people from outside the guild and town boundaries, which they had been reluctant to do before the Black Death. The plague increased the mobility of labor in Europe. In fact, some older theories held that the plague was a correction to overpopulation—prior to the Black Death, Europe's population had exceeded its resources, and it therefore suffered the resulting **Malthusian** check—a position no longer tenable.

Fewer students enrolled at universities; Oxford, the University of Paris, and Bologna all had reduced numbers for decades after the Black Death, perhaps because there was simply no superfluous population not needed for labor. There was also a reduction in the charitable economy of Europe, on which schools (including universities), hospitals, and churches depended. New universities were created; they were smaller, local institutions that did not require travel by the main roads, which were increasingly dangerous. This, too, was a result of the plague: an increase in violence and lack of order as a result of desperation and loss of civil stability.

The Black Death may have also diversified the economic culture of Europe, although there is some dispute among historians regarding exactly what changes occurred. Prices for basic commodities, especially grains and foodstuffs, immediately rose after the plague. This was partially the result of the reduction in labor; fewer people were available to work fields or mills for grinding grain. The decline in the supply of labor allowed for the surviving laborers to charge higher prices for their service or goods, at least immediately after the first outbreak. Wages also went up, whereas rents and other demands by those who hired laborers often went down. Rising inflation of prices and wages, together with lower rents, very quickly led rulers and governments to attempt to limit prices and wages. These laws, such as the Statute of Labourers in England in 1351, were only partially successful; commodities prices went down, wages were forced artificially low (set by law at pre-plague levels), but the laws also stirred up civil discontent which eventually led to rebellions, such as the Peasants' Revolt in 1381. *See also* Black Death and Late Medieval Christianity; Black Death, Flagellants, and Jews; Black Death: Literature and Art; Plague in Medieval Europe, 1360–1500; Plague in the Islamic World, 1360–1500.

Further Reading

Aberth, John, ed. *The Black Death: The Great Mortality of 1348–1350: A Brief History with Documents.* New York: St. Martins, 2005.

Bolton, James L. "The World Upside Down: Plague as an Agent of Economic and Social Change." In *The Black Death in England,* edited by W. M. Ormrod and P. G. Lindley, pp. 17–77. Stamford: Paul Watkins, 1996.

Byrne, Joseph P. *The Black Death.* Westport, CT: Greenwood, 2004.

———. *Daily Life during the Black Death.* Westport, CT: Greenwood, 2006.

Herlihy, David. *The Black Death and the Transformation of the West.* Cambridge, MA: Harvard University Press, 1997.

Horrox, Rosemary, ed. *The Black Death.* New York: Manchester University Press, 1994.

Platt, Colin. *King Death: The Black Death and Its Aftermath in Late-Medieval England.* Toronto: University of Toronto Press, 1997.

CANDACE GREGORY-ABBOTT

BLACK DEATH, FLAGELLANTS, AND JEWS. The first outbreak of the **Black Death** across Europe and the Mediterranean world in 1347–1352 disrupted the social world of European Christians, creating chaos and widespread fear across the continent. Whereas some blamed Jews for creating and spreading plague, others concluded that the plague was in fact an instance of divine judgment for their sins and those of their communities. Among the cultural legacies of the plague were the emergence of specific forms of lay religious organizations and the increased persecution of Jews, frequently by members of these organizations and by itinerant preachers.

The enormous casualties caused by the plague led many to conclude that divine judgment had fallen upon Europe for its sins, and some such individuals believed that the end of the world was upon them. Church doctrine taught that self-punishment and renunciation of pleasure could assuage the wrath of God, which was made manifest in the plague. In Germany, many laymen organized themselves into wandering bands of flagellants who practiced extreme asceticism: punishing their bodies as penance for sin by flogging themselves with multi-tailed whips called *flagella*. These organizations of penitents sought to cool God's anger and stave off further punishment, or at least to prepare themselves for the return of Christ, by renouncing worldly goods and punishing their bodies. Flagellation had been practiced for centuries as a form of extreme asceticism, but it had been largely confined to reformist orders of monks whipping themselves in their monasteries. The first known disciplinary confraternity (pious lay brotherhood) began around 1260 in central Italy. During the fervor caused by the plague, however, the number of flagellants spiked sharply as many confraternities adopted the practice, particularly in German states and the Low Countries.

The flagellants were groups of men from the general population who traveled in fairly large groups, singing penitential hymns, venerating a holy relic, and beating

POPE CLEMENT VI CONDEMNS THE PERSECUTION OF JEWS DURING THE BLACK DEATH (1348)

Recently, however, it has been brought to our attention by public fame—or, more accurately, infamy—that numerous Christians are blaming the plague with which God, provoked by their sins, has afflicted the Christian people, on poisonings carried out by the Jews at the instigation of the devil, and that out of their own hot-headedness they have impiously slain many Jews, making no exception for age or sex; and that Jews have been falsely accused of such outrageous behavior so that they could be legitimately put on trial before appropriate judges—which has done nothing to cool the rage of the Christians but has rather inflamed them even more. While such behavior goes unopposed it looks as though their error is approved.

Were the Jews, by any chance, to be guilty or cognizant of such enormities a sufficient punishment could scarcely be conceived; yet we should be forced to accept the force of the argument that it cannot be true that the Jews, by such a heinous crime, are the cause or occasion of the plague, because throughout many parts of the world the same plague, by the hidden judgment of God, has afflicted and afflicts the Jews themselves and many other races who have never lived alongside them.

We order you by apostolic writing that each of you, upon whom this charge has been laid, should straightly command those subject to you, both clerical and lay, when they are assembled in worship at mass, not to dare (on their own authority or out of hot-headedness) to capture, strike, wound or kill any Jews or expel them from their service on these grounds; and you should demand obedience under pain of excommunication.

Papal order to the Catholic clergy of September 26, 1348; from *The Apostolic See and the Jews*, vol. I, *Documents: 492–1404*, edited by S. Simonsohn (Toronto: Pontifical Institute of Medieval Studies, 1988), Doc. #373.

themselves bloody. When they arrived near a city and set up camp, they read a letter detailing a message from Christ or an angelic messenger validating their ascetic practices and exhorted everyone to repentance. Much of their preaching stirred audiences to prepare for the imminent apocalypse. Major condemnations of the flagellants began in 1349 with that of Pope Clement VI (r. 1342–1352) and other bishops and lay leaders who distrusted the self-led and very charismatic groups. Flagellant influence diminished by the late 1300s, as the church increased its censure of their more heretical teachings, and continued into the next century when large numbers were burned at the stake as heretics. Penitential confraternities based in parishes, operating in secret, and directed by clergy practiced flagellation past the sixteenth century. They were less associated with apocalyptic concerns and more with the everyday life of repentance and renunciation.

Many European Christians in the fourteenth century, and some modern scholars, believed that Jews suffered less from the plague than the Christian population, though this view has come under much academic scrutiny of late. Jewish ghettoes often had **water** supplies apart from the Christians and drank from their own wells. This raised concerns among many Christians who believed the plague was a waterborne poison planted by Jews (**poison libel**). These accusations caused sporadic but brutal attacks on Jewish individuals and communities. Itinerant preachers—particularly Franciscan friars—along with flagellants, and sometimes local clergy, preached against Jews on many occasions. Frequently, they claimed that the presence of unbelieving Jews in Christian communities was the cause (or at least, one cause) of God's judgment in the form of the plague. Older anti-Semitic accusations, such as the blood libel (the claim that Jews murdered Christian children on Passover) persisted, but most of the furor directed against Jews stemmed from the poison libel. On the shores of Lake Geneva many Jews were harassed, and some were killed because of these accusations. In February 1349, angry townspeople attacked the Jewish community in Strasbourg despite the efforts of local authorities; uncontrollable mobs burned to death many Jews in Alsace and exiled many more. In Avignon, however, the Jewish community was sheltered by papal command; Pope Clement VI, along with civil authorities from the Alps to the Elbe, condemned the disorder and random violence that pogroms caused. Even so, over the following year throughout the Rhineland, Jews were frequently drowned or burned. The poison libel moved northeast through Germany before reaching certain parts of Poland and the Baltic States. Violence against Jews by civil authorities was rarer, often involving the prosecution and execution of one or a few Jews for well poisoning. Some evidence suggests that communities targeted Jews who acted as moneylenders, to kill their creditors and escape paying their debts. Though incidents occurred in many regions throughout Europe, mob violence against Jews often clustered in specific regions, such as the Rhine valley.

The persecution of Jews triggered by the Black Death led to expulsions of Jews from some communities and the enlargement of Italian ghettoes as many Jews fled to Venice and Rome. The worst of the persecutions subsided by 1350, thanks at least in part to an assertion of political authority. Traveling groups of mendicants commanded respect for a long time afterward, often provoking public hostility against Jews, sometimes bullying the public into persecution of them. The plague had cleaved Jews away from some communities that had previously not quarreled with them. In consequence, the high medieval tolerance of Jews diminished even more quickly than it had before the plague.

The flagellants and various forms of violence against Jews were symptoms of the fear and chaos caused by plague outbreaks. Attempts by civil and ecclesiastical authorities to quell both problems culminated in Pope Clement VI's joint condemnation of the flagellants and the violence against Jews. These efforts were not very successful. Although the itinerant flagellant movement did fade away, persecutions of Jews associated with plague outbreaks continued into the sixteenth century. *See also* Bubonic Plague; Plague in Medieval Europe, 1360–1500; Religion and Epidemic Disease; Scapegoats and Epidemic Disease.

Further Reading

Byrne, Joseph. *The Black Death*. Westport, CT: Greenwood, 2004.

Cohn, Norman. *The Pursuit of the Millennium*. New York: Pimlico, 1993.

Herlihy, David. *The Black Death and the Transformation of the West*. Cambridge, MA: Harvard University Press, 1997.

Horrox, Rosemary, ed. *The Black Death*. New York: Manchester University Press, 1994.

Kieckhefer, R. "Radical Tendencies in the Flagellant Movement of the Mid-Fourteenth Century." *Journal of Medieval and Renaissance Studies* 4 (1974): 157–176.

Nohl, Johannes, and C. H. Clarke. *A Chronicle of the Black Death*. Yardley, PA: Westholme Publishing, 2006.

Ziegler, Philip. *The Black Death*. New York: Harper and Row, 1969.

DENNIS GREGORY CARAMENICO

BLACK DEATH: LITERATURE AND ART.   Devastation of the scale wrought by the **Black Death** produced wide-ranging cultural changes and reactions. Some of these caused pre-plague literary and artistic genres to focus on the plague and prompted the development of new plague-specific themes. The year 1347 marks the initial outbreak of the plague, which makes it the focus of the first literary reactions to the Black Death, and

1562 was the year in which the Flemish artist Pieter Brueghel the Elder (c. 1525–1569) painted his horrifying plague masterpiece, *The Triumph of Death*. These years bracket this article. The seeds of Brueghel's terrifying artistic vision, however, were planted in "popular" literature produced when the plague first appeared in 1347.

Italian poet Giovanni Boccaccio's (c. 1313–1375) introduction to the *Decameron* (c. 1351) is a famous example of "popular" plague literature. In 1348, Boccaccio informs his readers, the streets of once-beautiful Florence were covered with plague victims' corpses. All who were able either fled the city for a safer refuge in the country or locked themselves in their homes to escape the plague. Boccaccio mentions that the plague struck the Near East with a ferocity equal to that with which it hit western Europe. The *Report on the Pestilence* (1348), by Boccaccio's Syrian Muslim contemporary Abu Hafs Umar ibn al-Wardi (d. 1349), is written as a prayer to Allah, but it shares with Boccaccio's *Decameron* a keen eye for detail which allows the reader to understand just how terrible the plague was wherever it struck. Poetry by Boccaccio's friend Francesco Petrarch (1304–1374) (especially *Ad te ipsum*) painfully and intimately details the devastation caused by the plague. In England, poet Geoffrey Chaucer's (1343–1400) bawdy *Canterbury Tales* (c. 1387–1400), based largely upon Boccaccio's *Decameron*, contains important references to the Black Death.

The medical *consilia*, or physicians' advice pamphlets, existed before the era of plague, but the advent of Black Death prompted *consilia* authors to focus almost solely on the plague. The first and most often copied was that by the medical faculty at the University of Paris. These "plague tracts" contain an interesting blend of classical allusions, Christian and Muslim traditions, common sense strategies, and outrageous recipes to cure and avoid the Black Death. For example, plague tracts advise readers to close all of the doors and windows of one's home and then burn noxious herbs in an attempt to keep out "corrupted **air**." Thus, if one could avoid "bad air," and those stricken with the plague, one might be able to survive an outbreak.

Nearly everywhere the plague struck, local plague-tract genres developed. Fourteenth-century Spanish physicians such as Alfonso de Cordoba, and French and Moorish doctors such as Pierre de Damouzy and Abi Gafar Ahmed ibn Ali ibn Khatimah, contributed to the plague-tract genre. Each sought to provide remedies and treatments for the Black Death in his locale.

The obsession with plague found in some "popular" and most medical literature is mirrored in the emerging genres of "plague art," but the development of plague art is more hotly debated. Following the lead of scholar Millard Meiss (1904–1975), some art historians argue that Italian art appeared to "revert" to medieval themes of death and judgment because the plague radically changed the Italian and European artistic consciousness. Undoubtedly, the plague affected European art by killing nearly an entire generation of artists and their private and civic patrons, but the post-plague "reversion" to medieval themes was also the result of the influence of the Church. As the greatest patron of the arts, the Church had long used a fairly uniform iconography of the Last Judgment and Death to prompt repentance. With the advent of the Black Death in 1347, pre-plague themes such as the *Danse Macabre* quickly transitioned into symbols of the Black Death. With its writhing skeletons dancing arm-in-arm with soon-to-be-dead men, women, and children, the "Dance of Death" came to represent the need for repentance in the face of death by plague. In time, the *Danse Macabre* genre was joined by other "plague art" themes.

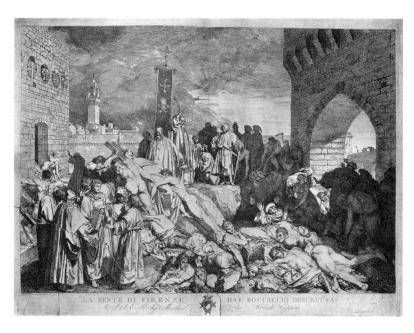

The plague of Florence in 1348, as described in Boccaccio's *Decameron*. Etching by L. Sabatelli after himself. Courtesy of Wellcome Library, London.

The *King Death* genre is an example of this type. It is "plague art" in the truest sense, developed in the post-1347 Black Death era. Paintings of *King Death* often depict a grinning skeleton—the Black Death personified—wearing a golden crown, mocking and torturing the living. *King Death* served as an effective reminder to the living that all would one day be subjects of his corpse-realm. Still other types of plague art depicted Death as an angel or demon, or even as God hurling plague-tainted arrows at unsuspecting mortals. Saints like Mary, Sebastian, and Roche (Rocco) became popular heavenly intercessors on behalf of mankind, as witnessed by hundreds of paintings and sculptures. Through plague art, the Church urged its adherents, faced with certain and perhaps untimely death, to repent before they too succumbed to God's wrath, the plague. However, repentance did not guarantee physical protection from the Black Death, and funeral paintings of plague victims show this. Early examples depict full funeral processions with priests presiding over individual funerals, whereas only slightly later scenes show bodies, priest and layperson alike, in makeshift coffins, being dumped unceremoniously into mass graves.

By 1562, the year in which Pieter Brueghel painted his masterpiece, *The Triumph of Death*, religious influence had waned and the promise of redemption had come to seem hollow. As skeletons romped over a wasteland strewn with corpses, living human beings failed to fend off random sword slashes, bony hands, and hangmen's gallows. Brueghel's vision of life is bleak, but it certainly serves to remind the viewer, following the earlier *Danse Macabre* and *King Death* traditions, that death "comes to us all." *See also* Black Death and Late Medieval Christianity; Black Death, Economic and Demographic Effects of; Plague in Medieval Europe, 1360–1500; Plague Literature and Art, Early Modern; Plague Memorials.

Further Reading

Boeckl, Christine. *Images of Plague and Pestilence: Iconography and Iconology*. Kirksville, MO: Truman State University Press, 2000.

Byrne, Joseph P. *The Black Death*. Westport, CT: Greenwood, 2004.

Grigsby, Bryon Lee. *Pestilence in Medieval and Early Modern English Literature*. New York: Routledge, 2004.

Horrox, Rosemary, ed. *The Black Death*. New York: Manchester University Press, 1994.

Lindley, Phillip. "The Black Death and English Art: A Debate and Some Assumptions." In *The Black Death in England*, edited by W. M. Ormond and P. G. Lindley, pp. 125–146. Stamford, UK: Paul Watkins, 1996.

Marshall, Louise J. "Manipulating the Sacred: Image and Plague in Renaissance Florence Italy." *Renaissance Quarterly* 47 (1994): 485–532.

Meiss, Millard. *Painting in Florence and Siena after the Black Death: The Arts, Religion, and Society in the Mid-Fourteenth Century*. Princeton: Princeton University Press, 1951.

WILLIAM LANDON

BLACK DEATH: MODERN MEDICAL DEBATE. Since the early twentieth century, the historical **Black Death** has been identified as the flea- and rat-borne bacterial **bubonic plague**. Specialists from several different academic fields, however, began challenging this diagnosis of the Black Death in the latter years of the century. These revisionists argue that the features of the Black Death that resemble modern bubonic plague are misleading and that the medieval environment and the behavior of the pestilence suggest a different disease altogether.

Bubonic plague is a disease of rodents, and the black rat (*Rattus rattus*) is deemed the most likely culprit of medieval epidemics, passing on the *Yersinia pestis* **bacteria** to humans through their fleas, who abandon the dead and dying rats. It is assumed, therefore, that the medieval world had the abundance of black rats needed to sustain the epidemics of the second pandemic (1347–1770) and that they were dying in droves immediately preceding human outbreaks. Historical sources from the fourteenth century, however, make little or no mention of the black rat's presence during times of plague. This issue has been thoroughly explored by several authorities, notably contemporary British medical historian J. F. D. Shrewsbury, who has concluded that because of the absence of evidence of rats in medieval Britain and the cold climatic conditions of northern Europe that suit neither rats nor their fleas, their populations must have been insignificant. He reasoned, therefore, that the Black Death, if it had been bubonic plague, could not have been particularly severe and that other diseases like **typhus** were acting in concert. More recently, British zoologist Graham Twigg took a similar tack, noting the lack of literary and archaeological evidence for the medieval black rat and suggesting anthrax as the cause of the Black Death. He emphasized historical descriptions of the disease spreading by touch or by contact with victims' possessions, the existence of rash-like symptoms, and the deaths of diseased animals. He also proposed the late medieval textile industry as a possible means of dissemination because human anthrax cases are commonly associated with contaminated animal products.

Proponents of bubonic plague respond that anthrax has never caused widespread **epidemics** and that medieval populations did not record the activity of rats or other vermin at any time. Others argue that the disease was not dependent upon the presence of sufficient rat populations or a climate hospitable for their fleas because bubonic plague could have been spreading from person to person via the human flea *Pulex irritans* or by the contagious variant **pneumonic plague**. Although several historical sources do mention that the disease manifested in different forms, including a more deadly type of lung infection that suggests pneumonic plague, these counter-theories remain questionable because the human flea is generally considered an unreliable vector and because pneumonic plague cases rarely occur outside a substantial bubonic epidemic.

The strongest evidence supporting the identification of Black Death as bubonic plague is the long list of references to the symptomatic buboes (lymphatic swellings). As contemporary historian Samuel Cohn argues, however, these references constitute only a minute percentage of the historical descriptions of the Black Death; myriad other symptoms also occurred. In addition, the bubo is not specific to bubonic plague; it also appears with numerous other infectious diseases.

Whereas the medieval pestilence took only five years to travel to almost every corner of Europe and the Middle East, modern bubonic plague took as long as forty years to spread outside of China during the **third pandemic** of the nineteenth century. This suggests the Black Death had a means of transmission much faster than the period needed for bubonic plague to spread among rat populations before being passed to humans. This is supported by numerous historical descriptions of the Black Death that attest to its almost instantaneous contagion. Additionally, whereas deaths caused by modern bubonic plague number around 13 million since the inception of the third pandemic a century ago, conservative estimates of the mortality inflicted by the Black Death suggest as much as 40 to 50 percent of the total population of Europe and the Middle East over five years. Problems of identification also stem from the nature of the historical data. For example, the extent of the mortality caused by the disease is still questioned because the population size of medieval Europe and the Middle East is unknown.

Revisionists such as British scientists Susan Scott and Christopher Duncan (d. 2005) have studied available mortality data (including wills, testaments, and burial records) from early modern plagues and suggest that the behavior of the Black Death more closely resembles that of a **virus**. They propose a hemorrhagic disease, similar to **Ebola**, as the possible cause.

Despite apparent differences between medieval and modern plague, bubonic plague is still commonly accepted as the cause of both. Recently, medieval skeletal remains of suspected pestilence victims from French burial grounds have tested positive for plague bacteria (*Y. pestis*) DNA. While this evidence has not been corroborated with data from other plague burial grounds, it seems to confirm the presence of the disease during the late medieval period. Medieval bubonic plague may have been a more virulent strain than the modern version, and the pathogen may have mutated into a more benign form, which would explain the apparent differences in speed, contagion, and mortality. The Black Death could possibly have been caused by marmot (a type of ground squirrel and common carrier of *Y. pestis*) plague—the only form of rodent plague known to be directly contagious—spreading to humans. *See also* Diagnosis of Historical Diseases; Historical Epidemiology; Insects, Other Arthropods, and Epidemic Disease; Plague: End of the Second Pandemic; Plague in Medieval Europe, 1360–1500.

Further Reading

Christakos, George, et al. *Interdisciplinary Public Health Reasoning and Epidemic Modelling: The Case of Black Death.* Heidelberg: Springer, 2005.

Cohn, Samuel K. *The Black Death Transformed: Disease and Culture in Early Renaissance Europe.* London: Arnold Publishing, 2002.

Drancourt, Michel, and Didier Raoult. "Molecular Insights into the History of Plague." *Microbes and Infection* 4 (2002): 105–109.

Gilbert, M. T., et al. "Absence of *Yersinia pestis*-Specific DNA in Human Teeth from Five European Excavations of Putative Plague Victims." *Microbiology* 150 (2004): 341–354.

Martin, A. L. *Plague? Jesuit Accounts of Epidemic Disease in the Sixteenth Century.* Kirksville, MO: Sixteenth Century Studies, 1996.

Scott, Susan, and Christopher J. Duncan. *Return of the Black Death.* Chichester, UK: John Wiley & Sons Ltd., 2004.

Shrewsbury, J. F. *History of Bubonic Plague in the British Isles.* New York: Cambridge University Press, 1970.

Twigg, Graham. *The Black Death: A Biological Reappraisal.* New York: Schocken Books, 1985.

KARL BIRKELBACH

BUBONIC PLAGUE.   Bubonic plague and its variants have killed millions of people in three devastating **pandemics**—including the **Black Death**—and countless regional **epidemics**, causing major social upheavals. The very work "plague" retains the power to terrorize people. Plague has inspired writers such as Giovanni Boccaccio (1313–1375; *The Decameron*), Daniel Defoe (c. 1660–1731; *A Journal of the Plague Year*), and Albert Camus (1913–1960; *La Peste*). Although **antibiotics** and public health measures have limited major epidemics, the threat of **bioterrorism** has brought plague back into the news.

Yersinia pestis is a rod-shaped **bacterium** classified as Gram-negative because it does not take up the purple dye of the classic Gram stain. With Wright, Giemsa, and other special stains, dye clumps at the poles, giving a "safety-pin" appearance. Working independently in Hong Kong, **Shibasaburo Kitasato**, a Japanese microbiologist who had worked with **Robert Koch** in Germany, and **Alexandre Yersin**, a Swiss microbiologist from the Pasteur Institute, identified the bacterium responsible for bubonic plague in 1894. Originally named *Pasturella pestis*, for **Louis Pasteur**, the bacterium was renamed in 1971 in honor of Yersin.

Infection with *Y. pestis* causes three symptom complexes, with incubation periods ranging from one to six days. Classic bubonic plague is characterized by swollen, intensely painful lymph glands or buboes (Latin for "groin swelling") in the groin, axilla, or neck, accompanied by fever, chills, and headache. The infection may spread quickly into the bloodstream; release of inflammatory toxins leads to circulatory collapse, organ failure, and death within days. Clotting defects cause purpura (bleeding into the skin), while blockage of small blood vessels leads to gangrene. Bacteria may also spread secondarily through the bloodstream into the lungs causing shortness of breath and bloody sputum. Untreated bubonic plague has a 50 percent mortality rate. It remains unclear whether survival of bubonic plague confers any lasting immunity. In primary **septicemic plague**, the bacteria invade the bloodstream directly at the site of the flea's injection of the bacteria. Primary **pneumonic plague** is transmitted from patient to patient through respiratory droplets.

Antibiotics must be started as soon as the disease is suspected based on the patient's history of exposure, results of physical examination, and evidence of plague bacilli in the blood, sputum, or fluid from buboes. Confirmatory testing by special staining techniques, growth of *Y. pestis* in cultures, or detection of plague antibodies in the blood takes several days. Efforts are under way to develop a rapid bedside screening test. The antibiotic streptomycin proved effective in the early 1950s. Today, less toxic drugs of the streptomycin class, such as gentamicin, are preferred. Tetracyclines and other classes of antibiotics are acceptable alternatives. People in close contact with infected patients or **animals**, as well as exposed laboratory personnel, are protected by prophylactic antibiotics. With prompt treatment, bubonic plague mortality is less than 10 percent.

Plague is a zoonosis, a disease transmissible from animals to humans. In 1898 experiments conducted in India and Pakistan by **Paul-Louis Simond** of the Pasteur Institute pointed to the rat flea *Xenopsylla cheopis* as a plague vector. Despite initial skepticism, further experimentation by other researchers led to general acceptance of the flea vector by about 1906. During plague epidemics, the black rat, *Rattus rattus*, is infected through the bite of the rat flea. The digestive tract of the flea becomes clogged with rat blood and bacteria. As the rat dies of plague, its fleas seek a new host. After an infected flea punctures human skin, its blocked digestive tract regurgitates thousands of plague bacilli under the skin. The bacteria enter the lymphatic channels or the bloodstream, causing bubonic or septicemic plague.

In the long intervals between epidemics, infected fleas retreat to wild rodents (sylvatic plague) which serve as reservoirs for *Y. pestis*. This enzootic cycle maintains the bacterium in nature until conditions are favorable for new epizootic and epidemic cycles. But black rats are not the only mammals that can support plague-carrying fleas: species of squirrels, prairie dogs, chipmunks, marmots, gerbils, and rats, as well as larger animals such as coyotes, rabbits, and even cats and dogs can also do so.

Historically, infected rats and their fleas traveled easily in **trade** caravans and ships' holds, and in **war** time accompanied moving armies and refugee populations. Domestic rats thrived in thatched roofs, granaries, and human refuse. Infected fleas survived for weeks in sacks of grain or woolen cloth.

The first recorded pandemic was the Plague of Justinian in the sixth century. The Black Death of the fourteenth century killed between one-quarter and one-half of Europe's population and similarly affected the Islamic world. In the 1890s pandemic, rapid steamship travel spread the plague from Chinese ports to much of the Pacific Rim, including Hawaii and the western coast of the United States.

Social Responses to Bubonic Plague. In the Middle Ages and well into the modern era, plague was seen as divine punishment for sinfulness. At various times, plague was blamed on contaminated food or water, foul **air**, witchcraft, unfavorable alignment of the planets, or climatic conditions. Minorities such as Jews were **scapegoated** for causing the plague and were exiled, persecuted, and murdered. Personal responses ranged from public displays of self-flagellation to fatalistic hedonism. Assigning blame for plague continued into modern times. During the third pandemic, heavy-handed interventions by the British colonial administration in the 1890s led some Indian citizens to suspect that the imperialists themselves were spreading plague. In San Francisco, the arrival of plague from Honolulu in 1900 created public panic. Because most of the early victims were Chinese immigrants, a harsh **quarantine** and other restrictions were quickly and irrationally imposed on all residents of Chinatown.

Early public health efforts to control plague included forced isolation of the sick and their families in locked and shuttered homes, appointment of plague **physicians**, establishment of health magistracies, enforcement of naval and land quarantines, erection of ***cordons sanitaires***, fumigation and **disinfection** measures, and forced removal to dreaded plague hospitals or **pest houses**. **Flight** from affected areas was a universal response.

The experience of **plague in San Francisco** between 1900 and 1907 reflected new developments in bacteriology, **epidemiology**, and public health. Plague, a bacterial disease that flourished in crowded, unsanitary neighborhoods, fit in well with the sanitarian belief that cleaning up filth and proper management of sewage could limit epidemics. Initial **sanitation** measures included fumigation with sulfur dioxide gas, disinfection with chloride of lime, and the burning of household refuse in the Chinese district. Residents of Chinatown understandably resisted efforts at forced **vaccination** with the plague vaccine developed in India in 1897 by Russian/Swiss microbiologist **Waldemar Haffkine**. The San Francisco epidemic caused 113 deaths over several years. Plague returned to San Francisco in 1907 during the sanitation crisis precipitated by the earthquake of 1906. The role of the rat flea was well accepted by that time, and health officials focused their efforts on destroying rats and their habitats.

Plague in Recent Times.   Between 1987 and 1998, the **World Health Organization** registered 26,000 plague cases with an overall mortality of 8 percent. Major epidemics were reported in Vietnam in the 1960s and 1970s, with limited outbreaks in the 1990s in India, Madagascar, Myanmar, and Peru. The Vietnam epidemic was linked to **environmental** and population disruptions as a result of war, underlining the close relationship between epidemic diseases and social factors.

Today, most plague cases in developed countries are sporadic rather than epidemic. In the rural western United States, infected rodents such as squirrels and prairie dogs transmit plague to rabbits and domestic animals. Ten to fifteen human plague cases are diagnosed annually in New Mexico and other western states. In the United States, all confirmed cases are reportable to the national **Centers for Disease Control and Prevention** (CDC). To protect those living in endemic areas, the CDC recommends rodent and flea control as well as public education about rodent habitats, insect repellents, safe handling of suspect animals, and indications for prompt medical attention. A vaccine offering limited protection was used in American military personnel in Vietnam and others at high risk, but was recently withdrawn. Research continues toward developing an effective plague vaccine.

Plague is a **bioterrorism** threat. During World War II, a Japanese **biological warfare** unit airdropped plague-infected fleas over China causing deadly local epidemics. Today, classic flea-borne bubonic plague is much less of a bioterrorism threat than aerosolized pneumonic plague. The United States and the Soviet Union conducted research on weaponized aerosolized pneumonic plague during the Cold War. Pneumonic plague is classified by the CDC as a Category A bioterrorism threat. The feared scenario is the introduction of aerosolized plague bacteria into a population. Although the bacilli would die within hours on exposure to sunlight, target populations infected with pneumonic plague would spread the rapidly fatal disease from person to person. Initially, doctors would logically suspect ordinary bacterial pneumonia rather than pneumonic plague, delaying mobilization of emergency public health resources. *See also* Black Death and related articles; Bubonic Plague in the United States; Historical Epidemiology; Insects, Other Arthropods, and Epidemic Disease; London, Great Plague of (1665–1666); Plague: End of the Second Pandemic; Plague in Britain (1500–1647); Plague in China; Plague in East Asia: Third Pandemic; Plague in Europe (1500–1770s); Plague in India and Oceania: Third Pandemic; Plague in Medieval Europe, 1360–1500; Plague in the Islamic World, 1360–1500; Plague in the Islamic World, 1500–1850; Plague of Justinian, First Pandemic; Public Health Agencies, U.S. Federal.

Further Reading

British Broadcasting Service. http://www.bbc.co.uk/radio4/history/voices/voices_salisbury.shtml

Centers for Disease Control and Prevention. *Plague.* http://www.cdc.gov/ncidod/dvbid/plague/index.htm

Cunha, Cheston B., and Burke A. Cunha. "Impact of Plague on Human History." *Infectious Disease Clinics of North America* 20 (2006): 253–272.

Dennis D. T., K. L. Gage, N. Gratz, et al. *Plague Manual: Epidemiology, Distribution, Surveillance and Control*. Geneva: World Health Organization, 1999.

Emmeluth, Donald. *Plague*. Philadelphia: Chelsea House, 2005.

Gregg, Charles T. *Plague: An Ancient Disease in the Twentieth Century*. Albuquerque: University of New Mexico Press, 1985.

Hirst, L. F. *The Conquest of Plague: A Study of the Evolution of Epidemiology*. Oxford: Oxford University Press, 1953.

Marriott, Edward. *Plague: A Story of Science, Rivalry, Scientific Breakthrough and the Scourge That Won't Go Away*. New York: Holt, 2002.

Orent, Wendy. *Plague: The Mysterious Past and Terrifying Future of the World's Most Dangerous Disease*. New York: Free Press, 2004.

Public Broadcasting Service. http://www.pbs.org/wnet/secrets/case_plague/

Scott, Susan, and Christopher Duncan. *Biology of Plagues: Evidence from Historical Populations*. New York: Cambridge University Press, 2001.

World Health Organization. *Plague*. http://www.who.int/csr/disease/plague/en/

SANDRA W. MOSS

BUBONIC PLAGUE IN THE UNITED STATES. Although the plague caused by the **bacterium** *Yesinia pestis*, and normally spread by rodent fleas within rodent populations, may have entered Latin America during the first century of contact with Europe, there were no signs of plague in the United States or Canada until the **third plague pandemic** at the end of the nineteenth century. It arrived at U.S. ports with shipborne rats and, predictably, sparked small **epidemics** along the West Coast. After a quarter of a century, researchers noted that the disease had established itself widely among local rodent populations in 14 western states. Human encroachment on this wide reservoir has accounted for most American plague cases since 1925.

Research into the *Y. pestis* genome has demonstrated that all plague found in the United States is of the Orientalis biovar and was introduced in the 1890s. This process began in San Francisco in June 1899, with the arrival of the Japanese freighter *Nippon Maru*, which contained stowaways and plague-infected rats. This was about four years into the third pandemic, which saw the dissemination of plague by steamship from East and Southeast Asia. It was also subsequent to the discoveries of the bacterial cause of plague, and its flea and rodent vectors. San Francisco's first victim was a Chinese man living in the squalor of Chinatown; he died on March 6, 1900. Officials erected a *cordon sanitaire* around the neighborhood's 12 blocks, while its Asian-American inhabitants did their best to hide further plague fatalities, and the press mocked public health efforts. On May 19 the presence of **bubonic plague** was officially admitted, and a wave of racist anti-Asian discrimination resulted. State and civic officials clashed, federal researchers investigated, and some called for the eradication of Chinatown itself. On April 8, 1901, the cleanup of Chinatown began, as **disinfectants** and fumigants flowed and some 14,000 rooms were cleansed. In the end, there were 121 reported cases in the city and 5 elsewhere, with 122 fatalities: a very high mortality rate of 97 percent.

Plague scares also struck New York City and Washington State's Puget Sound region in 1899 and 1900. The British ship *J. W. Taylor* had departed plague-struck Brazil and had lost its steward to plague, but docked in New York's harbor and underwent **quarantine** without incident. The Japanese *Nanyo Maru* was halted and quarantined at Port Townsend, Washington, as three on board had died of plague. In the fall of 1900 Seattle suffered three deaths of suspected plague, though only one was confirmed. Watchfulness and luck served American ports well.

The San Francisco Earthquake of April 18, 1906, reduced much of the city to rubble and set the scene for a second Bay Area epidemic. Infected and virgin populations of rats mixed, and stores of food aid lay carelessly about in the refugee-camp conditions about the Bay. On May 26 the first plague death was confirmed, but cases picked up only a year later, reaching epidemic levels in August 1907. By late in the year investigators found that 1.4 percent of captured rats had plague—a very high percentage—and reported cases rose to 190, with 96 fatalities. In February 1908 civic response was mobilized as incoming ships were fumigated and a plague hospital established. Incidence dropped, and by March 1909 the epidemic—America's worst—had ended. Of 205 known cases, 103 died. Second-year medical student Charles B. Hare took a sample of the bacteria back to his laboratory in Ann Arbor, Michigan, and accidentally contracted a case of **pneumonic plague** from a self-rolled, contaminated cigarette: the first American lab-acquired case of plague. He sustained heart damage but recovered, dying at age 50.

In 1908 the first domestic rodent with plague, a squirrel, was trapped in California. This set off a decade-long campaign during which 700,000 California squirrels were destroyed. Meanwhile plague had struck Cuba, and America's Gulf Coast began surveillance for plague. Investigators found plague-infected rats around New Orleans's docks beginning in 1912, and in June 1914 a man died of what could have been plague. This was quickly followed by 30 cases, with 10 deaths. Businesses, the press, and civic officials cooperated, and rat-trappers received a bonus for diseased rats. The diligence paid off and only a single case appeared in 1915, and another in 1916.

America's worst outbreak of pneumonic plague developed among Mexican nationals living in a Los Angeles neighborhood in 1924. In October 30 cases occurred among members of a family and boarders at their home. By month's end 11 were dead and 16 were dying. On November 2 civic authorities placed a cordon around the neighborhood, severely limiting contacts. Though more cases developed, the spread was contained. By its end, the epidemic had produced 33 cases of pneumonic plague, with 31 fatalities, and 8 cases of bubonic plague with 5 deaths.

Over the next quarter-century only 27 cases of plague were reported in the United States, with 14 fatalities. Sylvatic, or wild, rodents far from the West Coast became the most common vectors, whereas deaths from rat-borne fleabites became virtually unknown. A typical case was an Oregon sheepherder who contracted plague from a squirrel that lived with squirrels among whom plague was enzootic. Such geographically isolated cases were hard to treat, but they greatly reduced the likelihood of plague epidemics. Although the period saw the implantation of plague further and further eastward, it also saw the development of **Haffkine's** vaccine, **sulfa drugs** and later **antibiotics**, and effective **pesticides**. By the latter part of the 1950s, four Southwestern states—Arizona, Colorado, New Mexico, and Utah—accounted for most cases of plague in the United States, and until 1965 only two or three cases erupted during most years. An intertribal gathering of Navajo Indians at Gallup, New Mexico, became the focal point of a plague outbreak vectored by infected prairie dogs. Eight—possibly ten—cases occurred, but only one fatality was suffered, testimony to swift action on the part of public health officials.

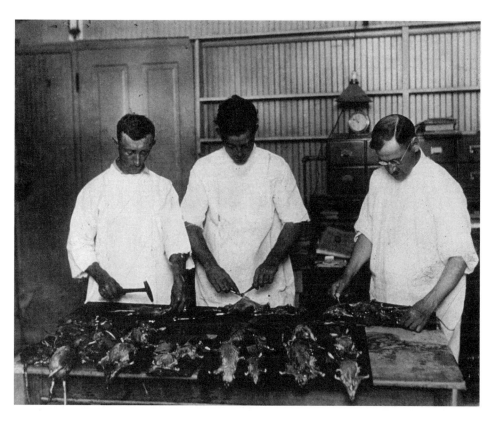

Examination in New Orleans of rats suspected of carrying bubonic plague in 1914. Courtesy of the National Library of Medicine.

From the mid-1960s the number of observed epizootics among wild rodents increased, as did the number of human cases. Growth in tourist traffic and **urbanization** in the Southwest would seem to account for much of this activity, as humans more frequently encroached on increasingly extensive plague reservoirs. From 1970 to 1991 there were 295 indigenous cases of plague in the United States, with 82 percent occurring in Arizona, Colorado, and New Mexico. Ground squirrels and, increasingly, domestic cats were the typical vectors. Fatality rates were 17 percent for men and 11 percent for women. Greater public awareness—including that among EMTs and primary care **physicians**—and stepped up public health surveillance may account for the decline in cases: from 1990 to 2005 only 107 cases were reported, of which 18 were primary septicemic and 5 primary pneumonic; 78.5 percent were primary bubonic plague. Despite years of human activity, a recent study shows that almost 15 percent of the so-called "four corners" region of the Southwest remains an area of "high risk" for plague infection. *See also* Animal Diseases (Zoonoses) and Epidemic Disease; Environment, Ecology, and Epidemic Disease; Insects, Other Arthropods, and Epidemic Disease; Kitasato, Shibasaburo; Plague in East Asia: Third Pandemic; Plague in San Francisco, 1900–1908; Plague in the Contemporary World; Public Health Agencies, U.S. Federal; Race, Ethnicity, and Epidemic Disease; Simond, Paul-Louis; Trade, Travel, and Epidemic Disease; Yersin, Alexandre.

Further Reading

Chase, Marilyn. *The Barbary Plague: The Black Death in Victorian San Francisco*. New York: Random House, 2003.

Echenberg, Myron. *Plague Ports: The Global Urban Impact of Bubonic Plague, 1894–1901*. New York: New York University Press, 2007.

Gregg, Charles T. *Plague: An Ancient Disease in the Twentieth Century*, Revised edition. Albuquerque: University of New Mexico Press, 1985.

Orent, Wendy. *Plague: The Mysterious Past and Terrifying Future of the World's Most Dangerous Disease*. New York: Free Press, 2004.

JOSEPH P. BYRNE

BUBONIC PLAGUE, SECOND PANDEMIC.   *See* Black Death and related articles and Plague-related articles.

C

CAPITALISM AND EPIDEMIC DISEASE. Capitalism is an economic system in which *the means of production*—or the tools, land, materials, and ideas used to create products and services—are generally privately owned and operated for profit by individuals or groups that form a corporation. In theory, individuals and corporations work (investing, producing goods, trading, etc.) in a free market, meaning that all parties mutually agree to prices and terms of exchange with minimal coercion or laws regulating supply or pricing. In application, though, capitalism is often regulated by society, either through public processes or laws. Capitalism and **epidemic** diseases have a complex relationship, each affecting and influencing the other in a number of ways.

Epidemics Can Impede Capitalism. People are the backbone of capitalist economies, as producers, innovators, and consumers. Epidemics impede the ability of capitalist economies to function and grow by negatively affecting people. First, epidemics decrease productivity by making people unable to work. For example, in parts of Africa where **malaria** is endemic, parents often miss weeks of work each year in order to care for suffering children. In addition, malaria may hurt the cognitive development of children and prevent them from attending school, often making them less able to work in the future.

Second, human capital, or the labor, skills, knowledge, and connections people use to carry the economy forward, is decreased when adults are sickened or die from epidemics. In Botswana, for example, life expectancy has fallen from 64 years of age in 1990 to 35 years of age in 2004, primarily as a result of the high number of deaths due to **AIDS**. The actual number of adults alive and well enough to work and start businesses has fallen dramatically. Their human capital is also lost to the economy and to future generations of entrepreneurs. In such a society, there is also an increased dependency burden, or a higher proportion of elderly, children, and sick individuals for whom adults must care, which results in decreased amounts of time and energy that can be devoted to economic activities. Similarly, a family may spend most or all of its disposable income on medicine or medical care. This decreased purchasing power slows consumer spending and the economy as a whole.

Stewardship of Resources.   Capitalism impacts the trajectory of epidemics through stewardship of key resources. For example, **water** is the most common vector for epidemic diseases such as **cholera** and **schistosomiasis**. A capitalist monopoly over water provision in South Africa in 2003 raised prices to cover the cost of new pipes. Poor families that could not pay their water bill had their service shut off and turned to unsanitary rivers and gutters for drinking water. This resulted in a deadly cholera outbreak affecting thousands. The public cost of treating these scores of sick reached into the millions of dollars by the time the epidemic was controlled.

Medical Care and Capitalism.   Access to adequate medical care includes access to health-care practitioners and infrastructure such as nearby hospitals and clinics with diagnostic technology. Modern capitalist states recognize the importance of wide access to at least basic emergency care for the public good. Monitoring, isolation, and treatment of infectious diseases have been in public hands for over a century, supported by taxes on private enterprises and with the products of profit-motivated pharmaceutical firms. Historically, capitalist societies, often influenced by Judeo-Christian moral and ethical codes, have made the greatest strides in human health and longevity; have provided the widest range in health-care options; and, given the profit motive, have shared these globally. Capitalism's economic surplus has been plowed back into basic and technical education, as well as into both basic and applied research that continues to benefit the world population.

Access to health-care practitioners in low-income countries is compromised by a worldwide "brain drain" driven in part by the global capitalist economy. Thousands of health practitioners from poor countries immigrate to developed countries each year in part because of vastly higher salaries and job security. In some African countries, for example, over 90 percent of medical school graduates lack incentives to remain and go on to practice medicine in the United States or Europe. Another factor is that low income countries often lack the infrastructure necessary for **physicians** and **nurses** to put their skills to use fully and care for patients. Many of these countries suffer from political and economic systems that misallocate resources toward self-aggrandizing individuals or elites, or toward bloody factional wars.

Investment in infrastructure, such as hospitals, diagnostic equipment, ambulances, laboratories, and so on, is also influenced by capitalism. Low-income areas that have the greatest burden of epidemic disease do not represent a profitable investment of capital because the potential consumer base simply cannot afford the product and because local instability makes the risks of investment too high. Unlike many other goods and services, however, inability to afford health-care has the serious consequences of sickness, disability, or death. Some countries have attempted to overcome the problem of access by using various combinations of taxes and public and private insurance systems to pool health-care risks and costs so that care is more affordable and accessible. Unfortunately, even these systems have significant gaps in reach or quality, and in many parts of the world they simply do not exist. Capitalism and its benefits will thrive where there are clearly recognized property rights and the rule of law.

Development and Access to Treatments.   Capitalism often impacts epidemics by directing how treatments for these diseases are developed and accessed. In a capitalist economy, the central function of any company is to make a profit in the free market. **Pharmaceutical** companies research and produce treatments for diseases. Eighty percent of drugs are purchased by people in North America, Europe, and Japan—wealthy, developed areas which together account for only 19 percent of the world's population. Following this market demand, pharmaceutical companies have generally focused their efforts on developing and marketing drugs for the diseases that are most common in these countries, such as cancer and ischemic heart disease. Indeed, such advances may help people all over the world suffering from such diseases. However, common epidemic diseases in poorer, tropical regions, such as malaria, **Chagas's disease**, and leishmaniasis, have spawned little research and therefore have few, or in some cases no, treatment options. In fact, a mere 16 of 1,393 new drugs or medicines registered in the United States and Europe between 1975 and 1999 were for the treatment of diseases from which people in developing countries typically suffer.

Developing a new drug involves enormous financial investments in researchers, labs, materials, along with large-scale human studies to test safety and efficacy. These investments carry financial risk. Experiments may repeatedly fail to yield a successful drug, or a competitor may develop a better or more popular product. Companies are willing to make a risky investment because they are confident that if there is a positive result, the profits will belong solely to them. This is because international organizations such as the World Trade Organization and national government agencies such as the U.S. Patent Office protect intellectual property (such as scientific discoveries) with patents. If a company has a patent on a new drug in the United States, for example, it has the rights to all manufacture, use, and sales of that drug for 20 years. During this period the company may set any price it chooses, which sometimes prevents access to the drug for the largest number of people who would benefit. In addition, though it significantly increases development costs, pharmaceutical companies also advertise drugs widely to increase consumer demand that may allow for a higher selling price.

Although capitalist enterprises produce many life-saving drugs, by no means does capitalism ensure that these drugs reach everyone. Access to treatment and care continues to be a persistent problem in areas with the highest burden of epidemic disease. This is particularly salient in the case of drugs that control **HIV**. Pharmaceutical companies, with the help of publicly funded universities, have transformed HIV from a death sentence to a survivable disease for those able to access Highly Active Antiretroviral Treatment (HAART). However, the price of a HAART regimen (also known as a "drug cocktail") even at a special discount from one major pharmaceutical company for the 30 poorest countries in the world, or "Low Development Index" countries, is still over $1200 per person per year. In these countries 50 to 90 percent of the population lives on less than $2 per day, or a total of $600 per year. Some companies have illegally broken patents to create cheaper, generic "copycat" HAART drugs that have significantly increased access—but, some argue, they have endangered intellectual property rights. Around the world fewer than one in four of the 35 million people living with HIV who require HAART drugs receive them. The consequence for many poor people suffering from epidemic disease is that, because they are not viable consumers, their lives are simply outside the capitalist market altogether. By being priced out of the market, their diseases have also been priced out of effective prevention and treatment. *See also* AIDS in Africa; Colonialism and Epidemic Disease; Cordon Sanitaire; Diet, Nutrition, and Epidemic Disease; Geopolitics, International Relations, and Epidemic Disease; Industrialization and Epidemic Disease; Industrial Revolution; International Health Agencies and Conventions; Malaria in

Africa; Medical Ethics and Epidemic Disease; Personal Liberties and Epidemic Disease; Poliomyelitis, Campaign Against; Poverty, Wealth, and Epidemic Disease; Race, Ethnicity, and Epidemic Disease; Sanitation Movement of the Nineteenth Century; Trade, Travel, and Epidemic Disease; Vaccination and Inoculation.

Further Reading

Avorn, Jerry. *Powerful Medicines: The Benefits, Risks and Costs of Prescription Drugs*. New York: Vintage, 2005.

Kim, Jim Yong. *Dying for Growth, Global Inequality and the Health of the Poor*. Monroe, ME: Common Courage Press, 2000.

People's Health Movement. *Global Health Watch: An Alternative World Health Report*. London: Zed Books, 2005.

United Nations Development Program. *Human Development Report 2006: Beyond Scarcity: Power, Poverty and the Global Water Crisis*. New York: Palgrave McMillan, 2006.

LINDSAY BROOCKMAN AND DANIEL PALAZUELOS

CENTERS FOR DISEASE CONTROL AND PREVENTION, U.S. *See* Public Health Agencies, U.S. Federal.

CERVICAL CANCER. *See* Human Papilloma Virus and Cervical Cancer.

CHADWICK, EDWIN (1800–1890). Edwin Chadwick, the architect of the public **sanitation movement**, was born in Longsight, near Manchester, on January 24, 1800. His mother died when he was young, and his father remarried, moving the family to London. Chadwick studied law at Middle Temple in 1832 and supported himself through journalism; both occupations brought him into contact with the ravages of **poverty** in the slums, courts, fever dens, prisons, and workhouses of London. He also worked as an assistant to political philosopher Jeremy Bentham (1748–1832) from 1830 to 1832.

The **cholera epidemic** of 1831–1832 prompted a governmental inquiry, and Chadwick, who disagreed with the report, conducted an investigation into the relationship between disease and sanitation. He presented his findings in *The Sanitary Conditions of the Labouring Population of Great Britain* (1842), demonstrating the necessity of public health reform. The report, which became the leading text on sanitation in the nineteenth century, concluded that disease and life expectancy were directly related to social conditions, calculating that the average lifespan of the working class was one-third that of the gentry and professional classes. Chadwick's report raised awareness of the need for action to improve living conditions to curtail premature death and disease amongst the poor. A healthy population would work longer and harder thus requiring less relief. Remedial suggestions included a constant supply of fresh, clean water; water closets in every residence; ventilation; and a system of transporting sewage to outlying farms that would be an inexpensive source of fertilizer.

Chadwick was responsible for the formation of the first Board of Health in 1848, which established central and local governing bodies to oversee regulation. Opposition to public health reform came from **water** companies and landlords who had vested interests in preserving the current system. Chadwick's unpopular views culminated in his forced resignation in 1854 to ensure the advances he achieved would be maintained. He wrote numerous reports and pamphlets, and he continued to campaign for legislative reform in the areas of tropical hygiene, poor law, drainage and sewage systems, army sanitation, burials in urban areas, public space, child labor, water supply, education, transportation, and sanitation.

Chadwick presided over the Sanitary Institute and the Association of Sanitary Inspectors in 1878, and he was a corresponding member of the Societies of Medicine and Hygiene in Belgium, France, and Italy. His insistence on the relationship between poverty and disease and the importance of state regulation of sanitation made him a pioneer in the history of public health reform. Chadwick was knighted in 1889 by Queen Victoria. *See also* Cholera: First through Third Pandemics, 1816–1861; Environment, Ecology, and Epidemic Disease; Epidemiology, History of; Industrialization and Epidemic Disease; Public Health Agencies in Britain since 1800; Public Health Agencies in the West before 1900; Snow, John; Urbanization and Epidemic Disease; Virchow, Rudolf.

Further Reading

Brundage, Anthony. *England's Prussian Minister: Edwin Chadwick and the Politics of Government Growth, 1832–1854.* College Park, PA: The Pennsylvania State University Press, 1988.

Chadwick, Edwin. *Report on the Sanitary Conditions of the Labouring Population of Great Britain.* Edinburgh: University of Edinburgh Press, 1965.

Hamlin, Christopher. "Predisposing Causes and Public Health in Early Nineteenth-Century Medical Thought." *Social History of Medicine* 5 (1992): 43–70.

HEIDI M. RIMKE

CHAGAS'S DISEASE.   *See* Sleeping Sickness.

CHILDHOOD.   *See* Children and Childhood Epidemic Diseases.

CHILDREN AND CHILDHOOD EPIDEMIC DISEASES.   Until the 1930s, health perils were a hallmark of childhood in every area of the world. In the United States alone in 1900, 13 percent of children died before their first birthday and 18.5 percent died before their fifth birthday. Children in western Europe fared no better; the infant mortality rate in Britain was 15 percent in 1906. The medical and lay communities in both Europe and the United States viewed these deaths fatalistically, contending that children were weak by nature and thus unusually vulnerable to illness. Not until the late nineteenth century did public health officials begin to view the high rate of childhood morbidity and mortality as preventable.

The publication in 1906 of *Infant Mortality: A Social Problem* by Sir George Newman (1870–1948), a British **physician** and pioneer in public and child health, ensured that the infant mortality rate—the number of deaths before age one in a particular population per 1,000 live births—would become the international measure of societal welfare. Newman argued that because babies were wholly dependent on others for care, infant mortality represented the state of everyone's wellbeing. This use of infant mortality as a communal gauge ensured that alleviating illness and death among children would become the focus of significant interest and investment in all societies.

Special attention to diseases affecting children was, and remains, necessary. Children have always been more susceptible to certain diseases than adults, by virtue of their lack of immunological experience, their anatomy, and their vulnerability in inhospitable **environments**. The traditional childhood diseases—which include **measles**, mumps, rubella (German measles), varicella (chicken pox), and **diphtheria**—confer lifelong **immunity** and thus, once experienced, cannot be contracted as an adult. Prior to the mid-1960s, when inoculating infants and children against these diseases became routine in most countries, the traditional childhood illnesses were so endemic (and occasionally **epidemic**) that most people had contracted them before age 15.

Of the infectious diseases now prevented by **vaccination**, diphtheria and pertussis (**whooping cough**) were the most deadly, each killing many hundreds of children annually in every large American and European city. In 1890 in New York City alone, diphtheria caused almost 2,000 deaths, mostly of children under the age of five; in some areas of the world between 45 and 55 percent of children who contracted diphtheria died of the disease. In England and Wales as recently as 1937, diphtheria was second only to pneumonia as a cause of death in childhood, killing 32 per 100,000 children under the age of 15. Campaigns to inoculate children against diphtheria were highly successful; by 1930 in New York City hundreds of thousands of children had been immunized.

Measles was also a serious illness because of its occasional tendency to cause deadly complications, including pneumonia and **encephalitis**. Rubella, although not dangerous to the sufferer, caused fetal defects in 25 percent or more pregnancies when contracted by a mother in the first trimester of pregnancy. Defects could include deafness, cataracts, microcephaly, mental retardation, congenital heart defects, miscarriage, and stillbirth. The worst recorded rubella epidemic in the United States occurred in 1965, resulting in 11,250 miscarriages and stillbirths, 2,100 newborn deaths, 11,600 cases of infant deafness, 3,580 cases of infant blindness, and 1,800 cases of infant mental retardation.

Another infectious disease disproportionately affecting children was **poliomyelitis**, an intestinal **virus** that had caused only a mild, inconsequential illness for most of human history. Between 1840 and the 1950s, however, polio became epidemic worldwide with the worst outbreaks of the twentieth century occurring in North America and Western Europe. Most victims were children under 15. During the epidemic, about 1 percent of polio cases attacked sufferers' central nervous systems and destroyed nerve cells, causing temporary paralysis or, in more severe cases, permanent paralysis or death. To this day, scientists do not know why polio affects mostly children, especially boys, and why the illness is most virulent in the summer. Outbreaks of polio still occur among nonimmunized groups, particularly in Nigeria, India, Pakistan, and Afghanistan.

Today, immunizations have largely eliminated the endemic and epidemic childhood diseases of yesteryear. Public health systems around the world strive to vaccinate as many children as possible to confer "herd immunity"—that is, because not all immunizations are wholly effective in every child, the higher the population's vaccination rate, the more everyone, even the un- and under-vaccinated, is protected. When public health systems break down—which does happen in areas affected by **war**, civil unrest, political turmoil, famine, drought, or poverty—and a significant percentage of children go unvaccinated, traditional childhood illnesses often return with devastating results. After the breakup of the Soviet Union in the early 1990s, for example, a once well-established childhood vaccination program faltered, and a diphtheria epidemic ensued; more than 140,000 cases resulted in more than 4,000 deaths. Epidemics such as measles have also returned to some communities in the United States. As an increasing number of American parents balk at getting their children immunized for fear that some immunizations cause autism (a suspicion not supported by studies to date), herd immunity wanes, and children, as well as some adults, are once again susceptible to the life-threatening diseases of yesteryear.

As lethal as the traditional childhood illnesses have been historically, they were by no means the biggest killers of children. Because of children's anatomy and their occasional exposure to toxic environments, the most deadly disease affecting children has always been diarrhea. Compared to adults, small children have meager water reserves. Faced with even a mild case of diarrhea, children dehydrate quickly. Infant diarrhea became epidemic in Europe and the United States as rapidly burgeoning cities became sanitation nightmares in the nineteenth century. Before the advent of sewers to separate human waste from drinking water and the passage of laws governing the production and distribution of cows' milk, children in urban areas died of diarrhea by the thousands each summer when milk and other food spoiled quickly. More than half the infants who died in late-nineteenth-century United States and Europe died of diarrhea. Today, diarrhea continues to be the main cause of death among children in developing countries where the recommendations for the prevention of the illness remain the same as they were more than 100 years ago: breastfeed, and if breastfeeding is not possible, provide infants with clean water and milk, keep food fresh, use latrines, and wash hands often.

Infant deaths from diarrhea began to ebb in the twentieth century only after urban reformers, public health departments, physicians, and urban newspapers joined forces to lobby for the passage of laws to ensure pure milk for children. The milk crusades, which lasted in some American cities for up to three decades or more (from roughly the 1890s through much of the 1920s), were highly visible and served to edify the public about the primary cause of infant death. In an era before refrigeration, pasteurization, and pure food laws, milk was shipped in 8-gallon uncovered vats and traveled for up to 72 hours in railroad cars before reaching the urban consumer. Milk spoilage was only one cause of infant diarrhea—the vat system of milk distribution also facilitated the adulteration of milk. To increase profits, shippers and merchants often added myriad substances to the content of vats—plaster, for example, to make skimmed milk look rich with cream, and powdered chalk to whiten milk dirtied by the open vat system. Consumers contributed to the disaster. Understandably wary about the milk they purchased, they often dipped their fingers into vats for sampling before ladling milk into vessels. In this way, diphtheria, scarlet fever, **tuberculosis**, and infant diarrhea all became milkborne diseases.

The seasonal incidence of deadly diarrhea among babies disappeared in most areas of the United States by the 1930s, thanks to reformers' successful efforts to improve the production, shipping, and sales practices of the dairy industry. Chicago was typical in that deaths from diarrhea went from 53.7 percent of all infant deaths in 1897, to 40.9 percent in 1905 (after milk vats were sealed by law), 39.4 percent in 1912 (after cows' milk had to be shipped and sold in individual, sealed bottles), 35.9 percent in 1918 (after cows' milk had to be pasteurized), 16.9 percent in 1924 (after milk had to be kept cold during shipping), and 11.1 percent in 1930 (after cows' milk had to be tested for bovine tuberculosis). As was typical throughout most of the United States and Western Europe, by 1939 in Chicago only 1.4 percent of the babies who died, died of diarrhea. As the general urban environment improved, the infant mortality rate in urban areas went from roughly 18 percent in 1897, to 12 percent in 1912, 8 percent in 1924, and 3 percent in 1939. This dramatic lowering of the infant death rate long before the availability of antibiotics and routine childhood immunizations is a prime example of how improvements in the environment contributed far more than medical treatment to declines in mortality.

After diarrhea, respiratory ailments were the second most significant cause of death among children. Those most at risk for infection were children younger than two and those already weakened by another health problem. This latter factor ensured that the youngest children were highly susceptible to respiratory disease—by the early twentieth century, urban health departments admitted that for decades many of the infants listed as dying from pneumonia or bronchitis likely died from opportunistic respiratory infections facilitated by a weakened condition as a result of diarrhea.

Sexually transmitted infections among adults also affected children. In the pre-**antibiotic** era, mothers with **syphilis** passed the disease to their children in utero. Children with congenital syphilis were predisposed to **meningitis**, severe mental retardation, and hydrocephalus and often died in infancy. **Gonorrhea** could be passed from mother to baby in the birth canal, affecting an infant's eyes and resulting in permanent blindness. In the nineteenth-century United States, gonorrhea was the most common cause of blindness among children, prompting physicians to often remark that this was a classic case of the "sins of the father" being visited on the children.

Change in daily habits occasionally triggered other diseases in children. Rickets, which causes softening of the bones and severely stunted growth in infants and children, was epidemic in late-nineteenth-century European and American cities. The disease is caused by insufficient calciferol, a hormone that helps balance calcium in the body. Sunlight triggers the body's manufacture of calciferol, also known as Vitamin D (despite not being a vitamin). In the nineteenth century, changes in human living patterns and behaviors prompted the illness: tenements had no windows, soft coal polluted cities and blocked sunlight, and unpaved urban roadways were so full of mud and muck that mothers kept their children indoors for fear they would drown in the deep puddles dotting city streets. In the 1930s, the addition of calciferol to infant formula and cows' milk (hailed as "Vitamin D fortified milk") eliminated rickets in Europe and America but unfortunately perpetuated the notion that rickets is a disease of dietary deficiency rather than of sunshine deficiency. Today the disease has appeared once again, mainly in breastfed infants, because concern about skin cancer has prompted mothers to cover infants from head to toe and slather sunscreen on any exposed skin. The growth in the number of working mothers has also contributed to the problem; many daycare providers tend to keep children indoors during daylight hours.

Today the leading cause of death among infants in the developed world is no longer diarrhea or any infectious disease but congenital abnormalities, premature birth, and Sudden Infant Death Syndrome. Among older children, the leading causes of death are unintentional injury, homicide, and suicide. In the developing world, however, as in the United States and Western Europe in the nineteenth and early twentieth centuries, diarrhea remains the leading cause of childhood death. That entirely preventable illnesses such as infant diarrhea and traditional childhood diseases are still ongoing threats in some areas of the world signifies that the root cause of infant and child mortality remains: some parents are still denied access to the resources they need to properly care for their children. *See also* Heredity and Epidemic Disease.

Further Reading

Garret, Eilidh, Chris Galley, Nicola Shelton, and Robert Woods, eds. *Infant Mortality: A Continuing Social Problem.* Burlington, VT: Ashgate, 2006.

Hammonds, Evelynn Maxine. *Childhood's Deadly Scourge: The Campaign to Control Diphtheria in New York City, 1880–1930.* Baltimore: Johns Hopkins University Press, 1999.

Klaus, Alisa. *Every Child a Lion: The Origins of Maternal and Infant Health Policy in the United States and France, 1890–1920.* Ithaca, NY: Cornell University Press, 1993.

Meckel, Richard A. *Save the Babies: American Public Health Reform and the Prevention of Infant Mortality, 1850–1929.* Baltimore: Johns Hopkins University Press, 1990.

Preston, Samuel H., and Michael R. Haines. *Fatal Years: Child Mortality in Late Nineteenth-Century America.* Princeton: Princeton University Press, 1991.

Wolf, Jacqueline H. *Don't Kill Your Baby: Public Health and the Decline of Breastfeeding in the Nineteenth and Twentieth Centuries*. Columbus: Ohio State University Press, 2001.

JACQUELINE H. WOLF

CHINESE DISEASE THEORY AND MEDICINE.   Archeological evidence for scientific and technological knowledge in China extends back at least to the **Neolithic** period (c. 6000 BCE), and written material is available from as early as the Shang period (c. 1700–1025 BCE). Early artifacts, dating from the Shang, include divinations written in the precursor to modern Chinese script on flat bones and turtle shells ("oracle bones"), as well as technically advanced bronze castings. The Zhou dynasty (1122–256 BCE) was characterized by the development of the dominant philosophical schools of traditional Chinese thought: Daoism, Confucianism, Moism, and Legalism. By the Han dynasty (206 BCE–220 CE) comprehensive cosmological views of the universe had been developed by the Daoists. These were based on a few universal principles: *yin* and *yang* complementarity, the relations and correspondences of *wu xing* (the five phases of the universe: wood, fire, earth, metal, and water), and the notions of *qi* (pronounced "chee"—vital force, or "matter–energy") and *li* (natural order or organizing principle). Traditional Chinese understanding of illness, disease, and healing is framed in terms of this worldview.

Two of the most important texts in Chinese medicine are *Huang di nei jing* and *Ben cao gang mu* ("The Yellow Emperor's Classic of Internal Medicine" and "The Great Pharmacopoeia"). These texts are still used as the bases for Chinese Traditional Medicine. The *Huang di nei jing* is a multi-authored text compiled between the second century BCE and the second century CE, in which a dialog between the mythical Yellow Emperor and one of his chief ministers explores many aspects of medicine: the concept of the body and its function; the detection, causes, and treatment of illness; and the way remedies act. The *Ben cao gang mu*, the life's work of Li Shizhen (1518–1593), is a compendium of medication (in the broad sense) that gives the historical background for the drugs, much botanical information, and the indications for the uses of the materials. The literary tradition of such treatises on drugs (*Ben cao*) gives a good idea of Chinese understanding of those areas now identified as botany, geology, and mineralogy, as well as pharmacology and physiology.

Chinese medical theory views the body as a microcosm of the cosmos, and its concepts are particularly rich in political metaphors. The body and its functions are likened to the government, with the need for storage depots, transportation routes, officials high and low, and regulations. Thus, the vital energy of the body, *qi*, must be regulated in its flow by the organs, with analogies to government officials; there are depots and storage sites for *qi*. Disease is often viewed in terms of the faulty regulation of *qi* flow, either too much or too little, and treatments are designed to help the internal regulators to do their jobs. This political conception of bodily function is joined to a system of regular correspondences that relate organs, symptoms, points on the body surface, and therapeutic approaches. This system of correspondences is universal and is not just part of medical thought. For example, the *yin-yang* and *wu xing* theories provide ways to think about the heart's correspondence to fire, and hence, because fire is overcome by water, the role of diuretics in treating heart disease is explained and rationalized. Not all such correspondences, however, are so clearly congruent to Western views. Therapeutic approaches to influence and regulate *qi* flow can involve insertion of needles (acupuncture), pressure, or heat (moxibustion) applied at specific places related to *qi* channels.

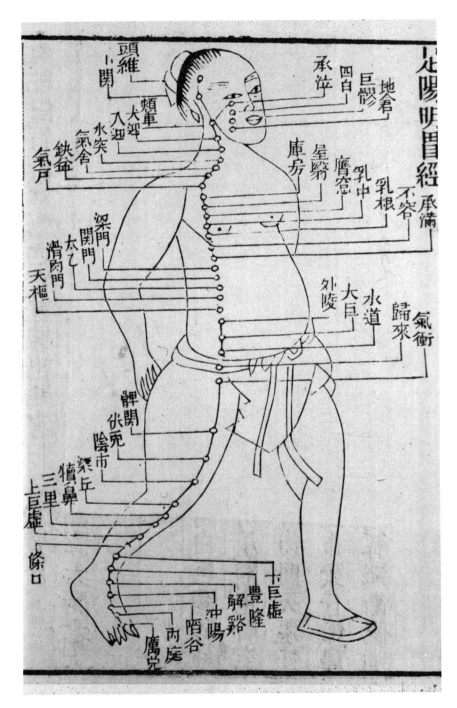

Full-length figure with acupuncture points and meridian in Chinese characters for stomach and foot disorders, 1875. Courtesy of the National Library of Medicine.

Another concept that is crucial in Chinese medical thinking is the distinction between internal and external aspects of the body and its relation to illness. Some illnesses arise from internal imbalances, for example in *qi* distribution. Other illnesses arise from external influences such as wind, dampness, or demons. A precise correlation between these Chinese concepts and Western categories, however, is not entirely successful. For example, to a Westerner the Chinese concept of the "triple burner" might seem to refer to some anatomical structure, but it actually refers to internal bodily functions, and is really much closer to the Western concept of "metabolism."

Because basic Chinese cosmological thinking allows both for action at a distance and for local variations, Chinese medicine searches for "patterns of disharmony" that are specific for a given patient. Thus, **astrological** as well as social and geographical factors influence both diagnosis and therapy. **Epidemic** diseases are often characterized as being the result of "External Pernicious Influences." Weather, external dampness, diet, exercise, sexual activity (or the lack of it) all have both internal and external aspects and are used to explain and avoid epidemic diseases or pestilences.

The available Western literature on science and medicine (both of which are Western analytical categories, not Chinese) in China is of two types: scholarly work and popularized works on exoticism. Western readers have been fascinated with tales of the exotic East at least since the days of Marco Polo in the late thirteenth century. Even today, there is a large market for uncritical accounts and explanations of the "mysteries of the East." Much of this is published under the rubric of health advice or "Eastern Religion." The serious student of the history of science and medicine in East Asia should evaluate this literature with the same level of criticism as any other scholarly work, that is, based on its documentation and argumentation. *See also* Ayurvedic Disease Theory and Medicine; Folk Medicine; Greco-Roman Medical Theory and Practice; Humoral Theory; Islamic Disease Theory and Medicine; Physician; Plague in China; Religion and Epidemic Disease; Severe Acute Respiratory Syndrome (SARS).

Further Reading

Kaptchuk, Ted J. *The Web That Has No Weaver: Understanding Chinese Medicine.* New York: Congdon & Weed, 1983.

Lloyd, Geoffrey, and Nathan Sivin. *The Way and the Word: Science and Medicine in Early China and Greece.* New Haven: Yale University Press, 2002.

National Library of Medicine. http://www.nlm.nih.gov/hmd/chinese/chinesehome.html

Scheid, Volker. *Chinese Medicine in Contemporary China: Plurality and Synthesis.* Durham, NC: Duke University Press, 2002.

Unschuld, Paul U. *Medicine in China: A History of Ideas.* Berkeley: University of California Press, 1985.

Veith, Ilza. *The Yellow Emperor's Classic of Internal Medicine.* Berkeley: University of California Press, 2002.

WILLIAM C. SUMMERS

CHLAMYDIA.   *See* Gonorrhea.

CHOLERA.   Cholera is an acute diarrheal disease caused by the **bacterium** *Vibrio cholerae*—short, curved, anaerobic, motile, Gram-negative rods. Spread by food and **water** supplies contaminated with the fecal discharges of cholera sufferers, cholera's violent symptoms tend to run a rapid course; once ingested, the incubation period for cholera can be as

CHOLERA'S MANY ALIASES

Originally, the term *Cholera-morbus* came from the time of **humoral theory** and denoted an illness or combination of gastric symptoms. It derives from the Greek word *chole,* which means bile, and the Latin *morbus,* meaning illness. In 1832 J. Kennedy noted other designations: epidemic cholera, spasmodic cholera, cholera asphyxia, and malignant cholera. French authors called it the *maladie noire* (black illness), *maladie bleue* (blue illness), *trousse-galant* (popular name), as well as the more clinical *choléréé, cholerragie,* and *cholarée lymphatique* (lymphatic cholera). Arabic and Hindi share the name *hyza;* Iranians call it *tokhmu.* In Sanskrit cholera is *dissochtau,* and in Maharatta it is *fural.* The Japanese use an adverb that indicates brutality, *korori,* and in Chinese the characters for tiger and wolf are used to compose the word, a reference to the aggressiveness of the illness.

Donato Gómez-Díaz

short as 12 hours or as long as 72. Although clearly an ancient disease that resided in South Asia for hundreds of years before becoming pandemic in 1816, cholera is considered the quintessential **epidemic** disease of the nineteenth century. The disease killed with such vivacity that it probably helped provide the major impetus for modern developments in public health such as clean water, hygiene, and sanitation. Cholera is still a formidable public health problem around the world, as there is currently a seventh world pandemic that began in the early 1960s. Cholera continues to thrive where systems of public health fail to provide basic sanitation and an adequate source of clean, unpolluted water.

The exact origins of cholera are unclear. **Historical epidemiologists** are uncertain of the pre-1816 history of cholera, but most agree that the disease was endemic to India for hundreds of years. Ancient Indian texts describe a disease that is most likely cholera. Cholera gets its name from the Greek words for "bile" (the brown fluid secreted by the liver) and "to flow." Before the nineteenth century, cholera was used to describe any severe vomiting and diarrhea. Epidemic cholera did not begin to extend pandemically until 1816, reaching England in 1831 and North America in 1832. It was only in the nineteenth century that the deadly and specific epidemic disease caused by *Vibrio cholerae* began to be called cholera. To avoid confusion, many medical authors added the prefixes "Asiatic" or "Indian." Others simply called it "cholera morbus," with specific reference to social fears generated by the **Black Death** (see sidebar).

Knowledge about cholera outbreaks after 1816 is far more substantial. Commonly used dates for the seven pandemics are as follows: the first pandemic lasted from 1816 to 1825; the second from 1827 to 1838; the third from 1839 to 1861; the fourth from 1862 to 1879; the fifth from 1881 to 1896; the sixth from 1899 to 1947; and the seventh from 1961 to the present. What makes cholera particularly elusive are the abilities of the bacterium to adapt to changing **environmental** conditions and of the host to develop resistance to otherwise effective **drugs**. Although only three strains of cholera are recognized to be epidemic, over 200 serogroups exist. The three known epidemic strains are *V. cholerae* O1 of the classical biotype, *V. cholerae* O1 of the El Tor biotype, and *V. cholerae* O139. All cholera strains are divided between the O1 group antigen (*V. cholerae* O1) and the non-O1 group (*V. cholerae*). Although laboratory evidence has confirmed that the fifth and sixth pandemics were caused by *V. cholerae* O1 of the classical biotype, the strains that caused the first four pandemics are unknown. Presumably, if the illnesses labeled **cholera before the pandemics** were indeed the disease currently recognized, a variety of strains and virulence levels existed. The El Tor biotype first emerged during the seventh pandemic in

Indonesia in 1961, creating a wave of fear around the globe. Although the O1 strains were thought to be the exclusive cause of epidemic cholera, the O139 serogroup emerged in southeastern India in 1992 as the first non-O1 *V. cholerae* strain to cause an epidemic outbreak.

The clinical and epidemiological features of *V. cholerae* O139 are identical to *V. cholerae* O1 of the classical biotype and *V. cholerae* O1 of the El Tor biotype. However, **immunity** to the O1 group is not protective against the new O139 strain. Horizontal gene transfer is probably responsible for the two newest strains of cholera. The genetic makeup and virulence levels of *V. cholerae* O139 are nearly the same as those of the O1 El Tor strains, which appear similar to the classical O1 stains as well. The appearance of the O139 strain led many public health authorities to believe it replaced the El Tor biotype. However, by 1994 the El Tor strain was responsible for a series of outbreaks in Bangladesh and currently resides endemic in most regions of Southeast Asia. As of 2007, in some areas of the world the O1 *V. cholerae* remains dominant, and in others the O139 periodically reemerges.

Cholera enters the body via the fecal-oral route of **transmission**—the cholera bacillus is passed on in the excreta of sufferers and enters new hosts through the mouth and digestive system. After a 24- to 48-hour incubation period, the bacterium synthesizes an exotoxin that triggers the massive secretion of water and electrolytes into the small intestine. Acute diarrhea, spasmodic vomiting, and severe cramps mark the onset of symptoms, and fever is usually absent. The clinical manifestations are a result of the amount of water and electrolytes lost: after losing 3 to 5 percent of normal body weight, thirst develops. After 5 to 8 percent loss, the victim suffers bodily weakness and postural hypotension, the face turns a blue-gray color, and the extremities become cold and darkened. After 10 percent weight loss, the pulse becomes weak, the eyes sunken, the skin wrinkled, and coma and somnolence are present. Although in the early stages of the disease the stools of cholera patients may contain fecal matter, the stools quickly become white and opalescent, the characteristic "rice-water" stools of cholera (termed because of the resemblance to water to which rice has been added). If not treated properly, profuse diarrhea and vomiting eventually lead to the near complete depletion of body fluids, dehydration, and death—a quarter of the body's fluids and vital body salts may be lost within a few hours. Feces from persons acutely infected with cholera are the main source of explosive epidemics. In a single day, a single cholera patient may produce up to 20 liters of stool containing as many as 10,000,000 vibrios per milliliter.

Cholera treatment is simple and inexpensive. Oral rehydration therapy (ORT), which constitutes the rapid replacement of fluids and electrolytes, is the most common and effective treatment. **World Health Organization** statistics show that the mortality rate for appropriately treated disease is usually less than 1 percent. Alternative treatment options include cereal-based formulations, intravenous fluid replacement for the initial management of severely dehydrated persons, and **antibiotic** treatments (usually tetracycline or doxycycline). Several types of cholera **vaccines** are under clinical trial.

Like other waterborne disease such as **dysentery** and **typhoid**, cholera is spread along the various pathways leading to the human digestive tract. Case-controlled investigations of cholera transmission since the nineteenth century have identified a wide range of water and food vehicles. Water clearly plays the most important role in spreading cholera. When urban water supplies have become contaminated with sewage that harbors the excreta of cholera victims, the most severe and widespread epidemics have ensued. Even immobilized persons can infect large numbers if basic **personal hygiene** and public sanitation are not followed. Other routes can be just as fatal. Uncooked fruits and vegetables, soiled linens, and unwashed hands have all frequently contributed to the spread of the disease. Recent research has also shown that cholera can live for extended periods in aquatic environments, adhering to crustaceans, zooplankton, and phytoplankton. This research also indicates shellfish as potential carriers of cholera and helps explain the ecology of the disease, its seasonal occurrence, and its endemic tendencies.

As a result of a combination of massive **urbanization, industrialization**, and an underdeveloped public health infrastructure, cholera ran rampant in Western countries for most of the nineteenth century. However, not everyone who ingests cholera contracts the disease, and many people probably ingested the disease without harm, as high concentrations of stomach acid often kill the organism before it is able to reach the small intestine. Only recently has the host-parasite relationship and full epidemiological picture of cholera become clear. Recent epidemiological and experimental studies have revealed that levels of gastric acidity and ABO blood group status are two leading factors that predispose individuals to cholera. People with relatively low levels of gastric acidity and type O blood are at the greatest risk.

Historically cholera has played an important role in the history of diseases that have affected civilization generally and public health specifically. When cholera struck the western world in the nineteenth century, lay and medical opinion alike disagreed on its defining features. Society looked at cholera with relentless fear; the debilitating symptoms of a disease that could strike and kill within a number of hours led to social unrest and summoned fears about plague. Although mortality rates from cholera at times approached those of the medieval plague epidemics, the morbidity rates were much lower. Cholera's morbidity trends were even lower than those of nineteenth-century **tuberculosis**, a much more dangerous disease that was feared much less than cholera.

Until the end of the nineteenth century, most of the western world believed in the miasmatic theory that cholera was transmitted through the **air**. Having roots in the **Hippocratic** medical tradition and having been refined throughout the medieval and early modern periods, this theory held that epidemics were transmitted through the putrefaction of the air by rotting **corpses** or animal or vegetable material. Victorians also ascribed moral and religious value to cholera; the disease was a punishment from God or a consequence of the neglect of natural laws. Indeed, the correlation among cholera, morality, and **poverty** persisted throughout the nineteenth century, reinforced by social reformers and religious zealots.

Recent research has expanded the understanding of cholera. The most important findings have been the emergence of the previously unrecognized strain, *V. cholerae* serotype 0139. Other research has shown that the El Tor biotype appears to be more resistant to adverse environmental factors and better adapted to foodborne transmission than the classical biotype. Cholera remains a global threat. Although it no longer poses a threat to countries with proper hygienic practices and basic sanitation, it poses a serious threat where access to safe drinking water and adequate sanitation are not guaranteed. *See also* Cholera: First through Third Pandemics, 1816–1861; Cholera: Fourth through Sixth Pandemics, 1863–1947; Cholera: Seventh Pandemic, 1961–Present; Disease, Social Construction of; Epidemiology, History of; Germ Theory of Disease; Historical Epidemiology; Koch, Robert; Public Health Agencies in the West before

1900; Sanitation Movement of the Nineteenth Century; Snow, John; Trade, Travel, and Epidemic Disease.

Further Reading

Centers for Disease Control and Prevention. *Cholera*. http://www.cdc.gov/ncidod/dbmd/diseaseinfo/cholera_g.htm

Hardy, Anne. *The Epidemic Streets: Infectious Disease and the Rise of Preventive Medicine, 1856–1900*. Oxford: Oxford University Press, 1993.

Hunter, Paul. *Waterborne Disease: Epidemiology and Ecology*. New York: John Wiley & Sons Press, 1997.

Mayo Clinic. http://www.mayoclinic.com/health/cholera/DS00579

National Library of Medicine. http://www.nlm.nih.gov/exhibition/cholera/

Pelling, Margaret. *Cholera, Fever, and English Medicine, 1825–1865*. Oxford: Oxford University Press, 1978.

Rosenberg, Charles. *The Cholera Years: The United States in 1832, 1849, and 1866*. Chicago: University of Chicago Press, 1987.

Vinten-Johansen, Peter, et al. *Cholera, Chloroform, and the Science of Medicine*. New York: Oxford University Press, 2003.

Wachsmuth, I., P. Blake, and O. Olsvik. *Vibrio cholerae and Cholera: Molecular to Global Perspectives*. Washington, DC: American Society of Microbiologists Press, 1994.

World Health Organization. *Cholera*. http://www.who.int/topics/cholera/en/

JACOB STEERE-WILLIAMS

CHOLERA BEFORE THE PANDEMICS.   Many early sources record the presence of **cholera** before the nineteenth century. It was described in China in the first century CE, and later in the seventh century by Wong and Wu Lien Teh. Both **Hippocrates** and **Galen** described an illness resembling cholera, and various European authors considered it one of the gravest **epidemic** diseases in ancient history.

India is without doubt cholera's place of origin, with an endemic pocket on the delta of the Ganges River. There, Hindu **pilgrimages** and festivities attracted large crowds that were exposed to cholera, creating a noticeably high correlation between cholera and holy days. In Bengal, Oola Beebee, the goddess of cholera, was worshipped, and a temple in her honor has stood in Calcutta since the end of the nineteenth century. Some Indian descriptions date as far back as 2,500 years ago, and fifth-century CE Sanskrit scriptures detail the spread of an illness with cholera-like symptoms. The disease periodically overextended its natural limits, probably being carried by ships.

After the arrival of the Portuguese in India in 1498, various Europeans documented the presence of cholera. Gaspar Correa (1496–c. 1563), a Portuguese historian in Goa, wrote of a new sickness that he called "moryxi" in his book *Legendary India* (1543). He described vomiting and cramps that could kill a man by the end of the day. Other names for this condition evolved, such as the French term *mort de chien* (a dog's death). In the spring of 1503, 20,000 men in the army of the Sovereign of Calcutta came down suddenly with a disease that struck the belly very painfully, so that many died in less than eight hours.

In 1563 another Portuguese doctor in Goa, García da Orta (1501–1568), published *Conversations on Simples and Drugs and Medical Materials from India*, a volume that contained the first modern description of cholera. In 1585 a French observer noted that the epidemic fired up once again. In 1629 a physician of the Dutch East India Trade Company reported in his *On Medicine of the Indies* that the General Governor of Batavia (present-day Jakarta, Indonesia) died of an acute dehydrating diarrheal illness. Goa was once again invaded by an outbreak in 1683.

The English and French colonial presence in India was marked by numerous cholera epidemics. Around 1760 the Scotsman James Lind (1716–1794) described a condition called "mordechin," and a Frenchman wrote of an epidemic that occurred from 1768 to 1771, taking the lives of 60,000 people (it is probable that this extended into Burma and Malaysia in 1770). Cholera appeared in Calcutta in 1781–1782, and the following year in the holy city of Hardwar, at which time 20,000 pilgrims died in eight days. At the same time, the Maratha armies, fighting for Tipu Sahib (1750–1799), Sultan of Mysore, were also afflicted. In 1787 another observation of the illness was described by an English physician, "Dr. Paisley," and in 1796 a Catholic friar recorded yet another. Sixty-four additional references to major cholera outbreaks in India date from 1503 to 1817, but the limitations in transportation probably contained the spread of the disease. *See also* Cholera: First through Third Pandemics, 1816–1861; Colonialism and Epidemic Disease; Contagion Theory of Disease, Premodern; Diagnosis of Historical Diseases; Environment, Ecology, and Epidemic Disease; Trade, Travel, and Epidemic Disease; Water and Epidemic Diseases.

Further Reading

Longmate, N. *King Cholera: The Biography of a Disease*. London: Hamish Hamilton, 1966.

Donato Gómez-Díaz

CHOLERA: FIRST THROUGH THIRD PANDEMICS, 1816–1861. Cholera was one of the most feared illnesses of the nineteenth century. The great **pandemics** started in India, and their spread coincides with the increase of **trade** and communication and with the **Industrial Revolution**. The first pandemic essentially had an Asiatic expanse, whereas the second and third reached Europe and the greater part of the Americas. The effects of cholera cast doubt on the power of science because theoretical approaches had little to offer against its unstoppable transmission. A bitter controversy arose between those who believed it was contracted by direct human contact (**contagion**) and those who believed it was produced by environmental factors. In England, this dichotomy erupted into the political debate in which Conservatives (Contagionists) disputed Liberals (Anticontagionists) on not only matters of public health but of free trade as well. Lastly, to solve the sanitary problem that private ventures had failed to accomplish, governments strengthened public health in a bid to control transmission factors by means of public hygiene.

Sources on **cholera before the pandemics** are fragmented. Most are descriptions of historians, travelers, and **physicians**, who since ancient times recorded instances in which symptoms indicated the presence of cholera. There are also accounts from the arrival of the Portuguese in India and the subsequent incursions in the colonial period by the Dutch, French, and English, and even references in Italian literature, that contain information about contagious epidemics that resemble cholera. After the first cholera pandemic (1816–1825), efforts were made to study and compile information, first by means of diverse English military-medical reports, and later through the use of Indian literature. The extension of cholera into Europe during the second (1827–1838) and third pandemics (1839–1861) left many accounts and studies that described its catastrophic course, as well as medical literature about prophylactic measures that governments adopted. In contrast, there was less information about what had happened in the Far East and Africa.

Nature of Disease Involved.   Cholera is an acute illness caused by the bacterium *Vibrio cholerae*. In its most fatal form, after an average incubation period of two to three days—and in some cases five hours to five days—the illness propagates, resulting in painful symptoms and a high likelihood of death. Acute nausea provokes violent vomiting and diarrhea; stools turn into a whitish liquid described as "rice water," until fragments of the intestines are passed. Afterwards, victims endure ferocious cramping and an insatiable thirst, followed by a state of prostration. Dehydrated and close to death, a patient shows the classic physiognomy of cholera: a sunken and withered face with wrinkled and cyanic lips.

Although other microorganisms can have similar clinical manifestations, the term cholera is reserved exclusively for the toxigenic species of *V. cholerae* 01 (two strains: Classical and El Tor) and 0139, regardless of the intensity of symptoms shown. The bacterium of cholera is transmitted by the oral-fecal path, primarily by water contaminated by fecal sediment and sometimes by the ingestion of contaminated food. For the prevention of cholera it is necessary that a community be outfitted with an adequate supply of clean, drinkable water and an effective sewage elimination system.

Two main positions emerged with respect to the nature of the cholera found in the outbreak of 1817. One interprets it as a form that existed since ancient times but with a newly aggressive transmission. The second agrees that the illness existed in forms of "cholera morbus" or "sporadic cholera" before the nineteenth century, but posits that the cholera of 1817 had new characteristics. With respect to the first position, Europe had suffered epidemics that doctors of the time described as resembling cholera. For example, a Flemish physician described in 1643 what he called *flux de ventre* (abdominal flow). The English doctor **Thomas Sydenham** documented the clinical manifestions and treatment of an epidemic of cholera in London in 1669. Nicolas Philibert Adelon (1782–1862), a specialist who edited a nineteenth-century French medical encyclopedia (1822), continued to use the traditional definition of cholera current since **Galen**. In his *Plagues and Peoples* (1984), William McNeill (b. 1917) claims that the only change was that in 1817 the illness stretched its usual boundaries and flourished in new and nonhabitual territories completely lacking resistance and accustomed reactions to its presence.

Many English physicians who tried to understand the first pandemic were aware of cholera's existence and asserted that the epidemic of 1817 had its own characteristics. In 1829 James Annesley (d. 1853) also maintained that he did not find prior references in Indian medical literature that coincided with the cholera suffered in 1817 and concluded that there existed two different types of cholera. One called "cholera morbus," which was typical in Europe, and the Indian "cholera sporadic." He also observed that neither form, as previously experienced, had manifested all of the characteristics of the new, pandemic form.

There was not a consensus among Indian physicians who wrote about what the causes were or how cholera was transmitted. Following traditional medical principles, it was believed that cholera was related to meteorological factors such as torrential rain or a fall in temperature, or to **air**-related factors such as poisonous and pestilent emissions from decomposing vegetal and human waste in dwellings. Europe initially adopted the same set of theories when it found itself in the same situation. Eventually, an effort was made to systematize a single theory involving various causes: the nervous, which attributed the disorder to infective illnesses of a cerebrospinal type; the humoral, which attributed changes in the blood from airborne causes to the illness; and the gastroenteric, which claimed it as gastroenteritis accompanied by other factors, the causes of which were essentially unknown.

Mortality.   Although cholera has been called the most significant epidemic in the nineteenth century, from a demographical viewpoint it can be seen as having had limited repercussions for multiple reasons. First, the most severe outbreaks lasted five or six years. Second, the percentage of the total population affected was quite low. In France the percentage of the population affected between 1832 and 1854 was 0.4 percent, which is far less than the 2 or 3 million victims of the plague from 1600 to 1870. There were widespread locations with significant mortality from cholera—the Cité quarter of Paris in 1832 had a 10 percent mortality rate, and Ariège in 1854 had a rate of 20 percent— but the outbreaks in these areas did not have a significant effect on the population. In other locations, like India, the situation was much more grave when cholera broke out in 1818 and affected 7.5 percent of its population; from 1817 to 1865, 15 million people perished.

The mortality rate varied. In the beginning of an epidemic the mortality rate was quite high, varying from 50 to 60 percent; later, the number of milder cases rose, and the mortality rate fell to between 25 percent and 30 percent. In 1876 the Spanish author Sánchez Merino set the rate of mortality between 36 and 40 percent, which was calculated to be 3 to 5 percent of the population. Hamburg, Germany, was battered by successive cholera epidemics. In 1832, 1.13 percent of the city's population perished, in 1848 1.06 percent, and in 1859 0.65 percent.

The pandemics also had a social and urban geography. Belgium's working class was especially hard hit in urban and industrial centers. In France during the 1832 epidemic, the poorest died in a ratio of 1.5 to 1 in comparison to upper classes, though the situation did improve over the course of the century. The epidemic was particularly fatal for the young and elderly compared to adults: French children and seniors were four times more likely to die than were adults.

Origins and Spread: The First Pandemic (1817–1825).   Though the Greeks and Romans may have suffered from cholera, it was endemic in parts of Asia and the Indian Ocean. European merchants and colonists first described contact with it in India at the end of the fifteenth century. Eighteenth-century **colonialism** in India brought England and France into close and lasting contact with South Asia and its cholera reservoirs. The Asian cholera epidemic of 1816–1821, however, is considered the first of the pandemics. Earlier accounts refer to the existence of some cases of cholera in Eastern India in 1814 and in August 1817 in Jessora, a village close to Calcutta, where 10,000 perished in a few months. Afterward, English soldiers stationed at Fort William in Calcutta fell victim. It rapidly spread; 5,000 soldiers died in a few weeks, devastating the army of General Francis Rawdon-Hastings (1754–1826). In a few months, 25,000 were treated for cholera in Calcutta, and 4,000 died; the following year, epidemic cholera propagated throughout India.

Advances in commercial exchange and navigation contributed to cholera's dispersion. Trade and maritime traffic brought the sickness northward. It hit China first, through the western port of Canton in 1820, and between 1822 and 1824 it sprawled through the

Yangtze Valley. Korea lost 10,000 to 100,000 in 1821. It entered Japan through Nagasaki in 1822 and was confined to the west. Cholera struck Sri Lanka in 1818, the Philippines in 1820, and Borneo in 1821; Java suffered 100,000 victims in 1820. Land routes brought it to western Afghanistan, to Shiraz in Persia (1821), to Basra (15,000 died in three weeks), and to Baghdad by way of the Tigris and Euphrates river valley. At the limits of the Mediterranean, it reached Syria in November 1822. The march proceeded to Anatolia and the port of Astrakhan in Russia where an exceptionally harsh winter (1823–1824) impeded its transmission beyond the Caspian Sea. It arrived at Africa's eastern coast and was carried by British troops stationed to help the Sultan of Oman in 1821. In the Persian Gulf, the slave trade directed it along the coast to Zanzibar. It also reached Egypt in 1823.

The Second Pandemic (1826–1838).   Scholars dispute the date of origin of the second pandemic. Some assign the years 1826 to 1838 and others 1829 to 1851. Beginning with the earliest accounts, it originated in the northeastern province of Bengal in India with diverse outbreaks in the Ganges delta in 1826. This sets it apart from the typical points of origin. From Lahore in the northeast, cholera followed along the caravan routes to Kabul and Balkh in Afghanistan and crossed into Russian territory at Bukhara in 1827. It reached Chiva in 1827 and was carried by Kirgis hordes to Chkalov (Russia) in the southern Ural Mountains in 1829; Tehran (Iran) was suffering by the end of 1829. Moscow was stricken in August of 1830, and before the end of 1831 the epidemic had spread to other main cities and towns of Russia. In 1831, Cossack troops were ordered to Poland, and they brought the disease with them. Hungary was affected in June of 1831 (100,000 deaths), and the spread extended to Germany (Berlin in August and Hamburg in October of 1831). In 1831 it reached Finland and Sweden, and Vienna was affected the same year. In October of 1831, England, Wales, and Scotland were stricken (31,474 victims) despite **quarantines** for people and freight. London and Glasgow were particularly punished. Before March of 1832, cholera was detected in Ireland, leaving 25,000 dead. Panic pushed governments to take measures against the disaster.

France was hit in 1832, killing 102,000 people. That same year, Irish immigrants brought cholera to Canada and the United States. Quebec, Philadelphia, and New York (3,000 victims in July and August) were simultaneously affected. It reached New Orleans in October, and in the course of three weeks, 4,340 residents were left dead. Passing through small cities and towns, the West was not spared cholera's spread. In the United States, the pandemic lasted from 1832 to 1849 and killed 150,000 people.

In February 1833, Havana, Cuba was left with 9,000 dead. The rate of mortality was almost 60 dead for every 1,000 inhabitants. In the rural areas, the total number of victims was three times that in the capital. Mexico followed with 15,000 dead in August. By 1837, it reached Nicaragua and Guatemala, and as a final lashing, it hit Colombia in 1850.

In the spring of 1831, **pilgrims** traveling through Mesopotamia and the Arabian Peninsula brought cholera to Mecca during the annual *hajj*. In three weeks, almost 3,000 pilgrims perished returning to their homes—a situation that would repeat itself throughout the nineteenth century. Another branch of the epidemic passed toward Syria and Palestine, while a third headed to Cairo (July, 1831) affecting the Nile delta. Muslim pilgrims brought cholera to Tunisia in 1831, and in the following years Ethiopia, Somalia, Zanzibar, Algeria, and Sudan were all stricken.

LIVING CONDITIONS IN ENGLAND AT THE TIME OF THE SECOND CHOLERA PANDEMIC, AS REPORTED IN EDWIN CHADWICK'S *REPORT ON THE SANITARY CONDITION OF THE LABORING POPULATION OF GREAT BRITAIN* (1842)

Mr. Robert Atkinson, Gateshead, states that: It is impossible to give a proper representation of the wretched state of many of the inhabitants of the indigent class, situated in the confined streets called Pipewellgate and Killgate, which are kept in a most filthy state, and to a stranger would appear inimical to the existence of human beings, where each small, ill-ventilated apartment of the house contained a family in number from seven to nine, and seldom more than two beds for the whole. The want of convenient offices in the neighborhood is attended with many very unpleasant circumstances, as it induces the lazy inmates to make use of chamber utensils [chamber pots], which are suffered to remain in the most offensive state for several days and are then emptied out of the windows. The writer had occasion a short time ago to visit a person ill of the cholera; his lodgings were in a room of a miserable house situated in the very filthiest part of Pipewellgate, divided into six apartments, and occupied by different families to the number of 26 persons in all. The room contained three wretched beds with two persons sleeping in each; it measured twelve feet in length and seven in breadth, and its greatest height would not admit of a person standing erect; it received light from a small window, the sash of which was fixed. Two of the number lay ill of the cholera, and the rest appeared afraid of the admission of pure air, having carefully closed up the broken panes with plugs of old linen.

From Edwin Chadwick's *Report on the Sanitary Condition of the Laboring Population of Great Britain,* reprint edition by M. W. Flinn (Edinburgh: University of Edinburgh, 1965).

Portugal fell victim in 1833, when an English ship of Polish volunteers arrived to fight for the liberal cause in the Portuguese civil war. In light of this event, Spain applied a rigid system of quarantines but was infected in August of 1833 and 1834, suffering 100,000 victims. By means of Catalonia it entered France and over the next two years passed through southern France and much of Italy, leaving 236,473 victims from 1834 to 1837. In 1837, it killed close to 3,000 people on the island of Malta.

It spread over China from 1826 to 1835, entering Malaysia and Singapore in 1826, and Japan in 1831.

The Third Pandemic (1845–1859). The third pandemic occurred during the years 1845 to 1859, although some authors list it from 1839 to 1861. In 1845 cholera broke out again in Bengal with a bidirectional projection towards Arabia in 1846 (Aden and Djeddah), arriving in Mecca in November, Mesopotamia (Baghdad, September 1846) and at the coast of the Black Sea (Tibilissi, July 1847). From there it propagated towards Turkey, hitting Istanbul in autumn 1847 and principalities of the Danube and Central Europe in 1848. In the spring of 1848, it was found in Norway, Finland, and the north of Germany; it then reached Berlin, and later Holland. From Rotterdam the illness passed through Belgium and Ireland in 1848. A ship from Hamburg, a port that suffered 5,400 victims, brought the disease to England in 1848–1849 (62,000 dead), to which it returned in 1854. In 1849 it appeared in Austria, Switzerland, and France (110,000 victims). From there it passed to Algeria. Austrian troops brought it to northern Italy (24,000 victims) in 1848–1849.

In the beginning of the 1850s, the pandemic resurged with new strength. In 1852 it invaded regions that had escaped its wrath, for example, the south of Germany. During the years 1854–1855, France and Italy were left with 146,000 and 248,514 dead, respectively. The Crimean War permitted cholera's arrival at major Mediterranean ports like Ancona and Naples in Italy. The mobilization of English, French, and Italian troops towards the Black Sea brought cholera to Bulgaria, Greece, and Turkey. In Spain, the spread of the epidemic in 1855 was one of the most lethal of the nineteenth century. It extended from the Mediterranean coast to the interior (236,744 victims; 1.5 percent of the population). From there it arrived again in Morocco and Algeria.

In December 1848, cholera appeared in the port cities of the United States and affected 5,000 New York residents. From the ports it spread rapidly along the rivers, canals, railroad lines, and stagecoach routes, bringing it to far-reaching areas. The main outbreak was in 1848 and 1849 and was followed by a series of sporadic outbreaks over the next six years. New Orleans, for example lost 5,000 people from 1850 to 1855. It went up the Mississippi, toward California, and toward southeastern Mexico, where it claimed 200,000 victims. In 1854 and 1855 it entered Venezuela; Brazil also suffered in 1855.

From Bengal, cholera arrived at Singapore in 1852, and from there it spread to China and Japan in 1854, the Philippines in 1858, and Korea in 1859. It ravaged Egypt from 1853 to 1858 and advanced towards Sudan and Eritrea. In 1859 Zanzibar, Mozambique, and Madagascar were affected.

Factors in Cholera's Spread.   Cholera's origin was in Bengal where it endemically appeared every year. Water was the fundamental vehicle of transmission, as a result of the persistent pollution of the Ganges's water, the abandonment of large ancient hydraulic works, the custom of leaving cadavers in the river, the general lack of hygenic conditions, and the domestic use of water reservoirs that were exposed to the air and contaminated with excrement and urine. Even these factors, however, do not explain the expanse it reached in the nineteenth century. Military expeditions and English attempts to extend colonial influence in India were fundamental during the first pandemic of 1817. The routes taken by the British East India Company's army were similar to those along which cholera spread. Troop movements also permitted the extension of cholera throughout the world. For example, when British troops participated in the war in Burma (1823) cholera appeared; when Russian troops marched toward Poland (1831), cholera infected their path until their arrival in Warsaw; Polish troops arriving to fight in the Portuguese civil war introduced the illness; General J. R. Rodil (1789–1853) advanced through Spain spreading cholera; and troops dispatched to fight in the Crimean War spread the disease toward Eastern Europe. But military campaigns are only part of the story. It is undeniable that cholera is an indicator of hygienic sanitation of a population. In this sense, the English conquest affected Indian society because it disrupted ancient systems of living, changing social solidarity and making survival more difficult.

Another argument for cholera's rapid and wide dispersion was the creation of new markets. Cholera was a great example of the diffusion of an illness along international trade routes, especially those connected with British imperial activity. The rise of British naval commerce in Bombay after 1815, which converted the city into the hub of many important maritime routes, allowed the advance of cholera toward the Persian Gulf and the Mediterranean, Caspian, and Baltic Seas. When ships from cholera-affected ports reached their destinations, cholera quickly spread. This is what occurred in the Mediterranean in 1854, with the arrival of ships at Messina for the invasion of Sicily and the ships moored in the port of Piraeus that infected Greece, which, after stopping in Gallipolis left cholera to be spread to the Dardenelles, Istanbul, and Varna. British control in the ports of Calcutta and Madras produced similar results in China, Taiwan, the Philippines, Tonkin, Vietnam, Java, Sumatra, Thailand, and Myanmar. As the means of transportation grew faster, the speed of disease propagation directly corresponded.

Cholera's spread was also facilitated by migration and temporary displacements like pilgrimages to Mecca and Medina, which allowed pilgrims to afflict places along their journey home.

Reactions.   During the nineteenth century, cholera was more than just an illness. It was also a social and political question because the diffusion of germs and subversive ideas went hand in hand. The epidemic revealed as much social animosity as it caused political confrontation.

After cholera arrived in England in October of 1831, a famous riot took place at the Swan Street Hospital in Manchester. Several thousands of people freed cholera patients believed to be the targets of homicidal doctors. This situation was repeated in other places in Europe. In the United States, in 1832 initial medical reports in New York City were ignored because of fear of the social and economic problems they would cause (although sanitary measures were adopted later). The sickness affected the poor above all, and **poverty** was popularly associated with vice. Hence, the idea emerged that cholera attacked those who were immoral. For this reason, religious leaders from the entire country appealed for prayer and fasting in hopes of a divine intervention. This approach was repeated in the epidemics of 1849 and 1854, although by then Americans were associating cholera with the poverty of Irish immigrants spurred by the **Irish potato famine**. What many overlooked was that these people were not affected by cholera because they were immigrants but because of they lived in deficient conditions. Finally, however, many resorted to the age-old response to epidemic disease: **flight**.

Historical Effects.   From the beginning of the eighteenth century, the number of doctors defending a contagion model for the spread of cholera increased. From this emerged the clash between supporters of this theory (contagionists) and the defenders of another, the anticontagionists, who believed its spread was airborne and was the result of environmental causes. Contagionists believed in the transmission of the illness through human-to-human contact or animal-to-human contact (as **Girolamo Frascatoro** had described in 1546 with his idea of invisible seeds). They believed that isolation, quarantines, and *cordons sanitaires* were adequate measures to avoid its spread. On the contrary, the anticontagionists held that the illness was propagated by respiratory emissions of the patient into environmental agents like air and water, from which others contracted it. They therefore opposed quarantines and proposed public sanitation and hygiene as an alternative.

When the affliction reached Europe in 1831, doctors tried to identify the manners of propagation and specify the nature and treatment they should adopt for cholera. They also advocated for public adoption of the measures dictated by their opinions on the nature of the disease. This led to constant conflict between contagionists like William Budd (1811–1880) and **John Snow** (at least initially) and anticontagionists like **Edwin Chadwick**, Southwood Smith (1786–1861), and **Rudolf Virchow**, though the opinion of the second group prevailed for much of the century.

Medical and political positions were allied. Wealthy merchants who worried about delivering their merchandise and governments in post-revolutionary Europe that sought to avoid alarming the population, allowed anticontagionism to triumph momentarily. Quarantine and all measures that impeded the liberty of exchange were abolished until the agent of transmission was identified.

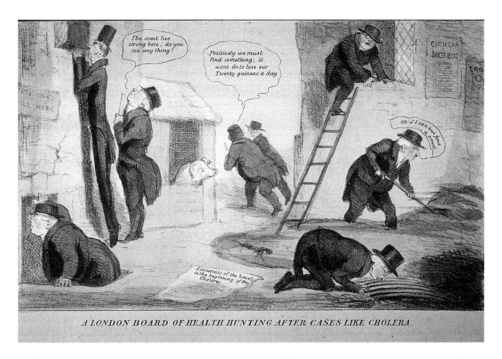

A LONDON BOARD OF HEALTH HUNTING AFTER CASES LIKE CHOLERA.

Officials from the London Board of Health "sniff" out the causes of cholera. Courtesy of the National Library of Medicine.

Though investigators like Budd, Snow, and Filippo Pacini (1812–1883) suspected the existence of a specific germ that caused the disease, it was not until 1883 that Robert Koch isolated and cultivated *V. cholerae*. In 1854, the Florentine Pacini discovered that various infected intestines contained a type of bacteria that he considered the cause of the epidemic. However, because he published his conclusions in a journal with only limited circulation, the significance of his discovery remained hidden.

The English physician John Snow already suspected during the epidemic in London of 1834 that cholera was transmitted essentially by water, but he lacked conclusive evidence. When cholera broke out again in 1848, he started an investigation that he published the following year. He explained his belief that poor sanitation and unclean water were tied to the epidemic. The Industrial Revolution increased the amount of urban housing and had terribly deteriorated the sanitary conditions of large cities. In 1854 he was able to demonstrate a common denominator between deaths from cholera in London, with his famous study of the Broad Street well. The discovery of the relationship between contaminated water and cholera created a model for explaining the transmission of the disease. It also demonstrated the necessity of public intervention with regard to general sanitation.

Determination of the factors affecting the contraction and spread of cholera during the nineteenth century began to be an obsession for Europeans and Americans because they were important elements for the investigation and solution of more general public

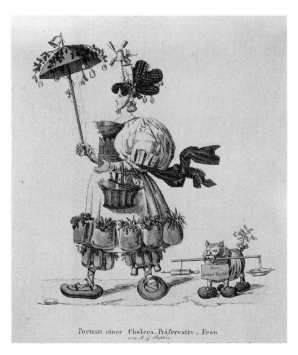

Portrait einer Cholera-Präfervativ-Frau
von M. y. Sophie.

A woman extravagantly equipped to deal with the cholera epidemic of 1832; satirizing the abundance of dubious advice on how to combat cholera. The animal's sign reads "Only no fear." German etching, c. 1832. Courtesy of Wellcome Library, London.

health problems. The consequences were significant because they consolidated the convictions of the sanitationists, who gained increasing influence over governments. They carried out the fight against the unhealthiness of cities with regular collection of refuse, the enclosure of open sewers, water filtration, and the progressive reform of housing conditions. These measures were accompanied by campaigns that strengthened a growing sense of the importance of **personal hygiene** in the battle against disease. The early cholera epidemics constituted a spur for practical conduct that was channeled through every nation and on an international level. For example, in England, after the outbreak of 1848, the General Board of Health was created, and in the United States, the quarantine officially established in ports in 1878 was a direct result of the 1873 epidemic. Action alone was not effective unless it was met by collaboration from other countries, and therefore a series of international conferences was convened. In 1851 the sanitary authorities of 14 European nations gathered to hold the world's first Sanitary Conference, a predecessor of the **World Health Organization**. *See also* Cholera before the Pandemics; Cholera: Fourth through Sixth Pandemics, 1862–1947; Cholera: Seventh Pandemic, 1961–Present; International Health Agencies and Conventions; Public Health Agencies in Britain since 1800.

Futher Reading

Arnol, Davis. *Science, Technology & Medicine in Colonial India*. New York: Cambridge University Press, 2000.

Baldwin, Peter. *Contagion and the State in Europe, 1830–1930*. New York: Cambridge University Press, 1999.

Bewell, Alan. *Romanticism and Colonial Disease*. Baltimore: Johns Hopkins University Press, 2000.

Evans, Richard J. *Death in Hamburg: Society and Politics in the Cholera Years, 1830–1910*. New York: Penguin, 2005.

Harvard University Library. *Contagion*. http://ocp.hul.harvard.edu/contagion/cholera.html

Hempel, Sandra. *The Strange Case of the Broad Street Pump: John Snow and the Mystery of Cholera*. Berkeley: University of California Press, 2007.

Kudlick, Catherine J. *Cholera in Post-Revolutionary Paris: A Cultural History*. Berkeley: University of California Press, 1996.

McGrew, Roderick E. *Russia and the Cholera, 1823–1832.* Madison: University of Wisconsin Press, 1965.

Morris, Robert John. *Cholera, 1832: The Social Response to an Epidemic.* Teaneck, NJ: Holmes and Meier, 1976.

Rosenberg, Charles E. *The Cholera Years: The United States in 1832, 1849, and 1866.* Chicago: University of Chicago Press, 1987.

DONATO GÓMEZ-DÍAZ

CHOLERA: FOURTH THROUGH SIXTH PANDEMICS, 1862–1947. Modern usage reserves **cholera** as a term to describe the acute diarrheal disease caused by *Vibrio cholerae*, the comma-shaped **bacterium** first recognized by the Italian scientist Filippo Pacini (1812–1883) in Florence in 1854, and discovered by **Robert Koch** to be the cholera's causative agent during January 1884 in Calcutta, India. Contemporary Europeans after 1816 labeled what for them was a new disease "Asiatic cholera," though a variety had probably been endemic from ancient times in the Ganges Delta. Before 1920 it was still a lethal disease, although in the most industrialized countries it later became a nuisance no longer to be feared. From the time of the fifth **pandemic** (1881–1896), improved sanitation in Europe and the Americas began to diminish cholera's global impact, a trend that continued until the sixth pandemic (1899–1947) began to wane in the 1920s. The last major international cholera emergency of the sixth pandemic occurred in Egypt in 1947.

Documentary evidence for the fourth through sixth pandemics in the West is rich. For the fourth pandemic (1862–1879), cholera's terrible trajectory in West Africa has left almost no documentary trace. But East Africa, Zanzibar, and the Indian Ocean are well served by means of the remarkable, horrific eye-witness account (1876) left by James Christie (fl. 1865–1873), who was then physician to the Sultan of Zanzibar.

With no effective treatment for classic cholera, nineteenth-century case fatality rates (CFRs) of 50 percent and mortality of over 100 per 1,000 population were common. Human susceptibility to this spectacular disease varied widely. People with blood types other than O and those with high levels of acidity in the digestive tract were less vulnerable and often asymptomatic, but their opposites were subject to alarming sickness. Immunity rarely persisted longer than a year or two.

Cholera's cause is the ingestion of an infectious dose of a serogroup of the *V. cholerae* bacterium present in **water** or food that has been contaminated either by fecal matter from an infected person or from free-standing bacteria present in plankton or seafood living in infected brackish water. The bacteria then multiply and attach themselves to the lining of the human bowel, producing an enterotoxin poison that interferes with the absorption of water, salts, and other electrolytes into the large intestine. In 20 percent of cases, a severe illness results, manifested by profuse watery diarrhea and repeated vomiting, leading to rapid loss of body fluids and salts. Feces and vomit easily infect water, soil, or food and result in a highly contagious stage. Severe dehydration, circulatory collapse, and death can result in a matter of hours without treatment.

The worst of diarrheal infections, cholera remains a fearful disease, deeply embedded in the collective memory of many societies globally. The serotype probably responsible for the first six cholera pandemics was *V. cholerae* O1, called "classical." A new strain, *V. cholerae*

O1 El Tor, less virulent but producing more asymptomatic infections, was responsible for the seventh cholera pandemic, which began in Sulawesi, Indonesia, in 1961.

For most of the nineteenth century, medical remedies for cholera remained as varied, and often downright harmful, as they were ineffective. Instead of replenishing fluids and electrolytes, misguided treatments often involved accelerated loss through purging, and the administration of alcohol, morphine, and other undesirable practices. Since the 1960s, fortunately, the development of improved rehydration techniques has reduced CFRs well below 20 percent, and often even below 1 percent. Even before, beginning with the fifth pandemic in 1881, cholera had begun to retreat from the most industrialized societies. This retreat, moreover, became a virtual disappearance as a result of improvements in standards of living that included welfare state reforms in housing, public health, and nutrition.

Origins and Spread.   The first pandemic (1817–1825), after spreading havoc in India during 1817, had reached throughout Asia soon after. Europe and the Americas were spared, and the impact on the regions of the Middle East and Africa was probably milder than subsequent visitations. Diffusion took place by land and sea, and was closely linked to **trade** and to **warfare**. The second (1827–1838) and third (1839–1861) pandemics followed a similar path, crossed over to the Americas, and were far more devastating.

Innovations in transportation like the railway and faster ocean navigation assisted cholera's spread after 1862, as did numerous annual **pilgrimages** and fairs related to the Hindu and Muslim faiths. Once the Suez Canal opened in 1869, Muslim pilgrims could board a passenger vessel taking them through the Canal and to the southeastern corner of the Mediterranean at Alexandria in a week.

In what retrospectively became the start of the fourth pandemic in 1862, cholera once again left the Ganges Delta, heading this time for Indonesia. By 1864 cholera had again exploded on the world scene in what was one of its most devastating decades until it burned itself out by 1873. With the exception of China and Japan from 1877 through 1879, the world was once again free of cholera. The worst pilgrimage outbreak ever in Mecca during 1865 marked the fourth pandemic when 15,000 of the estimated 90,000 pilgrims died. Also severe was cholera's association with the Hindu pilgrimage to Hardwar, India, two years later, when half of the quarter of a million visitors succumbed. Another feature was that cholera reached Europe not through Russia and overland, but by water via the Mediterranean into southern France and Italy.

The fourth pandemic probably killed more people than any other, and the years between 1865 and 1867 were exceptionally devastating in all corners of the globe. East Asia, the Middle East, and Europe reeled from successive blows, and the pandemic was Africa's worst of the nineteenth century. Cholera not only revisited sites in North and East Africa, but also made its maiden voyage to West Africa. The African invasions came from a variety of sources. Ships carried cholera from Bombay via Aden to Eritrea and Somalia, and then caravans transported the pathogen into the Ethiopian highlands from the port of Massawa on the Red Sea coast. In Ethiopia, cholera was indirectly responsible for a large shift in the distribution of the population.

From 1865 through to 1871, cholera worked its way down the East African coast by a variety of means. Overland, it reached the Great Lakes of Africa through Masai country in Kenya, and then moved south to Tanzania and the bustling city and island of Zanzibar, devastating that great market city with an estimated 70,000 deaths in 1869–1870. Indian Ocean sailing vessels engaged in coastal trade also carried cholera down through the Swahili ports to its southern limits just short of Delagoa Bay at Quelimane. Cholera also journeyed southeast to the Indian Ocean islands of Mauritius, the Seychelles, the Comoros, Nossi-be, and the Malagasy port of Majunga.

Beginning in 1865, cholera traveled across North Africa all the way west to Morocco, spreading from both Mecca and southern Europe. Tunisia's 1867 outbreak began with smugglers returning from Sicily. That same year, cholera traveled from France to Algeria and killed 80,000.

In November 1868, cholera spread from Algeria to Senegal (whether overland or by sea is not clear). In this, its first call ever to West Africa, cholera wreaked havoc in the small French colonial capital of Saint-Louis, and then reached inland to the Upper Senegal Valley. There, its arrival coincided with the rise of an Islamic messianic movement called *madiyanké*. Its leader pointed to the deaths of Fulbe tribal notables as punishment for collaborating with the French infidels. From the Senegal Valley, cholera traveled south through village after village among the Wolof states, reached Malinke country in the Upper Gambia River Valley in 1869, and penetrated south on the Atlantic coast as far as Portuguese Guinea.

In western and northern Europe, cholera casualties were lower, but by no means insignificant. In the dreadful year 1866, Sweden, Britain, Holland, and Belgium lost tens of thousands each. Even though it had not been the first visited, Russia eventually recorded significant deaths during the fourth pandemic. In the Mediterranean, Italy became infected through its eastern port of Ancona, France through Marseilles, and Spain through Valencia and Murcia. From these launching points, cholera easily made its way into the continent, facilitated by the significant movement of troops involved in a series of conflicts in the 1860s. Austria's war with Prussia in 1866 led to widespread outbreaks and deaths.

High death rates were also noted in the Americas. In the aftermath of the American Civil War (1861–1865), while large numbers of soldiers were still in military camps such as the one in Newport, Kentucky, cholera invaded the United States in May of 1866 through the ports of New York and New Orleans. That year, an estimated 50,000 persons died from cholera from the East Coast and the Gulf of Mexico as far west as Texas and New Mexico. Though it was not perceived at the time, these would be cholera's final visits to North America. Meanwhile, Canada and Mexico were almost entirely spared from cholera during the fourth pandemic.

Death tolls in the Caribbean, on the other hand, were high. Cholera made its way to Guadaloupe from Marseilles in 1865–1866, claiming 12,000 victims among a population of only 150,000. In South America, war abetted *V. cholerae*'s spread. Paraguayan troops engaged in a conflict against combined forces from Argentina and Brazil were overwhelmed by an outbreak in April of 1866. The war's victors also suffered epidemics, as did Uruguay and Peru.

The fifth pandemic was far less widespread globally. Especially in the North Atlantic world, many countries, applying hard-won lessons of sanitarianism concerning prevention through improved water systems, had seen the last of classic cholera during either the third or the fourth pandemic. Yet where cholera did strike after 1881, it continued to do so with great intensity, indicating that treatment had not improved at all.

Cholera launched its fifth escape from its endemic home in the Ganges Delta in 1881. In East Asia, unlike Europe and the Americas, the fifth pandemic was the worst on record. In Japan, where epidemiology was emerging as a discipline and where registrations of cholera infections were now being accurately tallied, seven separate outbreaks between 1881 and 1895 produced 340,000 cases. Anxious to respond with Western sanitary tools, the Meiji government addressed urban drinking water and sewage in legislation between 1878 and 1890. Numbers are not available for Japan's neighbors, but most endured multiple outbreaks between 1881 and 1895. China had six; Indonesia and Korea had five each; the Philippines had two; and Sri Lanka, Thailand, and Malaysia might have considered themselves fortunate to have suffered one visitation each.

The fifth pandemic arrived in Mecca from India's Punjab in 1881 and struck again the following year. Once again, the toll was terrible, estimated at over 30,000 dead among 200,000 pilgrims. From there, the infection quickly spread to Egypt, which experienced two waves. Over 16,000 Egyptians died during the second wave in 1895–1896, the last visitation of the disease until after the Second World War. Foreigners were not immune. In 1895, before the British garrison could withdraw from Cairo to Suez, it suffered through a nightmarish 139 deaths among its 183 cases. Only then did the British dramatically improve the water supply for troops in Cairo and Alexandria.

This second wave disseminating directly or indirectly from the Mecca pilgrimage meant almost certainly that pilgrims would again carry cholera back to North Africa. The pathogen appeared across North Africa spreading to Morocco in the early 1890s. From Morocco, cholera was able to make its way by caravan across the Sahara and into the Senegal Valley of West Africa in 1893–1894. The fifth pandemic also touched the Horn of Africa in this same period when it followed a terrible famine in the Ethiopian highlands and Eritrea. Known in Amharic as *ye nefas beshita*, "the disease of the wind," cholera added its misery to what was already a devastating rinderpest epizootic which was then killing most of the draft animals in Ethiopia.

By 1884 the Mediterranean ports of Toulon, Marseilles, Palermo, and Genoa were infected. In 1885 there were serious epidemics throughout Spain. Italy tried a **quarantine**, but a major outbreak at Naples claimed over 5,000, and the disease remained widespread for the next two years. In central Europe the fifth pandemic brought cholera only to Germany. Hamburg in 1892 suffered 7,582 deaths among 19,891 cases in an infamous epidemic that was directly traced to the city's poor water supply. Sporadic cholera struck another 250 German communities.

The cholera scene in Russia remained grim in the 1890s, and its victims possibly included the illustrious composer Peter Ilyich Tchaikovsky (1840–1893). Entering from Afghanistan and Persia, cholera reached Moscow and St. Petersburg, and moved on to the empire's western borders. Only in Russia did a phenomenon of earlier pandemics persist—peasant revolts against authority. Cholera in 1892 followed a famine the previous year and brought with it a familiar trail of riot, murder, and angry attacks on government and medical officials. Tsarists were still rigidly enforcing quarantine, isolation, and **disinfection** on the shoulders of an impoverished peasantry, and the medical profession had little success in educating peasants about the value of preventive measures.

Rare as well as mild outbreaks were the norm in the Americas during the fifth pandemic. The closest North America came to disaster was when eight badly infected ships arrived in the port of New York in 1892, but careful inspection and control resulted in only ten cases in the city. In the far south of the Americas, between 1893 and 1895, mild outbreaks occurred in Brazil, Uruguay, and Argentina.

The sixth pandemic began in 1899, after a hiatus of three years, and continued to be benign in the West and more sporadic elsewhere than earlier visitations. Arguably fewer people were dying from cholera, and effective rehydration treatments were just beginning to be developed.

In Europe the new pandemic proceeded from east to west following a pattern identical to previous visitations. Most Europeans never saw the dreaded disease; only Italy and Russia were exceptions. In Italy, a cholera disaster coincided with efforts at political consolidation in the new Republic. Both the epidemics of 1884 and 1910–1911 were implicated in such national issues as the "Southern Question," mass emigration, organized crime, and urban renewal. Cholera in Russia was more continuous. Turmoil, revolution, and civil war abetted cholera enormously during the years from 1902 to 1925. The cities of St. Petersburg, Jekaterinoslav, Kiev, and Orenburg all suffered terribly during the civil wars. Outside of South Asia, no region suffered greater losses from cholera than the vast Russian Empire. Its recorded total of 5,537,358 cases and 2,140,558 deaths, undoubtedly under-reported, included cholera outbreaks in no less than 58 of the 103 years between 1823 and 1926. Nevertheless, as the Red Army consolidated political power after the Bolshevik Revolution in 1917, cholera began to wane. The last bad year was 1922.

War was also cholera's handmaiden in central and southeastern Europe. Beginning with the Balkan Wars of 1912–1913 and continuing through the First World War and its aftermath, Romania, Serbia, Bulgaria, and Turkey all had to cope with the unwelcome presence of V. cholerae.

Triumphs there clearly were. Newly sanitized Japan mastered control of the disease, and North Africa, the Indian Ocean, Sub-Saharan Africa, most of Europe, and the Americas were virtually cholera-free during the sixth pandemic. The Second World War did not cause much cholera anxiety, despite the dramatic increase in air travel. The Egyptian cholera outbreak of 1947 may have been an exception as it did have a link to aviation. Cholera's sudden appearance in Egypt during September 1947 caught cholera experts everywhere by surprise. Its origins are obscure, but returning pilgrims were not involved this time. Some authorities suspected air travelers from India to Egyptian airfields run by the British. Among the first cholera victims were laborers working at the airfields near El Korein. The town of 15,000 on the eastern fringe of the Nile Delta and close to the Suez Canal was also the site of an annual fair, when thousands of date merchants gathered from all over Egypt and beyond. Also billeted there in 1947 were the 6,000 workmen from the British airfield. The panicked departure of laborers, together with merchants, helped spread cholera throughout Egypt before any local controls could be enforced.

Others who suffered terribly, this time at the beginning of the sixth pandemic, were the people living in the Philippines archipelago of over 7,000 scattered islands. Although no stranger to cholera, this locale suffered its worst cholera experience between 1902 and 1904 when it lost as many as 200,000 of its population of 7.6 million to the dreaded disease. The outbreak struck just as a three-year insurrection against American annexation was ending. The Philippine-American War took 800,000 additional Filipino lives and played a key role in exacerbating the impact of cholera. It is difficult to draw a line between the American war to subdue the Philippines and efforts to "conquer" cholera.

After the 1920s, with a few exceptions, cholera again retreated to its home waters in the Ganges Delta. Many medical historians in fact date the end of the sixth pandemic to the year 1923.

Reactions.   In Eastern Europe and Russia, so deeply embedded did cholera become in collective memory that the very term *kholera*, or *kholeria*, became a synonym for disaster in the Russian, Polish, and Yiddish languages. What was remarkable was that, as the rest of Europe steadily moved away from irrational and panic-inspired responses, in Russia little change occurred. The government reforms in all spheres, including public health and cholera control, remained sporadic and uninspired.

The final watershed for cholera in Europe was the devastating cholera outbreak that struck the major German port of Hamburg in 1892. This sad story demonstrated the risks involved in postponing the improvement of water services. Ironically, Hamburg had been a pioneer in sanitarianism, and was one of the first cities in Europe to introduce a centralized water supply and a sewage system in 1842. By the 1880s, however, Hamburg and Munich were the only holdouts against contagionist and bacteriological approaches in Germany. An old free city and self-governing in the new Second German Reich, Hamburg continued to draw its drinking water from the Elbe without treatment. Adjacent Altona, part of the Prussian State, had by 1892 introduced a modern water filtration plant. Altona was entirely spared during the 1892 epidemic, whereas Hamburg suffered roughly 7,500 deaths among over 19,000 cases in slightly over six weeks. After this dramatic confirmation of **germ theory**, Hamburg city fathers could no longer thwart public health reforms.

The tragedy at Hamburg also helped reinforce the American public health movement, which was already moving forward at full speed. As Hamburg was enduring its disaster, public health officials used their testing and quarantine powers to identify the first carriers arriving in New York that summer from Europe. A handful escaped but were tracked down by an army of health department staff and volunteers. Health workers also filled toilets and privies with disinfectants. As a result, only 10 people died of cholera in New York in 1892.

In Italy, a cholera disaster early in the sixth pandemic evoked popular emotions only seen in Europe almost a century earlier. The summer of 1910 saw cholera riots, attacks on physicians, mass panic and flights from cities, a return of religiosity and superstition, and sometimes furious rage directed against gypsies, who were the favorite **scapegoats** for the medical disaster.

Historical Effects.   As the fourth pandemic raged, the growth of scientific knowledge about cholera proved disappointing. A British physician, **John Snow**, in a remarkable epidemiological undertaking, used London's cholera epidemic of 1853 to argue that contaminated drinking water was the cause of this dread disease. But Snow's reasoning was not anchored in scientific proof, and scoffers at his waterborne theory remained long in the majority. Advances in technology, whether for shipping or warfare, seemed only to have benefited cholera's diffusion. Rapid sea transport led to major cholera outbreaks aboard ships and in quarantine stations at points of entry in the new world like New York, New Orleans, or Halifax, Nova Scotia. Faster travel only made the consequences of the Muslim pilgrimage worse. Meanwhile wars in Europe and the Americas continued to serve as cholera's allies.

Efforts to contain and control cholera were, however, not hopeless. Sanitarian successes in the United States were impressive, and smaller initiatives in Europe, India, China, and Japan were bearing fruit. In the Western enclave of Shanghai, China, cholera was much reduced through precautions such as the boiling of water. In 1870 the wealthy expatriate community there also invested in a 10-year campaign for a pure water supply. In Japan under the Meiji Restoration, the government by 1879 had modernized sanitary surveillance and created an improved water supply according to the Western model.

Scientific understanding finally began to advance with a breakthrough achieved by Robert Koch and his German research team in Egypt and India in 1883–1884. However, although the team succeeded in isolating the cholera bacillus, many in the scientific community remained unconvinced by Koch's research. Koch's opponents were able to neutralize his arguments, but they could not for long refute them. His identification of the bacillus was a major advance because it made possible the use of the laboratory to test for the disease even among asymptomatic carriers. He was also a strong advocate of state intervention in public health, and a believer in quarantine, isolation, disinfection, and the policing of the water supply.

Treatment and therapy based on the new epidemiology of cholera mushroomed in the 1880s and 1890s, even if success was elusive. Vaccine therapy, owing much to the enthusiasm for immunization generated by **Louis Pasteur**, began in Spain during a major cholera outbreak in 1885 when a Catalan physician named Jaime Ferrán y Clúa (1851–1929) became the first to apply Pasteurian principles when he inoculated over 40,000 Spaniards. A French commission of investigation impugned Ferrán's vaccine and methods. Although shortcomings certainly existed, theirs was an excessively harsh judgement on a pioneering medical microbiologist working in the very early days of **immunology**.

Experiments did not stop in Spain. Most successful of these early microbiologists was **Waldemar Haffkine**, a Jewish Ukrainian Pasteurian. From 1890 he began working at the Pasteur Institute in Paris on a live anticholera vaccine that required two doses. Between 1893 and 1896 in India, he was the first to conduct genuine field trials, mainly among laborers on tea estates, British troops, children in boarding schools and orphanages, and inmates of nine civil jails.

Haffkine's results were also mixed. His vaccine produced immunity against acquiring cholera but was of no therapeutic value if the disease had already been acquired. One serious problem was his difficulty in producing the vaccine in large quantities and standardizing it. The problem which haunted vaccine therapy then and now was that it could not eradicate cholera by producing the herd immunity effect, achieved when a threshold of 80 percent immunity makes the disease unable to persist.

In Europe, studies of the effectiveness of cholera inoculations during conflict in the Balkans and among First World War armies found that **vaccination** was not statistically significant either in preventing cholera or in shortening the length of time that recuperating patients remained carriers. New studies in Calcutta by 1928, however, came out more strongly in favor of cholera vaccination. By the late 1940s, international health experts recommended vaccination, especially in times of pilgrimage, war, or social breakdown, when regular sanitary measures could not be used.

Mass vaccination during the first half of the twentieth century became a popular, easily grasped, and visible indication that health authorities were doing something. Yet this very popularity became a danger insofar as it instilled a false sense of security. Vaccination could neither eradicate cholera nor provide herd immunity, and it was less effective than the provision of safe water in controlling the disease.

Improved international surveillance and cooperation did slowly evolve during the sixth pandemic. The good offices of International Office of Public Hygiene (IOPH) under the League of Nations, and of the **World Health Organization** (WHO) through the United Nations after its creation in 1948, were the chief agencies of this improved approach. Two control elements were safety of the water supply and surveillance of potential carriers. The first was associated with chlorination, a standard procedure where more permanent guarantees of safe water could not be met. The second, sometimes problematic, involved stool examination of suspected carriers, a procedure that only developed with the advance of a scientific means of carrying out the laboratory work. Yet even as early as 1926, the scientific consensus of the cholera subcommittee of the IOPH in Geneva declared this procedure to be of dubious value. Later, the WHO agreed. In its 1951 revision of International Sanitary Regulations, it dropped stringent rules for stool examination.

Without doubt, potentially the most important breakthrough in treatment of cholera patients was the advance in rehydration therapy during the sixth pandemic. Sir Leonard Rogers (1868–1962) of the Indian Medical Service pioneered in the administration of a hypertonic saline supplement with alkali and potassium combined with purified water. In some instances, this new technique reduced mortality by one-quarter to one-third. Rogers lent his services to the city of Palermo during the Italian cholera emergency of 1910 and was able to reduce CFRs to below 20 percent, something of a miracle compared with alarming rates in Naples and other Italian cities of the day. Later recognition that glucose added to salts helped stricken patients keep down orally administered solutions was yet another milestone.

Nevertheless, potential cholera victims would have to wait half a century until rehydration became a widespread therapy. Only with the development of simple orally administered rehydration solutions to replace more technically complicated intravenous procedures during the seventh cholera pandemic after 1968 did CFRs fall to 1 percent and below, making cholera no longer a fatal disease, provided treatment was timely.

Cholera continued as a serious endemic disease in colonial India, but it seemed no longer to be spreading internationally as the twentieth century progressed. A congratulatory note sounded internationally as the sixth pandemic faded almost from sight by mid-century, and some even declared that new knowledge of the etiology of disease and effective controls meant that the sixth cholera pandemic would be the world's last. Few in the WHO or in research institutions envisioned how a changing global ecology would permit a modified cholera pathogen to establish a free-standing and permanent niche in marine habitats not just in the Ganges Delta but in brackish water environments on several continents, and launch the seventh pandemic in 1961, one that shows little sign of abating at the present time. *See also* Cholera before the Pandemics; Cholera: First through Third Pandemics, 1816–1861; Cholera: Seventh Pandemic, 1961–Present.

Further Reading

Arnold, David. *Colonizing the Body: State Medicine and Epidemic Disease in Nineteenth-Century India.* Berkeley: University of California Press, 1993.

"Cholera Morbus" advertisement printed in *Harper's Weekly*, July 17, 1863. Courtesy of the National Library of Medicine.

De Bevoise, Ken. *Agents of Apocalypse: Epidemic Disease in the Colonial Philippines*. Princeton: Princeton University Press, 1995.

Evans, Richard J. *Death in Hamburg: Society and Politics in the Cholera Years*, 2nd edition. New York: Penguin, 2005.

Harrison, Mark. "Quarantine, Pilgrimage, and Colonial Trade: India 1866–1900." *Indian Economic and Social History Review* 29 (1992): 117–144.

Hays, J. N. *The Burdens of Disease: Epidemics and Human Response in Western History*. New Brunswick: Rutgers University Press, 1998.

Howard-Jones, Norman. *The Scientific Background of the International Scientific Conferences, 1851–1938*. Geneva: WHO, 1974.

Pollitzer, Robert. *Cholera*. Geneva: WHO, 1959.

Snowden, Frank M. *Naples in the Time of Cholera, 1884–1911*. New York: Cambridge University Press, 1995.

MYRON ECHENBERG

CHOLERA: SEVENTH PANDEMIC, 1961–PRESENT.   The seventh **pandemic** has coincided with the phenomenon of globalization, with which it is intimately linked. **Cholera epidemics** have become for some a litmus test of whether a national state possesses a modernized public health system. Alternative explanations would suggest that when cholera has been absent from one place for a century but present elsewhere, international connections to its etiology, not unsanitary practices in the region, constitute a more profitable area of investigation. Second, a wider historical perspective reveals how the economic restructuring of the 1980s weakened populations and helped make the outbreak in Peru and elsewhere so severe.

The seventh cholera pandemic was different from the first six in several respects. Its agent was a new variant of the cholera pathogen *Vibrio cholerae* 01 El Tor. El Tor held lower virulence for humans, enabling less severely ill patients to be more mobile and, therefore, to have the capacity to infect others over a longer period of time. Moving more slowly than cholera pandemics of the nineteenth century, the seventh pandemic had the greatest geographic span and made use of the fastest new technology (air travel), yet lasted longer than any earlier pandemics. At present, it shows no signs of abating.

The mildness and diminishing impact of the sixth cholera pandemic (1899–1947) had led many to believe that they had seen the last of this terrible scourge. Suddenly, in January of 1961, *V. cholerae* O1 El Tor began to spread from its starting point around Makassar on the large island of Sulawesi, Indonesia.

El Tor moved slowly, first through southern Chinese and Southeast Asian locales, and then to India in 1964. Over the rest of the decade, it followed a familiar nineteenth-century route to western Asia. By 1966 it was present on the borders of the Asian republics of the Soviet Union. The first global phase began in earnest in 1970 when cholera El Tor reached everywhere in the Middle East, struck the Soviet Black Sea ports of Odessa and Kerch, and hit West Africa hard. At this stage, the new wave of cholera spared the Americas and most of Europe, though it infected such old haunts of southern Europe as Lisbon, Barcelona, and Naples, allegedly carried from North Africa by seasonal workers and tourists. In the early 1990s, Russia, Romania, and a few other former Soviet bloc countries saw cholera's return.

A mild appearance of cholera at the Islamic holy site of Mecca, Saudi Arabia, in 1974 aroused concern from health authorities with historical memories of how **pilgrims** had involuntarily helped spread the disease in the nineteenth century. Fortunately, only a few cases were diagnosed among the 1 million Mecca pilgrims, and the disease did not spread from there. Sporadic but serious outbreaks occurred in the Kathmandu valley of Nepal. **War** zones like the Kabul region of Afghanistan also produced cholera flare-ups, but on nothing like the African scale.

The Americas, beginning with Peru in 1991, experienced a public health shock from which they are only now recovering: the first appearance of cholera in almost a hundred years. This time, the disease spread widely in South and Central America, and was present for a decade in Peru. Health officials everywhere were aghast at the force of cholera's impact on the Americas. A watershed in the seventh pandemic, the year 1991 was by far the worst since the nineteenth century, with 595,000 cases worldwide, over half of which were reported by Peru, although that country suffered a remarkably low 4,002 deaths and a CFR (case fatality rate) of only 1 percent. Peru and other locations in the Americas continued to face perils from cholera after 1991. Though rates fell, Peru continued to record cholera cases each year, which some researchers have attributed to local effects of the strong El Niño weather phenomenon. Devastation caused by Hurricane Mitch (1998) and other manifestations of extreme weather destroyed basic services and infrastructure in Central America as well.

Cholera's spread through the Americas by discontinuous leaps and sudden introductions from the far south in Argentina as far north as central Mexico encouraged rumors and fears about potential carriers. Culprits included migrant shrimp farm workers voyaging from Peru to Ecuador, itinerant preachers moving from El Salvador to Honduras, and drug smugglers flying with cocaine shipments from Amazon jungle bases to airstrips in Mexico.

Although Venezuela did not suffer huge losses to cholera overall, the differential impact of the disease on a concentrated region and ethnic group held many lessons. Cholera struck in the Orinoco Delta, in the remote State of Delta Amacuro, far to the east of the national capital of Caracas. Worst hit were the native peoples called the Warao living along the Mariusa River, a tributary of the Orinoco. After suffering terribly in 1992, the Warao faced second and third visitations of cholera in 1996 and 1997. The Venezuelan government deliberately downplayed cholera, underreporting cases and deaths by as much as a factor of 10.

For Africa, the seventh pandemic proved to be especially devastating. Unlike the localized, if severe, experiences with cholera that the continent witnessed in 1868 and 1893, this time almost every African state reported cholera to the **World Health Organization** (WHO). Even worse, free-standing cholera developed in the coastal lagoons and large river valleys of West Africa, in Lake Chad, on the coast and in the oases of Somalia, in the Great Lakes of East and Central Africa, and throughout Mozambique. Newly created reservoirs permitted the entrenchment of endemic cholera, which usually attacked affected regions at the start of the rainy season and died away at its end.

Africa's continuing struggle with cholera came in two waves. A dramatic beginning occurred in August 1970 when a group of Guinean students returned to the capital of Conakry from the Soviet Union, carrying this unwelcome visitor with them in what was possibly the first time cholera had used air transport to gain a significant new foothold. From Guinea, cholera spread like wildfire along the West African coast as far as Nigeria and north to the Niger Valley and Lake Chad. Its eastward journey continued to the Horn of Africa, and then down the East African coast to southern Africa.

After waning in the 1980s, the seventh pandemic surged in 1991. It struck 21 African states and continues to be a menace today. Political instability and state collapse in Central Africa were features of the postcolonial era, and cholera certainly profited. In 1994 war and terrible violence in Rwanda triggered a huge mass migration to the refugee center of Goma, in the Democratic Republic of the Congo (then called Zaire), where cholera exploded.

Southern Africa has also encountered serious cholera epidemics and has become an endemic focus since the 1970s. Official reporting of cholera along with much else changed as South Africa went over to majority rule by 1994. Nature, however, was not kind to the new South Africa. In 2000, endemic cholera from Mozambique spread to the state of Kwazulu-Natal. In 2001, South Africa reported the alarming figure of 106,151 cases, which was roughly 58 percent of the global total. Also reporting regional cholera were Swaziland, Zambia, and Malawi.

Although cholera exacted a terrible price in the nineteenth century, the Indian Ocean area and the neighboring East African coast has not been a hotbed for modern cholera. Off the coast of Tanzania, the Comoros Islands endured a major outbreak beginning in January 1998, its first experience with cholera in 20 years. Two years later, the large island of Madagascar, cholera-free for decades, suffered an outbreak in three provinces that would spread throughout the island the following year.

Latin American and African reactions to the seventh cholera pandemic were closely monitored by the WHO and by international cholera experts. Despite facing terrible morbidity, Peruvian health authorities responded quickly and efficiently to the pandemic and were able to keep CFRs remarkably low. Crucial elements in their success were the advance preparations: experience and confidence in oral rehydration therapy, an epidemic field investigation service for diarrhea, and laboratory resources to identify the cholera organism early in the outbreak. They were simultaneously criticized, however, for their reluctance to reinvest in **water** and sewage systems and for their continuing public health emphasis on curative rather than preventative programs.

The Venezuelan experience confirms that cholera stigmatization in Latin America was instrumental in further marginalizing the poorest inhabitants of society. One favorite explanation focused on culture and food preparation, just as had been the case in Peru with *ceviche*, marinated fish and seafood. Crabs were a diet mainstay not only of the Warao but of everybody in the Orinoco Delta, but it became a powerful belief that the Warao often ate them raw and that this was how cholera contamination began. The story was entirely mythical, as the Warao boiled crabs, a preparation that killed the bacteria. This invented discourse was widespread in the press and was even shared by professional health workers.

Although no one would deny that standards of public sanitation had been breached in many parts of the Americas, what was so striking was how many scientists avoided the central point: that the cholera pandemic of the Americas spread by means of drinking water contaminated with feces, not because of "cultural" practices, and that the poor could not afford to turn to more reliable but costly sources of potable water. The experiences of Peru, Venezuela, and so many other countries during the seventh pandemic demonstrated clearly that cholera is an excellent mirror of inequalities.

At the time, blaming of victims in Africa was also common. The issue was frequently both quantity and quality of water. So too was the singling out of African cultural practices, including allegedly unsanitary behavior of people at funerals, nomadic lifestyles, and the use of waterways for travel and **trade**. Clearly, Africa absorbed terrible death tolls not seen since the days of classical cholera in the nineteenth century. In the Lake Chad region, some villages lost as many as half to three-quarters of their populations. But blaming culture for these terrible outcomes did not explain how behavior made African people any more exposed than those in other parts of the globe.

A more fruitful area of explanation turned on natural factors, such as **environment**. Severe droughts drove hungry migrants to concentrate around fewer sources of water and food, which could quickly become contaminated. Conversely, unusually heavy rains could cause makeshift latrines to pollute water sources, and in cities, crumbling sanitary infrastructure to collapse. Such was the case during 2004 and 2005, which saw large increases in cholera cases in Senegal, for example.

Coinciding with natural phenomena has been the decline or collapse of African civil societies. As in the past, cholera profited from political instability. In the 1990s, war refugees from Liberia and Sierra Leone, who were often subjected to especially unsanitary living conditions, raised cholera rates there and in neighboring countries.

Occasionally, cholera's explosion had more to do with misguided government policy. In 2000, as the South African state was in transition under majority rule, local government authority in KwaZuluNatal, under pressure from the World Bank to reduce spending as part of their so-called "structural adjustment policy," or SAP, ceased providing free water to local residents. The very poor people living in the squatter settlement on the fringes of the town of Empangeni were forced to use local rivers for drinking water and sanitation, and a nasty cholera outbreak spread rapidly. *See also* Cholera before the Pandemics; Cholera: First through Third Pandemics, 1816–1861; Cholera: Fourth through Sixth Pandemics, 1862–1947; Colonialism and Epidemic Disease; Poverty, Wealth, and Epidemic Disease; Race, Ethnicity, and Epidemic Disease; Scapegoats and Epidemic Disease.

Further Reading

Barua, D., and W. B. Greenough III, eds. *Cholera*. New York: Plenum, 1992.

Briggs, Charles L., and Clara Martini-Briggs. *Stories in the Time of Cholera: Racial Profiling during a Medical Nightmare*. Berkeley: University of California Press, 2003.

Cueto, Marcos. "Stigma and Blame during an Epidemic: Cholera in Peru, 1991." In *Disease in the History of Modern America: From Malaria to AIDS*, edited by Diego Armus, pp. 268–289. Durham: Duke University Press, 2003.

Hays, J. N. *The Burdens of Disease: Epidemics and Human Response in Western History*. New Brunswick: Rutgers University Press, 1998.

Stock, Robert F. *Cholera in Africa*. London: International African Institute, 1976.

World Health Organization, Annual Reports on Cholera in *Weekly Epidemiological Record* 36 (1961) to 82 (2007).

MYRON ECHENBERG

CINEMA AND EPIDEMIC DISEASE.   During the first decades of the 1900s, disease and messages about its meaning to society began to find their way onto the big screen with the growing popularization of film as a medium of mass entertainment and information. Diseases and epidemics, real and fictional, have long served as both backgrounds and important elements of plot in feature dramas and thrillers and have provided metaphors for societal ills and fears. Filmmakers have also produced a large number of movies of an educational or informative nature, whether documentaries, newsreels, or discussions of personal hygiene and disease.

As a tool of preventive health, films have been used to disseminate information and warnings about disease outbreaks to the general public and to specific groups (e.g., school children, military inductees). From the early decades of the twentieth century, in the years before television, it was common for movie theaters to screen such productions along with newsflashes and official messages. These films were also presented in outdoor locations, particularly in more sparsely populated rural communities. During the First World War (1914–1918) the International **Red Cross** Society produced and screened preventive health films, such as those on epidemic prevention in **war** zones, and after the war the **Rockefeller Foundation** followed with movies on hookworm disease, which for many were their first exposure to the new medium.

Filmmakers quickly tapped the entertainment potential of adding disease and disaster to feature films, however, relegating educational movies to classrooms and military induction centers. Although disease had long had a place in fiction, the portrayals on film reflected deeper sociocultural anxieties arising from the vicissitudes of the era, ranging from **industrialization** and **urbanization** and the globalized conflicts of the First (1914–1918) and Second (1939–1945) World Wars to the even deadlier threats of the early Cold War (1945–1989) era.

In general, the thematic trends of popular cinema on epidemics can be categorized into those belonging to the first half of the twentieth century and those produced after 1945. Early in the century, audiences would have been familiar—and perhaps even have identified—with diseases like **tuberculosis** (*The Red Cross Seal*, 1910; *White Terror*, 1915) and **syphilis** (*Dr. Ehrlich's Magic Bullet*, 1940) that accompanied increasingly polluted workplaces and residences and changing social norms. In films of this era, hope for success over epidemics lay in the revolutionary advances of **germ theory** and biomedical sciences. Researchers such as **Louis Pasteur, Paul Ehrlich,** and **Robert Koch** were hailed and depicted as modern saviors of humanity (*Arrowsmith*, 1931; *The Story of Louis Pasteur*, 1935; *Citadel*, 1939).

Diseases and epidemic outbreaks in cinema took on more apocalyptic dimensions after 1945. New fears were spawned not just by the threat of weapons of mass destruction, but also by apprehensions over increasingly fluid borders brought about by innovations in transportation and communications as well as accelerating patterns of **trade** and migration. According to the cinematic world, governments and corporations have been responsible for generating epidemics by flirting with evil from highly dangerous but grandiose and promising experiments that they failed to control and contain (*Virus*, 1980; *Pandora's Box*, 1996; *Resident Evil*, 2002). Hence, epidemics on screen have resulted from accidental leaks in major biomedical projects, contagions released deliberately by sophisticated bioterrorists (*12 Monkeys*, 1995; *Winds of Terror*, 2003), or unidentified foreign germs imported unwittingly from exotic lands through primates, planes, and people themselves (*Outbreak*, 1995; *Fatal Contact*, 2006). Unlike the depictions of more limited and personalized scales of suffering from epidemics of the first half of the twentieth century, more recent depictions of the destruction from diseases have become increasingly rapid, overwhelming, and spectacular. Cinematic germs have the tendency to lay waste to entire cities, countries, and even civilizations. The microbe is visualized through and embodied

SELECTED THEATRICAL FILMS DEALING WITH EPIDEMIC DISEASE

The Andromeda Strain (Robert Wise, 1971)
Arrowsmith (John Ford, 1931)
Awakenings (Penny Marshall, 1990)
Cabin Fever (Roth Elis, 2002)
Cassandra Crossing (George Kosmatos, 1976)
The Citadel (King Vidor, 1939)
City of SARS (Steve Cheng, 2003)
Code Name Trixie (George Romero, 1973)
Contagious (Joe Napolitano, 1997)
The Crazies (George Romero, 1973)
D.R.E.A.M Team (Dean Hamilton, 1999)
Dawn of the Dead (George Romero, 1978)
Day of the Dead (George Romero, 1985)
Daybreak (Stephen Tolkin, 1993)
Deadly Outbreak (Rick Avery, 1995)
Dr. Bull (John Ford, 1933)
Dr. Ehrlich's Magic Bullet
    (William Dieterle, 1940)
80,000 Suspects (Val Guest, 1963)
Epidemic (Las Von Trier, 1987)
Fatal Error (Armand Mastoianni, 1999)
Gypsy Fury (Jacques Christian, 1949)
Hei Tai Yang 731 (Tun Fei, 1988)
I Am Legend (Francis Lawrence, 2007)
Infection (Ochial Masayuki, 2004)
Intimate Agony (Paul Wendkos, 1983)
Isle of the Dead (Dwain Esper and
    Mark Robson, 1945)
Jericho Fever (Sandor Stern, 1993)
The Killer that Stalks New York
    (Earl McEvoy, 1950)
Last Man on Earth (Sidney Salkow, 1964)
Longtime Companion (Norman René, 1990)
The Missing are Deadly (Don McDougall, 1975)
Mission Impossible II (Brian De Palma, 2000)
Morte a Venezia (Luchino Visconti, 1971)
Mosquito Man (Tibor Takacs, 2005)
The Navigator: A Mediaeval Odyssey
    (Vincent Ward, 1988)
Night of the Living Dead (George Romero,1968)
Nineteen Eighteen (Ken Harrison, 1985)

Nosferatu: Phantom der Nacht (Werner
    Herzog, 1979)
The Omega Man
    (Richard Fleischer, 1971)
Operation Delta Force
    (Sam Firstenberg, 1997)
Outbreak (Wolfgang Petersen, 1995)
The Painted Veil (John Curran, 2006)
Pandora's Clock (Eric Laneuville, 1996)
Panic in the Streets (Elia Kazan, 1950)
The Periwig Maker
    (Steffen Schäffler, 1999)
La Peste/The Plague
    (Louis Puenzo, 1992)
Die Pest in Florenz (Fritz Lang, 1918)
Philadelphia (Jonathan Demme, 1993)
Plague (Ed Hunt, 1978)
Plague Fighters (Ric Bienstock, 1996)
Quiet Killer (Sheldon Larry, 1992)
Rats (James Felter, 2006)
Resident Evil (John Anderson, 2002)
The Satan Bug (John Sturges, 1965)
The Seventh Seal
    (Ingmar Bergman, 1957)
Sister Kenny (Dudley Nichols, 1946)
The Stand (Mick Garris, 1994)
The Story of Louis Pasteur (William
    Dieterle, 1935)
Trollsyn (Ola Solum, 1994)
12 Monkeys (Terry Gilliam, 1995)
28 Days Later (Danny Boyle, 2003)
28 Weeks Later (Juan Carlos Fresnadillo,
    2007)
Virus (Kingi Fukasaku, 1980)
Virus (Armand Mastroianni, 1995)
Voyage of Terror
    (Brian Trenchar-Smith, 1998)
Winds of Terror (Robert Mandel, 2001)
Yellow Fever/La Fièvre Jaune
    (Glen Pitre, 1978)
Yibola Bing Du (Herman Yau, 1996)

Compiled by Liew Kai Khiun and Lesley Henderson

in infected, mutated, and hostile human bodies (*28 Days Later*, 2003; *Mosquito Man*, 2005), animal hosts, and delicate test tubes, as well as in the minds of scheming conspirators. Just as importantly, the saviors in films on epidemics are not prominent historical personalities in medicine but usually a motley crew of accidental heroes frantically racing against time to avert doomsday either by finding the vaccine or containing the spread of the virus. The staging of such desperate acts to overcome these unprecedented public health emergencies have become what Carl Elliot describes as "public health thrills" for the consumer market.

Since their deployment almost a century ago in public health films, cinematic portrayals of epidemic disease have shifted from providing history lessons to generating high-tech entertainment. Feature films' production costs far outstrip those of official notices and other means of disseminating public service information on the transmission of diseases, yet they may well serve to educate viewers about epidemic threats and official responses. Cinema now provides for audiences the virtual experiences of unfolding dramas of public health emergencies on biblical scales from the comfort of their seats. *See also* AIDS, Literature, and the Arts in the United States; Capitalism and Epidemic Disease; Popular Media and Epidemic Disease: Recent Trends; Scapegoats and Epidemic Disease.

Further Reading

de Lacerda, Antonio Pais. "Cinema as Historical Document: Aids in the 25 Years of American Cinema" in *Journal of Medicine and Movies* 2 (2006). http://www.usal.es/~revistamedicinacine/Indice_2006/OBRA/PRINCIPAL21.htm

Elliot, Carl. "Thrills of Public Health." *British Medical Journal* 310 (1995): 1015.

Foertsch, Jacqueline. *Enemies Within: The Cold War and the AIDS Crisis in Literature, Film and Culture.* Urbana: University of Illinois Press, 2001.

Journal of Medicine and Movies. http://www.usal.es/~revistamedicinacine/index.htm

Lederer, Susan E., and Naomi Rogers. "Media." In *Medicine in the Twentieth Century*, edited by Roger Cooter and John Pickstone, pp. 487–502. London: Harwood, 2000.

Lynch, Lisa. "The Neo/Bio/Colonial Hot Zone: African Viruses, American Fairytales." *International Journal of Cultural Studies* 1 (1998): 233–252.

Ostherr, Kirsten. *Cinematic Prophylaxis: Globalization and Contagion in the Discourse of World Health.* Durham, NC: Duke University Press: 2005.

———. "'Invisible Invaders:' The Global Body in Public Health Films." In *Cultural Sutures: Medicine and Media*, edited by Lester D. Friedman, pp. 249–314. Durham, NC: Duke University Press, 2004.

Pappas, George, et al. "Infectious Disease in Cinema: Virus Hunters and Killer Microbes." *Clinical Infectious Diseases* 37 (2003): 939–942

Picon, Onstoso. "The Plague: From Albert Camus to Luis Puenzo." *Journal of Medicine and Movies* 2 (2000) at http://www.usal.es/~revistamedicinacine/Indice_2006/OBRA/PRINCIPAL21.htm

Reagan, Leslie J., et al., eds. *Medicine's Moving Pictures: Medicine, Health and Bodies in American Film and Television.* Rochester, NY: University of Rochester Press, 2007.

Tomes, Nancy. "Epidemic Entertainments: Disease and Popular Culture in Early-Twentieth-Century America." *American Literary History* 14 (2002): 625–652.

Urbanski, Heather. *Plagues, Apocalypses and Bug-Eyed Monsters; How Speculative Fiction Shows Us Our Nightmares.* Jefferson, NC: McFarland, 2007.

LIEW KAI KHIUN

COLONIALISM AND EPIDEMIC DISEASE.   Colonialism may be defined as a relationship in which one population's government assumes political and economic control and authority over another population, usually with the intention of subjugating that population and carrying out resource and revenue extraction. Colonialism is thus an unequal relationship in which the colonized are subject to considerable forms of exploitation and in which colonizing groups justify their activities with the belief that they benefit colonized groups, which are in turn seen as culturally distinct or different, and often inferior. These underlying beliefs take a variety of forms. In the case of Spanish colonists, for example, they believed they were serving a just and benevolent mission in the Americas because they sought to carry out the evangelization of native populations. Alternatively, more modern forms of colonialism in the nineteenth and twentieth centuries depended on the idea that colonists engaged in a "civilizing mission" in the colonies at great personal cost and sacrifice. Like earlier Spanish versions, such convictions were founded on the unfortunate belief that non-European populations were culturally and racially inferior and thus needed the tutelage of Europeans. Racism and the denigration of cultural difference formed the cornerstones of the colonial project, and colonists justified their work with the argument that colonialism would serve the best interests of conquered groups.

Colonialism, however, often involved more than just political domination and contact between different groups. In many cases it also involved the unintended exchange of diseases, much to the detriment of colonized populations. **Epidemic** diseases, in particular, played a prominent role in shaping the experience of colonization and the transformation of colonial societies in different parts of the world. They also led colonial states to undertake various endeavors to understand and prevent disease.

Disease in Latin America.   Devastation as a result of colonialism and disease was particularly notable in Latin America, where contact with Spanish and Portuguese explorers beginning in the late fifteenth century devastated populations. Combined with labor exploitation and the violence of conquest and early colonial settlements, disease wiped out nearly the entire indigenous populations of the Caribbean islands settled by Spain between 1492 and 1519. On some Caribbean islands fewer than 100 indigenous people remained by the time Spanish colonists' attention shifted to the exploration and conquest of Mexico in 1519.

More generally, historians estimate that in much of the Americas, upwards of 90 percent of the indigenous population died in a massive demographic collapse after the Spanish Conquest. The collapse was largely the result of disease, and most of the population drop took place within decades of Spanish invasion. This process of depopulation was more dramatic in some regions than others, but after the first decades it transformed into a slow process of population decline punctuated by epidemics. Population loss was also more extreme in particular kinds of **environments** and climates. Diseases such as **smallpox** and **measles** flourished in warm, low altitude, tropical climates. They were relatively less destructive in dry, highland areas such as the Andes and Central Mexico, where a larger portion of indigenous populations survived.

The initial demographic collapse was so severe in Latin America's coastal lowland regions that it fuelled the initial extension of the **slave** trade to the Americas. African slaves provided labor for colonists in areas where diseases had wiped out the supply of indigenous labor, enabling the rise of plantation agriculture and fuelling the ascendancy of a rural landed elite. Colonists, however, frequently expressed concern about diseases they wrongly associated with Africans and the slave trade. For example, in the capital of colonial Peru, Lima, residents believed African slaves had brought **leprosy** to the colony, even though evidence now suggests Hansen's disease had existed in the Americas prior to colonization.

During much of the Spanish colonial period **physicians** and other colonists thus neglected their own roles as trans-Atlantic disease carriers, incorrectly blaming African populations for a variety of epidemic diseases. These beliefs among colonists about diseased African populations were, of course, unfounded. We know that African populations suffered high rates of illness during the colonial period and were susceptible to epidemics, but this susceptibility was the result of several factors including the brutal conditions of the slave trade, the poor provision of food by masters, and the harsh conditions of work and daily life. There is no evidence to suggest that Africans brought any more diseases to the Americas than the Spanish did.

As with slavery, labor conditions and malnutrition among indigenous populations in colonial Spanish America increased the overall susceptibility of such populations to both epidemic and endemic diseases. Rates of respiratory infections such as **tuberculosis** were very high among indigenous groups forced to work in mines such as Bolivia's infamous silver mines of Potosí. The mining of mercury and the use of mercury to process silver also caused high rates of disease and other conditions related to mercury poisoning. Epidemic diseases such as measles were not uncommon among miners either, and life expectancy tended to be very low. For much of the colonial period authorities expressed concern about such rates of disease, yet they also saw indigenous people as crucial for providing the labor to produce silver, which generated lucrative revenue for the colony. These conflicting interests would gradually lead colonists to implement disease prevention measures in the eighteenth century.

Disease in Later Colonial Societies.   Problems with diseases and epidemics were not by any means exclusive to the Spanish Empire or to early modern forms of colonialism. Rather, similar cases can be found in the British, French, and Dutch colonies of South Asia, Southeast Asia, and Africa during the nineteenth and twentieth centuries. Even in areas where colonization did not expose populations to virgin-soil epidemics, the changes in life brought on by colonization often exposed colonized people to new disease problems.

Writing about colonial Africa, the historian Megan Vaughan suggests that colonialism furthered the transmission of epidemic diseases by increasing the mobility and migration of populations, leading migrants to cities in southern Africa. Such groups would return to their communities with "the new diseases of **industrialization**, including tuberculosis and venereally transmitted **syphilis**, and facilitating the spread of other diseases." Colonialism also led to the introduction of epidemic diseases like measles that were new to many African societies and led to high mortality rates, while the broader process of conquest and colonization disrupted the rituals, practices, and beliefs indigenous people had traditionally followed in treating disease. More generally, in the modern period, forced migration, new labor requirements in extractive industries such as mining, and the requirement that subjects live in close residential quarters in cities furthered disease transmission in many colonies. Such changes often created venues in which disease could spread more easily, and they also required levels of exertion and potential hunger that weakened subjects' **immune systems**.

Problems with disease were also especially severe in colonial India. The historian David Arnold estimates that **cholera** alone led to the deaths of 15 million people in

British India between 1817 and 1865, and a further 23 million between 1865 and 1947, the year in which Britain relinquished colonial rule. Cholera constituted a source of tremendous administrative concern in the nineteenth century because it was difficult to control, it ravaged indigenous populations, it spread in epidemic form among colonial soldiers living in crowded barracks, and it threatened to spread among the colony's British settlers. Other diseases wreaked havoc on European colonies in Southeast Asia and Australia, where populations often had little or no previous exposure to certain diseases.

Understanding and Explaining Epidemic Disease. In many parts of the world, understanding and correctly diagnosing epidemic disease and other diseases constituted a problem for both the colonized and the colonizers. For colonizers, diseases generated all sorts of concerns about the viability of living for extended periods in foreign environments different from their own. The historian Warwick Anderson has documented these anxieties and fears of disease among colonial authorities and settlers in both the U.S. Philippines and British Australia in the nineteenth and early twentieth centuries. He shows that colonial officials and settlers theorized about the effects of tropical or harsh climates on their bodies. In some cases colonists even imagined that they suffered from unfamiliar diseases in the colonies, reasoning that this was the result of an incompatibility between their bodies and such climates and environments. They claimed settlers suffered from diseases that natives tended not to experience, although they sometimes also saw natives as potential sources of epidemic and endemic diseases that could spread among colonizers. In some cases colonists even imagined diseases and created conditions that we now know did not exist. In doing so, they imagined native bodies as adapted to environmental conditions, whereas their own bodies were seen as delicate and vulnerable.

For colonists seeking to explain epidemics, a central concern was thus the question of how disease varied or differed between the metropolis and the colonies. In the Spanish colonial period, a variety of theories abounded suggesting that environment and climate made the New World fundamentally different from the Old World. New World populations were thus also different from Old World populations and were subject to a variety of diseases, some of them in epidemic form. In British colonial Australia settlers grappled with the idea that the warm, dry environments of much of the territory would give rise to health problems different from those found in damp and muggy Britain. Likewise, Jennifer Seltz has shown that as the United States colonized and expanded into the West, settlers saw the environments of Texas, the Puget Sound region, and the San Francisco Bay Area as presenting distinct problems of disease and poor health. In all these cases it is worth noting that colonial attempts to understand disease predated the rise of **germ theory**, which posited that **bacteria** and **viruses** served as the sources or causes of most disease. Given the absence of a clear set of beliefs about germs, colonists employed a wide range of strategies to talk about and explain disease.

Colonists also saw the regions they had colonized as ideal locations for the investigation and study of disease. Making assumptions about the differences of nature and culture in regions such as Africa, they attempted to use their power to understand the unique workings of disease and its prevention in such settings. In the case of British colonial Africa, the historian Megan Vaughan argues that the British saw the continent as a wild and uncontrolled environment, and "the observations of early colonial medical men contributed to this larger European perception of Africa as a continent waiting to be tamed." In addition, anxious colonial administrators in Africa feared that indigenous populations served as reservoirs of diseases that could spread into settler communities.

Preventing Epidemics.   Colonial officials generally believed disease prevention was vital to carrying out colonial rule and resource extraction successfully in many parts of the world. This was because they tended to link the health of indigenous subjects to labor output and revenue production. By increasing population size in the colonies through disease prevention, officials thought they would increase overall productivity. To do this required transforming the environment in the colonies, controlling the movement of populations, and modifying popular customs to hinder disease transmission. Attempts to refashion colonies to achieve these goals extended as far back as the colonial period in Spanish America. They continued well into the twentieth century in British colonial Africa and South Asia.

In Spanish America, eighteenth-century officials worried for decades that the diminishing size of indigenous populations would lead to fewer workers to serve in the mines. In this way, they saw disease as a direct hindrance to colonial productivity and the success of the colonial enterprise. Engaging **Malthusian** notions of demography, which focused on calculating the population size and carrying capacity of different societies and environments, these colonists believed they could maximize population growth by preventing the diseases that had increased infant mortality and reduced life expectancy. As a result, in the late eighteenth and early nineteenth centuries, in particular, representatives of the Spanish crown and settlers in the colonies themselves took unprecedented measures to prevent epidemic diseases from wreaking havoc on their populations.

The most dramatic example of these measures was the transfer of the newly discovered smallpox vaccine from Spain to Latin America in 1803. Given the particular difficulties of keeping vaccine fluid alive outside of the bodies of humans or cows for extended periods, authorities opted to use orphans to transport the vaccine across the Atlantic. Loading orphans onto a ship under the care of a Spanish doctor, Francisco Xavier Balmis, authorities planned to transfer the fluid from orphan to orphan over the course of the journey. They did this because the vaccine took about a week to produce an immunological response and create pustules on patients' arms. By draining pus from these pustules each week and injecting it as a vaccine into the arms of other orphans, they would maintain the vaccine's potency until they reached land.

Known as the Balmis Expedition, this campaign to bring the smallpox vaccine across the Atlantic to the Spanish colonies was perhaps the most ambitious attempt of its kind to prevent disease in the colonial world by the early nineteenth century. Divided into two groups in the Caribbean, the expedition traveled through Mexico, Central America, and South America, forming local vaccine brigades and training local doctors and healers in the procedure along the way. The group in Mexico would eventually acquire new orphans and set sail from the colony's west coast, cross the Pacific Ocean, and deliver the vaccine to the Spanish Philippines and China. The other branch of the expedition reached Peru and eventually Bolivia. In Peru the expedition formed a series of vaccine brigades and juntas, and local doctors quickly took control of their administration. Encouraged by the possibility of eliminating smallpox epidemics, local doctors even made calculations to estimate how quickly the vaccine would accelerate population growth in the colony's capital, Lima.

As with the Spanish, British colonists also made smallpox control and prevention central to their colonial project. In many parts of the British Empire, however, colonial efforts at mediating disease led to conflict with indigenous peoples because the latter held very different views of the workings of disease and the relationship between medicine and broader beliefs. For example, in colonial India British smallpox **vaccination** efforts largely failed for several reasons. First, people were generally reluctant to receive the vaccine, which appeared to offer very little immunity and had been difficult to store. Second, Hindus considered the transfer of vaccine fluid from arm to arm a form of pollution, and they often objected on religious grounds to the use of calf lymph for cultivating the smallpox fluid. Furthermore, smallpox had long formed a complex part of Hindu religious beliefs before colonization, and in the nineteenth century it continued to possess clear spiritual overtones. It was directly linked to a Hindu deity named Sitala, who was seen not only as the source of smallpox, but also as a means to gain protection from the disease through worship. Because the vaccine contradicted these beliefs and was associated with both foreign rule and the intrusion of secular medicine, it became suspect in popular thought.

Given that colonies were places in which societies with widely divergent concepts of religion, cosmology, and the body all converged and mixed, the interpretation and treatment of diseases such as smallpox became a hotly contested act. Moreover, many cultures that were colonized by European societies possessed rich medical traditions of their own, creating situations in which different kinds of healers competed over who should have authority to speak about disease. Writing about India, David Arnold has documented the various ways in which epidemic diseases such as cholera generated conflict and acquired new meanings for both British settlers and Indian natives. For the British, cholera was a troublesome disease that was difficult to treat and thus "not only challenged attempts to establish the superiority of Western medicine but also emphasized the physical frailty and political vulnerability of colonial rule." The British saw cholera's spread as linked to Hindu rites and **pilgrimages**. The importance of these rituals and the abundance of cultural and religious interpretations of the disease frustrated their efforts to introduce sanitary measures and anticholera serum. Ultimately, for the British the inability to control cholera and the destructive, terrifying nature of the disease cast doubt on the ability of colonizers to reorganize, sanitize, establish order, administer, and exert political control over India. On the other hand, for indigenous people the unabated spread of cholera led them to question British rule and the authority of Western secular medicine. In many regions they held "a widely shared belief that the British were in some way responsible, whether through direct violation of Hindu taboos or indirectly through the disruptive effects of their military intervention on the Hindu cosmos." In this way, disease could form a very real hindrance to the establishment and forging of colonial rule.

Finally, since the colonizing European countries adhered to one or another branch of the Christian religion, with its imperative to "spread the Gospel," colonization—especially by majority Catholic countries and by others from the nineteenth century—was rarely unaccompanied by missionaries, who often possessed medical skills. Whether among Jesuit priests or nursing nuns, pious Protestant families or evangelical physicians, care for the soul and care for the body were symbiotic processes. The equation of Western medicine with Western Christianity by Hindus, Muslims, animists, or shamanists resulted in complex reactions, ranging from rejection of both to acceptance of both. Whether in New Spain or nineteenth-century British Africa, religion, medicine, and colonial political authority often formed a trinity that simultaneously aided and subjected, freed and enslaved native colonial populations. Control of effective healing and imposition of religion helped stabilize political authority, benevolent political authority and the Gospel message helped spread Western medicine, and Christian missions relied on both just colonial government and a monopoly on sophisticated medicine. These patterns played key roles in shaping the postcolonial health-care systems, especially in Sub-Saharan Africa.

See also Diet, Nutrition, and Epidemic Disease; Disease in the Pre-Columbian Americas; Disease, Social Construction of; Historical Epidemiology; Hospitals since 1900; Latin America, Colonial: Demographic Effects of Imported Diseases; Leprosy, Societal Reactions to; Malaria in Africa; Measles Epidemic in Fiji (1875) and Eugenics; Measles in the Colonial Americas; Non-Governmental Organizations (NGOs) and Epidemic Disease; Poverty, Wealth, and Epidemic Disease; Religion and Epidemic Disease; Sanitation Movement of the Nineteenth Century; Scapegoats and Epidemic Disease; Smallpox in Colonial Latin America; Smallpox in Colonial North America; Smallpox in European Non-American Colonies; Trade, Travel, and Epidemic Disease; Typhus and Poverty in the Modern World; War, the Military, and Epidemic Disease; Yellow Fever in Colonial Latin America and the Caribbean; Yellow Fever in North America to 1810.

Further Reading

Alchon, Suzanne Austin. *A Pest in the Land: New World Epidemics in a Global Perspective.* Albuquerque: University of New Mexico Press, 2003.

Anderson, Warwick. *Colonial Pathologies: American Tropical Medicine, Race, and Hygiene in the Philippines.* Durham: Duke University Press, 2006.

————. *The Cultivation of Whiteness: Science, Health, and Racial Destiny in Australia.* New York: Basic Books, 2003.

Arnold, David. *Colonizing the Body: State Medicine and Epidemic Disease in Nineteenth-Century India.* Berkeley: University of California Press, 1993.

Bashford, Alison. *Imperial Hygiene: A Critical History of Colonialism, Nationalism and Public Health.* New York: Palgrave Macmillan, 2004.

Cook, Noble David. *Born to Die: Disease and New World Conquest, 1492–1650.* New York: Cambridge University Press, 1998.

Harvard University Library. *Contagion.* http://ocp.hul.harvard.edu/contagion/colonialism.html

Kunitz, Stephen J. *Disease and Social Diversity: The European Impact on the Health of Non-Europeans.* New York: Oxford University Press, 1994.

Packard, Randall. *White Plague, Black Labor: Tuberculosis and the Political Economy of Health and Disease in South Africa.* Berkeley: University of California Press, 1989.

Seltz, Jennifer. "Embodying Nature: Health, Place, and Identity in Nineteenth-Century America." Ph.D. Dissertation, University of Washington, 2005.

Vaughan, Megan. *Curing Their Ills: Colonial Power and African Illness.* Stanford: Stanford University Press, 1991.

ADAM WARREN

CONJUNCTIVITIS.   Conjunctivitis is an inflammation of the conjunctiva and is the most common eye disease in the world. The conjunctiva is the thin, transparent mucus membrane that covers the posterior surface of the eyelids and the anterior surface of the eye (cornea or sclera). One of the most common symptoms of conjunctivitis is inflammation that causes a pinkish-red coloration (hyperemia), and because of this coloration conjunctivitis is frequently referred to as "pink eye."

Most nonmedical people tend to think of conjunctivitis as one disease, but it is actually a group of diseases with many causes and even more manifestations. The major categories are conjunctivitis caused by infectious agents, immunological (allergic) conjunctivitis, conjunctivitis caused by autoimmune disease and/or chemical irritation, and conjunctivitis of unknown cause. The category of conjunctivitis covered in this article includes those manifestations caused by infectious agents such as **viruses, bacteria**, rickettsia, chlamydia, and parasites, because these are the causes of conjunctivitis **epidemics**.

Viral Conjunctivitis. Viral conjunctivitis is the most common inflammation of the eye. Most children have at least one episode during their childhood years. Conjunctivitis is not limited to children, but the spread of the virus from child to child is especially common because of the natural tendency of children to touch each other while playing. Viral infections are frequently responsible for epidemics of conjunctivitis within families and military units, and among people in schools, offices, and factories. In addition to direct contact, the virus can be spread by contaminated materials (fomites) and microscopic particles.

Adenoviral (viruses that usually invade the upper respiratory tract) conjunctivitis is the most common form of viral conjunctivitis. So far there have been 19 different subdivisions (serotypes) of adenovirus identified as causative agents for adenoviral conjunctivitis. Once a patient (who is not immunodeficient, as an **AIDS** patient is) has conjunctivitis caused by one serotype, that person develops immunity to that serotype but remains susceptible to the other 18.

Pharyngoconjunctival fever is a triad of pharyngitis, fever, and conjunctivitis caused by an adenovirus. The conjunctivitis is usually identified with a watery discharge, redness, and swelling (edema) of the conjunctiva and frequently involves swelling of the eyelids. It is most commonly seen in children less than 10 years of age. There are at least three different serotypes of adenovirus that have been identified as etiological agents. This condition usually resolves spontaneously in two weeks.

Epidemic keratoconjunctivitis is a more severe form of conjunctivitis; there are at least three serotypes of adenoviruses identified as causative agents. It is called keratoconjunctivitis because it affects both the conjunctiva and the transparent anterior portion of the sclera (cornea). This form usually lasts 14 to 21 days with some symptoms lingering for months. There is a watery discharge and swelling of the conjunctiva (chemosis), hyperemia, and swelling of the lymph glands in front of the ear (preauricular adenopathy). Treatment of the symptoms is the only care currently available.

A well-documented incidence of epidemic keratoconjunctivitis was reported in Germany in 2004. The epidemic broke out among people serving in the German Armed Forces. Eventually it spread over 197 barracks and affected 6,378 soldiers. The civilian population outside of the barracks was also affected. The infection spread to the young adult male population first, followed by the young adult female population, and finally to children. Transmission was from person to person, and a clear and consistent strategy for dealing with the disease had to be adopted. If the soldiers were restricted to the barracks, there would be an increased risk to the other soldiers, but sending them home would increase the risk of spreading the infection to the civilian population. Thirteen barracks were completely closed down and twenty-eight were partially closed. Control measures were implemented, including **disinfection** of rooms and an isolation period of 21 days for soldiers with conjunctivitis.

Acute hemorrhagic conjunctivitis was first identified in 1969, around the time of the first lunar landing, and is therefore sometimes referred to as the "Apollo disease." This disease is associated with two strains of the coxsackievirus. The conjunctivitis is painful, is of rapid onset, and features chemosis and bleeding under the conjunctiva (subconjunctival hemorrhage). The conjunctivitis clears in four to six days, but the hemorrhages may last longer. This disease tends to erupt into epidemics involving up to half of the population of a city or region. There is only symptomatic treatment available.

There are several other forms of conjunctivitis-causing viruses. Each by itself is considered rare, but when combined they form a significant cause of conjunctivitis. A partial list of these viruses includes the viruses that cause fever blisters (Herpes simplex), chicken pox (varicella), shingles (Herpes zoster), **smallpox** (variola), German measles (rubella), **measles** (rubeola) and flu (**influenza**).

Chlamydial Conjunctivitis.   Conjunctivitis caused by chlamydial infections can take multiple forms. The most severe form is trachoma. Trachoma is endemic in many developing countries and is the most common cause of preventable blindness in the world. It was first described in the Egyptian "Ebers Papyrus" written some 3,600 years ago. It is most often found in areas of **poverty**, overcrowding, and poor public sanitation. Trachoma is usually the result of multiple untreated or under-treated episodes of chlamydial conjunctivitis, rather than a single infection. There are 400 million persons worldwide affected by trachoma, making it the most common of all chronic diseases. It usually affects both eyes. The advanced stage of trachoma is known as trichiasis—the inward turning of the eyelashes that causes corneal scratching (abrasions) and eventual blindness. The victim develops extreme pain; sunlight, dust, and smoke all irritate the eyes. The disease is three times more likely to affect women than men. In some cultures, when married female victims are not able to perform their traditional domestic duties they are rejected by their husbands. Transmission is by direct contact, through fomites, and via insect vectors such as flies.

Chlamydial trachomatis conjunctivitis of the newborn (sometimes referred to as infant inclusion conjunctivitis) is frequently caused by *Chlamydia* from the mother's cervix that infects the eyes of the newborn. The word "inclusion" was used because microscopic cyst-like structures (inclusions) were found in specimens of this disease in the early 1900s. It took almost 60 years before the *Chlamydia* organisms were isolated from these inclusions. The serotypes responsible for newborn conjunctivitis are usually the same as those responsible for adult inclusion conjunctivitis.

Adult inclusion conjunctivitis usually occurs in sexually active young adults and affects both eyes. Transmission of the *Chlamydia trachomatis* organism is commonly caused by oral-genital sexual practices or hand-to-eye contact. There have been reported outbreaks of indirect transmission in inadequately chlorinated swimming pools. The chlamydial agent is usually found in the urethra of the male and cervix of the female.

Bacterial Conjunctivitis.   Because most western physicians tend to treat all conjunctivitis with **antibiotics** and seldom culture the material that seeps from the eye, the actual incidence of bacterial conjunctivitis is unknown. Many bacteria have the ability to cause conjunctivitis; the most common are *Streptococcus pneumoniae*; *Corynebacterium diphtheriae*; enteric Gram-negative rods; and *Haemophilus*, *Moraxella*, and *Neisseria* species. Most cases start unilaterally but soon spread to the other eye.

Hyperacute bacterial conjunctivitis is marked by copious yellow pus (purulent exudate). Any severely purulent exudate should be cultured and treated immediately with antibiotics because it may indicate an early stage of meningococcal conjunctivitis in children. Delay could result in septicemia and/or severe injury to the eye. The most common organisms for hyperacute conjunctivitis are *Neisseria gonorrhoeae*, *kochii*, and *meningitides*.

Acute bacterial conjunctivitis, sometimes called catarrhal (inflammation of mucus membrane with increased mucus) conjunctivitis, frequently occurs in epidemic form. In temperate climates, the most common etiological organism is *Streptococcus pneumoniae*, but in warmer climates it is usually caused by *Haemophilus aegyptius*. Chronic bacterial conjunctivitis is caused by acute or subacute conjunctivitis that was untreated or inadequately treated.

Ophthalmia neonatorum is a general term used to describe conjunctivitis of the newborn from multiple causes such as gonorrhea and chlamydia infections from the mother's vagina. All newborn infants should receive preventive treatment (prophylaxis) against this form of conjunctivitis. Silver nitrate eye drops have traditionally been used and are very effective against gonococci conjunctivitis, but they are not effective against *Chlamydia trachomatis* infections, which are more common in the United States. In recent years, treatment with tetracycline or erythromycin eye ointments has replaced treatment with silver nitrate. Povidone-iodine eye drops are used in many areas of the world.

Parasitic Conjunctivitis.   In underdeveloped areas of the world, parasitic diseases Leishmaniasis and Microsporidiosis cause parasitic conjunctivitis. The tsetse fly, famous for causing **sleeping sickness**, can cause conjunctivitis. Previously uncommon **protozoa** have recently been found in the conjunctiva of patients with **AIDS**.

Infectious conjunctivitis runs the gamut from "simple pink eye" (uncomplicated viral and/or bacterial conjunctivitis), which can be irritating but self-limiting, to trichiasis, a painful, debilitating blindness leading to rejection by society. Many forms of conjunctivitis have no effective treatment or are traditionally over-treated in western society, whereas millions of people in underdeveloped societies lose their eyesight for lack of simple, effective, and inexpensive treatments. *See also* Children and Childhood Epidemic Disease; Contagion and Transmission; Meningitis; Personal Hygiene and Epidemic Disease; Poverty, Wealth, and Epidemic Disease.

Further Reading

Mayo Clinic. *Pink Eye: Conjunctivitis*. http://www.mayoclinic.com/health/pinkeye/DS00258

National Library of Medicine. *Medline Plus*. http://www.nlm.nih.gov/medlineplus/ency/article/001010.htm

Nelson, Leonard. *Harley's Pediatric Ophthalmology*, 4th edition. Philadelphia: W. B. Saunders Company, 1998.

Schrauder, A., et al. "Epidemic Conjunctivitis in Germany, 2004." *European Surveillance* 11 (2006): 185–87; online at: http://www.eurosurveillance.org/em/v11n07/1107-224.asp

THOMAS QUINN

CONSUMPTION.   *See* Tuberculosis.

CONTAGION AND TRANSMISSION.   The *Dictionary of Epidemiology* defines "contagion" as "the transmission of infection by direct contact, droplet spread, or contaminated fomites." Strictly speaking, rabies is a contagious disease, but by convention we usually do not refer to human rabies as such because it is uncommonly transmitted from human to human. "Transmission" refers to the specific means by which infectious agents cause infection. Contagion is thus a particular type of infectious disease transmission. Unfortunately these terms are often used loosely.

Because "transmission" implies either two hosts or an **environmental** source and a host, the host/source that transmits and the host that acquires infection, and because the means of transmission may be different from the means of acquisition (e.g., so-called fecal-oral spread) it is helpful to speak of "transmission/acquisition," or at least to keep the concept in mind. Some epidemiologists separate mechanisms of transmission into direct and indirect, based not only upon how the infection is transmitted, but also on how it is acquired (e.g., **inoculation** of cytomegalovirus during passage through the birth canal [direct transmission], or acquisition of **yellow fever** from the bite of an *Aedes aegypti* mosquito [indirect transmission]). Confusingly, transmission of diseases through large "droplet nuclei" that may arise from coughing or sneezing has been categorized as direct transmission, whereas acquisition of infectious agents from small aerosolized particles has been categorized as indirect transmission without regard to source. Moreover, respiratory agents such as "common cold" **viruses** that can be spread by droplet nuclei (direct transmission) can also be spread via contaminated fomites (indirect transmission). Many infectious agents can be transmitted by both direct and indirect means.

In general, when a human infection is acquired from another human by touching, kissing, sexual relations, passage through the birth canal, transplacentally (across the placenta), or via inhalation of infectious particles emitted from another person in close proximity (usually less than 1 to 2 meters)—all examples of direct transmission—we refer to the disease as being contagious. As noted, this provisionally sets aside as a special case animal to human spread, which by convention we usually do not refer to as contagious. Nevertheless, diseases such as rabies are said to be contagious when transmission occurs from animal to animal. When a human infection is acquired from an insect or environmental source (i.e., when the infectious agent is being maintained or is amplified in that source) we speak of noncontagious (indirect) spread. Noncontagious spread is usually broken down into vehicle-borne (e.g., **water**borne, foodborne, fomite-mediated) and vector-borne, with the latter category referring to either mechanical or biological transmission by ticks, mosquitoes, sandflies, or other **insects**. (Biologic transmission refers to the support of replication and usually amplification of the infectious agent.)

Examples of contagious diseases include those acquired by direct inoculation (e.g., **syphilis** and other sexually transmitted diseases), by droplet acquisition (e.g., **influenza, measles, pneumonic plague**), and transplacentally (e.g., rubella). Examples of noncontagious infectious diseases include vector-borne diseases (e.g., yellow fever, **malaria, Lyme disease**, and flea-borne **bubonic plague**), vehicle-borne diseases (e.g., waterborne **cholera**, fomite-borne acute hemorrhagic **conjunctivitis**, foodborne salmonellosis), and **air**borne infection (e.g., coccidiomycosis, New World **hantaviruses**).

Development of Concepts of Contagion in the Twentieth Century.   The discovery of the microbial causes of many diseases in the last quarter of the nineteenth century, stimulated by Casimir Davaine (1812–1882) and **Robert Koch's** anthrax "co-discovery" (i.e., identification of the organism, characterization of its life cycle, and experimental determination of the natural history of infections) led to rapid advances. During this period there was a series of microbiological triumphs (e.g., establishment of the etiologies of **tuberculosis**, plague, and cholera) that led to epidemiologic understanding of infectious diseases' transmission and acquisition. By the early 1900s, when the vector-borne etiologies of malaria, yellow fever, and **dengue** had been established, and when "filter-passing" infectious agents (particularly viruses) had been identified, the framework was largely complete, and our understanding of the principles and mechanisms of infectious disease transmission were recognizably similar to those of the very early twenty-first century. With this knowledge came new public health control measures and clinical therapies, including vaccines (e.g., rabies, 1885), passive immunotherapies (e.g., **diphtheria** antitoxin, 1890), and environmental control (e.g., controls for yellow fever).

Yet it was not a time of complacency. A variety of methods and standards had to be worked out. For example, immunologic research led to serologic (blood) tests of **immunity** to infectious agents, and these tests led to the realization that **bacteria** and viruses were incredibly diverse antigenically. Such diversity had profound implications for treatment and prevention. Treatment of life-threatening pneumococcal disease with immune serums was complicated by the fact that different immune serums had different abilities to treat disease caused by different pneumococcal capsular polysaccharide types. In the first two decades of the twentieth century, four different polysaccharide types were identified, with a fifth category (pneumococcus Type IV) representing a number of different organisms that would have to be (and eventually were) distinguished from each other.

Among other important concepts established in this era was the realization that the presence of an infectious disease did not exactly correspond to the potential for contagion. Humans and animals could transmit a number of infectious diseases before they themselves became ill (i.e., during incubation), as well as after they had gotten better. Moreover, people could become carriers of some organisms, potentially transmitting disease directly or by shedding into the environment, continually or intermittently, over long periods of time.

Related to this was a better understanding of environmental introduction and persistence of infectious organisms such as *Vibrio cholerae* in drinking water. Indeed it was during this era that scientists came to understand why it had taken so long to understand and accept contagionism. Looking for general principles that would apply to all of the important epidemic diseases (e.g., cholera, **typhoid**, and plague), they had not appreciated the complexity of the problem. The same diseases could be transmitted directly from person to person but at the same time transmitted indirectly and at a distance between persons who had had no contact (e.g., via contaminated water [cholera, typhoid] or insects [plague]). Anthrax, an extreme example, was transmitted to humans by three distinct mechanisms to cause three distinct diseases (cutaneous, gastrointestinal, and pulmonary anthrax).

Taken as a whole, this new understanding of contagion and disease transmission/acquisition created many challenges for public health. That healthy people could transmit deadly diseases to others, for example, created a difficult new role for public health, as illustrated by the case of "Typhoid **Mary**" **Mallon**, whose involuntary incarceration by public health officials created a highly charged controversy that reverberates today in cases of **AIDS**, XDR **tuberculosis**, and other transmissible diseases.

Also of note was the development in the early twentieth century of the concept of microbial coinfection. Studies of immigrants housed at Ellis Island in New York, for example, revealed that crowding predicted not only attack rates from specific infectious diseases, but also mortality rates. Subsequent research demonstrated the interaction of different diseases in producing mortality: for example the mortality from measles was much higher in children who also had diphtheria. This phenomenon was shown most dramatically in

1917 during the epidemics of measles in U.S. Army training camps. In a number of camps the high death rates of healthy young men from measles were directly attributable to previously asymptomatic carriage of streptococci. A year later, during the **influenza pandemic of 1918–1919**, the identical phenomenon was found and exhaustively studied, leading to the almost universal conclusion that most deaths during the influenza pandemic were associated with, and probably caused by, severe secondary bacterial pneumonias (largely pneumococcal and streptococcal, with a smaller number of outbreaks associated with staphylococci, *Bacillus* [*Haemophilus*] *influenzae*, or other pathogens). Concepts of transmission and contagion as they related to actual disease risk had thus become bewilderingly complex; preventing diseases required not only public health knowledge but also immunologic and microbiologic efforts backed up by considerable experimental **animal research**.

Contemporary Concepts and Usages.   During the last century, a solid understanding of disease transmission allowed identification and characterization of a number of new and newly recognized diseases. For example, the infectious nature and the several modes of transmission of AIDS (e.g., sexual, needle-borne) made it clear that AIDS was caused by an infectious agent several years before Human Immunodeficiency Virus (HIV) was identified. The 2003 SARS outbreak featured an epidemiologic picture so clear in indicating respiratory and/or close-contact transmission of an infectious agent that the epidemic was quickly stopped by familiar public health measures even before the causative virus was identified. Many similar examples can be given.

Contagion itself, and many other aspects of infectious disease transmission, have become common knowledge to almost everyone, including children, who after a certain age readily accept the wisdom of parental proscriptions against eating something that has fallen on the floor or kissing an aunt with a cold, and in favor of washing their hands after using the bathroom.

In his famous 1943 book, C. E. A. Winslow asked why it had taken so long to establish contagion as a mechanism for disease acquisition. There are probably a number of answers, not the least compelling of which is that events often look clearer in hindsight. Other factors probably include inability to imagine subclinical infection, transmission that occurs either before disease onset or after disease resolution, and the fact that a number of infectious agents can be transmitted by multiple means (e.g., cholera by contaminated water and by contaminated bed linens; **smallpox** by exhaled droplets and by contaminated clothes; plague by flea bites and by exhaled droplets; anthrax by inhaled spores, by ingested meats, and by direct skin inoculation).

From the organism's point of view, survival ultimately depends on access to animal or human hosts, and there may be many different roads and byways to get there. Direct person-to-person contagion via a single mechanism of transmission/acquisition (e.g., measles, influenza) may at first seem ideal, but it can be problematic if the organism in question kills or incapacitates its host, encounters uncrowded populations, or can be defeated by mechanical means (e.g., face masks). Organisms that cause human disease generally exist in complex microbial ecosystems in which survival may depend on flexibility and on ability to adapt to new hosts, to survive environmental differences of temperature and humidity, and to infect by more than one route. Each major infectious disease—plagues, pestilences, and inconsequential diseases alike—represents a complicated interaction between the host, microbial agent, and environment, in which the mode of transmission is but one facet of the negotiated picture. *See also* Immunology.

Further Reading

Bashford, Alison, and Claire Hooker, eds. *Contagion: Epidemics, History and Culture from Smallpox to Anthrax*. London: Pluto Press, 2002.

Jarcho, Saul. *The Concept of Contagion in Medicine, Literature, and Religion*. Malabar, FL: Krieger, 2000.

Winslow, C. E. A. *The Conquest of Epidemic Disease: A Chapter in the History of Ideas*. Princeton: Princeton University Press, 1943.

DAVID M. MORENS

CONTAGION THEORY OF DISEASE, PREMODERN.   Long before the emergence of modern bacteriology, the idea of **contagion** (from "contact") was generally recognized by many human societies. Where groups accepted the idea that illness could be transmitted by "contact," there developed a certain wisdom that shaped practices for protecting the health of the community against the dangers of diseases. But premodern concepts of contagion, and the customs they underpinned, showed a great deal of variation. In ancient Mesopotamia, for instance, taboos against touching the sick were based on a religio-magical belief that evil spirits possessing the ill could be transferred to a new victim by touch, whereas Indian medicine held that merely looking at a person might constitute contact enough for transferal. Although the transmissibility of **epidemic** diseases like the plague and the danger of remaining in a disease-stricken area were accepted, contagion played a minor role in India's **Ayurvedic** epidemic disease theory and medicine. A survey of traditions illustrates the variety of possible beliefs and practices of contagion.

Ancient Hebrew medicine recognized the transmissibility of certain diseases, which led to the adoption of regulations regarding personal and public cleanliness; for instance, those who suffered from **leprosy** were considered unclean, and their clothing was burned.

Traditional **Chinese disease theory and medicine** revealed a degree of awareness about contagion. During the **smallpox** outbreaks in premodern China, it was observed that close contact with the sick caused infection. The Qing imperial family built shelters of isolation to prevent contagion. Medical texts recommended staying away from the sick bed, the corpse, and the coffin; avoiding noxious odors; and covering the nostrils and ears to prevent the penetration of poisonous vapors into the body.

Greco-Roman medical theories and practices also display an understanding of contagion. In his account of the **Plague of Athens**, Thucydides (c. 460–395 BCE) mentions the transmission of disease from one person to another. **Galen** warned against the dangers of having contact with the sick. Despite awareness of contagion, however, epidemic diseases were usually blamed on corruption of the **air** and **miasma**, or on exhalations rising from putrefying ditches, city garbage, human **corpses,** and rotting animals. Postulated by **Hippocrates** and further developed by Galen, this theory was combined with the **humoral theory** to explain the occurrence of epidemics. Belief in the association between **air and epidemic disease** was firmly established, holding that when air lost its normal composition, its substance and qualities putrefied, and it consequently posed a risk of disease to all who inhaled it.

Islamic disease theory and medicine embraced a vaguely defined awareness of contagion, both through direct person-to-person contact and through **heredity**, though Muhammad (570–632) explicitly denied its role in disease transmission. **Avicenna** observed that visible contact was not necessary for transmission in all cases: someone who

ENGLISH NURSE FLORENCE NIGHTINGALE AGAINST CONTAGION THEORY (1859)

The idea of "contagion," as explaining the spread of disease, appears to have been adopted at a time when, from the neglect of sanitary arrangements, epidemics attacked whole masses of people, and when men had ceased to consider that nature had any laws for her guidance. Beginning with the poets and historians, the word finally made its way into medical nomenclature, where it has remained ever since, affording to certain classes of minds, chiefly in the southern and less educated parts of Europe, a satisfactory explanation for pestilence and an adequate excuse for non-exertion to prevent its recurrence.

And now, what does "contagion" mean? It implies the communication of disease from person to person by *contact*. It presupposes the pre-existence of certain germs like the sporules of fungi, which can be bottled up and conveyed any distance attached to clothing, to merchandise, especially to woolen stuffs, for which it is supposed to have an especial affection, and to feathers, which of all articles it especially loves—so much so that, according to quarantine laws, a live goose may be safely introduced from a plague country; but if it happens to be eaten on the voyage, its feathers cannot be admitted without danger to the entire community. There is no end to the absurdities connected with this doctrine. Suffice it to say, that in the ordinary sense of the word, there is no proof, such as would be admitted in any scientific inquiry, that there is any such thing as "contagion."

From her "Notes on Hospitals," quoted in *Medicine and Western Civilization*, edited by David J. Rothman, et al. (New Brunswick, NJ: Rutgers University Press, 1995) pp. 362–363.

stared at a victim of **conjunctivitis** might catch the ailment. Islamic medical writers adopted and developed Galenic ideas of disease transmission rooted in the idea of miasma. Leprosy, elephantiasis, scabs, **consumption**, smallpox, **measles**, and various forms of plague were cited as transmissible diseases in Islamic medical literature.

After the Crusades (begun in 1096), Europe came to be devastated by leprosy, **typhus**, smallpox, and especially **bubonic plague**. Starting from the mid-fourteenth century, several waves of plague struck Europe, killing at least a quarter of the population during the initial outbreak called the **Black Death** (1347–1352). The idea that plague was transmitted through contact was widespread. But it was also believed that talking to or looking at the sick or the dead, or encountering their clothing or dwellings, could confer the disease. This prompted the establishment of public health boards or health magistracies and the implementation of precautions such as the *cordons sanitaires* and practices of **disinfection**. **Quarantine** measures were adopted in several Mediterranean port cities, requiring that all arriving ships and immigrants wait 30 or 40 days before entering a city. Starting from the fifteenth century, **pest houses** were constructed to isolate those who suffered from the plague. These were clearly meant to isolate sick individuals from the healthy public.

During the sixteenth century, **diphtheria, measles**, and, especially, **syphilis** and **gonorrhea** became common in Europe. The first major epidemic of syphilis broke out among the sailors of Columbus returning from the New World, and then spread to Europe. It was understood that syphilis was transmitted through contact. **Girolamo Fracastoro**, a **physician** from Verona, speculated about the nature of contagion and suggested that syphilis spread through sexual contact. In 1546 he wrote a treatise (*De Contagione*) in which he explained disease transmission by invisible "seeds" of disease, which he called *seminaria*. He suggested that *seminaria* were transferred to the air from the sick, where they would multiply and move to another person. According to Fracastoro, there were three different types of contagion. The first occurred only through direct contact (e.g., scabies, tuberculosis). The second occurred through indirect contact with fomites deposited on intermediary objects used by the sick. The third occurred at a distance (e.g., pestilential fevers, tuberculosis, smallpox). Although the ideas of contagion through contact with the ill and contagion through contact with clothing or wood touched by the sick were hardly new, Fracastoro was among the first to advance an account of indirect contagion in terms of a substance deposited on intermediary objects.

Until the microbiological and microscopic revolution of the nineteenth century, ideas along Fracastoro's lines were widely accepted. In fact, up until the mid-seventeenth century, disease was broadly considered to result from a set of causes drawn from a systematic hierarchy, and these causes could be combined in various ways. At the top of the hierarchy of causes there was God, without whom neither epidemics nor cures would be possible. After God, cosmic influences of the stars and astronomic events were accepted as causes of disease. God, stars, and planets all exercised indirect influences through a more direct agent: the air, a substance that, once corrupted, could damage the vital powers of the living when breathed. At the bottom of the hierarchy were people, who, either through natural dispositions or through lifestyles, were capable of falling prey to a disease.

Around the mid-sixteenth century, when Fracastoro wrote his work on contagion, a lively discussion was going on in learned medical circles regarding the nature of contagion, its mechanisms, its degree in different diseases, and its relationship to putrefaction. Although Fracastoro used the concept of seeds innovatively to explain contagion, the concept itself was nothing new to his contemporaries, as such ideas were available through the printed versions of ancient and medieval works. In fact, in ancient Greco-Roman medical writings, seeds of diseases were believed to remain as residuals in the body of the sick, even after the symptoms disappeared, and they could be reactivated as a result of a wrong regimen of diet and exercise.

Within a generation Fracastorian principles began to circulate among the learned, partly in the context of the plague of Venice in 1555–1557. Although most plague treatises written immediately after the Black Death said nothing about contact or contagion, a majority of later authors discussed plague in the terms set by Fracastoro. His views and terminology were quickly integrated into mainstream knowledge about epidemics, especially regarding the plague, measles, and typhus. What would become a modern theory of contagion became possible with the invention of the **microscope** and its use, initially by **Antony van Leeuwenhoek**, to investigate what are now called microbes. However, it was only to be two centuries later that a relationship between microbes and diseases would be accurately established. The **germ theory of disease**, proposing that small organisms were responsible for causing infectious diseases, acquired general acceptance with the pioneering research of **Louis Pasteur** and **Robert Koch**. Soon afterwards, the **bacteria** causing **tuberculosis, cholera, plague** and many other diseases were discovered. *See also* Astrology and Medicine; Leprosy, Societal Reactions to; Magic and Healing; Mallon, Mary; Personal Hygiene and Epidemic Disease; Religion and Epidemic Disease; Scientific Revolution and Epidemic Disease; Syphilis in Sixteenth-Century Europe.

Further Reading

Aisenberg, Andrew. *Contagion: Disease, Government, and the 'Social Question' in Nineteenth-century France.* Stanford: Stanford University Press, 1999.

Baldwin, Peter. *Contagion and the State in Europe, 1830–1930.* New York: Cambridge University Press, 1999.

Carlin, Claire L., ed. *Imagining Contagion in Early Modern Europe*. New York: Palgrave Macmillan, 2005.

Carmichael, Ann G. "Contagion Theory and Contagion Practice in Fifteenth-century Milan." *Renaissance Quarterly* 44 (1991): 213–256.

Conrad, Lawrence I., and Dominik Wujastyk, eds. *Contagion: Perspectives from Pre-Modern Societies*. Burlingotn, VT: Ashgate, 2000.

Harvard University Library. *Contagion*. http://ocp.hul.harvard.edu/contagion/index.html

Jarcho, Saul. *The Concept of Contagion in Medicine, Literature, and Religion*. Malabar, FL: Krieger, 2000.

Nutton, Vivian. "The Seeds of Disease: An Explanation of Contagion and Infection from the Greeks to the Renaissance." *Medical History* 27 (1983): 1–34.

———. "The Reception of Fracastoro's Theory of Contagion: The Seed that Fell among Thorns?" *Osiris* 2nd series 6 (1990): 196–234.

Pernick, Martin S. "Contagion and Culture." *American Literary History* 14 (2002): 858–865.

Rosenberg, Charles E. "Florence Nightingale on Contagion." In *Explaining Epidemics*, edited by Charles E. Rosenberg, pp. 90–108. New York: Cambridge University Press, 1992.

Zuckerman, A. "Plague and Contagionism in Eighteenth-century England: The Role of Richard Mead." *Bulletin of the History of Medicine* 78 (2004): 273–308.

NÜKHET VARLIK

CORDON SANITAIRE.   *Cordon sanitaire*, a French phrase meaning "protective line," is a barrier designed to prevent the spread of a disease by severely restricting the movement of people and goods between areas affected by disease and those where the disease is not present. The cordon may be intended to contain an outbreak of disease within its boundaries or to keep an epidemic out of the enclosed area. The earliest known *cordons sanitaires* were established during the late fifteenth century as Italian city-states tried a variety of methods, including **quarantine**, to battle the **bubonic plague**. *Cordons sanitaires* became a common tool to combat not only plague, but also **sleeping sickness, cholera, typhus, influenza, yellow fever**, and a host of other **epidemic** diseases.

For hundreds of years, the theory behind the sanitary cordon was that infected people and objects that had been in contact with them could spread the targeted disease. In most cases, the disease in question, such as bubonic plague, was not actually being spread by contagious individuals, but cordons were often nonetheless effective because they inadvertently blocked the passage of the actual vectors of disease, such as rat fleas.

Once the etiology of such epidemic diseases as plague, yellow fever, and cholera was understood, cordons became far less common, replaced by less burdensome, more cost-effective disease management tools. They did not disappear entirely, however, because they could be effective against diseases such as influenza that were actually spread by human contact. In other instances, cordons were modified to be more useful in the prevention of epidemic disease. For example, after World War I (1914–1918), an Allied sanitary cordon on Poland's eastern border was designed to thwart the spread of lice-borne typhus, which was then raging in the new Soviet Union. Travelers were not allowed to pass through the cordon without being bathed and deloused and having their clothing sterilized. The delousing was an effective component in the campaign against typhus, as it attacked the actual carrier of the disease.

European **Cordons Sanitaires.**   Perhaps the best-known *cordon sanitaire* is the voluntary isolation of the English village of Eyam during a seventeenth-century epidemic. Late in 1665, during the **Great Plague in London**, plague struck the village, supposedly brought in from the capital by fleas hitchhiking on a shipment of cloth delivered to the village tailor, who was the first to die. When casualties started to rise in the spring of 1666, the villagers, at the urging of their young minister, Reverend William Mompesson (d. 1709), and his predecessor, Rev. Thomas Stanley (d. 1670), made the noble decision to isolate themselves in hopes of preventing the spread of plague to other communities in the Derbyshire area. A few wealthier residents left or sent family members away before the village closed itself off, but approximately 350 shut themselves in. A perimeter of stones was laid out surrounding the village and no one passed the boundary in either direction until November, when the pestilence had run its course. Neighboring communities provided food for Eyam, leaving supplies in designated locations along the boundary cordon and receiving payment in coins "disinfected" by running water or vinegar. Mompesson's wife Catherine died during the epidemic, but he survived to raise their children, who had been sent from the village prior to the imposition of the cordon. Only one in four residents survived, but the plague did not spread to the rest of the district.

Historically, such self-imposed cordons were exceptional; usually a *cordon sanitaire* was imposed by a government authority that used military forces to enforce the boundary restrictions. Because of their burdensome nature, sanitary cordons were usually temporary affairs, targeting a particular outbreak of disease. In the mid-1700s, however, the Habsburg rulers of Austria set up the first permanent military *cordon sanitaire* along its long frontier with the Ottoman Empire. By 1770 soldiers were stationed in sentry posts located no more than a musket-shot apart for a thousand-mile stretch, with larger forts situated at strategic locations. People and goods could only cross into Austrian territory at designated checkpoints with quarantine stations. Cotton and wool were held in storehouses for weeks, with peasants paid to sleep on the bales and monitored to see if they showed signs of disease. Other goods, including letters, underwent **fumigation** with burning sulphur before passing through the checkpoint. Travelers were quarantined for 21 days under ordinary circumstances and up to 48 days when there was confirmation of plague being active in Ottoman territory. The cordon was maintained until 1871, despite decades of complaint that the travel restrictions were an economic burden with little medical justification. There were no major outbreaks of plague in Austrian territory after the *cordon sanitaire* was established, whereas the Ottoman Empire continued to suffer frequent epidemics of plague until the mid-nineteenth century.

Europeans used *cordons sanitaires* as part of their strategy to fight other epidemic diseases besides plague. For example, the French response to an outbreak of yellow fever in Spain in the 1820s was to set up a cordon in the Pyrenees Mountains, manned by 30,000 troops, to prevent the disease from sweeping north. Travelers could only cross the barricade at three approved quarantine sites. During the 1830 cholera outbreak in Russia, Moscow was surrounded by a military cordon, most roads leading to the city were literally dug up to hinder travel, and all entrances to the city save four were sealed. Moscow and other cities found cholera immune to the barrier approach, strengthening a growing sense that the psychological and economic hardships presented by a sanitary cordon outweighed the health benefits.

Colonial **Cordons Sanitaires.**   When Europeans began to establish colonies around the globe, they applied familiar tactics such as quarantine and establishment of *cordon sanitaires* against the epidemic diseases they encountered, even though there was considerable debate over the relative efficacy of the contagionist and sanitarian approaches to public health. In colonial Asia and Africa, there were accusations that *cordon sanitaire* was imposed as a means of social control of native people, rather than as a truly effective medical tool. For example, the cordon utilized in an attempt to control sleeping sickness in the Belgian Congo in the early 1900s played havoc with native African social and economic life, whereas Europeans living in the region were largely unaffected by its strictures. In China, the French and other European powers established colonial enclaves surrounded by *cordons sanitaires* designed to protect themselves against diseases endemic in the native population. The British seemed to rely heavily on cordons and quarantines in both Egypt and India to combat such diseases as plague and cholera, until the measures proved overly disruptive of their economic interests.

American Cordons Sanitaires.   Bubonic plague struck the American territory of Hawaii in 1899, triggering a *cordon sanitaire* around Honolulu's Chinatown district, where the disease first appeared. The Hawaiian National Guard was tasked with maintaining a cordon around a 35-acre area that housed 10,000 Chinese, Japanese, and native Hawaiian residents, a quarter of Honolulu's population. Commerce in the city was in turmoil, as immigrants could not reach their jobs. Food shortages soon developed within the quarantined area because residents were unable to fish or get to their farms. Asians working as live-in servants were not allowed to visit relatives or friends in the Chinatown district and were further required to take a daily public shower at a "disinfection station," a humiliation that illustrates the racial prejudice that underlay many of the quarantine regulations.

When cleansing the homes of plague victims with carbolic and sulfuric acid proved ineffective, unsurprisingly, in halting the spread of the disease, the Honolulu Fire Department began the controlled burning of buildings. On January 20, 1900, a fire set in a building where a plague victim had died got out of control and most of Chinatown was destroyed. As Asians rushed to escape the fire, they were at first turned back by the National Guard and white vigilantes maintaining the cordon. Finally, one exit from the district was opened, allowing terrified residents to evacuate the fire zone. Eight thousand people left homeless spent the next several months living in churches or warehouses as white city officials decided whether to rebuild their community or to turn the land over for commercial development. Many bitterly insisted that the government had deliberately allowed the fire to spread, a conviction only strengthened when one local newspaper printed an editorial celebrating the fire for wiping out the plague while simultaneously clearing off valuable real estate.

As the third plague pandemic reached the shores of the western United States, Asians were again singled out for special treatment. On March 6, 1900, a Chinese immigrant was found dead of bubonic plague in a hotel in San Francisco's thriving Chinatown. Members of the city's Board of Health moved with surprising swiftness; the very next day, March 7, they established a *cordon sanitaire* around the 12-block Chinatown district. Police officers manning the cordon allowed whites living or working within the quarantined area to leave while forcing more than 10,000 Asians to remain inside its boundaries. Negative press and vocal complaints by Chinese business leaders convinced city officials to drop the cordon after only two days. However, it was reinstated in May when more cases of plague began to appear among Chinese workers.

Between March 1900 and July 1901, there were 39 confirmed cases of death from bubonic plague in San Francisco, with 35 of the deceased being Chinese. Although health

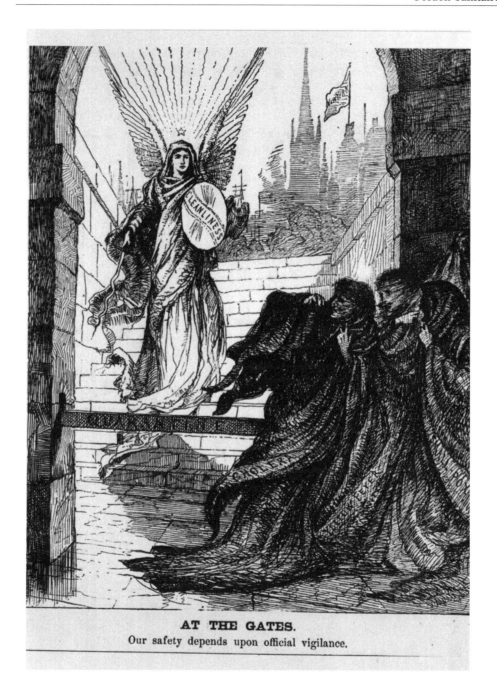

AT THE GATES.
Our safety depends upon official vigilance.

"At the Gates: Our safety depends upon official vigilance." The specters of cholera, yellow fever, and smallpox recoil in fear as their way through the Port of New York is blocked by a barrier reading "quarantine" and an angel whose shield reads "cleanliness." New York, Harper and Brothers, September 5, 1885. Courtesy of the National Library of Medicine.

officials argued that the blockade was necessary to prevent outbreaks of the disease from spreading beyond Chinatown, race, rather than residency, seemed to be the determining factor regarding whether someone was subject to quarantine, as white Chinatown residents were free to travel outside the cordon. Asians living within the cordon were particularly alarmed when the Board of Health announced it had purchased land on an island in San Francisco Bay and was considering a plan to relocate Chinese and Japanese residents there and to raze Chinatown in the interest of public health. Leaders of the Chinese community went to court in June, complaining about the selective enforcement and suggesting that city officials had not made adequate arrangements to provide food and other essentials to those inside the *cordon sanitaire*. Judge William Morrow (1843–1929) ruled in their favor, ordering an end to the discriminatory cordon and to any plans to evacuate or demolish Chinatown. No major outbreak of plague subsequently developed in the city, although there continued to be deaths from the disease, particularly in the Chinese community.

In 1882, in response to a virulent outbreak of yellow fever in Brownsville, Texas, and northern Mexico, a *cordon sanitaire* was established 180 miles north of the city, terminating at the Rio Grande to the west and the Gulf of Mexico to the east. People traveling north had to remain quarantined at the cordon for 10 days before they were certified disease-free and could proceed. Similar cordons were used elsewhere in the United States to combat the spread of yellow fever, such as in Jacksonville, Florida, in 1888 and Brunswick, Georgia, in 1893. During the **influenza pandemic of 1918–1919**, sanitary cordons were part of the quarantine measures employed by many American communities, including Fairbanks, Alaska; Princeton University; and tiny Gunnison, Colorado (population 1,329).

Whether sanitary cordons will play a role in future pandemics is a matter of controversy. The ease of modern travel increases the speed at which carriers can unwittingly transmit disease before an effective cordon could be established, and maintaining a *cordon sanitaire* around a large modern city for any length of time would be a complex logistical nightmare. However, although both the **World Health Organization** (WHO) and the U.S. Department of Health and Human Services advise against the use of cordons except in unique circumstances, many local and national emergency preparedness plans for communicable diseases still contain provisions for *cordons sanitaires*. *See also* Capitalism and Epidemic Disease; Cholera: First through Third Pandemics, 1816–1861; Colonialism and Epidemic Disease; Contagion Theory of Disease, Premodern; Disease, Social Construction of; International Health Agencies and Conventions; Medical Ethics and Epidemic Disease; Napoleonic Wars; Personal Liberties and Epidemic Disease; Plague and Developments in Public Health, 1348–1600; Plague in San Francisco, 1900–1908; Race, Ethnicity, and Epidemic Disease; Severe Acute Respiratory Syndrome (SARS); Trade, Travel, and Epidemic Disease; War, the Military, and Epidemic Disease.

Further Reading

Baldwin, Peter. *Contagion and the State in Europe, 1830–1930*. New York: Cambridge University Press, 1999.

Echenberg, Myron. *Plague Ports: The Global Urban Impact of Bubonic Plague, 1894–1901*. New York: New York University Press, 2007.

Rothenberg, Gunther E. "The Austrian Sanitary Cordon and the Control of Bubonic Plague: 1710–1871." *Journal of the History of Medicine and Allied Sciences* 28 (1973): 15–23.

TERESA LESLIE

CORPSES AND EPIDEMIC DISEASE.   During and in the wake of an outbreak of **epidemic** disease, dealing with excessive numbers of human corpses can prove problematic. As the numbers of the dead increase, the task of burying or otherwise disposing of bodies can overwhelm those who survive. Traditional funeral customs may become impossible or be deemed dangerous to follow. Corpses left unburied or hastily dealt with can become a threat to public sanitation. Likewise, diseased human and animal corpses can be a vector for the further spread of disease. Under epidemic conditions, corpses must be managed carefully in order to prevent conditions from worsening. For physicians, they have also proven to be important sources of information about specific diseases.

During the **Black Death** and subsequent outbreaks of **bubonic plague** in Europe, the number of corpses overwhelmed urban areas in particular. In Tudor and Stuart London, the task of determining whether a person had died of the plague fell to "searchers," usually older women, dependent upon pensions, who were paid a small amount by their parish to inspect the bodies of those who died. If the searcher determined that a person had indeed died of plague, authorities would **quarantine** the rest of the victim's family, locking them in their home, which often meant that they would also contract the disease and die.

Historically, the capacity of corpses to spread epidemic disease—real or imagined—was exploited for purposes of **biological warfare**. Among the most infamous stories of such activity was an account reported by Gabriele de Mussis (fl. c. 1345), whose work *Historia de Morbo* is the principal contemporary source on the arrival of plague in Europe. De Mussis claimed that the plague entered Europe through the city of Kaffa in 1346 (now Feodosia in the Ukraine), when the Mongol army attacking the city was struck by **plague**. Although they were losing the siege, the Mongols allegedly used catapults to fling the corpses of those who had succumbed to plague into the city. De Mussis reported that the **air** and **water** in Kaffa became infected, and the townspeople succumbed to the plague. According to some plague historians, it is more likely that the town's population was infected when rats carrying the plague entered the city and triggered an epizootic, causing the rat fleas to move on to human hosts and infect them. However, without doubt, the plague-corpse missiles caused substantial terror and concern among Kaffa's populace and may have carried plague-ridden fleas.

Burial practices during major plague outbreaks also shifted radically. In preparation for the arrival of plague in the late 1340s, Sir Walter Manny (c. 1310–1372) and Ralph Stratford (c. 1300–1354), bishop of London, each purchased fields outside of the city of London in which tens of thousands of corpses were buried. Mass graves became the norm in later outbreaks of the plague as well. English novelist Daniel Defoe (c. 1660–1731) reported that during the **Great Plague of London** (1665–1666), just one of the enormous pits dug by the buriers or "bearers" of the dead measured 40 feet by 18, and was 18 feet deep. Defoe wrote that more than 1,100 bodies were thrown into it. Plague outbreaks such as the Great Plague disrupted customary mourning rituals or interrupted them altogether. During the 1665 outbreak, the orders issued by the city magistrates included stipulations that no one was to accompany a corpse to the churchyard and that an infected corpse could not lie in the church itself. No sermon was to be delivered, and the bodies were to be buried only between sunset and sunrise.

Other epidemic diseases have caused similar disruptions to burial practices. Ebola, an extremely lethal strain of **hemorrhagic fever**, is known to be active for several days after its host has died. The U.S. **Centers for Disease Control and Prevention** recommend that

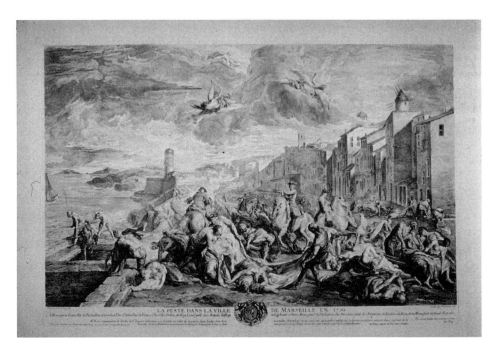

"The Plague in the City of Marseille in 1720." Depiction of a waterfront scene with victims, dead and dying, and the removal of infected corpses. Original painting by J. B. De Troy. Courtesy of the National Library of Medicine.

burial practices be radically altered in cases of Ebola virus. Recommended practices include spraying the body with bleach and burying it in a hole at least 2 meters deep. Researchers have determined that although Ebola might not be readily transmitted during certain funeral rituals, sharing a meal with fellow mourners at funerals creates a strong risk factor for acquiring the disease.

Certain other cultural practices have aided the spread of epidemic disease. Some epidemic diseases are spread through the practice of eating corpses. Among the Fore tribe in Papua New Guinea, the disease *kuru*, related to "mad cow disease" or bovine spongiform encephalopathy (BSE) is known to have spread through the practice of eating the dead. Because women among the Fore have traditionally eaten the brain tissue of the dead, they have suffered from a higher rate of the disease than men. There are also indirect ways to consume human remains. Some researchers argue that BSE entered Britain with the importation of animal bone and tissue from India for use as cattle feed. Human remains, believed by some researchers to include tissue from sufferers of vCJD or Creutzfeldt-Jakob disease, the human variant of BSE, was thought to be mixed with the animal tissue. Human remains commonly wash up on the shores of the major river systems in India. Although burial practices there tend to involve cremation, many families are too poor to afford enough wood to burn the entire bodies of their loved ones and must settle for partial cremation. Bone collectors who work along the river shoreline then gather the human remains along with those of dead animals. Bones exported from India are ground up and included as a major ingredient in commercial cattle feed. The disease agent (an infectious protein called a *prion*) spreads throughout the nerve tissue of the cattle, concentrating in the brain and spinal cord. Humans who consume beef infected with BSE are at risk for developing the disease themselves, especially if they consume the brain and spinal cord (often used in ground beef).

Corpses of epidemic disease victims have also provided Western doctors with important insights into effects of the disease on the body, and later of the pathogens themselves. During the Black Death, Pope Clement (r. 1342–1352) understood this and encouraged otherwise rare autopsies of plague victims. During later plague outbreaks, physicians and surgeons conducting risky dissections of victims contracted the disease. **Alexandre Yersin's** breakthrough insights into the bubonic plague pathogen followed his successful struggle to obtain corpses from British authorities in Hong Kong. *See also* Hospitals and Medical Education in Britain and the U.S.; Hospitals since 1900; Medical Education in the West, 1100–1500; Medical Education in the West, 1500–1900; Plague and Developments in Public Health, 1348–1600; Public Health in the Islamic World, 1000–1600; Religion and Epidemic Disease; Urbanization and Epidemic Disease; War, the Military, and Epidemic Disease.

Further Reading

Centers for Disease Control. *Infection Control for Viral Hemorrhagic Fevers in the African Health Care Setting.* Online Manual, CDC Special Pathogens Branch. http://www.cdc.gov/ncidod/dvrd/spb/mnpages/vhfmanual.htm#content

Eamon, W. "Cannibalism and Contagion: Framing Syphilis in Counter-Reformation Italy." *Early Science and Medicine* 3 (1998): 1–31.

Klitzman, Robert. *The Trembling Mountain: A Personal Account of Kuru, Cannibals, and Mad Cow Disease.* Cambridge, MA: Perseus Publishing, 1998.

Wheelis, Mark. "Biological Warfare at the 1346 Siege of Caffa." *Emerging Infectious Diseases* 8 (2002): 971–975.

MELISSA SMITH

D

DEMOGRAPHIC DATA COLLECTION AND ANALYSIS, HISTORY OF.   The study of infectious disease is largely the study of demography, of patterns of human settlement and population characteristics that promote or inhibit the propagation and subsequent spread of this or that disease agent. It was in the collection of demographic data on disease incidence in populations that causes of disease were first studied and the social characteristics of disease events revealed.

A very early example of the systematic accumulation of national population data in Europe is the famous *Domesday Book* commissioned by William the Conqueror (1028–1087) in 1086 to assess patterns of land ownership for taxation purposes. It was so named because it was said to be as comprehensive as the definitive records that would be used to call all to account on Judgment Day: "there was no single hide nor a yard of land, nor indeed one ox nor one cow nor one pig which was left out."

From the fourteenth to the eighteenth century, most European birth and death records were kept at the parish level and were at best haphazard, though record keeping tended to improve over time. By the eighteenth century, several trends were transforming both the relationship of the state to its population and the relationship between the state and the then-evolving science of disease studies. Mercantilism and the early **Industrial Revolution** prompted vast population shifts from the countryside to the city. Rapid **urbanization** resulted in population centers of previously unimaginable sizes. The densely packed cities that resulted became centers of **epidemic** disease propagation as well as commerce, reservoirs whose effect increased as the cities grew. The result was seen as an economic threat to the extent disease limited the available labor pool. As a result, the health of citizens became a subject of economic and political interest.

At the same time, English chemist Robert Boyle's (1627–1691) program for establishing matters of fact through the social construction of assent created the context in which science, including medical science, would seek to understand disease. This new concept of science demanded new systems of analysis in which social and medical data were to be analyzed mathematically.

In the 1600s William Petty (1623–1687), a London **physician** and economist interested in the health of populations, coined the phrase "political arithmetic" to describe "the art of reasoning by figures upon things related to government," and especially population health as a critical barometer of the health of the state. His friend John Graunt (1620–1674) demonstrated patterns of regularity in mortality based on a study of London's "Bills of Mortality." These were systematic, parish-based weekly tabulations of mortality and causes of death that began in the mid-sixteenth century and were meant to signal the onset of plague. When the numbers rose beyond an expected norm, civic and royal authorities enacted public health precautions. Published from the early seventeenth century, they also informed the public when to flee the capital and when it was safe to return. The Dutch mathematician Christian Huygens (1629–1695) took up the problem of creating a table of life expectation and, in 1693, Oxford astronomer Edmund Halley (1656–1742) published an analysis of age-at-death statistics compiled in Breslau, a German town known for its record keeping, that marked the beginnings of actuarial science.

With increasingly precise public records of births and deaths came a series of practical applications that in retrospect are the beginnings of medical demography. In 1760, Daniel Bernouli (1700–1782) analyzed **smallpox** mortality in a manner demonstrating the increased lifespan that resulted from inoculation. In the next century, the French mathematician Adolphe Quetelet (1796–1874) collected the statistical applications of his contemporaries and predecessors to create a systematic structure that could be applied to biological and social phenomena.

The ability to analyze datasets numerically was married to improved record keeping by the state. In France, a *méthode numerique* developed with increasingly accurate public records to permit an unprecedented description of disease events within national and regional populations. In England economists and moralists like Jeremy Bentham (1748–1832) argued for both the collection of health-related data and a numerical approach to its analysis. These arguments became the life's work of Bentham's former secretary, the barrister **Edwin Chadwick**, perhaps the single most significant figure in the public health movement in England in the first half of the nineteenth century.

In the 1830s a series of legislative changes in England began the transformation of the traditional, local system of reportage to one based on a national system of registration districts and registration sub-districts whose registrars would be responsible for the collection of demographic and health-related data. Chadwick championed these changes, along with a modern census of all British households. **William Farr** was hired by the General Record Office in 1839 and was deeply involved with England's first comprehensive, modern national census in 1841.

Chadwick used the resulting data in his landmark 1842 *Report* on the sanitary condition of the laboring population of Great Britain, which demonstrated the relationship between health and social circumstance in the evolving metropolitan city. Beginning with Chadwick's, a series of seminal studies relied on nationally collected data to analyze the nature of disease and its effect on populations. In 1852, for example, during the second **cholera pandemic**, William Farr used national population data and data on cholera mortality collected by London registrars, to argue the nature and origin of cholera. In this, he was the first to demonstrate a clear relationship between regional water supplies and epidemic cholera at the metropolitan scale.

The data was sufficient to advance local studies of disease incidence as well. This data was critical, for example, to **John Snow's** famous 1855 study of an 1854 cholera outbreak in his neighborhood of St. James, Westminster, in London. Thus by the mid-nineteenth century, demographic data had become a principle medium for both studies of disease causation, and more generally, the health of populations at a range of scales. *See also* Cholera: First through Third Pandemics, 1816–1861; Plague and Developments in Public Health, 1348–1600; Sanitation Movement of the Nineteenth Century.

Further Reading

Koch, Tom. *Cartographies of Disease: Maps, Mapping, and Medicine.* Bridgewater, NJ: Esri Press, 2005.

Rosen, George. 1993. *A History of Public Health.* Expanded first edition. Baltimore: Johns Hopkins Press, 1993.

Rusnock, Andrea A., ed. *Vital Accounts: Quantifying Health and Population in Eighteenth-Century England and France.* New York: Cambridge University Press, 2002.

Scott, Susan, and C. J. Duncan. *Human Demography and Disease.* New York: Cambridge University Press, 1998.

Shapin, S., and S. Schaffer. *Leviathan and the Air-Pump: Hobbes, Boyle, and the Experimental Life.* Princeton: Princeton University Press, 1985.

TOM KOCH

DENGUE FEVER.   *See* Hemorrhagic Fevers; Hemorrhagic Fevers in Modern Africa.

DIAGNOSIS AND DIAGNOSTIC TOOLS.   Health care practitioners work every day like detectives with many diagnostic tools to help treat a patient's illness. The process begins when a patient presents to a clinic with a symptom or problem. By asking him questions, performing a physical exam, and running diagnostic tests, the health care practitioner will be able to construct a list of possible diagnoses, called the differential diagnosis. Depending on what is found through the diagnostic tests, a single disease process from the list may prove to be most probable. The diagnosis can sometimes be made immediately, but often a trial treatment will be necessary to decide whether the diagnosis was correct or a new diagnosis needs to be sought.

Sensitivity and Specificity.   No diagnostic test is perfect. The usefulness of a given test is described in two ways: how sensitive it is and how specific it is. A sensitive test will detect a positive result in someone who has the disease. Therefore, if a very sensitive test is negative, then the disease is very likely absent. A specific test reliably detects those cases in which the disease is not present, so if the test is positive, the disease becomes more likely. A sensitive test helps to "rule out" a disease (put it lower on the list of possible diseases), whereas a specific test helps to "rule in" a disease (move it higher on the list). Each test has its own sensitivity and specificity, depending on the inherent qualities of the test itself. Another concept called pretest probability refers to the likelihood that the patient has the disease—given other known factors—before the test is even ordered. It helps to put the sensitivity and specificity of a test in context. Each factor helps determine the probability that a diagnosis is correct.

The Clinical History.   Any element of a person's past history, family history, or daily life may be considered a risk factor for a potential diagnosis. Smoking, for example, is a risk factor for lung cancer, whereas traveling in the Amazon is a risk factor for contracting exotic tropical diseases. Asking a patient to explain the story surrounding her illness, along with any mitigating factors relating to her symptoms, is central to understanding these risk factors. Similarly, an effort should be made to list and understand the patient's past medical history, including the history of diseases she has had, chronic disease she still suffers from, **vaccinations** she has received, and the history of diseases that have affected her family members. Elements of a good social history include where she lives and works; whether she is sexually active and with whom; and whether she smokes, drinks alcohol, or uses illegal drugs. Many health care practitioners believe that the vast majority of diagnoses can be made from a good history alone. In certain situations, such as during a **cholera epidemic**, in which many people are gravely affected at once, the clinical scenario and the patient's symptoms are often the only elements needed to make the diagnosis and get the patient the treatment she needs in time to save her life.

Physical Exam.   For centuries, the physical exam was the only diagnostic tool that doctors had, so new and descriptive terms were invented to describe their observations: bowel sounds were called "borborygmus"; unusual sounds in the lungs were called "crackles"; sounds in the heart were called "murmurs, rubs, or gallops." New tools were developed to aid in gathering this information, such as the stethoscope, reflex hammer, and tongue depressor. Sometimes tests pioneered by a certain doctor would take on the doctor's name; for example, the multicolored spots on the inside of the mouth of a patient infected with **measles** are called "Koplik spots." The physical exam thus can be seen as a series of hands-on tests that, like laboratory tests, provide data that is only as useful as the test's sensitivity, specificity, and pretest probability. It provides important clues to what disease process is occurring, and sometimes the diagnosis can be made with these tests alone. Many of the viral exanthemas, such as measles, mumps, or rubella, can be diagnosed alone by the skin's appearance and the clinical story of how the rash developed.

Laboratory Tests.   A wide variety of tests can be performed on various body samples to aid in making a diagnosis. The following describes the most useful test categories in epidemic diseases.

Body Fluid Tests.   Urine, stool, cerebrospinal, abdominal, lung-pleural, joint, amniotic, and vaginal fluid can all be collected from the body and studied. The analysis of these fluids is central to the diagnosis of many epidemic diseases. For example, the chemical composition of the fluid can be quantified, leading to important clues regarding what disease process may be affecting it. Similarly, it can be observed under a **microscope** to qualify what types of blood cells predominate, or what types of pathogens are infecting it.

Chemistry Tests.   Countless chemical compounds, such as electrolytes, vitamins, lipids, and drug and hormone levels, can be tested for in most body fluids. In the metabolic panel, for example, multiple key electrolytes in the serum of the blood are quantified. How each falls within or varies from the normal range will help paint a picture of how the body's metabolic functions are operating. Similarly, the presence of various proteins called enzymes in the bloodstream implies that damaged cells in the body have lost their structural integrity and are leaking their contents into the blood. These tests are particularly useful when looking for liver, muscle, or heart damage. Epidemic diseases are usually not diagnosed with chemistries alone, but the damage that they do to the body is. For example, liver function tests may be greatly elevated when someone is infected with viral **hepatitis**. Finding the cause of the damage and treating the patient accordingly is critical to his survival.

Immunodiagnostic Tests.   Another group of proteins called antibodies, generated by the body's immune system to fight off infections, can also be tested for in the blood. If a specific antibody is present, then there is proof that the person was once infected or may still be infected. Immunodiagnostic tests study the reaction between these antibodies and the substances with which they interact, called antigens. These tests are critical in diagnosing many infectious diseases, but are also used for detecting autoimmune diseases (in which the body attacks itself), and also in diagnosing some cancers. The ability to detect the antibody against **Human Immunodeficiency Virus** was crucial to helping curb its spread. In fact, it is so important to be sure that this antibody test is as accurate as possible that it is composed of two tests. The first is very sensitive and will detect HIV quite well but will also produce some false positive results (showing up positive when HIV is not really present). All these positive results will then undergo a second test that is very specific and will help clarify which positives are truly HIV and which are mistakes.

DNA and Genetic Testing.   Ever since the discovery of DNA in the 1950s, countless new techniques have been developed that can detect and describe the genetic material within human beings or within the pathogens that are infecting them. By using lab methods such as the polymerase chain reaction, or PCR, which can amplify even small amounts of DNA so that there will be more material to work with, and gel electrophoresis, which is used to separate various segments of the DNA on a gel plate, labs can now manipulate the genes of both humans and pathogenic agents. For example, a form of PCR called reverse transcriptase PCR can be used to quantify the viral load in HIV infections. Similarly, genetic tests in humans can help predict how a person's inherited genetic make up, or genes, predispose her to certain diseases, such as in certain types of cancer.

Hematological Tests.   Much can be learned about the body through the blood. The complete blood count, or CBC, quantifies and qualifies the white blood cells (WBCs), red blood cells (RBCs), and platelets in the blood. A hematocrit, for example, is a common test used to describe the portion of the blood made up of RBCs. The blood is then put on a slide, stained, and observed under a microscope in order to determine the characteristics of the different blood elements. RBCs will be studied carefully for the presence of certain infections, such as in **malaria**, in which the diagnosis is actually made by observing the organism in the RBC. The WBCs can also be differentiated. The type of WBC that predominates may suggest the type of infection in the body: neutrophils may be elevated in bacterial infections like **meningitis**, lymphocytes in viral diseases, and eosinophils in parasitic diseases, such as in intestinal worms. Coagulation factor tests, such as the PT-INR and PTT describe how well the blood can coagulate, or become solid to form scabs and stop bleeding. In **Dengue fever**, the body's blood may get "thinner" thereby putting the body at risk for severe bleeding.

Histology and Cytology (Pathologic Examination of Body Tissues).   A pathologist examines microscopic samples of potentially diseased body parts to help diagnose diseases. These samples could include a scraping of cells (cytology), such as from a "Pap smear" testing for **cervical cancer**, or a solid tissue biopsy (histology), such as the biopsy taken from an abnormal growth found in the body. Once removed, the sample will first be inspected grossly with the naked eye. It will then be stained with special dyes and sliced paper-thin so that when inspected under the microscope, many pathologic characteristics of the cells and tissue can be identified, such as whether the cells look cancerous or appear infected.

Microbiologic Tests.   Various methods exist to grow and characterize the **viruses, bacteria**, and fungi that infect humans. Most samples are first stained with a dye, such as the Gram Stain or Giemsa Stain, and then examined under a microscope. Cultures can be made by placing any body fluid sample on a culture medium in a Petri dish that allows the pathogen to multiply so it can be more easily identified. **Bubonic plague**, for example, can be diagnosed by drawing out pus from an infected "bubo," staining it, and then culturing it to look for the bacterium *Yersinia pestis*. Cultures will often be tested to discover the sensitivities of the pathogens to various **antibiotics**. Diagnosing active **tuberculosis** still requires microscopic examination and/or subsequent cultures of sputum smears coughed up by an infected person. In areas where exposure to tuberculosis (TB) is not very common, a skin test called a Tuberculin PPD Test can be performed by injecting a small sample of TB protein under the skin and seeing if the body reacts to it. If it does, then the patient has been exposed to TB, but it may still be dormant in the lungs. A chest x-ray or sputum smear will help to distinguish whether the TB is active.

Radiology.   Before imaging technologies were widely available, it was common to perform an "exploratory surgery" by opening a person's abdomen from top to bottom to look inside for the problem with the naked eye and bare hands. Luckily, ever since the first x-rays, there has existed the ever increasing ability to take pictures of the deepest parts of the body without having to actually go inside. First, the x-ray is a common and affordable method used to create a two-dimensional image by penetrating the body part under study with radiation and then developing the picture that is made. In many parts of the world where tuberculosis is endemic, the chest x-ray is often the only radiology study readily available. For more detailed pictures, the computed tomography scan (CT scan) may be available. With this technology, the part of the patient under diagnosis is put into a donut-shaped machine that takes a series of x-rays all around the body. Then a computer synthesizes these many images to create a three-dimensional picture of what is inside. Magnetic resonance imaging, or MRI, provides greater clarity by using magnetic energy instead of radiation to draw the internal landscape. Ultrasound technology is an alternate imaging method that uses supersonic echoes to make a picture that is less clear. It has its advantages, though: it can be used at the patient's bedside and can look at moving body parts in real time, such as the heart in an echocardiogram.

Nuclear Medicine Studies is a relatively new field within radiology that determines not only what a patient's body looks like anatomically but also how it is functioning physiologically. In the WBC Scan, a sample of WBCs from the patient's body are collected and labeled with a radioactive marker. When reinserted into the body, the cells travel to areas of inflammation or infection, thereby helping provide important clues to where exactly an infection is located. This could be critical when one suspects that there is an abscess causing a patient to be febrile, but traditional methods cannot reliably locate it.

Electrocardiogram, Electroencephalogram, Electromyogram.   Much of the body works by electricity. As charged ions move across the membranes of nerves, heart cells, and muscle cells, the electrical charge that is produced can be measured by a probe that is placed on the skin directly above. If these probes are placed above the heart, the test result produced is called an electrocardiogram, or ECG; if above the brain, it is called an electroencephalogram, or EEG; if above or within a skeletal muscle, it is called an electromyogram, or EMG. Because the movement of these cells' electricity produces recognizable patterns as they print out on a computer, any change in the functioning of the cells will also produce recognizable patterns of those diseased states. This technology provides doctors with a relatively inexpensive and noninvasive method of understanding how various parts of the body are functioning.

Endoscopy, Bronchoscopy, Otolaryngoscopy, Laproscopy, Cystoscopy.   The human body has a number of openings to the outside world. The ears, nose, mouth, urethra, vagina, and anus are all gateways to internal hollow spaces that can be explored with a camera on the end of an extension. The names of these techniques will usually begin with a Greek or Latin word naming the organ, which is then followed by the suffix "–scopy." In this way, endoscopy is the exploration of the upper gastrointestinal (GI) tract; colonoscopy is the exploration of the colon, or lower GI tract; bronchoscopy is exploration of the lung's bronchi, and so on. Newer equipment can also use extensions to take tissue biopsies and fluid samples, inject medicines, and even remove some cancers. Because this technique allows doctors to perform minimally invasive procedures on patients, it has improved the screening and treatment of many diseases. In AIDS, for example, immunocompromised patients can sometimes suffer a serious lung infection from an organism called PCP. A positive diagnosis is made by finding the pathogen in the sputum, but patients are often not able to produce a good sample by simply coughing. A bronchoscope greatly increases the sensitivity of this test because it can often collect a sputum sample from deep within.

An emerging field of diagnostic technology known as biomedical informatics involves the use of computers and other new information technologies to integrate, contextualize, and assess the diagnostic findings of multiple tests in support of the process of differential diagnosis and decisions based upon it. *See also* Corpses and Epidemic Disease; Diagnosis of Historical Diseases; Heredity and Epidemic Disease; Human Body; Human Immunity and Resistance to Disease; Medical Ethics and Epidemic Disease.

Further Reading

Fischbach, Frances. *A Manual of Laboratory and Diagnostic Tests*, 6th edition. Hagerstown, MD: Lippincott Williams and Wilkins, 2000.

Fox, Stuart Ira. *Human Physiology*. Boston: McGraw-Hill, 2005.

Hoffbrand, Victor, et al. *Essential Haematology*. New York: Blackwell, 2006.

Mettler, Fred A. *Essentials of Radiology*. St. Louis: Saunders, 2004.

Swartz, Mark H. *Textbook of Physical Diagnosis: History and Examination*, 5th edition. St. Louis: Saunders, 2005.

Wu, Alan. *Tietz Clinical Guide to Laboratory Tests*, 4th edition. St. Louis: Saunders, 2006.

DANIEL PALAZUELOS

DIAGNOSIS OF HISTORICAL DISEASES.   Modern researchers have diagnosed historic diseases according to their similarities to modern illnesses. Medical historians obtain the evidence for the associations between past and present diseases by studying all types of literary, medical, administrative, and ecclesiastical (church) records, as well as relevant artwork and archaeological evidence from the period in question. For example, the numerous plague **epidemics** of the **second plague pandemic**, starting with the medieval **Black Death** and continuing well into the eighteenth century, have been mostly diagnosed as the **bacterial** disease **bubonic plague** because historical accounts mention lymphatic swellings (buboes) and the coughing of blood, which is believed to indicate the concurrent presence of the pulmonary variation of the disease, **pneumonic plague**. However, advances in theory and methodology of modern medicine have gradually altered the approach to afford less credible face-value diagnoses, especially when the nature of the disease in question is uncertain.

Nineteenth-century discoveries and advances in laboratory science proved **germ theory**, ushering in the modern age of medicine. This changed not only the understanding, prevention, treatment, and **diagnosis** of present diseases, but also the understanding and diagnosis of historic plagues. As the theory gradually became accepted, and the pathogens which cause some of the most infamous plagues, such as bubonic plague, **cholera, tuberculosis, typhus**, and anthrax were studied extensively, a renewed interest in the history of diseases was provoked, especially between the late nineteenth and mid-twentieth centuries, when the **third plague pandemic** gripped the world with the fear of another Black Death catastrophe.

As more information concerning current disease pathogens was amassed, specifically their behavior, ecology, and transmission vectors, the more such knowledge was applied to the diagnosis of historic plagues. For example, when it was proven that modern bubonic plague was spread by rats and that their fleas were the vectors by which humans were infected, historians easily saw rats and fleas as the cause of famous plague outbreaks like the **Plague of Justinian** and the Black Death.

For the most part, the matching of historic plagues with modern diseases remains popularly accepted and, in many cases, unchallenged. There is little doubt, for instance, that the disease which struck London in 1854, meticulously investigated and documented by the English physician **John Snow**, was an epidemic of **cholera**. We can be similarly certain that the great mortalities suffered by the natives of the New World after contact with Europeans in the sixteenth century were the result of the introduction of viruses like **measles** and **smallpox**. Diseases such as these have persisted into modern times and affected almost every area of human settlement at one time or another, engendering both a familiarity and reputation that serve to identify them almost beyond doubt.

However, history is full of many examples of plagues that modern medicine cannot diagnose with any real certainty. The mysterious plague that struck a Carthaginian army as its soldiers were laying siege to the Greeks of Syracuse in 396 BCE (Carthaginian Plague) remains unidentified. Similarly, medical historians have suggested that the Great **Plague of Athens** was variously measles, smallpox, bubonic plague, anthrax, typhus fever, or one of many others, without any consensus. The **Antonine Plague**, believed to have been brought back by Roman troops after campaigns in the East, was documented by the great **Galen**, but its nature remains a mystery. Similar in pathology was the Plague of Cyprian of the 270s. The medieval period is similarly dotted with mysterious illnesses, such as the unnamed epidemic that took disastrous tolls on the French army of King Louis VII (1120–1180) during the Second Crusade (1147–1149), whereas the early modern period witnessed another puzzling case for modern historians: the English **Sweating Sickness**. This malady appeared in the late fifteenth century, causing several terrible epidemics, most notably in England but also in Germany and parts of northern and eastern Europe, before disappearing completely by 1551.

Although several diagnoses have been suggested for these unknown plagues, none of them has been clearly identified. This is mainly the result of a lack of historical information or, as in the case of the English Sweats, the disease's apparent extinction. In the case of the Black Death, contention has recently developed because of the apparent marked differences between the medieval pestilence and the behavior of modern bubonic plague. Dilemmas such as the above have provoked new approaches to the diagnosis of historic diseases.

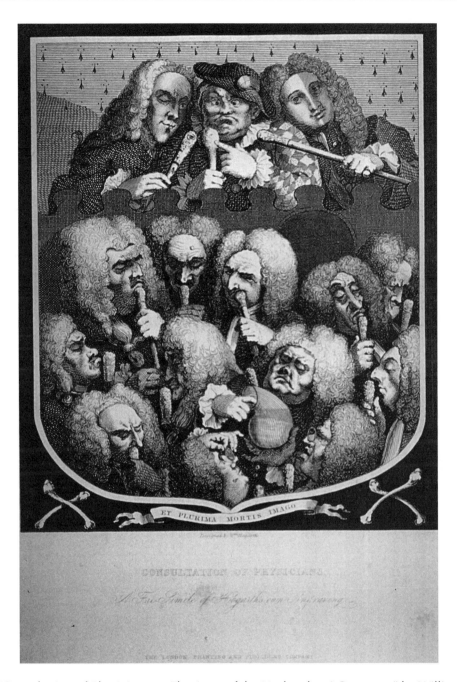

"Consultation of Physicians, or The Arms of the Undertakers' Company," by William Hogarth, 1736. Caricature of twelve physicians consulting on the contents of a urinal. Pictured above the group are, left to right, Dr. "Spot" Ward, Mrs. Mapp (known as "Crazy Sally"), and Chevalier Taylor (a well-known quack). Courtesy of the National Library of Medicine.

Since the mid-twentieth century, the theoretical approach to identifying historic diseases has changed considerably, albeit without significantly altering the traditional diagnoses already in place. Sir Frank MacFarlane Burnet (1899–1985), a prominent specialist in **immunology**, stated that historical diseases are best assessed by **epidemiology** rather than by interpreting the descriptions of symptoms contained in historical sources. This entails a move towards diagnosis by studying disease behavior in populations rather than in individuals.

Because epidemiology is a very broad discipline, including elements of mathematics, statistics, demography, and biology, as well as medicine and history, interdisciplinary approaches have been characteristic of recent attempts to diagnose historic diseases. In some cases, mathematical functions have been applied to historic population data to calculate accurately the transmission rates, incubation, and infectious period of the diseases that affected them. For example, an investigation of the parish records of baptisms, marriages, and deaths for the small northwest English town of Penrith during a sixteenth-century plague outbreak has revealed vital epidemiological information concerning the disease's behavior, indicating that it was most likely a virus—as opposed to bubonic plague, as previously diagnosed. Studies like this tend to be more localized, focusing on specific outbreaks as opposed to a whole series of epidemics, and they prove that with the right type of historical information and focus, the principles of epidemiology can ascertain the type of infectious disease affecting an historic population at any one time.

Because medicine and history are fields that are constantly evolving, the theories and tools by which historic diseases are diagnosed will continue to change as well. In recent laboratory tests, dental pulp from plague-era skeletons has been analyzed in the hope of finding traces of bubonic plague **bacterium** that could definitively prove the identity of the Black Death. To date, the results have been inconclusive, but if the technology is perfected, the future of historical diagnoses could be in the laboratory. *See also* Black Death: Historical Epidemiology, Modern Medical Debate.

Further Reading

Cunningham, Andrew. "Transforming Plague: The Laboratory and the Identity of Infectious Disease", *The Laboratory Revolution in Medicine*, edited by Andrew Cunningham and Perry Williams, pp. 245–294. New York: Cambridge University Press, 1992.

Gilbert, M. T., et al. "Absence of *Yersinia pestis*-specific DNA in human teeth from five European excavations of putative plague victims." *Microbiology* 150 (2004): 341–354.

Morens, D. M., and R. J. Littman. "Epidemiology of the Plague of Athens." *Transactions of the American Philological Association* 122 (1992): 271–304.

Scott, Susan, and Christopher Duncan. *Biology of Plagues: Evidence from Historical Populations*. New York: Cambridge University Press, 2001.

KARL BIRKELBACH

DIAGNOSTIC TOOLS.   *See* Diagnosis and Diagnostic Tools.

DIET, NUTRITION, AND EPIDEMIC DISEASE.   Diet and nutrition are linked to epidemic or infectious diseases in two main ways. First, foods can be vehicles for infections. Second, the quality of diets may influence the state of nutrition of the body, which may impact upon susceptibility to infections.

Foods as Vehicles for Disease.   There are many different food infections, which differ greatly in terms of severity of the symptoms and in other ways. Food infections may amount to relatively mild forms of food poisoning involving vomiting and diarrhea, which are frequently dealt with domestically, without referral to a doctor. Therefore food poisoning statistics, where they are collected, usually only record a small proportion of cases. The symptoms of the milder forms of food poisoning usually arise from the irritation of the intestines by toxins produced by **bacteria** such as *Salmonella*. This organism was first identified in 1888, and since then the importance attached to food poisoning as a public health problem has varied geographically and over time. During the Second World War in Britain, for example, when the state became heavily involved in the purchasing and distribution of food, and in communal feeding, interest in food poisoning increased. In another example, upon the establishment of the British National Health Service in 1948, when, for the first time, all patients could consult a general practitioner free of charge about minor ailments, there appeared to be a rapid increase in food poisoning, leading to a series of food safety initiatives.

The incidence of food poisoning is closely related to food production, handling, and consumption methods. For example, during the post–World War II period, factory farming of poultry meat and eggs led to an increase in the consumption of these foods, whereas the advent of frozen poultry, microwave ovens, and fast food outlets, increased the risk of poisoning from infected products. In particular, by the late 1980s it was apparent that there was widespread contamination of poultry meat and eggs with *Salmonella enteriditis* phage type 4 (*S. enteriditis* PT4), a bacterium that is harmless to poultry but pathogenic to humans. Recent policies aimed at eliminating *S. enteriditis* PT4 in flocks (notably **vaccination**) have led to a decline in this form of food poisoning. Health education campaigns have also encouraged consumers to boil their eggs and cook their poultry meat thoroughly. At the same time, however, a new form of food poisoning, caused by *Campylobacter jejuni*, which was first discovered in the 1970s, has become widespread. Campylobacteriosis, like salmonellosis, is often a mild disease, but because of biological differences between the organisms, countering *Campylobacter* is currently proving problematic.

Common strains of *Salmonellae* can produce systemic disease (infection spread through the body), and even death, in the young, elderly, and immunocompromised, but such infections are usually associated with the microorganisms that cause the enteric fevers, and such organisms as *Escherichia coli* 0157. The latter was first identified as a threat to human health in 1982 and became known as the "burger bug," in view of its association with ground beef. *E. coli* 0157 can cause hemolytic uremic syndrome, kidney failure, and death, and survivors may be brain-damaged or otherwise permanently disabled.

Other food-transmitted diseases include some that may only become apparent years or decades after consumption of the infective agent. These include bovine **tuberculosis**, which was common before measures were taken to eliminate the infection from dairy herds and to enforce the pasteurization of milk. Since the 1990s, much publicity has been given to variant-Creutzfeldt-Jakob Disease (vCJD), which is believed to be caused by an unusual infectious agent—a prion protein present in beef from cattle infected with Bovine Spongiform Encephalopathy (BSE). Only just over 200 known cases had occurred worldwide by April 2007, so, in spite of the massive disruption caused to the British and other national beef industries by measures to counter the spread of BSE and reduce the risk of vCJD, the disease can hardly classified as "epidemic" in the usual sense of the term.

Diet, Nutrition, and Susceptibility to Epidemic Disease.   The existence of these associations is widely assumed, yet the precise relationship between food intake and susceptibility to infection is unclear. Famine situations rarely provide clear-cut evidence as, quite apart from hunger, they usually involve large movements of people, overcrowding, and unsanitary conditions. Human feeding experiments often prove difficult to replicate, the relevance of **animal experiments** to humans can always be debated, and there are often alternative interpretations of epidemiological studies.

In 1902, Robert Hutchison (1871–1960), in *Food and the Principles of Dietetics,* opined that an insufficient supply of protein, as well as general underfeeding, lowered resistance to disease, citing the epidemics that followed the **Irish potato famine** as an example. He also remarked that exposure to infection was especially dangerous on an empty stomach, such as before breakfast, and that "the tubercle bacillus seems to find a specially-favorable soil in ill-nourished persons." This latter point reflects general medical opinion of the period. During the late nineteenth and early twentieth centuries, a plentiful diet (along with fresh air and graduated exercise) was an important component of the new "open air" **sanatorium** treatment for tuberculosis. Sanatoria for wealthy, fee-paying patients were established at first, but later facilities were also created for working class people. Tuberculosis patients lost weight as the illness progressed, but gained weight as their condition improved. It was therefore assumed that the well nourished were less susceptible to the disease, and that a plentiful diet would enhance the resistance of the infected.

Certain foods, such as dairy products, cod liver oil, and fresh fruits and vegetables, were often regarded as being of special importance in the prevention and treatment of tuberculosis. But from the 1910s, such foods were also celebrated for other reasons by advocates of the "newer knowledge of nutrition," who discovered that such foods could prevent specific noninfectious deficiency diseases such as rickets, beri-beri, and scurvy. These diseases, they believed, were caused by an inadequate intake of small quantities of certain organic constituents, which became known as "accessory food factors" or "vitamins," which were only present in significant amounts in certain foods. Most of the early vitamin pioneers, including Frederick Gowland Hopkins (1861–1947), who shared a Nobel Prize for the discovery of vitamins, also considered that low vitamin intakes decreased resistance to infectious disease. Edward Mellanby (1884–1955), who was credited with showing that rickets was a vitamin deficiency, argued that vitamin A should be regarded as an "anti-infection" vitamin and claimed to have demonstrated its value in the treatment of puerperal fever and in animal experiments.

The notion that vitamins were connected with infectious as well as deficiency diseases was linked with the vitamin pioneers' view that, in general, the role of nutrition in preventative and curative medicine had been neglected since the late-nineteenth-century bacteriological revolution. This view created common ground among the interwar nutrition enthusiasts, not all of whom thought that vitamins were of great practical importance. John Boyd Orr (1880–1971), for example, at the Rowett Research Institute in Aberdeen, considered that minerals were of greater importance than vitamins. And his research program included attempts to explore links between mineral intake and infections in both animals and humans.

Later in the interwar period, as others tested Mellanby's and Orr's hypotheses, it became clear that the links between nutrition and infection were not as simply demonstrated as these scientists had imagined, and evidence provided by practical experience during the

Second World War and its aftermath seemed only to confuse the issue further. In 1949 an editorial in the British medical journal *The Lancet* declared that "Every mother of a family, and every doctor in practice, firmly believes that the best bulwark against infection is good wholesome food." However, in spite of the "appallingly low nutritional standards in Germany" at the end of the **war**, there had been no major epidemics, whereas experiments on antibody production by starving people also suggested that malnutrition did not "play as large a part in widespread epidemics as is generally supposed." Similarly, children living in admirable conditions contracted childhood diseases, and the well fed were susceptible to colds and influenza. In addition, **poliomyelitis** seemed more common among young adults in excellent physical condition, in well-fed countries. But not all analysts of wartime health records failed to find links between diet, nutrition, and infectious disease. Isabella Leitch (1890–1980) showed that in populations in which energy and protein intakes were restricted, mortality from tuberculosis increased, reinforcing the rationale for the sanatorium dietary regimen and popular views of the benefits of a good diet.

Since the 1940s, the advent of **antibiotics** reduced the significance of many bacterial infections, but most "mothers" and "practicing doctors" have no doubt continued to regard good food as a precaution against infection. Popular nutritional preventative and curative strategies among Western populations, however, have increasingly involved vitamin supplements bought from **pharmacists**, health food shops, or supermarkets, as much as they have "healthy eating." Besides multi-vitamin preparations and cod liver oil, large doses of vitamin C were commonly swallowed in the hope of combating the common cold and influenza, viral diseases that antibiotics are powerless to counter. This practice was encouraged by the publication of *Vitamin C and the Common Cold* by Nobel Prize winner Linus Pauling (1901–1994), in 1970.

Mainstream medical and scientific opinion never moved in favor of Pauling's views, but there was, however, no practical and effective conventional treatment for the common cold and influenza with which the "megavitamin C therapy" competed. The situation was different in the case of the more recent Pauling-inspired approaches to **HIV/AIDS**. While official health agencies emphasised that good nutrition could help to preserve the qualify of life of HIV-positive individuals, the claims of Matthias Rath (1955–), an associate of Pauling, that cocktails of micronutrients can combat HIV/AIDS as or more effectively than antiretroviral drugs, have been highly controversial. Rath accused the multinational pharmaceutical companies of profiteering from HIV/AIDS, and the approach of South African Health Minister, Manto Tshabalala-Msimang (1940–) to the prevention and treatment of the disease was much influenced by Rath. In 2003, after much criticism, the South African government agreed to make antiretrovirals available in the public sector, but Tshabalala-Msimang has been slow to implement this policy.

At the beginning of the twenty-first century the precise links between nutrition and susceptibility to epidemic disease remain unclear, although **historical epidemiology** is now beginning to provide some suggestive data—for which biomedical explanations are required. A recent analysis shows that during the Second World War, mortality from infectious diseases such as **diphtheria**, tuberculosis, **measles, whooping cough, dysentery**, bronchopneumonia, diarrhea, **typhoid**, and **influenza** increased in the Netherlands, especially in the younger age groups, but remained stable in neighboring Denmark. Both countries were occupied by Nazi Germany, but whereas the energy and animal-food content of the Dutch diet declined during the war, the Danish diet was relatively unaffected.

It has been suggested that the richer micronutrient (i.e., vitamin and mineral) content of the Danish wartime diet accounts for the difference, but a century after Frederick Gowland Hopkins published the first articulation of the vitamin concept, the precise nature of the links between diet, nutrition, and epidemic disease remain elusive. *See also* Animal Diseases (Zoonoses) and Epidemic Disease; Bioterrorism; Ergotism; Germ Theory of Disease; Greco-Roman Medical Theory and Practice; Human Body; Human Immunity and Resistance to Disease; Humoral Theory; Islamic Disease Theory and Medicine; Mallon, Mary; Pharmaceutical Industry; Poison Libels and Epidemic Disease; Protozoon, –zoa.

Further Reading

Atkins, P. J. "White Poison: The Health and Consequences of Milk Consumption." *Social History of Medicine* 5 (1992): 207–227.

Hardy, Ann. "Food, Hygiene and the Laboratory: A Short History of Food Poisoning in Britain, circa 1850–1959." *Social History of Medicine* 12 (1999): 293–331.

Leitch, I. "Growth and Health." *British Journal of Nutrition* 5 (1951): 142–151. Reprinted in *International Journal of Epidemiology* 30 (2001): 212–216, available online at http://ije.oxfordjournals.org/cgi/reprint/30/2/212.pdf

Pennington, T. H. *When Food Kills: BSE, E. Coli and Disaster Science.* New York: Oxford University Press, 2003.

Trentmann, F., and F. Just, eds. *Food and Conflict in the Age of Two World Wars.* Basingstoke: Palgrave, 2006.

DAVID F. SMITH

DIPHTHERIA.   Diphtheria is a **bacterial** upper respiratory disease with high mortality rates in young **children**. At the end of the nineteenth century, microbiologists and public health experts successfully applied the principles of **germ theory** to the diagnosis, treatment, and prevention of diphtheria.

Diphtheria is caused by *Corynebacterium diphtheriae*, an organism with no known **animal** reservoir. *C. diphtheriae* is a thin rod that stains purple with the Gram stain (Gram-positive). With special stains, the bacteria show a characteristic club-like appearance with heavy uptake of dye at one or both ends (Greek *korynee*, club). With some stains, metachromatic granules (clumps of dye) are seen within the bacteria. *C. diphtheriae* will not grow on the usual agar medium used to diagnose streptococcal throat infections; special growth media are required. Four strains or biotypes of *C. diphtheriae* form distinct colonies called gravis, intermedius, belfanti, and mitis. As they divide in laboratory cultures, the bacteria arrange themselves at angles to one another, giving a "Chinese-ideogram" appearance under the microscope. Toxin-producing strains of *C. diphtheriae* produce an exotoxin responsible for most of the life-threatening symptoms of diphtheria; nontoxigenic strains cause less severe symptoms.

C. diphtheriae is spread through airborne respiratory droplets and nasal secretions or by direct contact with infected skin ulcers. During epidemics or in endemic areas, asymptomatic carriers can transmit the disease, presenting a public health risk. *C. diphtheriae* can live for weeks on fomites (inanimate objects capable of transmitting germs) such as dust particles, although this is rarely a route of human infection. A diphtheria-like illness has been linked to a related bacterium, *C. ulcerans*, transmitted through unpasteurized milk.

Clinical Picture and Treatment.   In classic childhood diphtheria, toxigenic C. *diphtheriae* invades the upper airway, attaching to the mucosa (superficial membrane) of the nasopharynx, tonsils, pharynx, larynx, and/or trachea. After an incubation period of two to seven days, the child develops a sore throat with little or no fever. The bacteria release exotoxin, which binds to receptors on nearby tissues, causing localized inflammation and cell necrosis. In this environment, the bacteria continue to multiply and produce toxin, with the formation of pus-like exudate. The exudate congeals into a characteristic tough, grayish membrane that adheres to the tissues of the throat, soft palate, and larynx. Efforts to lift the membrane cause bleeding. Enlarged lymph glands in the neck may cause a characteristic "bullneck" appearance. In severe cases, the membrane and tissue swelling extend downward toward the trachea and bronchi, causing airway obstruction. In mild cases, the membrane begins to slough off after a week, and the patient recovers rapidly. In severe cases, the victim suffers death from asphyxiation within days of the onset of symptoms.

The spread of diphtheria exotoxin through circulation causes two major complications. In 10 to 25 percent of cases, exotoxin may attack the heart muscle causing myocarditis (inflammation of the heart). Untreated myocarditis has a high mortality rate as a result of irregularities in heart rhythm. Early in the illness, the diphtheria toxin may attack the myelin sheath that coats the nerves, causing muscle weakness in the face, eyeballs, and throat. Weeks to months later, transient paralysis may develop in the arms and legs. Recovery from neurological complications is usually complete.

Much of the diphtheria found in the United States today involves the skin (cutaneous diphtheria), often in adults. In these cases, C. *diphtheriae* invades neglected skin wounds or areas of infection, causing a deep, nonhealing ulcer with a grayish-brown membrane. Complications are rare, but the skin ulcers are a reservoir of infection and constitute a public health risk.

Laboratory confirmation of diphtheria takes several days, but **antitoxin** should be administered as soon as the disease is suspected. In the United States, antitoxin is obtained through the **Centers for Disease Control and Prevention** (CDC). Delay in administering antitoxin increases complications and mortality. The dose of antitoxin depends on the severity of the infection. Because the antitoxin is prepared in horses, there is a risk of severe allergic reactions to the serum; procedures have been established for desensitizing patients who require antitoxin. **Antibiotics** such as **penicillin** or erythromycin eliminate the bacteria and are used in conjunction with antitoxin. Antibiotics without antitoxin are used for asymptomatic carriers and for those with cutaneous diphtheria. In severe cases with airway obstruction, an endotracheal tube is inserted into the airway, or a tracheostomy performed surgically until the patient improves. In recent outbreaks, mortality has ranged between 10 and 20 percent. Many people have some residual **immunity** from previous immunizations that may modify the course of the illness.

History.   Diphtheria was probably recognized in antiquity, although distinctions among various types of throat infection were not clear at the time. In past centuries, deadly **epidemics** of childhood throat infections were referred to variously as *cynanche trachealis, angina* (inflamed throat) *maligna contagiosa, angina suffocativa,* sore throat distemper, membranous croup, putrid sore throat, *el garratillo* (Spanish, strangler), malignant ulcerous sore throat, and *morbus suffocans.* **Cotton Mather** described "a malady of bladders in the windpipe" in seventeenth-century Boston. A major epidemic swept the

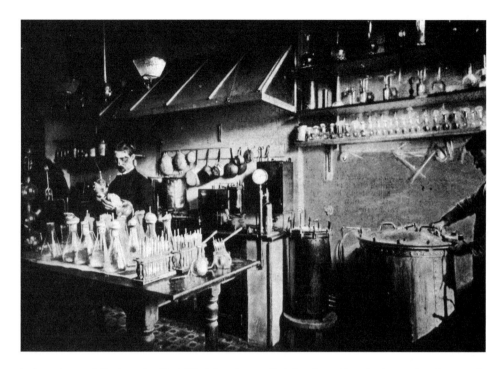

Laboratory of Pasteur Institut (Paris), where diphtheria antitoxin is made. A man is shown using autoclaves to sterilize chicken broth in which to grow the antitoxin. January 3, 1895. Courtesy of the National Library of Medicine.

northeastern American colonies in the late 1730s, killing up to one-third of all children. Often, all the children in a family would succumb within days. Applications of antiseptics and harsh cauterizing solutions added to the suffering of the child with little benefit. In 1826 Pierre Bretonneau (1778–1862) in France clarified the clinical picture, distinguished diphtheria from scarlet fever, and gave the disease its name (Greek *diphtheria*, leather). Bretonneau and others pioneered the use of tracheostomy for airway obstruction.

In the nineteenth century, diphtheria became **pandemic**. Over 1,000 children died of diphtheria annually in New York City, a pattern that continued to the end of the century. In the early 1990s, widespread diphtheria epidemics (150,000 cases) occurred in the Newly Independent States of the former Soviet Union, generally among older children and adults who had previously been at least partially immunized; case fatality rates exceeded 20 percent in the worst affected areas.

Research and Control.   Epidemic diphtheria was a terrifying prospect for parents and **physicians**. Progress in bacteriology and public health administration brought the disease under control within a few decades. In Berlin the bacterium was identified under the microscope by Edwin Klebs (1834–1913) in 1883 and grown on special culture media by his associate, Friedrich Loeffler (Löffler; 1852–1915) in 1884. Loeffler also identified the carrier state. *C. diphtheriae* was originally named the Klebs-Loeffler bacillus. In the late 1880s, bacteriologists Emile Roux (1853–1933) and **Alexandre**

Yersin at the Pasteur Institute showed that bacteria-free filtrates of diphtheria caused fatal disease in guinea pigs, proving that bacterial exotoxin was responsible for many of the symptoms of diphtheria.

In the 1890s, work by **Emil von Behring** and **Shibasaburo Kitasato** in Berlin, Roux in Paris, and other researchers led to the production of a diphtheria antitoxin in horses. The antitoxin-containing serum reversed the course of the disease and saved the lives of countless children. Health departments in New York and other American cities quickly began producing antitoxin in their own laboratories for distribution to physicians. A local diphtheria outbreak in Nome, Alaska, in the winter of 1925 was brought under control by serum rushed to the afflicted city by relays of dogsleds; the event is recalled by the annual Iditarod dogsled race from Anchorage to Nome.

In 1913, Hungarian pediatrician Bela Schick (1877–1967) developed a skin test for determining if a child was susceptible to diphtheria. In the 1920 and 1930s, research by Gaston Ramon (1886–1963) at the Pasteur Institute and by others led to the introduction of diphtheria toxoid (chemically modified toxin) and the development of an effective vaccine against diphtheria.

Immunization. Universal immunization with diphtheria toxoid has largely eliminated the disease in many countries. Despite universal childhood immunization recommendations, many children in the United States and other developed countries do not receive a full course of **vaccinations**. Many adults have waning levels of protective antibodies despite immunizations in childhood. Incompletely immunized travelers to endemic areas may contract diphtheria and become infectious to others.

Diphtheria vaccine is usually administered in a combined injection with tetanus and pertussis (**whooping cough**) vaccines. The CDC advises four doses of diphtheria toxoid in infancy with a booster at about age five and another at age twelve. Adults should receive booster shots, usually combined with tetanus toxoid, every 10 years for life. *See also* Contagion and Transmission.

Further Reading

Centers for Disease Control and Prevention. *Diphtheria.* http://www.cdc.gov/ncidod/dbmd/disease-info/diptheria_t.htm

Hammonds, Evelyn M. *Childhood's Deadly Scourge: The Campaign to Control Diphtheria in New York City, 1880–1930.* Baltimore: Johns Hopkins University Press, 1999.

Mayo Clinic. *Diphtheria.* http://www.mayoclinic.com/health/diphtheria/DS00495

National Library of Medicine. *Medline Plus.* http://www.nlm.nih.gov/medlineplus/ency/article/001608.htm

Overturf, Gary D. "*Corynebacterium diphtheriae.*" In *Principles and Practice of Pediatric Infectious Diseases,* 2nd edition, edited by Sarah S. Long, Larry K. Pickering, and Charles G. Prober, pp. 771–776. Philadelphia: Elsevier Churchill Livingston, 1997.

Pickering, L. K., ed. *Red Book: Report of the Committee on Infectious Diseases,* 27th edition. Elk Grove Village, IL: American Academy of Pediatrics, 2006; see pp. 277–281.

Salisbury, Gay, and Laney Salisbury. *The Cruelest Miles: The Heroic Story of Dogs and Men in a Race Against an Epidemic.* New York: W. W. Norton, 2003.

Vitek, C. R., and M. Wharton. "Diphtheria in the Former Soviet Union: Re-emergence of a Pandemic Disease." *Emerging Infectious Diseases* 4 (1998): 539–550.

World Health Organization. *Diphtheria.* http://www.who.int/mediacentre/factsheets/fs089/en/

SANDRA W. MOSS

DISEASE IN THE PRE-COLUMBIAN AMERICAS.   Prior to the arrival of the Spanish in the Caribbean in 1492, a variety of diseases endemic in the Old World were completely unknown among populations in the New World. These included **smallpox, measles,** and **bubonic plague.** After 1492 these three diseases and several others crossed the Atlantic into the Americas, devastating populations that had few immunological defenses as a result of lack of prior exposure. Within a century other diseases foreign to the New World would also arrive, leading to a massive population decline among indigenous peoples that did not subside until the mid-seventeenth century in Mesoamerica and the early eighteenth century in the Andes of South America.

The absence of Old World diseases from the New World was most likely the result of several factors. For one thing, many diseases could not survive or spread from person to person in the cold climate of the Bering Strait, the region through which the slow expansion of original populations from Asia into the Americas took place. To say that New World populations had no experience with certain diseases, however, should not be misunderstood to mean that they lacked disease altogether prior to 1492, or that they enjoyed an ideal of good health. For many years historians incorrectly believed that indigenous peoples in the Americas enjoyed exceptional health and had few problems with disease, but newer research in history, archaeology, and medical anthropology suggests that this was not so. We now know that such groups in fact suffered from a broad range of diseases and that epidemics periodically placed strains on many societies. Experiences with disease, moreover, varied widely according to the region and climate of the Americas where specific populations lived. Patterns of disease likewise varied according to whether populations were hunter-gatherers who migrated in search of food or sedentary agriculturalists who grew their own food and lived in relatively permanent settlements. Such populations grappled with disease in complex ways.

Diseases Present Before Contact.   Some diseases appear very clearly to have been indigenous and unique to the New World. These include several **protozoan** infections including leishmaniasis and Chagas's disease, a kind of tropical illness common in Brazil. Although these diseases are considered lowland tropical infections spread by mosquitoes, colder and higher altitude regions also had their own specifically New World illnesses. These included Carrion's disease in northern South America's mountain valleys, among others. In this way, New World populations may have lacked exposure to several virulent diseases common in the Old World, but that did not mean they were without their own set of maladies.

For hunter-gatherers, scholars have drawn on archaeological records as well as contemporary ethnographic studies to suggest that such populations prior to 1492 likely suffered from a series of gastrointestinal and respiratory diseases brought with early populations across the Bering Strait. According to the historian Suzanne Austin Alchón, gastrointestinal disorders included bacterial and parasitic infections such as shigellosis, salmonellosis, tapeworms, hookworms, whipworms, and pinworms. In addition, infections of staphylococcal and streptococcal bacteria also led to skin diseases and potentially fatal respiratory diseases such as pneumonia and meningitis. Pneumonia appears to have been a common cause of death among both hunter-gatherer populations and sedentary agriculturalists.

Scholars speculate that respiratory infections and gastrointestinal diseases also served as the leading causes of death before 1492 among sedentary groups dependent on agriculture. One such respiratory disease, **tuberculosis,** emerged as an especially problematic illness among dense populations. This is because the agent or bacillus that causes tuberculosis required the congregation of people in close spaces in order to spread from individuals who coughed to those in close proximity. Writing mainly about North America while discussing works on South America, the archaeologist Jane E. Buikstra (b. 1945) notes that skeletal remains reflect the presence of tuberculosis prior to the arrival of the Spanish. This is made evident by erosive spinal lesions, and some scholars such as M. J. Allison have also found pulmonary evidence of the disease on bodies excavated in Chile. The epidemiological patterning of these cases suggests that the disease was a mild form of tuberculosis.

Another disease that scholars believe was most likely present in the Americas before the Spanish arrived was **malaria**. Although there is some speculation that the Spanish brought malaria to the New World, it is also clear from native Mesoamerican sources that indigenous people were already familiar with the specific kinds of fevers associated with the disease. There are questions, however, as to how virulent malaria may have been among New World populations prior to 1492. If the mosquito-borne disease had been present in a particularly virulent strain, it would be reasonable to infer that the corresponding communities subject to infection would have had low population levels. But population density was in fact quite high in lowland coastal regions where mosquitoes transmit the disease, leading scholars to argue that the strain was mild.

Researchers have also long debated whether venereal **syphilis** was present in the New World prior to 1492, and whether it then spread into Europe via Spanish exploration and contact with natives. According to Jane Buikstra, certain lesions found on New World skeletons correspond to a set of related diseases known as treponematoses, which include venereal syphilis, yaws, and endemic syphilis. Disagreement persists, however, as to whether the skeletal evidence corresponds best with endemic syphilis and yaws or with venereal syphilis. Some scholars ask if venereal transmission of treponematoses originated in Europe after nonvenereal forms had spread there from the New World.

Pre-Columbian and early colonial texts suggest that indigenous populations experienced and feared epidemics in Mesoamerica and South America. Epidemics were a likely occurrence in North America as well. Often the writers of these texts and codices used vague language, discussing various "epidemics" and "plagues" that struck groups like the Aztecs in their early histories. As a result, we remain unable to identify many of these disease outbreaks. For example, the physiologist and historical demographer Sherburne Cook (1896–1974) wrote in 1946 that the Aztecs suffered from a disease they named *matlazahuatl*, which may have been **typhus**. Depictions of individuals suffering the fevers of *matlazahuatl* are present in one early colonial codex, but there is no way to link the condition to a modern disease typology with reasonable certainty.

Disease Variation across Populations.   Patterns of disease distribution in the New World depended in large part on variations between particular environments and the different ways human populations interacted with those environments. The tremendous variation in regions and climates of the Americas makes it very difficult to generalize about specific diseases across populations. Diseases of tropical lowland climates, for example, tend not to spread into high altitude regions, where environmental conditions and the absence of specific disease vectors make their transmission difficult. In addition, human populations that developed sedentary agriculture and lived in dense urban settlements tended to experience a set of problems with disease different from that of nomadic, dispersed hunter-gatherer groups. The presence of epidemics among the Aztecs and the

Incas, two populations that developed large cities and depended on agriculture and animal husbandry for survival, attests to this difference. Animals such as the turkey, guinea pig, and llama often served as vectors for the transmission of diseases to humans.

Disease patterns and frequencies also varied according to differences in nutrition levels in various parts of the Americas. That is to say, certain diseases were more common in times of drought and famine, and other diseases could be the result of chronic malnutrition or vitamin deficiencies among different groups. These processes weakened the body's immune system in many cases and left it more vulnerable to diseases such as tuberculosis. It is also worth noting that the kinds of foods populations consumed varied tremendously in the Americas, leading to different health problems. Food and other offerings, moreover, were central to how groups carried out healing and ritualized beliefs about disease.

Aztec and Inca Understandings of Disease. Both the Incas and the Aztecs saw the body as reflecting the structure of the universe through its own organization and the functions of its parts. Moreover, they saw the body and the universe as connected. As a result, phenomena such as diseases that affected the body were seen not only as particular episodes of individual suffering, but also as events related to broader cosmological processes.

Among the Incas the structure of the body reflected the structure of the Inca Empire, which was divided into four quadrants just like the four limbs of the body. The universe followed a similar structure. In the case of the Aztecs, the historian Bernard Ortiz de Montellano writes that "astronomical events could affect bodily functions and, conversely, human behavior could affect the equilibrium and stability of the universe." To treat, cure, or prevent disease thus often meant addressing both the specific afflictions affecting the individual patient and the wellbeing of the society through larger-scale rituals and cleansings. Moreover, both groups believed they could appeal to and appease their deities such that epidemics and illnesses could be prevented.

At the level of individual treatment, both the Aztecs and Incas relied on the expertise of herbalists, healers who drew on their knowledge of curative properties of plants and, to a lesser extent, animals to heal those suffering from disease. In the case of the Inca, different groups within the empire possessed knowledge of their own about medicinal herbs, though they also relied on traveling healers. One group in particular, a population known as the Kallawaya, possessed unusually effective medical knowledge of plants. As a result, they served as the official healers to the Inca state, traveling widely from the region around Lake Titicaca.

Like residents of the Inca Empire, the Aztecs and their imperial subjects also relied heavily on medicinal cures made from plants and animals. For the Aztecs milder diseases were treated with such medicines, whereas more severe conditions required complex, religiously based interventions. The emperor Motecuhzoma I (c. 1398–1469) established a botanical garden in 1467 for medical research, drawing on varieties of plants and knowledge about treatment from throughout the vast empire. General knowledge of herbal cures, however, predates that institution in Mesoamerica by centuries. It constituted a source of wonder for the Spanish, who wrote about Aztec medicine in works such as the *Florentine Codex* by Bernardino de Sahagún (1499–1590).

Both the Aztecs and the Incas also saw disease as reflecting relations between humans and the divine. For the Aztecs, diseases were caused by a mixture of supernatural phenomena linked to their religious beliefs and notions of deities, by magic or spells inflicted by sorcerers and others, and by natural or physical causes. Ortiz de Montellano argues, however, that the Aztecs did not see these categories of causation as separate, but rather combined and integrated them in their explanations. Curing disease thus required addressing the immediate physical symptoms of the patient as well as the larger social and cosmological processes that had brought disease on the society. They drew on specialists called *nahualli* and *paini* in the Aztec language of Nahuatl to diagnose magical and supernatural causes of disease. To make such diagnoses, Ortiz de Montellano claims, the *nahualli* or *paini* often consumed hallucinogenic substances to communicate with supernatural beings.

The Aztecs themselves often saw diseases as working in the human body by causing changes in the strength and form of three animistic forces central to human life. These animistic forces were known as *tonalli, ihiyotl,* and *teyolia.* Although each had a specific function and occupied a different part of the body, *tonalli* in particular was central both to human life and to establishing links between individual human beings and their gods and universe. The imbalance between *tonalli* and other animistic forces and the loss of *tonalli* itself, which occupied the head near the forehead, were thought to bring on weakness and illness. Curing disease thus often required reestablishing lost *tonalli* in the patient through a variety of means.

The Aztecs treated diseases associated with divine causation through communal rituals and individual acts such as offerings and confession. Often they directed rituals to particular deities they believed were tied to specific diseases. For example, those affected with skin and eye diseases attributed their ills to a god named Xipe-Totec. Ortiz de Montellano writes that during the spring they would participate in a ritual wearing "the flayed skins of men who had impersonated the god (according to the Aztecs the men had *become* the god) and had been sacrificed." Severe diseases were sometimes seen as having other kinds of complex causes (among them sin) that required ritualized treatments, such as confessions and incantations. The loss of animistic forces, in particular, could be interpreted as the result of immoral behavior. The treatment of disease thus often focused on establishing and practicing correct behavior to carry out therapy or preserve good health.

For the Incas, disease was also linked to questions of proper behavior, ritual purity, and relations between humans and the divine. The Incas saw disease as a source of significant concern that required both the healing of individual bodies and the healing of the body politic. This was in part because they believed disease was a reflection of sin, or *hucha* in their native language of Quechua. In order to cure people and eliminate disease, the sick had to confess their sins to special confessors known as *ychuri*, and a ritual cleansing known as a *citua* was carried out annually in the empire's capital, Cuzco. According to the famous Jesuit missionary Bernabé Cobo (1580/2–1657), who wrote a history of Peru in the seventeenth century, the Incas celebrated the *citua* in August because it marked the beginning of a period when levels of disease tended to spike in the Andean highlands. Through the ritual the Incas asked one of their deities, the creator god Viracocha, to prevent illness from affecting Cuzco and the empire as a whole in the current year. They did this by expelling all dogs and non-Incas from the city, as well as those Incas who possessed physical deformities (which the Incas interpreted as resulting from moral fault). On the following day, the Inca royalty and nobility congregated with soldiers at Cuzco's Sun Temple, where they held torches and waited for the new moon to rise. Cobo writes that upon seeing it, they cried out "diseases, disasters, and misfortunes, be gone from this land!" Others in the city left their homes and shouted repeatedly "May the evil go! Oh how we have wished for this festival! Oh Lord, let us live another year so that we may see another festival!" As they repeated these sayings, residents opened and shook their blankets and clothes, believing this would expel illness from their homes.

Different groups of Inca troops also congregated at Cuzco's Sun Temple and then in the city's main square as part of the *citua* festival of ritual cleansing. They did this to extend the process of cleansing and purification throughout the empire. At the temple they offered drinks in sacrifice before running from Cuzco in the direction of the empire's four quadrants, shouting as the moon rose "May the evil go!" Cobo claimed they ran in relays over long distances in the empire as an act of purification from disease. In this way, the rituals solidified the pre-Columbian belief that disease was to a large degree an expression of the relationship among mortals, the dead, and the divine. *See also* Astrology and Medicine; Diagnosis of Historical Diseases; Diet, Nutrition, and Epidemic Disease; Disease, Social Construction of; Environment, Ecology, and Epidemic Disease; Historical Epidemiology; Latin America, Colonial: Demographic Effects of Imported Diseases; Malaria in the Americas; Measles in the Colonial Americas; Religion and Epidemic Disease; Smallpox in Colonial Latin America; Smallpox in Colonial North America; Syphilis in Sixteenth-Century Europe; Yellow Fever in Colonial Latin America and the Caribbean.

Further Reading

Alchón, Suzanne Austin. *A Pest in the Land: New World Epidemics in a Global Perspective.* Albuquerque: University of New Mexico Press, 2003.

Allison, M. J., et al. "Tuberculosis in Pre-Columbian Andean Populations." In *Prehistoric Tuberculosis in the Americas,* edited by J. E. Buikstra, pp. 49–61. Evanston, IL: Northwestern University Archaeological Program, 1981.

Buikstra, Jane E. "Diseases of the Pre-Columbian Americas." In *The Cambridge World History of Human Disease,* edited by Kenneth Kiple, pp. 305–317. New York: Cambridge University Press, 1993.

Cook, Noble David. *Born to Die: Disease and New World Conquest, 1492–1650.* New York: Cambridge University Press, 1998.

Cook, Sherburne F. "The Incidence and Significance of Disease among the Aztecs and Related Tribes." *The Hispanic American Historical Review* 26 (1946): 320–335.

Cook, Sherburne F., and Woodrow Borah. *The Aboriginal Population of Central Mexico on the Eve of the Spanish Conquest.* Berkeley: University of California Press, 1963.

Crosby, Alfred. *The Columbian Exchange: Biological and Cultural Consequences of 1492.* Westport, CT: Greenwood Press, 1972.

Lopez Austin, Alfredo. *The Human Body and Ideology: Concepts of the Ancient Nahuas.* Salt Lake City: University of Utah Press, 1988.

Ortiz de Montellano, Bernard. *Aztec Medicine, Health, and Nutrition.* New Brunswick, NJ: Rutgers University Press, 1990.

Storey, Rebecca. *Life and Death in the Ancient City of Teotihuacan: A Modern Paleodemographic Synthesis.* Tuscaloosa, AL: University of Alabama Press, 1992.

Verano, John W., and Douglas H. Ubelaker, eds. *Disease and Demography in the Americas.* Washington, DC: Smithsonian Institution Press, 1992.

ADAM WARREN

DISEASE, SOCIAL CONSTRUCTION OF.   One of the keys to understanding the social construction of disease is the difference between illness and disease. Illness can be defined as the subjective physical process that people undergo, whereas a disease is the label that a person or group puts on that person's experience. In most of the Western world, the biomedical model of medicine is often seen as holding the key to the truth of many illnesses. In this system, the signs and symptoms of illness that a person presents with, such as cough and fever, can be studied and then defined as a type of disease, such as **influenza**. A skilled health care practitioner usually makes this **diagnosis**. Similar to the scientific method, the diagnostic method involves creating hypotheses and testing them against observable, measurable data. The doctor who correctly diagnoses influenza uses this method, hypothesizing that there is influenza based on the symptoms the patient complains of, and then using the exam, lab tests, and centuries of knowledge from the medical community to verify her hypothesis. In this model, because diseases are conceptualized to have a cause that can be discovered, isolated, and then treated, modern biomedical medicine has cured some forms of cancer, eliminated diseases that once killed people in **epidemic** proportions, and even found pills that help to ease the pain of those diseases that cannot be cured.

The social construction of disease perspective, however, argues that although the diagnosis may seem to be an objective truth, it is really only a concept constructed by doctors working within one framework to describe a given phenomenon. This position does not argue that the symptoms of the illness are imagined or that the achievements of the treatment are not impressive. Instead, a social constructionist attempts to understand how the complex interplay of society, culture, and politics influences the way diseases (and their sufferers) are named, understood, and treated. The realizations that result from these questions help to place the diseases in their cultural, historical, and political contexts.

What one personally trusts to be true is largely a product of past experience and learning. In many societies across the world, and throughout the history of humankind, the diagnostic method has not been the primary method of diagnosis leading to treatment. Instead, people learned from their understanding and observations how rationally to construct other systems that addressed their illnesses. In many places, sophisticated methods very different from modern biologic medicine developed and spread because people experienced sustained health with these methods.

For example, Traditional **Chinese Medicine** (TCM) began thousands of years before the Western world developed the scientific method. In biomedicine, the goal is often to understand a disease as unfolding in a straight line—as being linear: if the cause is a specific **virus**, then the result will be influenza. In TCM, the cause and effect of illnesses are considered to be more wide ranging. From this perspective, illness and the body work not linearly, but through what has been called "the web that has no weaver." Practitioners of TCM aim to consider all the factors that relate to the illness, such as diet, mental state, personality type, and so forth. The illness is not analyzed as a one-time problem, but as a result of patterns in the patient's life. In fact, the aim of TCM is not always to cure diseases, but rather to realign the potential energy of the body, the *qi* (pronounced "chee"), so that it can heal itself, and the illness can no longer exist. Because this method cannot, by definition, isolate one specific cause of a person's illness, TCM has not been as successful in treating specific diseases that have one cause, such as infections. But because it is more inclusive of many factors, it has been found to be very powerful in treating illnesses that have many factors, such as pain syndromes—diseases that western medicine is often unable to treat adequately.

There are countless other examples of different systems across the world that aim to define and treat illness. Sometimes, when people from different cultural perspectives are brought together to care for an illness, their separate mental constructions of what disease it is may collide. Anne Fadiman (b. 1953), in her book *The Spirit Catches You and You Fall*

Down, tells the story of a young Hmong girl who immigrated to the United States and was subsequently diagnosed with a brain disorder called epilepsy by her American doctors. Her family's cultural understanding of the illness differed radically, however, with the biomedical model proposed by the doctors. Whereas these doctors saw her illness as being caused by irregular electrical activity in the brain that could be medicated and controlled, the family saw her illness as a spiritual problem and attributed it to her wandering soul. Fadiman's story illustrates how the social construction of a disease can greatly affect a person's experience of her illness; the way that the reality of her illness weighed on them all, and their failure to comprehend the other's perspective, led to unfortunate consequences for the little girl.

Even within the same culture, however, conflict can occur when people of diverse genders, classes, or political standings construct diseases differently. As an example, when **AIDS** became prevalent in the United States, young homosexual men were affected first. The scientific medical system had not yet isolated the virus that causes the disease and the U.S. government avoided recognizing that people were dying from the disease. Gay men were often treated as shameful, second-class citizens. AIDS was socially constructed by many as a "gay disease," thereby enforcing the false belief that heterosexuals were safe. Some religious groups even claimed that the disease was a curse from God on homosexuals.

Feeling abandoned by their leaders and doctors alike, many homosexual men and other early infected groups, such as hemophiliacs, suffered tremendously at the sheer uncertainty of an awful disease that was quickly spreading. The play *Angels in America*, by Tony Kushner (b. 1956), explores this very question. In one scene, a powerful lawyer named Roy speaks to his doctor about his new and troubling symptoms. Roy has sex with men but does not want to call himself homosexual. In turn, what he chooses to call himself influences how he has constructed his relationship to not only the illness, but also the society in which he lives and has power:

> Doctor [Henry]: Nobody knows what causes it. And nobody knows how to cure it . . . AIDS . . .
>
> Roy [Lawyer]: Your problem, Henry, is that you are hung up on words, on labels, that you believe they mean what they seem to mean. AIDS. Homosexual. Gay. Lesbian. You think these are names that tell you who someone sleeps with, but they don't tell you that . . . . homosexual is what I am because I have sex with men. But really this is wrong. Homosexuals are not men who sleep with other men. Homosexuals are men who in fifteen years of trying cannot get a pissant antidiscrimination bill through City Council. Homosexuals are men who know nobody and nobody knows . . . And what is my diagnosis, Henry?
>
> Henry: You have AIDS, Roy.
>
> Roy: No, Henry, no. AIDS is what homosexuals have. I have liver cancer.

Many activist groups interested in social change and social justice argue that the definition of who is sick and who is healthy is not always based on healing the individual patient, but rather, on defining social order and maintaining power differences between groups and individuals. Sometimes written into the very language of medicine are the assumptions and prejudices of the people who have the power to define disease. If this process that allows mistaken prejudices to be tagged onto scientific thought goes unchecked, the disempowered individual or group will be isolated, as male homosexuals were during the first years of the AIDS epidemic. This may create a false sense of security for those who are considered "healthy," but it provides no real safety. History later proved this right, as AIDS quickly spread to the very heterosexual populations that did not suspect that they were at risk. This same process is at work in other cases. For example, **tuberculosis**, though potentially dangerous to entire populations, has often been written off as a disease limited to the homeless, immigrants, and criminals. Diseases like alcoholism and drug addiction are often socially constructed as only affecting those who are amoral and weak. Countless epidemics that could have been diverted early on grew out of control because of such shortsightedness.

The definition of a disease is not always a matter of conflict between groups and cultures; sometimes it is a conflict across history as knowledge increases and opinions change. Even within the same culture, diseases can be redefined in dramatic ways. Stomach ulcers were once thought by western biomedicine to be the result of stress and diet, but as further study showed a type of **bacterium** called *Helicobacter pylori* to be the cause, the old philosophy quickly became obsolete. **Malaria** was once thought by the Romans to be spread by bad air, not mosquitoes: hence the name "mala aria."

Understanding the social construction of disease is therefore a powerful way of analyzing how the phenomenon of illness is translated into the definition of a disease. It calls into question the very notions of truth, knowledge, power, and authority. A common criticism of this method is that it seems to imply that illnesses are imagined, but this is not accurate; it does not criticize people's symptoms but rather questions how these symptoms are interpreted. For those interested in clinical medicine, the key lesson of social constructionist thought is that the notion of who is sick and who is well, who is safe and who is at risk, should always be considered in its cultural, historical, and political contexts. By doing this, one can better understand how people interact with their bodies, each other, their health-care practitioners, and their illnesses. *See also* AIDS, Literature, and the Arts in the United States; Astrology and Medicine; Ayurvedic Disease Theory and Medicine; Black Death, Flagellants, and Jews; Black Death and Late Medieval Christianity; Cinema and Epidemic Disease; Epidemiology; Greco-Roman Medical Theory and Practice; Humoral Theory; Irish Potato Famine and Epidemic Disease, 1845–1850; Islamic Disease Theory and Medicine; Leprosy, Societal Reactions to; Literature, Disease in Modern; Magic and Healing; Poison Libels and Epidemic Disease; Popular Media and Epidemic Disease: Recent Trends; Race, Ethnicity, and Epidemic Disease; Religion and Epidemic Disease; Scapegoats and Epidemic Disease; Sexuality, Gender, and Epidemic Disease; Syphilis in Sixteenth-Century Europe; Tuberculosis and Romanticism.

Further Reading

Fadiman, Anne. *The Spirit Catches You and You Fall Down: A Hmong Child, Her American Doctors and the Collision of Two Cultures*. New York: The Noonday Press, 1997.

Gergen, Kenneth J. *Social Construction in Context*. New York: Sage Publications, 2001.

Kim, Kiheung. *Social Construction of Disease*. New York: Routledge, 2006.

Kushner, Tony. *Angels in America: A Gay Fantasia on National Themes*. New York: Theatre Communications Group, 1993.

Lorber, Judith. *Gender and the Social Construction of Illness*, 2nd edition. Lanham, MD: AltaMira Press, 2002.

DANIEL PALAZUELOS AND LINDSAY BROOCKMAN

DISINFECTION AND FUMIGATION.   Disinfection is the method of killing infectious disease agents outside the human body, typically with the use of chemicals. The related practice of fumigation is the use of gaseous chemical agents to kill microorganisms and pests (mosquitoes, body lice, rodents) that carry and transmit disease-causing microorganisms.

Early **miasma** theory identified filth and the noxious airs it created as the source of **epidemic** disease. During the **second plague pandemic** Europeans scrubbed the houses and furniture of victims with vinegar and fumigated houses by burning aromatic plants and firing guns. They also smoked tobacco to cleanse the air around them, held "plague infected" items—especially textiles—over fires, and set up smoky bonfires in city streets. The **sanitation movement** of the nineteenth century retained the theory and many of the processes. Sanitary hygienists emphasized cleanliness and the use of perfumes to neutralize the disease-causing foul airs. In the last decades of the nineteenth century, the laboratory work of **Louis Pasteur** and **Robert Koch** gave rise to the **germ theory of disease** which shifted attention from dirt and foul smells to microorganisms as the culprits in disease causation. Bacteriologists now emphasized that mere cleanliness was not enough, but that sanitation should employ disinfectants that would kill germs.

Following Pasteur's work, Joseph Lister (1827–1912), an English **surgeon**, sought to develop a disinfectant to kill the germs that caused wound infections in hospitals. He used carbolic acid to disinfect surgical implements, and he also sprayed a mist of carbolic acid into the air over the operating field while he performed surgery, with the intention of destroying airborne germs. Influenced by Lister, hygienists started advocating the use of disinfectants as a precaution against disease. People were advised to use disinfectants to wash the bodies of people suffering from disease, to purify the air in the sickroom, and to fumigate and cleanse any items an infected person had touched. Manufacturers began to market a range of chemical disinfectants that they touted as "germ-destroyers," although they were not necessarily effective. By the early twentieth century, manufacturers were also advertising products that could serve as personal disinfectants in the form of mouthwashes and skin cleansers that would kill the germs that cause disease.

As epidemiologists started to understand better the means by which germs were spread, they began to target those pests that were known as vectors or carriers of disease. For example, mosquitoes were known to spread the protozoa that caused **malaria** through much of the tropical world. In order to kill the insect vectors of disease and thus limit the potential for outbreaks of epidemics, public health officials fumigated homes and sprayed fields with insecticides in regions where malaria was prevalent.

Today, heat, radiation, and a variety of chemicals, including phenolic compounds and glutaraldehyde, are used as disinfectants and fumigants to kill germs and to disrupt vectors of disease. These methods of disinfection are employed widely in hospitals and agricultural and food production industries where infectious microorganisms could potentially spread quickly to a large population. *See also* Insect Infestations; Insects, Other Arthropods, and Epidemic Disease; Personal Hygiene and Epidemic Disease; Pesticides; Plague and Developments in Public Health, 1348–1600; Semmelweis, Ignaz; Yellow Fever Commission, U.S.

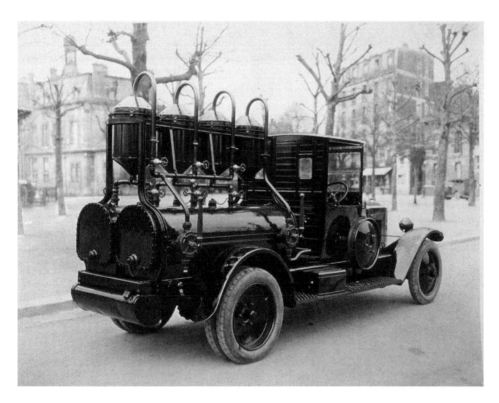

Truck equipped with disinfection tanks. Courtesy of the National Library of Medicine.

Further Reading

Corbin, Alain. *The Foul and the Fragrant: Odor and the French Social Imagination*. Cambridge, MA: Harvard University Press, 1986.

McDonnell, Gerald E. *Antisepsis, Disinfection, and Sterilization: Types, Action, and Resistance*. New York: ASM, 2007.

Tomes, Nancy. *The Gospel of Germs: Men, Women, and the Microbe in American Life*. Cambridge, MA: Harvard University Press, 1998.

WILLIAM H. YORK

DOCTOR.   *See* Empiric; Physician; Quack; Surgeon.

DRUG RESISTANCE IN MICROORGANISMS.   Killing disease-producing microorganisms with various substances is a major part of the battle against **epidemic** disease. Almost as soon as it was known that they could be killed, researchers discovered that some microbes could survive normally lethal doses of drugs. These microorganisms were commonly described as "drug-fast," from the German suffix *–fest*, meaning –proof). These early studies interpreted the microbes' resistance as "adaptation" to the toxic agents. By 1907, however, **Paul Ehrlich** focused on the concept of naturally resistant organisms, especially in the case of *Trypanosoma brucei* and p-roseaniline.

In 1913 Ehrlich clearly described drug action on microbes in Britain's *The Lancet*: pathogenic microbes are only killed by substances with which they have a certain natural relationship and through which relationship the germs are "fixed" (bound) by them. Once this "principle of fixation" was accepted, drug-fastness in a pathogen was readily explained as a reduction in receptiveness of the pathogen's "chemo-receptors" for certain chemical combinations in the drug. In other words, the chemical connection between the pathogen and the drug that normally proved fatal to the pathogen could not take place. Already in 1913, the problem of clinical drug resistance was confronting the **physician** and microbiologist. Ehrlich discussed the problem of "relapsing crops" of parasites as a result of the biological properties of the parasites.

One corollary of the specific chemo-receptor hypothesis was that combined chemotherapy was best carried out with agents that attack entirely different chemo-receptors of the microbes. Using a military metaphor, Ehrlich urged the use of a "simultaneous and varied attack" on resistant pathogens. From the earliest days of chemotherapy, multiple drug therapy using agents with different mechanisms for connecting to a given pathogen was seen as a way to prevent emergence of resistant organisms.

From the mid-1930s until the early 1960s microbiologists contested and debated the central problem of "adaptation versus mutation." Even those who viewed most microbial resistance (to chemicals and later to **antibiotics**) as some sort of inheritable change, or mutation, were divided on the issue of whether the mutations in pathogens arose in *response* to the chemical or antibiotic agent or occurred *spontaneously* and were simply observed after selection against the sensitive organisms.

As soon as a new antibiotic was introduced, reports of drug resistance appeared: sulfonamide resistance in 1939, **penicillin** resistance in 1941, and streptomycin resistance in 1946. Research focused on three major problems: (1) cross-resistance to other agents; (2) distribution of resistance in nature; and (3) induction of resistance.

In a major review in 1952, Bernard Davis (1919–1994) boldly (for the time) asserted that **bacteria** have nuclei, and that chromosomes within these nuclei apparently undergo mitosis. He went even further to note that some strains of bacteria are able to inherit qualities—including acquired drug resistance—from each of two parents, as do organisms generated by sexual unions. By mid-century, bacteria had come to be recognized as "real" cells, with conventional genetic properties, and it was only logical, Davis argued, to consider genetic mutations as the basis for inherited drug resistance.

The mid-century work in microbial genetics by Salvador Luria (1912–1991) and Max Delbrück (1906–1981), by Joshua (b. 1925) and Esther (1922–2006) Lederberg, and by David A. Newcombe (b. 1929) settled the matter of "induced versus spontaneous" mutations to drug resistance. They found that resistant organisms were already present in bacterial populations, having arisen by some "spontaneous" process; they were simply selected to survive and reproduce by the application of the drug. Because mutations to resistance to different agents were independent events (not resulting from use of a drug), Ehrlich's concept of multiple drug therapy could be refined and made precise.

In the 1950s, especially in Japan, researchers noted the emergence of many strains of pathogens with resistance to several different drugs. The patterns of resistance were complex and did not fit a simple single mutation model. Careful epidemiological and bacteriological studies of drug-resistant strains in Japan led Tomoichiro Akiba (b. 1903) and colleagues, and Kuniyasu Ochiai and colleagues, to suggest that multiple drug resistance may be transmissible between bacterial strains both *in vivo* and *in vitro* by plasmids known as resistance transfer factors (RTFs) or R-factors. Because of the promiscuous nature of R-factors, once a gene for drug resistance evolves, it can rapidly spread to the DNA of other organisms or even different species.

Knowledge of the mechanisms by which a drug worked with a pathogen often led directly to understanding the pathogen's mechanisms of resistance. Once it was known that penicillin killed bacteria by inhibiting the synthesis of certain cell-wall molecules that were found only in some bacteria (Gram stain-positive), one could understand that the Gram stain-negative bacteria were naturally resistant to penicillin. Likewise, inactivation of penicillin by a specific bacterial enzyme (beta-lactamase) aimed at a part of the penicillin molecular structure was discovered to be another key mechanism resistance to penicillin by certain bacteria. Such studies of antimicrobials have demonstrated the many ways in which microbial drug resistance evolves.

The production of antibiotics produces byproducts that are sometimes mixed into **animal** feed supplements, which therefore often contain the residues of the antibiotics themselves. The widespread use of such antibiotic-containing animal feed has led to a massive selection for resistant organisms in farm animals. The drug-resistance genes, unfortunately, are easily transmitted by R-factors into human strains leading to the widespread appearance of antibiotic resistance in human pathogens. This problem is especially common for the ubiquitous pathogen, *Staphylococcus aureus*, in which multiple drug-resistant isolates are frequently encountered.

Resistance emerges any time an antibiotic is used for any length of time, or is used in weak and clinically ineffective amounts. Widespread use of ineffective concentrations promotes emergence of drug-resistant populations. For these reasons, it is important to reserve application of new antibiotics to the infrequent cases where they are the only effective agents, as well as to employ sufficiently high and prolonged treatments to minimize the outgrowth of mutant bacteria with newly acquired resistance patterns. *See also* Hospitals since 1900; Human Immunodeficiency Virus/Acquired Immune Deficiency Syndrome (HIV)/AIDS; Immunology; Influenza; Malaria; Sulfa Drugs.

Further Reading

Arrow, Kenneth J., et al., eds. *Saving Lives, Buying Time: Economics of Malaria Drugs in an Age of Resistance*. Washington, DC: National Academies Press, 2004.

Davis, Bernard D. "Bacterial Genetics and Drug Resistance." *Public Health Reports* (1952): 376–379.

Ehrlich, Paul. "Chemotherapy: Scientific Principles, Methods, and Results." *The Lancet* 2 (1913): 445–451.

Levy, Stuart B. *The Antibiotic Paradox: How the Misuse of Antibiotics Destroys Their Curative Powers*, 2nd edition. Cambridge, MA: Perseus, 2002.

Mahajan, R. C., and Amu Therwath, eds. *Multi-Drug Resistance in Emerging and Re-Emerging Diseases*. New Delhi: Narosa, 2001.

Salvers, Abigail, and Dixie Whitt. *Revenge of the Microbes: How Bacterial Resistance Is Undermining the Antibiotic Miracle*. Washington, DC: ASM Press, 2005.

World Health Organization. *Anti-Tuberculosis Drug Resistance in the World: Third Global Report*. Geneva: WHO, 2005.

WILLIAM C. SUMMERS

DYSENTERY. Dysentery (derived from the Greek *dys* "bad" and *enteron* "intestine") is a generic term for a group of diseases that cause inflammation and necrosis of the large intestines. All of these diseases are associated with bloody diarrhea and can be deadly, depending on the source of the dysentery, as well as on available treatment. This type of diarrhea is distinctively different from the watery diarrhea commonly seen with **cholera**, not only in content but also with regard to the site of infection.

Dysentery is one of the most prevalent **epidemic** diseases in the world. Both infectious **bacterial** and **protozoan** agents, as well as certain chemical injuries, are associated with the development of dysentery. People throughout the world, of all socioeconomic classes and ages, are susceptible to developing dysentery; however, it is most often found in developing countries with poor waste management and inadequately treated water supplies. It should be noted that infected **children**, the elderly, and immunocompromised individuals have increased morbidity and mortality. Dysenteric epidemics affecting hundreds of thousands of people occur every year despite known effective treatments and preventive measures.

Biological Causes of Dysentery.   Infectious bacterial agents that cause dysentery are varied and include *Shigella*, *Campylobacter*, *Escherichia coli*, and *Salmonella* species. In addition to bacterial infections, dysentery is often caused by infection with the protozoan *Entamoeba histolytica*. Infectious agents display some regional variation but all result in frequent and often painful diarrhea that contains mucus, pus, neutrophils, and exfoliated colonic epithelial cells. *Shigella* and *E. histolytica* are the most common causes of epidemic outbreaks.

Shigella is a Gram-negative, nonmotile bacillus of the taxonomic family Enterbacteriaceae (a family which also includes *Escherichia coli* and *Salmonella*). Japanese physician Dr. Kiyoshi Shiga (1871–1957) discovered this strain of bacteria over 100 years ago. Four species compose the genus *Shigella*: *S. sonnie* (serogroup D), *S. flexneri* (serogroup C), *S. boydii* (serogroup B), and *S. dysenteria* (serogroup A). The basis for serogroup division is the differences detected in the O antigen which produces a variety of polysaccharide structures on the cell surface. These species can be further classified into 40 different serotypes.

Shigella infects and reproduces primarily in humans, but the organism has been recovered from the feces of captive primates. *Shigella* enters the body via fecal-oral transmission as a result of consuming contaminated food or water. Humans need only acquire 10 to 100 bacterial cells to become infected. Once in the digestive system, *Shigella* survives the low pH of the stomach as well as the immunological structures and digestive enzymes of the small intestine to reach the large intestine. Once in the colon, the bacteria are phagocytized by M cells found within the gut associated lymphoid tissue (GALT). The bacteria promptly escape the phagocytic vesicle, exit the M cell utilizing the cell's own cytoskeleton, and enter the surrounding epithelial cells via the basolateral surfaces of the cell. Additionally, *Shigella* invades local macrophages, thus evading the innate and acquired portions of the immune system. Within the epithelial cells, *Shigella* inhibits the cells' protein-producing machinery, effectively killing the cell while utilizing the space for reproduction. At this time, the more virulent *S. dysenteria* begins to produce the Shiga toxin, which is a potent cyto- and neurotoxin. Through this and other toxins, *S. dysenteria* causes the most clinically significant infectious complications. Both *S. dysenteria* and *S. flexneri* can cause extra-intestinal complications that include congestive heart failure and/or hemolytic-uremic syndrome that can progress to renal failure. **Physicians** see greatly reduced infectious symptoms with an *S. sonnie* infection (typically only moderate diarrhea).

Physicians' choice of treatment for *Shigella* infection has often included ampicillin and trimethoprim-sulfamethoxazole accompanied with oral rehydration and nutritional supplements. However, **antibiotic** resistance to these drugs has fluctuated since about 1980.

The National Antimicrobial Resistance Monitoring System (NARMS) branch of the **Centers for Disease Control and Prevention** (CDC) reported in 2004 that the *Shigella* samples tested were highly resistant to ampicillin (77.8 percent), streptomycin (61.0 percent), sulfisoxazole (52.4 percent), trimethoprim-sulfamethoxazole (51.4 percent), and tetracycline (49.2 percent). Additionally, multidrug-resistant strains have been reported. Currently, quinolones, cephalosporin derivatives, and azithromycin are the drugs of choice. At this time, there is no available vaccine.

Amoebic dysentery is caused by the protozoan *Entamoeba histolytica*. Russian biologist Friedrich Losch (1840–1903) discovered the presence of the amoeba in 1873 and utilized dog experimentation to establish the relationship between the parasite and the disease in dogs. The Egyptian outbreaks of dysentery in 1885 and 1896 led Greek researcher Stephanos Kartulis (1852–1920) to detect a similar relationship between the parasite and disease in humans. Most medical information concerning *E. histolytica* was established by the end of the 1800s.

Because of specific species virulence factors, *E. histolytica* is the only one of nine common human protozoa that causes disease. In fact, it is a single-cell parasite that is the third highest cause of death from parasitic infection. Transmission of *E. histolytica* occurs by ingestion of the cyst form of the amoeba. Cysts are capable of surviving for long periods of time outside of the body and can even produce viable trophozoites (the mobile form of the amoeba) following exposure to chlorinated **water**. Trophozoites are the infectious and reproductive form of the organism. Within the distal ileum, trophozoites shed their cysts and can then colonize the intestines, reproduce via the formation of novel cysts, or cause infection as a result of a variety of virulence factors.

Infection within the colon typically manifests itself acutely in one of four ways: dysentery or bloody diarrhea, toxic megacolon, amebic appendicitis, or ameboma of the colon. Invasion of the intestinal lining is thought to occur through the induction of apoptosis followed by phagocytosis of host cells. This proposed path of infection might allow the parasite to kill neutrophils and other pro-inflammatory cells resulting in a minimal inflammatory response. Additionally, this path of invasion would explain the bloody diarrhea associated with parasitic infection. Extraintestinal infection can occur throughout the body but is typically found as liver abscesses because of direct access to the liver via the hepatic portal vein.

Currently, 90 to 99 percent of infected individuals are asymptomatic, which means that the body is capable of clearing the infection (usually within 12 months) and that not all sub-species of histolytica are invasive. Treatment options vary but often include two amebicidal agents that will eliminate both the cyst and trophozoite forms. Additionally, supportive care is given to those with complications occurring because of infection.

Epidemiology. *Shigella* and *E. histolytica* are the most common causes of dysentery worldwide. In addition to causing similar symptoms, these organisms also share a common mode of **transmission**, via a fecal-oral pathway. Crowded areas in developing or socially disrupted countries with improper waste management and unsanitized water during times of drought and increased temperatures are the most likely places for epidemic dysentery. Until the late nineteenth century, dysentery was also very common in military camps and among troops on campaign, often taking more lives than action with the enemy.

The **World Health Organization** has estimated that 80 million cases of *Shigellosis* are contracted annually with 700,000 of these resulting in death. An overwhelming number of these cases are among children and the elderly. The most common cause of epidemic infection is *S. dysenteria* (Sd1) followed closely by infection with *S. flexneri*. Regional reports show that Sd1 ranges throughout the world with recent infections occurring in from 1969 to 1973 in Central America, from 1993 to 2000 on the African continent, and in 2000 in India. In North America, *S. sonnie* is the most common cause of *Shigellosis*. Infection with this serotype often produces acute, self-limited diarrhea but not deadly sequelae. In 2005 outbreaks in the United States occurred in Kansas, Kentucky, and Missouri daycare centers. Laboratory analysis confirmed close to 1,000 cases with a high degree of multiple antibiotic resistance.

A report in the *New England Journal of Medicine* suggested that there are 50 million cases of *Amebiasis* annually with 50,000 resulting deaths. One out of every ten infected individuals develops clinical symptoms. As with *Shigellosis* a large number of ill patients are represented by the young and the elderly. Southeast Asia and Central America are often plagued with outbreaks. In the United States, infections are often seen in immigrants. The last outbreak of *Amebiasis* as reported by the Centers for Disease Control and Prevention occurred in 1983 in Los Angeles, California, with close to 50 cases diagnosed but no common source of infection found. *See also* Drug Resistance in Microorganisms; Urbanization and Epidemic Disease; War, the Military, and Epidemic Disease.

Further Reading

Centers for Disease Control and Prevention *Amebiasis*. http://www.cdc.gov/ncidod/dpd/parasites/amebiasis/factsht_amebiasis.htm

Ravdin, J. I. *Amebiasis: Human Infection by Entamoeba histolytica*. New York: John Wiley & Sons, 1988.

World Health Organization. http://www.who.int/topics/dysentery/en/

NICK RAGSDALE

E

***

EARLY HUMANS, INFECTIOUS DISEASES IN. The long prehistory of infectious disease in humans extends back far beyond the pathogens that first emerged as infections in the hunter-gatherer ancestors of the *Homo* line around 2 million years ago. Those early prehumans bequeathed to us various "heirloom" infections, previously inherited from primate ancestors and retained by the early hominin line when it diverged 6 to 7 million years ago from the ancestral chimpanzee line.

The simplest category of heirloom infections comprised, presumably, the staphylococci, streptococci, and coliform **bacteria**—all families of bacteria that routinely coexist as commensals in and on humans. These bacteria can cause wound infections, throat infections, and diarrheal diseases when their micro-**environment** is disturbed or tissue is damaged. Soil-dwelling hookworms and the tetanus bacterium would also have been encountered often.

Over time, the succession of bigger-brained *Homo* species, eating increasing amounts of meat and using **animal** skins for rudimentary clothing and shelter, must have experienced new contacts with a wider range of bacteria and foodborne helminths (the various smaller enteric worms). Some evidence, though, indicates that nomadic humans are much less likely to harbor helminths, which depend on a fecal-oral transmission pathway, than are human communities living in settled, more crowded conditions. Larger gut-infesting worms, including tapeworms, are a very ancient group of commensal organisms with few retained independent capacities—they have evolved to be able, with minimal metabolic effort, to absorb nutrients passively through their outer coat. Early humans would have encountered them often in undercooked or raw meat from animal prey.

Various **viruses** able to persist or lie dormant for decades, such as the ubiquitous Epstein-Barr virus and a range of herpes and **hepatitis** viruses, also infected hunter-gatherers. The herpes virus group illustrates well a long parasitic history in both apes and hominins. These viruses could achieve unhurried vertical transmission, between generations, sometimes via processes of reactivation after several decades of dormancy. Later paleoanthropological evidence, from the past several hundred thousand years, suggests that our *Homo* cousins, the Neanderthals, who occupied Europe and western Asia for much of the last quarter-million years, were also afflicted with dental cavities and infective arthritis.

The majority of newly-evolved human infections come from animal sources, via initial zoonotic infection. Others come from soil, such as the **Legionnaires' disease** bacterium, or from **water**, such as the **cholera** bacterium. Zoonotic infections would have occurred sporadically in hunter-gatherers, from locally circulating infectious agents in wild animals. Predation by early hunters was one direct route of acquisition. Other pathogens, such as simian **malaria** (in monkeys) and **trypanosomiasis** in antelope and buffaloes, require an **insect** vector for transfer from animal to human. Most such infectious contacts would have been transient because few zoonotic agents have the innate capacity to persist within tiny nomadic bands. Further, most pathogens cannot persist within humans without a sufficient sustained supply of susceptible young hosts with immature immune systems. Nevertheless, recent scares over the **Ebola** and **Marburg** viruses, both apparently acquired from tropical forest animal sources, underscore the occasional potential virulence of such agents.

Most of today's well-known common diseases did not exist in hunter-gatherer times. Indeed, the "crowd" diseases (such as have become prominent in later millennia: **measles, smallpox, influenza,** and many others) did not enter human populations until their progenitor microbes had an opportunity to "jump" from domesticated and pest animals into humans in the new ecological setting of **Neolithic** settlements. Further, the early human hunter-gatherers, living in small, isolated, and mobile groups, could not have sustained the endemic circulation of acute infectious diseases of that kind.

This radical shift toward farming, herding, and settled living emerged gradually, from around 10,000 to 11,000 years ago. This occurred in the wake of the warming and environmental changes that followed the retreat of the last 80,000-year-long glacial period. Fossil and pollen records show that this transformation in global climate decimated and displaced many species of edible animals and wild plant foods. In low to middle latitudes, humans responded by relying more on growing plants and herding animals. As food yields slowly increased so, inevitably, did localized human populations increase in size, in accord with available food supplies.

Those settlements created a new ecological niche for microbes. Indeed, this was a major "transition" in the human-microbe relationship—it allowed the proliferation of rodents, mosquitoes, and other pest species that were able to contribute new infectious pathogens to the early agrarians, whereas the closer and repeated contact with animals allowed the emergence of many novel zoonotic infections. This process thus ushered in the consequent rise of various human-adapted infections (malaria, **schistosomiasis, tuberculosis, leprosy,** influenza, smallpox and many others). Roundworms (nematodes) also thrived as human intestinal parasites now that people in settled communities were much more likely to make contact with and ingest fecally infected material—soil (especially young children) and plant foods. In particular, the roundworm *Ascaris lumbricoides* has been a human pathogen for many millennia. Overall, this radical change in human ecology greatly affected the pattern of disease. **Paleopathological** studies, comparing preagrarian and postagrarian skeletal remains, have shown that the early farmers were shorter, and shorter-lived, than their immediate hunter-gatherer forebears; they were generally less well fed and more exposed to infectious diseases.

This gradual and multicentered agrarian transition was the dominant source of today's familiar infectious diseases—that is, diseases able to establish themselves as endemic infections within populations and, in many cases, able to move between populations in epidemic fashion. This category includes acute viral diseases like measles, mumps, chickenpox, and influenza, and bacterial diseases such as tuberculosis, leprosy, and **syphilis**. Today, we think of those infectious diseases as part of the "natural order."

The zoonotic origins of these "crowd" diseases are legion and fascinating. Smallpox arose via a mutant pox virus from cattle. Measles is thought to have come from the virus that causes distemper in dogs, leprosy from water buffalo, and the common cold from horses. Lesions in skeletons from the Middle East indicate that tuberculosis may have afflicted humans from at least 6,000 to 7,000 years ago. Dating from later millennia, tuberculosis-like lesions have been identified in the lungs of ancient mummies from Egypt and Peru. *Mycobacterium tuberculosis,* now adapted to humans, and *Mycobacterium bovis,* from cattle, are genetically very closely related, and this, and cross-infection from cattle to human, accords with the general thesis that the "crowd" infectious diseases of humans arose via zoonotic infection from cohabiting animals. In an uncomfortable reprise of this cattle-to-human transition, the bovine spongiform encephalopathy (BSE, or "mad cow disease") prion found its way into humans sometime in the 1980s.

The list of cross-species transfers from animal sources to humans is long—and lengthening, as we acquire new zoonotic infections such as **HIV, SARS,** and the Nipah virus. Some historians consider that Asia, characterized by early large agrarian populations, may have been the main source of the infectious diseases that derived from domesticated and pest animal species, whereas Africa was the cradle of vector-borne infectious diseases from wild animal sources, including malaria, **Dengue** fever, and African trypanosomiasis (sleeping sickness). Malaria most probably gained its foothold as a human infection from early forest clearing and farming in western Africa. Later, irrigated agriculture afforded increased opportunities for various disease vectors and intermediate hosts: water-breeding mosquitoes, the water snails that spread schistosomiasis, and the guinea worm.

The animal-to-human passage of zoonotic infectious disease occurred widely around the world, in centers of agriculture and **urbanization**. South America's **Chagas's disease**, for example, entered human populations several thousand years ago, probably in Brazil, via domestication of guinea pigs by Amerindians. Chagas's disease is transmitted by a trypanosome (a **protozoan** cousin of the African trypanosome) via the blood-feeding triatomine bug that lives naturally in the earthen walls of guinea-pig burrows where it transmits the infection among guinea pigs. Mummies from northern Chile provide evidence, dating back several millennia, of organ damage from Chagas's disease and of the presence of the triatomine bug itself. The bug adapts readily to the earthen walls and thatching in poor rural housing where it transmits the trypanosome between humans. Today it infects a huge 15 to 20 percent of the population in the "southern cone" countries of South America, causing thinning and, often, rupture of the walls of the heart, colon, and esophagus.

As villages evolved into larger towns, and higher-order city-states and civilizations followed, so did the skeletal evidence of social stratification become stronger. Rulers, priests, warriors, merchants, laborers, and peasant-farmers became the defining basis of political structures, power, and privilege. Much of the evidence indicates that infectious diseases took their greatest toll on the poor and the peasantry. Adult height, estimated from skeletal remains, was greater in the urban wealthy than in the rural workforce. Some of this differential reflected nutritional deprivation, some of it chronic and repeated infections.

It is important to remember that the many and various mutant microbes that early humans acquired from animal sources all have, themselves, very much longer ancestries. The mammals and **birds** from which we have recently acquired so many of our infectious diseases are themselves late-stage hosts in these long-running narratives. Indeed, bacteria and viruses predate the evolution of multicellular life by a billion years or so and spent eons learning, via the dispassionate processes of biological evolution, to infect one another and to acquire ways of adapting to hostile biochemical warfare (i.e., nature's **antibiotics**). They therefore have a genetic flexibility and fast-breeder survival capacity that we have only recently begun to fully recognize. *See also* Diagnosis of Historical Diseases; Historical Epidemiology.

Further Reading

Barnes, Ethne. *Diseases and Human Evolution.* Albuquerque: University of New Mexico Press, 2005.
Cockburn, Aidan. "Where Did Our Infectious Diseases Come From? The Evolution of Infectious Disease." *CIBA Foundation Symposium* 49 (1977): 103–112.
Karlen, Arno. *Plague's Progress: A Social History of Disease.* London: Gollancz, 1995.
McMichael, Anthony. *Human Frontiers, Environments and Disease: Past Patterns, Uncertain Futures.* New York: Cambridge University Press, 2001.
McNeill, William. *Plagues and Peoples.* New York: Penguin, 1976.

ANTHONY MCMICHAEL

EBOLA.   *See* Hemorrhagic Fevers; Hemorrhagic Fevers in Modern Africa.

ECOLOGY.   *See* Environment, Ecology, and Epidemic Disease.

ECTOPARASITES.   Ectoparasites are organisms that live on the surface of other animals and depend on their hosts in order to complete their own life cycle; hosts can range from other **arthropods** to birds, fish, and mammals. Ectoparasites with human hosts include mites, lice, fleas, and ticks. Though other arthropods, such as tsetse flies and mosquitoes, feed on human blood and may thereby transmit disease, they do not abide on or very near the skin and are therefore not considered ectoparasites. Although these creatures usually trigger only itching, rash, or allergic reaction to their saliva or feces, they are sometimes infected with parasites of their own that can cause diseases ranging from **typhus** to **bubonic plague**. As a result, ectoparasites are significant vectors of human disease.

Mites.   Mites are tiny arthropods related to spiders and ticks. Scabies, an infestation by the mite *Sarcoptes scabei*, causes great discomfort although not serious disease. Adult mites, less than half a millimeter in length, dig burrows in the outer layers of the epidermis, where they lay eggs that hatch in three to four days. Intense itching and burning is caused by the secretions of the parasites, which prefer to live in the moist folds of the body such as between the fingers and the toes and in the groin area. Scratching can sometimes lead to staph or other secondary infections.

Scrub typhus is caused by *Rickettsia tsuitsugamushi,* **bacteria** that live within the cells of mites or chiggers and are spread to humans through their bites. It occurs primarily in Southeast Asia and the Pacific, and affected thousands of Allied soldiers and marines during World War II (1939–1945). Symptoms include high fever, profuse sweating, and swelling of the lymph nodes. Another disease associated with mites, the rarer but less serious rickettsial pox (*Rickettsia akaria*), is also spread through mite bites and produces a skin rash and mild fever.

Lice.   Lice spend their entire life cycle on host animals, which can include birds and mammals. There are three varieties of lice that live on humans: *Pediculus humanus capitis*, or head lice; *Pthirus pubis*, or pubic lice; and *Pediculus humanus humanus*, or body lice. Although all cause severe itching and rash, the body louse can also serve as a vector of disease, spreading pathogens responsible for illnesses including epidemic typhus, trench fever (Werner-His disease), and louse-borne **relapsing fever**. Typhus and trench fever are spread through infected lice feces and relapsing fever through the body fluids of crushed lice. Lice are spread through close contact with an infested individual, or the sharing of clothing or bedding; infestations are most common under crowded, unsanitary conditions that make good hygiene difficult.

The adult body louse, a wingless insect from 2 to 4 millimeters in length, normally lives not on the skin of its host but on clothing, visiting the host only to feed. A female louse will lay nine or ten eggs per day, cementing them to clothing or bedding. The eggs, or nits, hatch within a week into nymphs, which grow to adulthood in about 16 days. Nymphs and adults feed on the blood of their hosts. Adults can live up to 40 days on a human host but will die within a few days if deprived of the ability to feed.

The most serious human disease transmitted by lice is **epidemic** typhus fever, which is caused by bacteria in the Rickettsia family, *Rickettsia prowazekii*. Although less well known than typhus, epidemic relapsing fever and trench fever have both caused millions of human deaths. An outbreak of relapsing fever in Eastern Europe killed an estimated 5 million people between 1919 and 1923. Trench fever, so named because it was first identified among soldiers in the trenches of the western front during World War I, killed more than 800,000 during the course of that **war**. The disease reemerged during World War II and then largely disappeared; a variant known as urban trench fever has become prevalent since the 1990s among urban homeless populations in Europe, Africa, and North America.

Fleas.   Fleas are small, hard-bodied wingless **insects** (order *Siphonaptera*) that subsist as adults on the blood of their mammal or bird hosts, although they can survive for long periods of time without feeding if no hosts are available. Their powerful legs allow them to jump from host to host and to avoid attempts by the host to remove them. Most fleas are not host specific, and there are more than a dozen species that will feed on humans.

Fleas are carriers of two major pathogens affecting humans. Infected rat fleas (particularly *Xenopsylla cheopis*) can transmit the bacterium *Yersinia pestis*, and thus bubonic plague, to humans. Murine (or endemic) typhus fever can also be spread by fleas infected by *rickettsia typhi* bacteria.

Ticks.   Ticks, small arachnids of the order *Acarina*, come in two varieties—hard ticks, or Ixodidae, and soft ticks, or Argasidae. Ticks spend a portion of their life cycle on a host animal, feeding on its blood. Hard ticks may remain attached to hosts for days as they continue to feed but soft ticks feed in a matter of minutes. Ticks, because they often harbor pathogenic parasites that are transferred to humans through their bites, are vectors of a number of human diseases, including **Lyme disease** (caused by bacteria), Rocky Mountain spotted fever (Rickettsia bacteria), **babesiosis (protozoa)**, Q fever (bacteria), Crimean-Congo **hemorrhagic fever (virus)**, and tick-borne relapsing fever (bacteria). Rocky Mountain Spotted Fever, the most serious tick-borne disease in the United States, is a sometimes-fatal disease characterized by flu-like symptoms—fever, chills, muscle ache—and a rash. Lyme disease, the most common disease transmitted by ticks in the United States, begins with flu-like symptoms and a characteristic circular rash. If left untreated, the infection can spread to the joints, causing arthritis and severe joint pain, and/or the nervous system, causing numbness, tingling in the extremities, and memory problems. *See also* Animal Diseases (Zoonoses) and Epidemic Disease; Colonialism and Epidemic Disease; Contagion and Transmission; Disinfection and Fumigation; Environment, Ecology, and Epidemic Disease; Hemorrhagic Fevers in Modern Africa; Personal Hygiene and Epidemic Disease; Pesticides; Typhus and Poverty in the Modern World; Typhus and War.

Further Reading

Buckman, Robert. *Human Wildlife: The Life that Lives on Us*. Baltimore: Johns Hopkins University Press, 2003.

Marshall, Adrian. *The Ecology of Ectoparasitic Insects*. New York: Academic Press, 1981.

Maunder, J. W. *Human Ectoparasites*. New York: Taylor and Francis, 1991.

TERESA LESLIE

EHRLICH, PAUL (1854–1915). Paul Ehrlich was the founder of modern chemotherapy and also made important contributions to the study of the immune system, blood, and cancer. Born on March 14, 1854, in Strehlen, Germany (now Strzelin, Poland), Ehrlich received his medical degree from the University of Leipzig in 1878. Upon graduation, he went to work at the Charité Hospital in Berlin, where he developed a method of staining the tubercle bacillus newly discovered by **Robert Koch**. In 1891, he joined the staff of Koch's newly founded Institute for Infectious Diseases in Berlin. Ehrlich became director of a laboratory for serum research and testing at Steiglitz in 1896. A new Institute for Experimental Therapy was created for him in Frankfurt in 1899, and he remained as its director until his death on August 20, 1915. From 1906 on, he was also head of the Georg-Speyer Haus, a laboratory for experimental chemotherapy built adjacent to the Institute.

From Ehrlich's days as a medical student, he was intrigued by the concept that drugs and chemicals had a particular affinity for specific organs and tissues. In the 1890s, his attention was focused on **immunology** when his colleague at Koch's Institute, **Emil Adolf von Behring**, discovered an antitoxin to combat the toxin produced by the **diphtheria** bacillus. Ehrlich played a significant role in assisting von Behring in the development of a standardized and sufficiently potent antitoxin preparation for use in the treatment of diphtheria patients. In order to explain the fact that the antitoxin specifically combined with the toxin molecule, Ehrlich developed his side chain theory. He theorized that the diphtheria toxin has the ability to combine with and poison specific molecular structures ("side chains" or "receptors") in the cell. As the cell compensates, some of the excess side chains produced are released into the bloodstream where they serve as antitoxins, specifically combining with and neutralizing the toxin. This concept paved the way for the emergence of the modern receptor theory of drug action. Ehrlich shared the Nobel Prize in Medicine or Physiology in 1909 for his contributions to immunology.

In the early twentieth century, Ehrlich began experimenting with dyes and other substances searching for chemical agents that could act with the same specificity as the antitoxins. He reasoned that one could cure infectious disease by finding chemicals that would specifically attack and destroy pathogenic microorganisms within the body without harming the human host cell. He and his coworkers synthesized and modified the structures of numerous chemicals, testing the activity of these compounds in experimental animals against diseases caused by microorganisms known as trypanonosomes. Later they also tested these compounds against **syphilis**. They soon focused on organic arsenic compounds. In 1909 they discovered that the 606th chemical that they tested, later trade-named Salvarsan, was effective against syphilis in animals. Although Salvarsan was not an ideal therapeutic agent because of its toxic side effects and the prolonged treatment required, it was the first drug that was truly effective in treating syphilis. It provided Ehrlich with a practical demonstration of the value of his concept of chemotherapy and helped to stimulate the search for other chemical agents against infectious diseases. *See also* Human Immunity and Resistance to Disease; Tuberculosis.

Further Reading

Bäumler, Ernst. *Paul Ehrlich: Scientist for Life*. Translated by Grant Edwards. New York: Holmes and Meier, 1984.

Parascandola, John. "The Theoretical Basis of Paul Ehrlich's Chemotherapy." *Journal of the History of Medicine and Allied Sciences* 36 (1981): 19–43.

Silverstein, Arthur M. *Paul Ehrlich's Receptor Immunology: The Magnificent Obsession*. San Diego: Academic Press, 2002.

JOHN PARASCANDOLA

EMPIRIC.   Empiric refers to a wide range of European medical practitioners—women as well as men—who lacked the formal university medical training and guild membership of physicians and were not **surgeons**. "Empirical" denotes their general method of learning, which depended upon the observation of medical practice (as well as a certain degree of trial and error) rather than on the reading and interpretation of medical texts, which was the standard mode of learning in the universities. More importantly, however, "empiric" can also be applied to those who devalued book-learning in favor of hands-on experience and medical knowledge acquired by doing, a stance taken by **Hippocrates, Galen,** and the controversial **Paracelsus** in the first half of the sixteenth century. These opposing philosophies led to a long-running antagonism between empirics and **physicians**, with the latter often labeling empirics as fraudulent **quacks** or charlatans. Nevertheless, empirics occupied an important niche in the medical marketplace, offering an alternative set of regimens and remedies that could differ markedly from the more traditional, Galenic **humoral** treatments and remedies offered by university-trained physicians. This became especially prominent in the sixteenth and seventeenth centuries, when empirics became almost synonymous with proponents of **Paracelsian** or chemical medicine.

Empirics were, in some ways, well situated to deal with **epidemic** diseases such as **smallpox, syphilis,** and **bubonic plague**. This was the result of their common presence in both urban and rural areas, of the much smaller fees they generally charged, and of the fact that wealthy traditional physicians were often among the first people to flee when plague struck. Because many empirics claimed proficiency in treating internal disorders—traditionally the prerogative of the physician—they were a logical choice for beleaguered towns and villages thus deprived of their local doctors (itself a label indicating formal education).

As this pattern was repeated during the sixteenth and seventeenth centuries, empirics established important footholds in many urban centers at the expense of their university-trained cousins. Their social and professional importance rose to such a degree that, shortly before the **Great Plague of London** (1665–1666), a number of English empirics banded together to establish the Society of Chemical Physicians in London, a short-lived rival to the Royal College of Physicians. Members of the Society openly advertised prophylactics and cures for plague during the epidemic. That they did a brisk business in treating plague victims may be inferred from the fact that 40 of the 50 practicing physicians in the Royal College fled London. Though the Society did not survive, its establishment was made possible in part by the repeated outbreaks of plague suffered by western Europe in the early modern period. Empirics continued to play a prominent role in the treatment of epidemic disease and made notable contributions to medical science and procedure well into the eighteenth century. *See also* Apothecary/Pharmacist; Folk Medicine; Medical Education in the West, 1500–1900; Paracelsianism; Plague in Britain, 1500–1647; Plague in Europe, 1500–1770s; Scientific Revolution and Epidemic Disease.

Further Reading

Furdell, Elizabeth Lane. *Publishing and Medicine in Early Modern England.* Rochester, NY: University of Rochester Press, 2002.

Gevitz, Norman, ed. *Other Healers: Unorthodox Medicine in America.* Baltimore: Johns Hopkins University Press, 1988.

Pelling, Margaret. *Medical Conflicts in Early Modern London: Patronage, Physicians, and Irregular Practitioners, 1550–1640.* Oxford: Clarendon Press, 2003.

Lingo, Allison Klairmont. "Empirics and Charlatans in Early Modern France: The Genesis of the Classification of the 'Other' in Medical Practice." *Journal of Social History* 19 (1986): 583–603.

MARK WADDELL

ENCEPHALITIS.   Encephalitis is a condition of the brain that involves swelling and inflammation. It can be triggered by non**epidemic** reactions to such things as complications following a **vaccination**, mumps, chicken pox, or herpes. However, in the twentieth century encephalitis also took on an epidemic form caused by a viral infection often carried by an **insect** vector, especially mosquitoes. This type of disease has been labeled an arbovirus or **arthropod**-borne virus. Its effects cover a wide and varying range of symptoms, but there is a basic pattern. Most types of encephalitis cause high fever, very severe headaches, stiff necks, irrationality, irritability, mental confusion, and a semi-comatose state that can continue for years. Because of this last symptom, encephalitis has been mistakenly called a "sleeping sickness." For some victims the infection can lead to death. The mortality rate for epidemic encephalitis can range from 5 to 75 percent, depending on the strain, with the normal range being roughly 15 to 20 percent.

Analysis of blood and cerebrospinal fluid collected with a lumbar puncture will determine the presence of the disease. Mild encephalitis may disappear rapidly with simple bed-rest and analgesics for the pains, whereas more serious infections, determined with encephalography and magnetic resonance imaging, may require observation in a hospital and treatment with appropriate antivirals such as amantadine or acyclovir, corticosteroids, or drugs to prevent seizures.

Two main types of the disease have been observed since World War I (1914–1918). The first broke out during the **war** and continued into the next decade. It was originally diagnosed by the Austrian medical researcher Constantin von Economo (1876–1931) who determined that it represented a new, but unidentified, viral infection that would soon be called "encephalitis lethargica." Its cause was, and still is, unknown. By the late 1920s it had disappeared as mysteriously as it had arrived. Although the Matheson Commission in New York City had systematically studied it during the decade, the **virus** was not isolated, so despite its virulent impact that caused thousands of deaths, its nature remained obscure. Its aftereffects were most disturbing, as many survivors continued on in a somnolent, trance-like state. This long-term condition would eventually be analyzed by Dr. Oliver Sacks (1933–) in the 1960s and would become the source material for both a book and a motion picture entitled *Awakenings* (1990).

In the early 1930s another form of epidemic encephalitis appeared, first in Paris, Illinois, but more spectacularly in St. Louis, Missouri. The 1933 St. Louis epidemic made headlines because it was an unknown disease that was similar to lethargica but had many different aspects. The new strain killed older people, occurred in the spring and summer, and did not have as many debilitating aftereffects as the earlier encephalitis strain. It would be given the name St. Louis encephalitis, and this form would continue to appear from the 1930s into the 1980s. Other strains of encephalitis were discovered in various parts of the world, such as Japanese B in Asia; Murray Valley in Australia; and a horse-based form, Venezuelan, in South America. The equine connection also has a history in North America, having been reported during the nineteenth century as an epizootic known as "blind staggers." This type, called eastern or western equine encephalitis depending on location, could infect humans on occasion. The first of the eastern outbreaks in humans took place in Massachusetts in 1938. This epidemic featured symptoms that differed from all the previous encephalitis types. Although the number of victims was relatively small, the mortality rate was a shocking 74 to 75 percent, and the primary targets of the disease were children under 10, including a significant percentage of infants. In addition, the effects on those who survived included severe brain damage and permanent mental retardation. Similar, but less virulent, attacks of this eastern equine strain continued to target humans on into the 1950s, especially on the east coast of North America.

The Virus and Its Transmission.   The viruses for all of the encephalitis strains since 1933 have been isolated, starting with the St. Louis type discovered by pathologist Margaret Smith (1896–1970) in that city. For many years, however, the disease's means of transmission were unclear. Back in 1933 a set of failed human experiments that had unsuccessfully attempted to prove a mosquito carrier was involved led public health officials to look elsewhere for a **transmission** medium. During the 1940s, however, the mosquito vector theory was reexamined and soon verified. What had been missed earlier was the presence of a necessary bird host that mosquitoes had to first bite in order to spread the disease. This discovery came about as a result of the work of William McDowell Hammon (1904–1989) and William C. Reeves (1917–2004) in the Yakima Valley of Washington state. Based on their research, the mosquito-bird-mosquito cycle of epidemic encephalitis transmission was accepted. Human beings, it was discovered, were simply occasional and accidental dead-end hosts who contracted the virus only under a very specific set of environmental conditions. Humans could not pass on the disease to other humans.

Therefore, by the 1950s and 1960s, the main outlines of the encephalitis arthropod-borne virus had been mapped. Health officials knew what they were dealing with and how to combat it, although certain questions about the disease still remained unanswered. For instance, it was never clear at the start of an epidemic which mosquito breeds were implicated, because the study of mosquito types and breeding places was still underdeveloped. Even more difficult to determine were the types of birds that served as hosts. They could be domestic fowl or endemic wild species or, even more likely, migratory birds just passing through the area. Migratory species might, it was believed, become infected in one geographic area, and then fly into another area that had, up to that time, been free of encephalitis virus. They would serve as the reservoir that would be bitten by local mosquitoes that would then spread the epidemic in its new location. Also unknown was the mechanism by which the virus could survive the cold winter months. It has been suggested that occurs in the body of a hibernating mosquito, but this remains a matter of scientific debate.

Because of its mosquito-bird-mosquito cycle, epidemic encephalitis is an environmentally driven disease. It requires a pattern of weather, bird, and insect interactions for it to spillover to either horses or humans. It needs a wet, rainy season followed immediately by a dry period that creates stagnant breeding pools for vector mosquitoes. There have to be very large numbers of mosquitoes emerging from these pools, as well as wind currents that can spread them to a wider geographic area. An equally large bird population must be available to act as hosts, and both the type of bird and the type of mosquito have to be carriers or reservoirs acceptable to the encephalitis virus. Epidemics can also take place in regions that do not at first appear likely, such as the High Plains of Texas, where human-made environmental changes can establish the necessary natural conditions. Thus, the digging of irrigation canals in an arid area or the creation of catch-basins from **water** drained out of sewerage treatment plants can provide the required breeding grounds for mosquitoes and even wetlands for birds. It is this general environmental nature of encephalitis that necessitates an epidemological investigation that includes a range of scientific specialties such as **ecology**, mammology, ornithology, veterinary medicine, and agricultural studies in addition to the expected fields of **epidemiology** and virology.

There is no cure for viral encephalitis nor is there any effective immunization. People who live in regions with high mosquito counts and a large bird population can protect themselves by wearing appropriate clothing and by applying insect repellent to ward off mosquitoes. The only systematic method of combating encephalitis either before or during an epidemic is to kill off either the bird hosts or the mosquito vectors. Because many different bird species may be involved in the infection cycle and because mass killing of birds is both unfeasible and socially unacceptable, it is the mosquitoes that are attacked. A typical anti-encephalitis campaign from the 1950s to the present involves the use of significant amounts of **insecticide**, originally DDT, now a diluted form of malathion, that is either sprayed from airplanes or, more likely, belched from the back of a slow moving street fogging truck. Also part of such a campaign is the draining of stagnant water from empty lots and receptacles in people's backyards that may serve as breeding pools. Ponds and ditches are usually treated with larvicide. Therefore, ironically, the methods to deal with an environmentally caused outbreak of encephalitis involve altering or destroying aspects of that environment, a fact that can sometimes lead both to natural degradation and to political controversy. *See also* Encephalitis, Epidemic Outbreaks in the Twentieth Century; Gorgas, William Crawford; Yellow Fever Commission, U.S.

Further Reading

Booss, John, and Margaret M. Esini, eds. *Viral Encephalitis, Pathology, Diagnosis and Management.* New York: Blackwell Scientific Publications, 1986.

Jarvis, Eric. "A Plague in Paradise: Public Health and Public Relations during the 1962 Encephalitis Epidemic in St. Petersburg, Florida." *Florida Historical Quarterly* 85 (2007): (at press).

Kroker, Kenton. "Epidemic Encephalitis and American Neurology, 1919–1940." *Bulletin of the History of Medicine* 78, 1 (2004): 108–147.

Sacks, Oliver. *Awakenings.* New York: Vintage, 1990.

ERIC JARVIS

ENCEPHALITIS, EPIDEMIC OUTBREAKS IN THE TWENTIETH CENTURY. Encephalitis is an inflammation of the brain occasionally triggered by such things as post-**vaccination** reactions, mumps, or herpes. Its symptoms can include sudden fever, severe headaches, irrationality, drowsiness, and at its worst coma that can lead to death. In the post–World War I era, encephalitis assumed a new viral **epidemic** form that led to outbreaks around the world.

Its first and most notorious form became known as *encephalitis lethargica*. It was originally noticed in 1915, while the war was still raging, and after the war it spread dramatically until roughly 1926, when it disappeared as mysteriously as it had appeared. It seemed to be linked somehow to the great **influenza pandemic of 1918–1919**, except that it had begun before the influenza outbreak, and its worst impact occurred in the winter of 1919–1920. It was initially studied by the Austrian medical scientist Constantin von Economo (1876–1931), who believed that the disease represented a new viral strain, even though the **virus** was never discovered. It eventually killed thousands of people and could affect survivors by placing them into a coma-like trance. This led to the disease often being incorrectly called "**sleeping sickness**," even though it had no relation to the African illness of that name. Lethargica has remained a controversial and unknown disease to this day.

In North America, viral encephalitis did not return until the 1930s. It, however, proved to be a type different from lethargica, with somewhat varied characteristics. This new type made a brief appearance in Paris, Illinois, in 1932 and then assumed an epidemic form in St. Louis, Missouri, during the late summer and fall of 1933. It became known as St. Louis encephalitis or SLE. Initially it was believed to be a return of encephalitis lethargica, but it struck at a different time of year, attacking different age groups with a set of less severe long-term effects. As a result, public health officials soon realized that they were dealing with a different strain. This time the virus was isolated, but the disease's cause and its mode of **transmission** could not be determined. It eventually spread throughout the city and its surrounding county until it ultimately ended with the advent of colder weather. The city suffered nearly 1,200 cases, with 221 recorded deaths.

In 1933 the speculation surrounding its transmission focused on the role of mosquitoes as probable carriers, especially since St. Louis was swarming with mosquitoes that summer. However, following a set of experiments utilizing **human subjects**, the mosquito theory was dropped. A group of physicians and then convict volunteers allowed themselves to be bitten by mosquitoes that had just bitten encephalitis victims. None of them contracted SLE. This led investigators to turn to other theories of contagion. What they had not realized was that the mosquitoes had to bite an infected **bird** host and that the disease could not spread from person to person directly. Only under a specific set of **environmental** conditions involving climate, mosquito breeds, and precise types of migratory birds could SLE spill over to infect humans, who served only as dead-end hosts.

This picture finally became clear during the 1940s, and as a result St. Louis encephalitis was placed into a group of similar viruses known as **arthropod**-borne viral encephalitis, or arboviruses. SLE continued to break out during the 1950s in cities such as Louisville, Kentucky, and in unexpected places such as the High Plains and the Lower Rio Grande Valley of Texas. By the time of the Texas outbreaks, the mosquito-bird-mosquito cycle theory was generally accepted but was still being tested. By the next major outbreak, in St. Petersburg, Florida, in 1962, the only unknowns were the types of mosquitoes and birds that were involved. Health authorities battled the epidemic the only way they could: by killing the mosquito carriers with the use of clouds of insecticides from mobile fogging machines. Similar outbreaks of SLE occurred in Houston (1964) and Dallas (1966), whereas it emerged in Memphis, Tennessee, in 1975, and in the Canadian provinces of Ontario and Manitoba in 1975.

Other strains of viral encephalitis evolved in various parts of the world. For instance, there was a type known as Japanese B encephalitis; it was discovered in 1924 and its virus isolated in 1935. It was similar to SLE but was more dangerous, with a death rate of 50 to 70 percent; the rate for SLE was generally 15 percent. Japanese B occurred in Japan in the 1930s and spread to other Asian nations such as Taiwan, Korea, and India right into the twenty-first century. Yet another type of encephalitis appeared in Australia in 1917 called Murray Valley encephalitis. It also had a high mortality rate and continued to break out during the 1920s, the 1950s, and into the 1970s. Beyond these varieties of the disease, there were also types that were known to attack primarily horses. These strains of equine encephalitis could, on occasion, attack humans also. One of the most serious was Venezuelan equine encephalitis that occurred throughout parts of Latin America. In North America another strain, Eastern Equine encephalitis, also claimed human victims, particularly among young **children**, for the first time in Massachusetts in 1938. It reoccurred in other parts of the eastern United States into the 1950s.

Epidemic viral encephalitis was never the killer that **yellow fever** had been, but it was yet another mosquito-carried disease that could kill and seriously injure. There is still no cure nor any preventative. The only method of combating viral encephalitis remains that of killing the insect carriers. *See also* Animal Diseases (Zoonoses) and Epidemic Disease; Disinfection and Fumigation; Pesticides.

Further Reading

Dourmashkin, R. R. "What Caused the 1918–30 Epidemic of Encephalitis Lethargica?" *Journal of the Royal Society of Medicine* 90 (1997): 515–520.

Jarvis, Eric. "A Plague in Paradise: Public Health and Public Relations during the 1962 Encephalitis Epidemic in St. Petersburg, Florida." *Florida Historical Quarterly* (at press).

Monath, Thomas P., ed. *The Arboviruses: Epidemiology and Ecology*, Vols. 1 and 4. Boca Raton, FL: CRC Press, 1988.

Eric Jarvis

ENDERS, JOHN FRANKLIN (1897–1985). The worst **poliomyelitis** epidemic in the United States occurred in 1952, when 57,000 people were stricken. John Enders and his team discovered that the **virus** that causes polio could be grown rapidly, and in a variety of different tissues, opening up the field of human virology. Medical historian John Simmons summed up their importance: "Their discovery of tissue culture technique is often lauded as a classic instance of scientific intuition combined with careful experiment leading to a medical breakthrough." These mass production techniques meant that American microbiologists **Jonas Salk** and **Albert Sabin** could go forward with their polio research and develop a vaccine.

Enders was born in Hartford, Connecticut. Though he was a graduate student in English, a friend who was in a microbiology program influenced him to change his major. He received a doctorate in bacteriology and **immunology** from Harvard University, where he was a student of microbiologist and **typhus** expert Hans Zinsser (1878–1940).

Enders, who began his career working with viruses in animals and developing animal vaccines, was asked to set up an infectious disease laboratory at Children's Hospital in Boston, Massachusetts, in 1946. In his early experiments, he found a way to grow the mumps virus in a tissue culture made up of fragments of chick embryos. During an experiment with the chicken pox virus, Enders and his team found that they had culture, composed of human embryo tissue, left over. So that the tissue would not go to waste, they tried growing polio viruses in it, using **antibiotics** to kill any contaminants. It had been previously thought that the polio virus would only grow in nervous system tissue, which had to be obtained from the brain or spinal cord of monkeys and could potentially be contaminated. But they found that they could use many different types of human tissue, including foreskin tissue from infant circumcisions and embryonic tissue from miscarriages. Using a new test tube technique, they were able to see how the polio virus killed the cells in the tissue.

Enders turned down the opportunity to develop a virus vaccine because his lab was not set up for vaccine production, and he felt that it would be better for private industry to develop a vaccine. Both he and Sabin believed that a live virus vaccine (made of live microorganisms that have been weakened but still maintain their ability to give immunity) would provide the best form of protection against polio.

Enders received the Nobel Prize in Physiology or Medicine in 1954 and was adamant that his team members Drs. Thomas Weller (1915–) and Frederick Robbins (1916–2003) share the honor equally with him. Enders developed a **measles** vaccine that was marketed in the early 1960s, and in his retirement, he investigated **HIV**, the virus that causes AIDS. *See also* Human Immunity and Resistance to Disease; Measles, Efforts to Eradicate; Poliomyelitis, Campaign Against; Vaccination and Inoculation.

Further Reading

Simmons, John G. "John Franklin Enders: Persuading Viruses to Multiply." In *Doctors and Discoveries: Lives that Created Today's Medicine*, edited by John G. Simmons, pp. 266–269. Boston: Houghton Mifflin, 2002.

Williams, Greer. "Enders: Polio Research's Debt to Mumps." In *Virus Hunters*, edited by Greer Williams, pp. 251–269. New York: Knopf, 1959.

MARTHA STONE

ENTERIC FEVERS.   "Enteric" means "pertaining to the intestines," and the historic term "enteric fever" refers to two diseases characterized by fever and intestinal symptoms. These are now known as **typhoid** and paratyphoid and are caused by different **bacteria** of the salmonella group, paratyphoid being the milder disease. They have probably been human diseases since prehistoric times and are still common in many less developed countries. Unlike other salmonelloses, these are not zoonoses: there is no **animal** reservoir of the microbes that cause these diseases. Excrements (usually feces, but occasionally urine) of either healthy carriers or active or recovering cases are always ultimately responsible for outbreaks, with the vehicle of infection normally being food or drink. Outbreaks are often small and localized, but they can also be large, as when public **water** supplies are contaminated, and they may occur far from the original source—for example, when contaminated foodstuffs are transported across or between countries. Where typhoid is endemic, the incidence of the disease tends to peak in the summer months. Enteric fevers can attack people at any age, but younger people and in-comers to endemic areas are often especially susceptible. The precise demographic characteristics of outbreaks are frequently understandable in terms of the vehicle of infection and the eating and drinking habits of the victims. Historically, typhoid outbreaks occurred when sanitary conditions were poor and **personal hygiene** difficult, such as in besieged cities or overcrowded prisons. Recently, it has been claimed that the **Plague of Athens**, which killed about a third of the population of the city and its leader, Pericles, was a typhoid **epidemic**. Historians debate the precise role of the outbreak in ending the war with Sparta, but it is generally agreed that the loss of the war was the beginning of the end of Athenian hegemony of the ancient world. Much later, sanitary conditions prevalent during the early period of European global colonization were conducive to the spread of typhoid. Between 1607 and 1624, over 6,000 settlers died from typhoid in Jamestown, Virginia. The unplanned or badly planned **urbanization** in the eighteenth and nineteenth centuries also created conditions favorable to enteric fevers, and their control was one of the aims of the public health and sanitation reforms that followed.

Evidence of typhoid in the ancient world appears in the Hippocratic corpus. In *Of the Epidemics* (400 BCE), a case is described in which "Silenus" developed small red spots, a classic sign of typhoid. The evidence that the Plague of Athens was typhoid comes from the analysis of ancient microbial DNA extracted from teeth recovered from the mass grave at the Kerameikos ancient cemetery in Athens. Although some features of the disease described by the historian Thucydides (460–400 BCE), such as its sudden onset, differ from those seen today, the DNA sequences observed are sufficiently similar to those of the modern typhoid germ to allow the conclusion that the plague was either typhoid or a very similar disease. It is recognized that there are many different strains of the typhoid germ, which cause outbreaks in which different symptoms are prominent, and that the impact of the disease also varies according to the population attacked.

The interpretation of the DNA as typhoid, however, has been challenged. On the basis of a description of symptoms by the Greek historian Arrian of Nicomedia (c. 87–147), it has also been suggested that typhoid was the cause of death of Alexander the Great (b. 356) in 323 BCE. The Roman Emperor Augustus (63 BCE–14 CE) also appears to have suffered from the disease, which was treated by cold baths by Antonius Musa, a first-century Roman physician, a treatment that was still used in the nineteenth century.

Enteric fevers are distinguished from ordinary microbial food poisoning in that the former generally have a longer incubation period—at least 7 and often 20 days—with microbes carried from the gut by the blood to invade and disrupt numerous organs. In other words, enteric fevers are "systemic" infections. The symptoms of microbial food poisoning, in contrast, can appear within hours of eating the implicated food and are usually confined to inflammation and irritation of the gut. The attack rate in enteric fevers (number of cases among the population exposed to the contaminated food or beverage) depends upon the number of bacteria ingested but also varies according to the strain involved. The main clinical features of typhoid are usually a slow-onset prolonged fever, along with such symptoms as abdominal pain and digestive problems (diarrhea or constipation), headache, cough, and lethargy. The characteristic "rose spot" rash and liver or spleen enlargement are present in a minority of victims. Those who recover normally do so in about 28 days, but about 2 percent continue to pass the typhoid organism in their feces, with the gall bladder and the tube that transfers bile from the gall bladder to the intestine being the usual site of continued infection. Older women are most susceptible to becoming carriers. Possible complications of typhoid include **meningitis** (inflammation of the lining around the brain and spinal cord), osteomyelitis (bone infection), endocarditis and myocarditis (which affect the heart), bleeding from or perforation of the gut, and pneumonia. Before the availability of **antibiotics**, some 12 to 16 percent of victims died from these complications.

The distinction between typhoid and paratyphoid was not made until the era of bacteriology. The bacterium associated with typhoid had already been described in 1880 (now known as *Salmonella typhi*). In 1896, however, another bacillus was isolated that caused an illness similar to typhoid, apart from variations in the clinical signs and source of infection. This disease was named paratyphoid, and the associated organism, *Salmonella paratyphoid*, of which three forms were subsequently identified, labeled A, B, and C, which have different geographical distributions. In paratyphoid, the intestinal changes are more diffuse than in typhoid, whereas the skin eruptions are larger and more extensive. Paratyphoid is also rarely spread by water.

Enteric fevers continue to be a serious health problem in less developed countries, where public sanitation and water filtration, treatment, and sterilization remain inadequate. Patients also tend to delay seeing a doctor, and antibiotics are often not easily available in these countries. Typhoid resistant to chlomaphenicol, the usual antibiotic treatment, and multiple **drug resistance** have caused increasing concern in recent years. Occasionally, chloramphenicol-resistant strains had been encountered from as early as 1950, but it was not until the early 1970s that a large outbreak of choremphenicol-resistant typhoid occurred. This took place in Mexico, where the incidence of typhoid had declined for some 20 to 25 years as sanitary conditions were improving. Nevertheless, a massive epidemic began explosively in 1972 in Mexico City and the State of Hidalgo, soon spreading to the Central Valley and beyond. There were an estimated 10,000 to 15,000 cases during 1972, and the fatality rate, 13 percent at first, was unusually high. It emerged that 96 percent of the strains involved in the epidemic were chloramphenicol-resistant. The authorities responded with health education and the regulation of food markets, along with some 5 million doses of vaccine. The epidemic subsided in 1973 but lasted until 1975. As time passed, for poorly understood reasons, the proportion of the chloramphenicol-resistant strains involved declined. It proved surprisingly difficult to pinpoint the vehicle of infection, although for some geographically self-contained

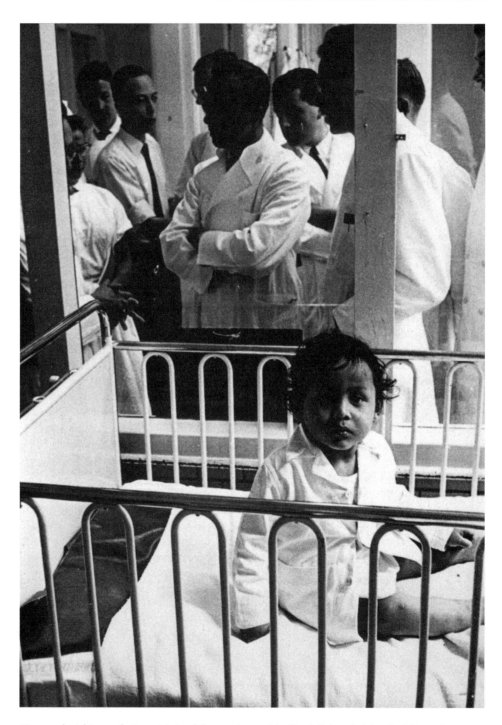

First typhoid inoculation. United States Army Medical School, March 1909. Courtesy of the National Library of Medicine.

outbreaks within the overall epidemic, contaminated water was certainly involved. Bottled beverages came under suspicion, but it was concluded that, unusually, direct person-to-person spread was an important feature.

In 1984 it was estimated that globally there were 16 million cases of typhoid illness and 600,000 deaths annually. It has been estimated that, during 2000, there were 21,650,974 cases of typhoid illness and 216,510 deaths, and 5,412,744 cases of paratyphoid illness. However, in view of the shortage of laboratory and surveillance facilities in many of the counties where typhoid remains endemic, the reliability of the methodology upon which these data are based is uncertain. In countries such as Egypt, India, and Chile, where sufficient data are available, a downward trend in the incidence in typhoid is apparent, consistent with improvements in sanitary conditions in these countries. But some regions, especially south-central and southeastern Asia, continue to have a high incidence of enteric fevers. *See also* Colonialism and Epidemic Disease; Diagnosis of Historical Diseases; Diet, Nutrition, and Epidemic Disease; Hippocrates and the Hippocratic Corpus; Sanitation Movement of the Nineteenth Century; Typhoid Fever in the West since 1800; Vaccination and Inoculation.

Further Reading

Crump, John A., Stephen P. Luby, and Eric D. Mintz. "The Global Burden of Typhoid Fever." *Bulletin of the World Health Organization* 82 (2004): 346–353.

Emmeluth, Donald. *Typhoid Fever*. Philadelphia: Chelsea House, 2004.

Papagrigorakis, Manolis J., et al. "DNA Examination of Ancient Dental Pulp Incriminates Typhoid Fever as a Probable Cause of the Plague of Athens." *International Journal of Infectious Diseases* 10 (2006): 206–214.

Shapiro, Beth, Andrew Rambaut, and Thomas P. Gilbert. "No Proof that Typhoid Caused the Plague of Athens (a reply to Papagrigorakis et al.)." *International Journal of Infectious Diseases* 10 (2006): 334–335.

"Typhoid Fever in Mexico." Editorial in *The Lancet* 305 (1975): 1230.

DAVID SMITH

ENVIRONMENT, ECOLOGY, AND EPIDEMIC DISEASE.   Like various other large mammals, *Homo sapiens* is a patch-disturbing species. Over tens of thousands of years, humans have encroached upon and changed the natural environment and have done so at an increasing scale and with growing intensity. This encroachment has, inevitably, disturbed or disrupted many ecosystems and interspecies relationships, thereby affecting the ecology, geographic range, and activity of infectious agents. There are, we presume, tens of millions of different species and types of **bacteria, viruses**, and other microbes "out there" in the natural world. Hence, a major part of human experience— both biological-evolutionary experience and cultural experience—has been to encounter an increasing number of these infectious agents as human populations have spread and diversified around the world.

History might be told as a series of major transitions in the ever-changing relationship between the human and microbial worlds: **Neolithic** agrarianism, contacts and conflicts between adjoining empires, transcontinental explorations and conquests, and **industrialization** and **urbanization**. Today we are adding a new and momentous layer to that story of environmental exploration and encroachment and microbial mobilization. Many of the large-scale environmental changes that humankind is now imposing on the biosphere, such as changes in the pattern and scale of land use, the use of waterways, and global climate change, have great implications for the pattern of infectious disease occurrence and **transmission**, now and in future.

Land Use and Environmental Change.   Several decades ago the eminent twentieth-century microbiologist Rene Dubos (1901–1982) noted that throughout history humans have always substantially changed the environment in which they live. Many of these changes, he pointed out, affected the ecology and the occurrence of infectious diseases. The main human-induced environmental changes that affect infectious disease risk today include the following: land clearing, especially tropical deforestation; road building; irrigation; dam building; changes to regional climate; intensified crop and animal production systems; urban growth and sprawl; continuation of poor sanitation practices; and the pollution of coastal **waters**.

In the early 2000s, a working group of several dozen scientists from around the world reviewed what is known from published research about how patterns of land use affect the emergence of new infectious diseases. They ranked the land-use activities with greatest impact, in descending order: agricultural development; urbanization; deforestation; population movement and displacement; introduced species/pathogens; biodiversity loss; habitat fragmentation; water and **air** pollution (including heightened respiratory susceptibility); road building; impacts of **HIV/AIDS** on human resources for farming and land management; climatic changes as a result of human generation of greenhouse gases; and hydrological changes, including construction of dams.

The following examples illustrate some of the different ways in which various human environmental impacts affect emerging infectious diseases.

Altered Environment and Habitat with Increased Population Sizes of Either "Reservoir" Host Species or Vector Species.   Forest clearance, with road building, ditch construction, and subsequent damming and irrigation, has diverse impacts on anopheline mosquito species—the species whose members are vectors for **malaria**. Cleared land and the creation of ditches often enhance breeding opportunities for local anopheline mosquitoes. Recent studies in the Peruvian Amazon have clearly shown a strong positive relationship between the intensity of forest clearance and the abundance of malaria-transmitting mosquitoes. On the other hand, land clearance and habitat disruption may eliminate some local mosquito species and thereby open a niche for an invasive anopheline mosquito species.

The rodent-borne **hantavirus** provides an illustration of how regional fluctuations in climate (whether natural or human-amplified) can disturb relationships among species within ecosystems. This virus occurs widely in rodent populations in agricultural systems in South America and East Asia and in arid grasslands in North America and elsewhere. In mid-1993, an unexpected outbreak of a mysterious viral infection occurred in humans in the Four Corners region of the southwestern United States. The infection caused acute respiratory distress and had a high fatality rate. This novel disease was eventually traced to infection with a previously unrecognized hantavirus, maintained primarily within the reservoir population of native deer mice. The disease was duly called "hantavirus pulmonary syndrome." Human infection by this virus can apparently occur by the inhalation of wind-blown dried excretions of infected mice.

Why did this disease emerge in 1993? Researchers surmised that the El Niño meteorological event of 1991–1992, with its unseasonably heavy summer rains in the American

Southwest, had caused a great increase in the local rodent populations and had thus made the 1993 outbreak possible. Populations of deer mice were reported to have been more than 10 times greater than the previous 20-year seasonal average.

Biodiversity Change and Habitat Fragmentation.   Deforestation with fragmentation of habitat increases the "edge effect" the extent of interspecies contacts at land-use boundaries—which increases pathogen-vector-host interaction. This process has contributed, in recent decades, to the emergence of a number of viral **hemorrhagic fevers** in South America: in Argentina (Junin virus), Bolivia (Machupo virus), and Venezuela (Guanarito virus).

These hemorrhagic fever infections typically occur in outbreaks ranging from a few dozen to thousands of cases. They are caused by arenaviruses for which wild rodents are the natural hosts. Outbreaks have mostly occurred in rural populations, when people become infected by contact with contaminated rodent excretions. This is well illustrated by the Machupo virus. The clearing of forest in Bolivia in the early 1960s, accompanied by blanket spraying of DDT to control malaria mosquitoes, caused both an infestation of the cropland by *Calomys* mice and the DDT poisoning of the usual predators of those mice (the village cats). The consequent proliferation of mice led to the emergence of a new viral fever, the Bolivian (Machupo) Hemorrhagic Fever, which killed around one-seventh of the local population.

Ecosystem Changes, Loss of Predators, and Host-Species Imbalance.   Tick-borne **Lyme disease** in the northeastern United States illustrates this type of complex influence on infectious disease occurrence. This bacterial disease was first identified in the American Northeast in 1976 in the town of Old Lyme, Connecticut. The disease is spread by black-legged ixodic ticks that are infected with the spirochete *Borrelia burgdorferi.* The ticks normally feed on mammalian species, especially deer and white-footed mice, with the latter being the more likely source of the infective agent; that is, the mice are considered the more "competent" host species for transmission of the spirochete.

The tick has a three-stage life cycle: larva, nymph, and mature adult. Transmission of the spirochete is influenced by temperature and rainfall, which affect both the geographic range of the intermediate host mammals and the speed of maturation of the immature (larval-nymphal) tick. The temperature-dependent synchrony of blood feeding by both the larval and nymphal stages of the tick is an important requirement for maintenance of infection within the maturing ticks. In the northeastern United States, the tick is predominantly infected by feeding on spirochete-infected white-footed mice.

The tick, however, can also feed on other small mammals, most of which do *not* carry the spirochete. Hence, in depleted local ecosystems with few mammalian species, the tick-nymphs will be more likely to feed on infected mice, and so the proportion of infected ticks will be much greater than when the ecosystem has a diversity of food sources for ticks. In fact, forest fragmentation and hunting in the northeastern United States have reduced biodiversity in this ecosystem. This has entailed the loss of various predator species—wolves, foxes, raptors, and others—and a resultant shift of tick-feeding from the less to the more competent host species (i.e., white-footed mice). This example illustrates how a range of environmental and ecosystem changes in response to land-use and species eliminations, along with middle-class suburban sprawl into woodlands, can combine to influence the occurrence of an infectious disease.

Niche Invasion.   The emergence of some infectious diseases results from a pathogen invading a newly created, or recently vacated, ecological niche. A good example of the former is the Nipah virus, which first emerged as a human disease in Malaysia in 1997–1998.

Human contact with this naturally bat-borne virus followed the establishment of pig farms, constructed in combination with fruit orchards within newly cleared areas of tropical forest in central-northern Malaysia. It is thought likely that the unusually intense El Niño event of those same years, 1997–1998, and the associated extreme forest fires and smoky haze in Southeast Asia, impaired forest fruit yields, and that this forced the fruit-bats to seek food further afield. This they apparently did, especially from the newly available fruit orchards. Consequently, thousands of pigs were infected, often fatally, and over 100 infected pig handlers and slaughterhouse workers died from this new zoonotic viral infection.

The emergence of the Nipah virus in humans was, in summary, associated with a combination of environmental changes—forest clearance, unusual fires, and smoke—that caused a marked decline in forest fruit yield. This caused a displacement of fruit bats to a new food-source niche, which opened up new cross-species opportunities for the fruit bat virus.

Global Climate Change.   The advent of human-induced global climate change is a major, momentous, new category of environmental change and ecological disturbance. Most infectious agents, their vector organisms, and their nonhuman reservoir species are sensitive to climatic conditions—as well as to many of the other environmental changes that will result (e.g., changes in vegetation and, hence, in vector-**insect** populations). Hence, it is widely expected that climate change will, via changes in both average climatic conditions and climatic variability, affect the spatial-temporal patterns of many infectious diseases.

The common microbial causes of food poisoning, including *Salmonella* and *Campylobacter* organisms, are known to be sensitive to temperature. Most food poisoning cases occur in the hotter months of the year and in the hotter countries of the world. The reported incidence of food poisoning has risen in many developed countries (which have systematic reporting of these diseases) in recent decades, but this has many plausible explanations. One possible contributor is the underlying warming that has occurred. There is a need for careful research on this topic.

Meanwhile, some tantalizing reports are appearing, as recently occurred for foodborne *Vibrio parahemolyticus*, a major bacterial cause of seafood-associated food poisoning. In summer 2004, a major outbreak of this disease occurred on a cruise ship off northern Alaska after passengers had eaten oysters. The record showed that mean coastal-water temperatures had increased by 0.2°C per year since 1997—and, in particular, that 2004 was the only year when the critical temperature of 15°C had been exceeded throughout the July–August oyster harvest season. Researchers concluded that "rising temperatures of ocean water seem to have contributed to one of the largest known outbreaks of *V. parahaemolyticus* in the U.S.," and they concluded that, with global warming, this elevated risk is likely to persist in the future.

Overall, there is increasingly suggestive evidence that the climate change that has occurred over the past three decades or so has influenced at least a handful of climate-sensitive infectious diseases. These include the northward extension of the tick that transmits tick-borne **encephalitis** in Sweden over the 1980s–1990s in association with warming winters, and an apparent increase in the human disease itself; the ascent of highland malaria to higher altitudes in parts of eastern and southern Africa in association with local warming; and the recent northward drift of the January winter "freezing zone" that limits the survival of the water snail that transmits **schistosomiasis** in eastern China.

Conclusion. Human intervention in the environment has been an age-old source of exposure to new microbes. The experience of the past several decades has underscored more clearly just how rapidly and adroitly microbes are able to take advantage of new environmental niches and altered ecological configurations. This newer understanding should have a steadying effect on our approaches to environmental disturbance, especially environmental changes now occurring on an unprecedented scale as we begin to change natural systems, such as climate systems, at regional and global scales. As we escalate our repertoire of environmental "patch disturbances," we can expect to see, and to experience, an increase in the rate at which new and resurgent infectious diseases appear and spread.

See also Animal Diseases (Zoonoses) and Epidemic Disease; Black Death: Modern Medical Debate; Colonialism and Epidemic Disease; Diet, Nutrition, and Epidemic Disease; Disease in the Pre-Columbian Americas; Early Humans, Infectious Diseases in; Epidemiology; Greco-Roman Medical Theory and Practice; Insect Infestations; Irish Potato Famine and Epidemic Disease, 1845–1850; Latin America, Colonial: Demographic Effects of Imported Diseases; Malthusianism; Pesticides; Poverty, Wealth, and Epidemic Disease; Sanitation Movement of the Nineteenth Century.

Further Reading

Barnes, Ethne. *Diseases and Human Evolution*. Albuquerque: University of New Mexico Press, 2005.

McMichael, Anthony. *Human Frontiers, Environments and Disease: Past Patterns, Uncertain Futures*. New York: Cambridge University Press, 2001.

Schwartz, Maxime. *How the Cows Turned Mad: Unlocking the Mysteries of Mad Cow Disease*. Translated by Edward Schneider. Berkeley: University of California Press, 2004.

Walters, Mark. *Six Modern Plagues, and How We Are Causing Them*. Washington, DC: Island Press, 2003.

Weiss, Robin, and Anthony McMichael. "Social and Environmental Risk Factors in the Emergence of Infectious Disease." *Nature Medicine* 10 (2004): 570–576.

ANTHONY MCMICHAEL

EPIDEMIC AND PANDEMIC. The *Dictionary of Epidemiology* defines the term "epidemic" as "the occurrence in a community or region of cases of an illness, specific health-related behavior, or other health-related events clearly in excess of normal expectancy." "Pandemic" is defined as "an epidemic occurring over a very wide area and usually affecting a large proportion of the population." A pandemic is thus simply a very large epidemic. The term "outbreak," on the other hand, usually indicates a small epidemic. Clearly there is a good deal of subjectivity in these terms; different authorities may refer to the same event using different designations, and it is not infrequent that a single authority, in a presentation or manuscript, will refer to an event as an "epidemic" in one place and an "outbreak" in another. Although, like its counterparts, "pandemic" is sometimes used loosely, it usually indicates an event that is either global or at least covers a continent or major region of the world (e.g., the 1918 "Spanish influenza" pandemic). Similarly, the term "outbreak" is used preferentially when the health event in question is localized in time or place and limited in its impact upon a larger population (e.g., an outbreak might occur in a school, factory, or military unit).

The word "epidemic" is derived from the Greek root words for "on or about" (*epi*) "the people" (*demos*). Samuel Johnson's 1755 dictionary (London) contains the word "epidemick," apparently a fairly new word at the time; by the early nineteenth century it had strongly taken hold in English (minus the terminal "k"). "Epidemic" eventually replaced the earlier term "epidemy," from the medieval "ipedemye," spelled in various ways, and related to the Greek "epidemia." Cognates of "epidemy" have been retained in other languages, for example, the German (*epidemie*) and the French (*épidémie*).

Corresponding terms referring to animal diseases are "outbreak," "epizootic," and "panzootic." Even epidemiologists occasionally refer to animal outbreaks as "epidemics," despite its nonsensical meaning, and also refer to epizootiological aspects of animal diseases as "epidemiological," perhaps because the latter is more easily pronounced or more widely understood. America's first great epidemiologist, Noah Webster, eventually became the nation's first prominent lexicographer. It is of interest to note that in early editions of *Webster's Dictionary* (e.g., New York, 1828) he defined the noun "epidemic" as "a disease generally prevailing," and one that "seizes a great number of people at the same time." He also listed two interchangeable adjectives, "epidemic" and "epidemical," to be used in distinction to "endemic or local." Before "epidemic" and its cognates became popular, an infectious epidemic disease might be called a "plague" or "pestilential disease" (*pest* and *peste* in German and French/Italian/Spanish, respectively) or a "*loimos*" (λοιμοζ) after the Greek term for plague.

In modern English usage, "epidemic" is commonly applied in a broad sense to refer to infectious, chronic, and lifestyle-associated diseases (e.g., SARS, diabetes mellitus, and obesity). It also enjoys popular usage as an all-purpose indicator of frequency (e.g., in referring to an epidemic of school tardiness). Until recent decades, however, an epidemic was almost always taken to mean a widespread acute disease, and in that sense it is the product of a long history of terms and concepts used to describe severe "pestilential" occurrences, almost all of which were infectious (with a few historical exceptions, such as outbreaks of **ergotism** or mercury poisoning).

History.   Under whatever terminology, epidemic infectious diseases have been recognized since ancient times. Indirect lines of evidence suggest that in **early humans'** hunter-gatherer days large epidemics were unlikely to occur for the simple reason that small nomadic kinship groups had only occasional contact with each other, limiting the spread of microorganisms. Crop cultivation and animal domestication, which began about 10,000 years ago with the **Neolithic Revolution**, supported early **urbanization** with large concentrations of stable populations capable of sustaining widespread **transmission** of microorganisms. Moreover, it is probable that during this era many epidemic infectious diseases arose when animal organisms learned to switch hosts to infect, and to be transmitted among, humans (e.g., **measles, smallpox,** and **tuberculosis**).

By Old Testament biblical times, epidemics and epizootics were apparently common (e.g., the Pharaonic "plagues" in the *Book of Exodus* [c. 1552 BCE], some of which are now speculated to have been infectious). An epidemic was also described in *The Iliad* (events occurring around 1250 BCE). By the fifth century BCE, epidemic descriptions entered a new era of sophistication with the **Hippocratic corpus**, which described a number of epidemic diseases, such as mumps. The **Plague of Athens** (430–426 BCE), which occurred during the Peloponnesian Wars and may have brought about the end of Greece's Golden Age, was vividly described by Thucydides (c. 460–400 BCE). Although the disease has not been conclusively linked to any disease known today, Thucydides' account is a landmark in epidemic history, representing the first disease characterized as a distinct entity on the basis of its clinical and epidemiologic pattern. Thucydides' description remained highly influential for centuries and formed the centerpiece of and often model for thousands of written histories of other epidemic diseases, which were typically compared to the Athenian disease, which served as a benchmark.

During the Renaissance and early Enlightenment (c. 1400–1800), it was common practice in writing treatises and dissertations to assemble epidemic chronologies that spanned recorded history, sometimes running into hundreds of entries. The Enlightenment featured attempts to distinguish one disease from another, at first on nosologic (naming) grounds that drew upon minor clinical and epidemiological differences to create charts that supposedly displayed relationships and differences among diseases and types of disease. Although ultimately unscientific, these nosologies did encourage rational observational study of epidemics and epizootics, a process aided by recognized epidemics of noninfectious diseases for which an etiology could be found (e.g., lead poisoning of wine and other drinks).

By the late 1700s infectious disease outbreaks and epidemics were being studied rationally and reported in the medical literature. Among these were naval outbreak investigations, delineation of complex diseases like anthrax by clinical-epidemiologic means, and investigation of cattle epizootics including rinderpest throughout the eighteenth century. In 1776 King Louis XVI (1754–1793) set up an international disease outbreak surveillance and investigation system in France and its overseas possessions, representing the first national governmental epidemic disease unit. During the 1832 cholera pandemic, epidemiologic methods based on statistical analysis of **demographic** risk factors (age, socioeconomic status, population density, etc.) finally brought the study of epidemics into a rational framework capable of contributing to the microbiologic breakthroughs that occurred in subsequent decades.

Modern Epidemic Concepts. A 1992 report of the U.S. Institute of Medicine has added a new concept and new vocabulary to epidemic diseases. Entitled *Emerging Infections*, this influential report has categorized epidemic diseases into those that have newly emerged and those that continue to reemerge (e.g., **HIV/AIDS** [newly emerging in 1981] and **Dengue** fever [reemerging/resurging over recent decades]). A third category "deliberately emerging" was later coined to address **bioterrorism**. More important than nomenclature, this report has reorganized scientific thought about infectious disease epidemics by emphasizing the many risk factors that influence emergence/reemergence, including risk factors related to the microbial agent (e.g., genetic mutation, host adaptation), the host (e.g., immunodeficiency), and the environment (e.g., crowding, travel).

Today epidemics and pandemics are routinely investigated and reported by local and national governments, and by international agencies such as the **World Health Organization** (WHO). For example, WHO has been involved in international planning for an **influenza** pandemic, recognizing that based upon historical evidence new pandemic strains arise periodically, on average every 30 years or so over the last three centuries. WHO also played a leading role in the 2003 SARS epidemic, which threatened to become pandemic when cases were exported from Hong Kong to a number of other countries. In the United States (for example) epidemic surveillance and outbreak investigation is conducted by all 50 states and by the Commonwealths and Territories, as well as by major cities and some county health departments. These activities are supported by, and to some extent coordinated by, the federal U.S. **Centers for Disease Control and Prevention** (CDC), which also provide epidemic response backup to states. In addition, the United States and many other developed countries assist other countries and the WHO in support of epidemic activities, including outbreak investigation, **diagnostic** assistance, and provision of laboratory materials. *See also* Animal Diseases (Zoonoses) and Epidemic Disease; Biblical Plagues; Chadwick, Edwin; Cholera: First through Third Pandemics, 1816–1861; Contagion Theory of Disease, Premodern; Diagnosis of Historical Diseases; Environment, Ecology, and Epidemic Disease; Epidemiology; Epidemiology, History of; Historical Epidemiology; Human Immunity and Resistance to Disease; Snow, John; Virchow, Rudolf.

Further Reading

Garrett, Laurie. *The Coming Plague: Newly Emerging Diseases in a World Out of Balance*. New York: Farrar, Straus, and Giroux, 1994.

Last, John M. A *Dictionary of Epidemiology*, 2nd edition. New York: Oxford University Press, 1988.

Lederberg, Joshua, Robert E. Shope, and Stanley C. Oaks, eds. *Emerging Infections: Microbial Threats to Health in the United States*. Washington, DC: National Academy Press, 1992.

Morens, David M., Gregory K. Folkers, and Anthony S. Fauci. "The Challenge of Emerging and Re-emerging Infectious Diseases." *Nature* 430 (2004): 242–249.

Winslow, Charles-Edward A. *The Conquest of Epidemic Disease: A Chapter in the History of Ideas*. Princeton: Princeton University Press, 1943.

DAVID M. MORENS

EPIDEMIOLOGY. Epidemiology has been eclectically defined over its brief—less than two-century—history, and its meaning is apparently still evolving. The *Dictionary of Epidemiology* (2004) defines epidemiology as "the study of the distribution and determinants of health-related states or events in specified populations, and the application of this study to health problems." It further adds, more coherently, that epidemiology is "that branch of medical science which treats of epidemics."

A wise and anonymous epidemiologist once observed that epidemiology "is all things to all men . . . The plethora of definitions is the very heart of the problem . . . a structure sturdy enough to . . . shelter **physicians**, dentists, veterinarians, and **nurses**; very small (micro) biologists and fat chemists; mammalogists, bugmen, birdmen, and spacemen; traffic directors and city planners; engineers mechanical, sanitary, electrical, stationary, and human; sociologists, psychologists, and anthropologists, cultural and otherwise . . . everything!" Indeed, the first of the above definitions, derived from earlier constructions, is steeped in the political correctness of modern public health (e.g., epidemiology should not study just diseases but also health). Moreover, it is often said (illogically) that epidemiology cannot really be epidemiology unless its findings are actually *applied* to health problems, casting it firmly as a proactive tool of public health. Epidemiology thus tends to be defined differently by those who wish to use it to achieve different aims.

The many and often tortured current definitions of epidemiology reflect confusion, particularly in the United States, where epidemiologic approaches are aggressively being taken up and adapted by professionals in a variety of disciplines, are being applied to new and different problems far removed from actual epidemics and infectious disease epidemics in particular, are being infused with methodological and theoretical complexities, and are being taught increasingly in graduate schools to students without grounding in the medical arts or biomedical sciences.

These changes have led to a diffused professional body of epidemiologists distanced from epidemiologists of earlier generations in their emphasis on mathematical and theoretical study of data sets, trying to tackle the arguably more complicated problems of chronic and lifestyle-related diseases, which have become the major causes of morbidity and mortality in developed nations. This has led also to a generational and professional divide within epidemiology; it is unclear how or whether this will be reconciled. The new era of genomics, proteomics, and bioinformatics is likely to affect the future evolution of epidemiology in ways that are yet unknown.

Without taking a position on how epidemiology should be defined, it is worth noting that the word and concept came largely out of the study of pestilential and other infectious diseases. The origin of the term "epidemiology" has not been identified, but it was first used in its modern sense in continental Europe in the 1830s and 1840s in forms such as *Epidemiologie* (in Germany) and *épidémiologie* (in France). Appearance of the cognate in English may have occurred around December 1849 during the first planning sessions for what became, several months later, the Epidemiological Society of London. As many of the founding members of that society read the French medical literature regularly, a plausible argument could be made that "epidemiological" and "epidemiology" were imported from the French language directly into English. It is curious to note, however, that during the early decades of epidemiology, its practitioners did not call themselves "epidemiologists." When "epidemiologist" did catch on, about a decade later, it was not in reference to a professional discipline but to a side-interest of physicians and occasionally others who drew upon their eclectic professional skills to serve the public health.

History.   Although "epidemiology" and its cognates may have been new in the 1830s, the idea of examining and recording the occurrences and patterns of epidemic diseases was by then at least 3,000 years old. An ancient example is the **biblical plagues** of Egypt recorded in Exodus, written circa 1552 BCE. The ancient Greeks made major conceptual contributions to what might best be called "proto-epidemiology" (epidemiological ideas and activities undertaken before the word and concept had come into existence). Such observations were recorded in the **Hippocratic corpus**, as outlined in *Airs, Waters, Places*. Here the author posits that epidemic diseases are distinct entities appearing in patterns of either pathognomonic (characteristic of a single disease) or constellationary (occurring together in a pattern) clinical signs/symptoms, and under particular conditions of season, weather, and geological events. Democritus (c. 460–370 BCE) proposed that contagious diseases are spread by tiny invisible particles. And the still-unidentified **Plague of Athens** (430–426 BCE), described by Thucydides (c. 460–400 BCE), is a recognized landmark in the study of epidemics because it represents the first known characterization of a disease as a distinct entity on the basis of its clinical and epidemiologic pattern.

Many other epidemics were described and catalogued between Greco-Roman times and the eighteenth-century Enlightenment. But without an understanding of modern **germ theory** or infectious disease etiology, or any rational way to distinguish one disease from another, proto-epidemiology had difficulty moving beyond mere descriptions. During these centuries, occasional proto-epidemiologic investigations of occupational outbreaks were conducted (e.g., of lead poisoning), but these seem to have had little influence on epidemiologic thought. Even so, progress was gradually made by recording the patterns and features of one disease at a time, without any awareness of movement toward overarching concepts of disease occurrence.

A critical first step in the development of epidemiology was disease distinction: without it there could be no basis for studying disease determinants or distributions. Persian-born physician **Rhazes** clearly distinguished **smallpox** from **measles**, and later observers eventually proposed other distinct contagious diseases (e.g., the Scot Bernard de Gordon [c. 1260–1318], who drew upon Rhazes and the Persian **Avicenna**, to list eight distinct diseases he thought were communicable [most of them correctly]).

During these many centuries there seems to have been no concept or term that corresponds closely to any modern concept of "epidemiology." "Loimologia," "loimology," and "loimographia," used in the seventeenth century, referred to the centuries-old chronicling of *loimos* (λοιμοζ), an ancient Greek term corresponding roughly to major epidemic/pandemic diseases. "Epidemical" and "epidemial," popular in the late 1700s and early 1800s, were adjectives applied to infectious disease epidemics. The Latin term *epidemiologia* appeared as early as 1802 (*Epidemiologia española*), but the book's subtitle (*ó Historia cronológica de las pestes, contagios, epidemias y epizootias*) makes clear that this "discourse about epidemics" applied only to the centuries-old practice of compiling chronological lists of important epidemics. This activity was, by the late eighteenth and nineteenth centuries, transformed into medical geography, as practiced, for example, by Noah Webster (1758–1843), August Hirsch (1817–1894), and Charles Creighton (1847–1927), and it spilled over into medical history, as practiced by physicians like Justus Friedrich Karl Hecker (1795–1850).

As the Enlightenment ended and the **Industrial Revolution** began, urban population concentration led to increasingly severe epidemics, but also to counteractive **sanitary movements**, to development of mortality, morbidity, and other **demographic data** systems, and to the appearance of vital statisticians and preventive medicine physicians. In the early years of this new industrial age, a generation of physicians returned to their European homes from the **Napoleonic wars**, many influenced by the radically new subjects of public health and social medicine, to address disease prevention in all segments of the population, prominently including the urban poor. These so-called "hygienists" studied the incidence and prevalence of various health conditions in populations, making use of census data and medical arithmetic, and identifying disease-specific demographic risk factors such as sex, age, locale, occupation, crowding, socioeconomic status, and others. In essence, these physicians systematically studied the distribution and determinants of diseases in open populations, the first true epidemiology. Their work can best be seen in the voluminous literature of the 1832 Parisian **cholera** epidemic. A generation later, the establishment of a national Register of Births and Deaths in England and Wales, coupled with the almost universal adoption of national censuses, led to further advances in epidemiology, as in the groundbreaking work of **William Farr**, William Budd (1811–1880), and **John Snow**. Snow's separate investigations of cholera incidence rates by contaminated and uncontaminated London **water** supplies, and of cholera contamination at Soho's Broad Street pump, were eventually recognized as landmarks in epidemiology and are taught to all epidemiologists today.

Modern Epidemiology. Throughout the nineteenth century, epidemiology was strongly oriented toward infectious disease outbreak/epidemic investigation and control, as it had been for centuries. The 1920s, however, saw epidemiology develop in new direc-

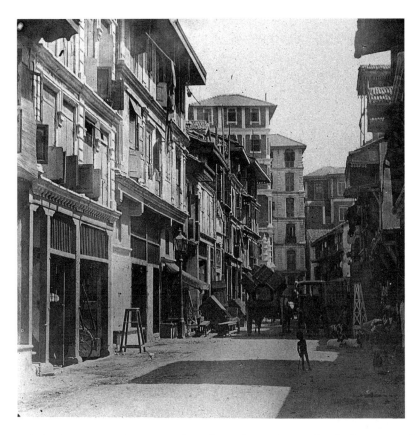

Lantern slide illustrating elements of epidemiology during third plague pandemic, c. 1900, Old Bengalpura Street, Mumbai, India. Wellcome Library, London.

tions, including such infusions of expertise from the social sciences as better standardized methodologies to link disease risk factors to diseases by comparing incidence rates in exposed and unexposed persons (cohort studies), and by comparing prior exposure frequencies in ill and well persons (case-control studies). In the United States, these developments were heavily influenced from about 1920 to about 1980 by the national experiment in establishing numerous schools of public health in universities. Throughout much of the twentieth century the United States was a leader in all forms of epidemiology, but this era now seems to be rapidly ending as the value of epidemiology has become more widely appreciated.

Although epidemiology is still subject to a bewildering array of definitions, it remains possible to identify some of its most visible practitioners. The term "epidemiologist" is generally used only to describe persons with doctoral degrees (M.D., Ph.D., Sc.D., Dr. P[ublic] H[ealth], etc.) who have had specific academic or practical training. Epidemiologists often work in national health agencies, such as the U.S. **Centers for**

Disease Control and Prevention and the U.S. National Institutes of Health, in state and local health departments, as faculty in Medical Schools and Schools of Public Health, as Preventive Medicine officers in the military, in industry (working with drug and vaccine development, and sometimes in occupational health), and in many other positions. People with masters and other degrees concentrating in epidemiology are often referred to in health department practice as "epidemiology specialists," or by a similar term. In addition to health department work, they are also employed by industry and in academic research support positions.

As epidemiology evolves, it is probably best to view it not as a professional discipline but as an approach to public health problem solving, in which the methods and approaches are less important than the ultimate effect on population health. Indeed, until recent decades, virtually all epidemiologists were credentialed in another discipline (often medicine) and tended to view epidemiology as one of a number of "tools" (alongside, for example, clinical skills, microbiology, biostatistics) to be drawn upon in order to solve practical public health problems. Epidemiologist David Fraser has proposed that epidemiology be viewed as a liberal art, an idea that has taken hold in some academic institutions, the subject and principles now being taught to undergraduates and even to high school students. Increasingly, epidemiology and epidemiologists are the subjects of books and films, with the diseases they study serving as plot devices. This phenomenon seems to reflect public awareness and interest, a desirable occurrence given that however far removed from the "real world," epidemiology must inevitably return to the problems of real human beings affected by real health problems. *See also* Epidemiology, History of; Historical Epidemiology; Measles, Efforts to Eradicate; Public Health Agencies in the West before 1900; Sanitation Movement of the Nineteenth Century; Smallpox Eradication.

Further Reading

Fraser, D. W. "Epidemiology as a Liberal Art." *New England Journal of Medicine* 316 (1987): 309–314.

Gordis, Leon. *Epidemiology*, 2nd edition. New York: Saunders, 2000.

Kenrad, Nelson. *Infectious Disease Epidemiology: Theory and Practice*. Boston: Jones and Bartlett, 2006.

Morabia, Alfredo Morabia, ed. *A History of Epidemiologic Methods and Concepts*. Basel: Birkhauser Verlag, 2004.

Rosen, George. *A History of Public Health*. Expanded Edition. Baltimore: Johns Hopkins University Press, 1993.

Rothmna, Kenneth J. *Epidemiology: An Introduction*. New York: Oxford University Press, 2002.

DAVID M. MORENS

EPIDEMIOLOGY, HISTORICAL.   *See* Historical Epidemiology.

EPIDEMIOLOGY, HISTORY OF.   Whereas the complex statistical methods and concepts in use by epidemiologists today are relatively new, the study of population-level disease phenomena can be traced back to ancient times. "**Epidemiology**" stems from the Greek "logos" (the study of) and "**epidemic**," which in turn is derived from "epi" (upon) and "demos" (people).

Greek **physician Hippocrates** is often described as the first epidemiologist. He reportedly traveled extensively, treating the sick, teaching young doctors, and meticulously recording his observations. His *On Airs, Waters, and Places* provides an early conception of epidemiology: "Whoever wishes to investigate medicine properly should proceed thus: in the first place to consider the seasons of the year, and what effects each of them produces for they are not at all alike, but differ much from themselves in regard to their changes. Then the winds, the hot and the cold," the qualities of the **water** and soil, as well as the behaviors of the inhabitants, including "whether they are fond of drinking and eating to excess." Extensive observation of these factors would, in turn, reveal patterns in the behavior of epidemics.

Although many of Hippocrates' conclusions appear erroneous today, his great innovations were in emphasizing observation as the primary route to scientific knowledge and the identification of natural, rather than supernatural, causes of epidemics. Greek philosophers were prone to reduce complex phenomena to the invisible actions of a few simple elements (earth, **air**, fire, and water), but Hippocrates rejected metaphysics in favor of empirical observation. This empirical approach was subsequently stifled, however, by dogmatic adherence to **Galen's humoral theory**, which dominated medical thinking for some 1,600 years.

Beginning in the sixteenth century, the early **Scientific Revolution** brought about a more robust empirical approach to scientific knowledge, rooted in observation and experimentation, and began the challenge to Galenic medicine. Meanwhile, an infrastructure for collecting census data was being developed in England and Wales; in 1538, Thomas Cromwell (c. 1485–1540), King Henry VIII's (1491–1547) chancellor, ordered all parishes to keep a register of baptisms, marriages, and burials. In London, death statistics were published as the London Bills of Mortality—a practice pioneered by Milan and Venice—which by 1629 began to include causes of death. Two seventeenth-century figures, shopkeeper and amateur scientist John Graunt (1620–1674) and economist and philosopher Sir William Petty (1623–1687), saw the value in such data and developed early methods for utilizing it. In his book *Natural and Political Observations . . . upon the Bills of Mortality* (1662), Graunt used this data to demonstrate that mortality was very high in infancy and higher in the country than in the city.

Two broader developments in the eighteenth century proved important for the development of statistical medicine. The growth of **hospitals** during this period greatly increased the opportunities for clinical investigation, as physicians could now observe a larger number of patients with similar ailments and make comparisons. At the same time, the mathematical theory of probabilities was being developed and applied to a wide range of phenomena, including medicine. French mathematician Pierre-Simon Laplace (1749–1827) published a series of papers in the 1770s that attempted to capture human judgment in mathematical terms, and he recommended that physicians apply the calculus of probability in making clinical decisions. Parisian clinician Pierre-Charles-Alexander Louis (1787–1872) at La Charitè hospital advocated what he called the "numerical method" of analysis, which consisted of systematic record keeping and statistical comparisons to evaluate different treatments. This theoretical framework was crucial for the development of statistical methods for epidemiology.

It was in the nineteenth century that epidemiology as a discipline came into its own, furthered by Victorian enthusiasm for both quantification and social reform. The General Register Office was founded in 1836 to carry out civil registration of births, marriages, and deaths in England and Wales. **William Farr**, who had studied medicine and statistics with Pierre Louis in Paris, joined the Office as a compiler of statistical abstracts. During his 40-year tenure at the office, he played an essential role in gathering and analyzing data for epidemic investigations and developed systems of disease classification. Additionally, during this time, in 1850, the London Epidemiological Society was formed "with the specific purpose of determining the causes of and methods of preventing cholera and other 'epidemic diseases.'"

Today, every introductory epidemiology textbook relates the story of how London physician **John Snow** demonstrated that cholera was transmitted through contaminated water, rather than by changes in local atmospheric conditions (or miasma). After an 1854 outbreak in London, Snow plotted the houses of cholera victims on a map, illustrating how they clustered around a water pump on Broad Street. But Snow's most ambitious and ingenious study—a model for the developing discipline of epidemiology—was a large-scale natural experiment in which he mapped out the source of the water supplied to neighborhoods in South London by rival water companies. Lambeth Waterworks Company took its water from the Thames upstream of London, beyond the reach of most of London's sewage. Snow found that households served by competitor Southwark and Vauxhall Company, which took its water directly from the Thames in central London, had six times as many cholera cases as did the households served by its rival.

Snow's evidence was indeed persuasive, but it was not the entire story. Critics pointed out that the neighborhoods served by the two companies differed in other ways as well—Southwark and Vauxhall served poorer households in more crowded areas closer to the river. Farr conducted the most thorough analysis of data from the cholera epidemic in nineteenth-century Britain, looking at age, **sex**, temperature, weather conditions, property values, and domestic crowding, along with countless other variables. His key finding was a consistent inverse relationship between cholera mortality and soil elevation. This finding supported the view of Farr and other leading public health experts at the time that cholera epidemics were precipitated primarily by changes in local atmospheric conditions. The ongoing debate provided the impetus for the development of novel methods for gathering and analyzing data and testing hypotheses, and Farr later came to accept Snow's theory based on the extensive evidence.

With the advent of **germ theory** in the late nineteenth century, the microbiologist in the laboratory became the center of medical discovery, as the **microscope** revealed causative agents of anthrax, **tuberculosis**, and other deadly diseases. German physician **Robert Koch's** postulates set out conditions for identifying pathogens with a particular disease: the organism must be found in all animals with the disease, but not in healthy animals; the organism must be isolated from a diseased animal and grown in pure culture; and the organism should cause disease when reintroduced into a healthy animal. With further study of **viruses** in the early twentieth century, however, it became clear that Koch's postulates could not be met for all diseases. **Wade Frost**, the first American professor of epidemiology, maintained that, in the absence of experimental evidence, epidemiologists must proceed "inductively," accumulating observations from a variety of sources and piecing them together into a coherent explanation of the role of a microorganism in a specific disease.

The debate over the relationship between smoking and health in the 1950s, although it focused on chronic disease, had an enormous impact on the discipline of epidemiology. In 1950 five case-control studies revealed that hospital patients with lung cancer, compared to individuals who were healthy or had an unrelated condition, were more likely to be smokers. However, skeptical scientists, including some prominent biostatisticians and epidemiologists, challenged the methods employed in these studies and suggested alternative interpretations of the results. For example, legendary statistician R. A. Fisher (1890–1962) hypothesized the existence of a common cause behind both cancer susceptibility and the urge to smoke. This debate, in turn, provided an impetus for the development of new statistical methods to analyze epidemiologic data and for the undertaking of large cohort studies, such as the American Cancer Society study that tracked 188,000 middle-aged male smokers and nonsmokers. By 1964 the evidence from over 30 case control studies and 7 large cohort studies was overwhelming, and the conclusions of the Surgeon General's committee on smoking and health affirmed that epidemiology could provide sufficient evidence of cause and effect to guide medical and public health decisions.

Epidemiology has evolved dramatically from its early development as a diversion for curious physicians into a highly specialized discipline. Epidemiologists today receive rigorous training both in statistical methods and in biomedical science, typically specializing in a particular disease area. Nevertheless, at the same time, the discipline remains inherently cross-disciplinary, as contemporary epidemiologists must understand and piece together information from the molecular and genetic level to that of human populations in order to understand the causes and determinants of patterns of disease. *See also* Cholera, First through Third Pandemics, 1816–1861; Demographic Data Collection and Analysis, History of; Plague in Britain, 1500–1647.

Further Reading

Hempel, Sandra. *The Strange Case of the Broad Street Pump: John Snow and the Mystery of Cholera.* Berkeley: University of California Press, 2007.

Hippocrates. *On Airs, Waters, and Places.* Translated by W. H. S. Jones. Cambridge, MA: Harvard University Press, 1923.

Kowal, Areta O. "Danilo Samoilowitz: An Eighteenth-century Ukrainian Epidemiologist and His Role in the Moscow Plague (1770–72)." *Journal of the History of Medicine and Allied Sciences* 27 (1972): 434–446.

Morabia, Alfredo Morabia, ed. *A History of Epidemiologic Methods and Concepts.* Basel: Birkhauser Verlag, 2004.

Parascandola, Mark. "Skepticism, Statistical Methods, and the Cigarette: A Historical Analysis of a Methodological Debate." *Perspectives on Biological Medicine* 47 (2004): 244–261.

Stolley, Paul, and Tamar Lasky. *Investigating Disease Patterns: The Science of Epidemiology.* New York: Scientific American Library, 1998.

MARK PARASCANDOLA

ERGOTISM. Ergotism is a generic term for three distinct human diseases resulting from the ingestion of cereal grains, most notably rye, that have been infected with the fungus *Claviceps purpurea*. *C. purpurea* produces spore bearing stalks (sclerotia) that contain a variety of chemicals, known as alkaloids, several of which are hazardous to humans and animals. The three best-known alkaloids are ergotamine, ergonovine, and lysergic acid hydroxyethylamine. Ergotamine can cause blood restriction to certain parts of the body producing a condition known as gangrenous ergotism. Ergonovine can cause spontaneous abortions in women. Lysergic acid hydroxyethylamine can cause a condition known as convulsive ergotism with symptoms ranging from hallucinations, to vomiting, diarrhea, and lethargy. All ergot alkaloids have been synthesized in the laboratory, with much of the early work done by Sandoz Pharmaceuticals.

C. purpurea is an ascomycete, a sac fungus. In the spring and early summer it produces the sclerotia, which may germinate into as many as a dozen stalks that contain pollen. Windblown pollen may land on grass or grain and there germinate. The spores quickly colonize the host. The fungus sclerotia then emerge where the grain would normally form. Harvested fields may contain both healthy grain and grain infected with the ergot fungus. Fields that are somewhat moist are especially conducive to infection. Grains such as rye or barley are particularly susceptible to colonization. When cleaned properly, the grain is suitable for consumption, but if not, then various ergot alkaloids will be present in the grain when it is consumed, even as baked goods.

Gangrenous ergotism often leads to a loss of blood in the extremities, which can lead to loss of nails or even of feet and hands. Before the loss of sensation, the disease often produces feelings of intense heat in the affected extremities. In the Middle Ages this latter sensation caused the disease to be referred to as St. Anthony's fire. There are several documented medieval outbreaks of ergotism, most often in central Europe, with the first occurring in the ninth century. Outbreaks continued well into the nineteenth century in central Europe with children being particularly affected. In the Middle Ages and early modern era, gangrenous ergotism was sometimes coupled to convulsive ergotism with its resulting hallucinations and bizarre behavior, a combination that further emphasized nonphysiological aspects of St. Anthony's fire.

Some folk medical practitioners recognized the hazard but also the benefits that ergot could produce, although using too much of an ergot compound could prove dangerous. From the eighteenth century, midwives often used ergot compounds that contained ergonovine to induce childbirth, a practice that found its way into orthodox medicine for a time. An increased dosage of the compound, however, could be used to induce an abortion earlier in a pregnancy. Other compounds containing ergotamine were used to lessen the chances of hemorrhaging after delivery.

The convulsive ergotism produced by lysergic acid has produced several episodes of mass hysteria, the most notable occurring in Pont-St.-Esprit, France in 1951. During this episode some people jumped off the roofs of their houses believing they were pursued by demons. Although the cause of this episode has never been conclusively determined, most investigators believe it was caused by ergot-infected rye flour from a nearby mill. Convulsive ergotism has also been advanced as an explanation for witch accusations in the early modern era, most notably the Salem, Massachusetts, episode in 1692. Although several of the girls who were accusers of the Salem witches ostensibly exhibited symptoms similar to those of convulsive ergotism, most scholars do not accept this explanation, turning instead to social and cultural explanations. The advocates of convulsive ergotism as an explanation for witchcraft accusations tend to focus solely on the medical symptoms of the accusers and ignore all other aspects of the witch panic.

During his work synthesizing ergot alkaloids in 1943, the Sandoz chemist Albert Hoffman (1906–) turned his attention to the lysergic acid compounds. As he progressed through the compounds, he found one, LSD-$_{25}$, that produced intense hallucinations when ingested, something that Hoffman first experienced as he rode his bicycle home from work. Sandoz patented LSD-$_{25}$ and initially marketed the new drug as an aid to medical health professionals. Several health care professionals began to engage in research using the new drug in the early 1950s, and it was prescribed in several mental hospitals for a variety of mental problems. Another group also took an interest in LSD-$_{25}$. The Central Intelligence Agency began experimenting with the new drug as an aid to interrogation or for use in creating chaos in a hostile population. In the 1960s the MK-Ultra program sponsored by the CIA and military intelligence soon progressed to field trials on sometimes unsuspecting populations. Some civilians also turned to LSD-$_{25}$ as a recreational drug calling it an aid to consciousness expansion. The Harvard psychologist Timothy Leary (1920–1996) became a noted exponent of the value of LSD. Both uses of LSD helped to produce a backlash, and Congress passed legislation criminalizing the manufacture or possession of LSD-$_{25}$.

Ergotism continues to pose a potential health hazard as *C. purpurea* remains in some grain supplies. Although present in all parts of the world, ergotism has been more of a problem in central Europe than elsewhere, and much of the work designed to control ergot infections is centered there. The principal means of preventing ergot infections continues to be rigorous cleaning of grain supplies to remove the ergot spores. Medical practitioners continue to be interested in ergot alkaloids. Ergotamine is marketed under several trade names as a means for controlling migraines. There is even some renewed interest in experimenting with LSD-$_{25}$ as a means of dealing with some mental disorders. Ergotism illustrates the old truisms that one amount of a drug can be a cure and another amount can be a poison. *See also* Biological Warfare; Diet, Nutrition, and Epidemic Disease; Environment, Ecology, and Epidemic Disease; Folk Medicine; Human Subjects Research; Pharmaceutical Industry; Social Psychological Epidemics.

Further Reading

Fuller, J. G. *The Day of St. Anthony's Fire*. New York: Hutchinson, 1969.

Hudler, George W. *Magical Mushrooms, Mischievous Molds*. Princeton: Princeton University Press, 1998.

Matossian, Mary Kilbourne. *Poisons of the Past*. New Haven: Yale University Press, 1989.

JOHN M. THEILMANN

ETHNICITY.   *See* Race, Ethnicity, and Epidemic Disease.

F

FARR, WILLIAM (1807–1883). A pioneering English statistician and health researcher, William Farr was a creator of the modern life table, a statistical tool for predicting the lifespans of groups of people, and an important advocate for the systematic collection and application of health statistics. He served for 40 years in the General Register Office (GRO), created in 1839 to collect birth and mortality data in Great Britain. Not only was he a seminal figure in the development of the state's collection of health-related data, but he was also a researcher who made important contributions to both medicine and statistics.

Born in 1807, the eldest son of a Shropshire laborer, Farr was apprenticed at the age of eight to a patron who encouraged him to professional studies. Aged 19, Farr was apprenticed to a **surgeon**, first as a wound dresser and then as a dispenser of drugs. Thanks to a bequest from his patron, in the 1820s Farr studied medicine in Paris where hygiene and medical statistics were evolving as cutting edge medical subjects.

Returning to England in 1832, Farr briefly practiced as an **apothecary** while writing articles on medical statistics and their collection and application. Hired by the GRO in 1839, Farr was intimately involved in a range of initiatives to assure the collection of accurate statistical data. The resulting data was used by Farr and other officials as well as made available to other researchers interested in the study of health and disease. His development of a new system for the classification of disease (nosology) for use on death certificates helped Britain reform its system of health reporting.

Farr's masterwork, a study of England's **cholera** outbreak in 1848, was described by the *Lancet*, then as now a preeminent British medical journal, as "one of the most remarkable productions of type and pen in any age or country." Titled *A Report on the Mortality of Cholera in England, 1848–1849* (1853), its 100 pages of dense type were complemented by 300 pages of supporting charts, diagrams, maps, and tables that describe the epidemic in terms of incidences of illness (morbidity) and of death resulting from it (mortality) cross-referenced economically, geographically, and socially. His conclusions on the 1854 cholera epidemic clashed with the insights of Dr. **John Snow**, and Farr's argument that cholera was airborne rather than waterborne was eventually proved incorrect. Even so, his work remains a model of epidemiological research and perhaps the most rigorous study of the potential for atmospheric diffusion of pathogens in the nineteenth century. During the 1866 cholera outbreak in East London, Farr harnessed his earlier lessons, accepted Snow's finding of waterborne causation, and quickly exposed the source of the pollution. He served as Compiler of Abstracts at the GRO until 1880. *See also* Cholera: First through Third Pandemics, 1816–1861; Demographic Data Collection and Analysis, History of; Public Health Agencies in Britain since 1800.

Further Reading

Eyler, John. "The Changing Assessments of John Snow's and William Farr's Cholera Studies." *Sozial- und Präventivmedizin* 46 (2001): 225–232, online at http://www.epidemiology.ch/history/papers/eyler-paper-1.pdf
———. *Victorian Social Medicine: The Ideas and Methods of William Farr*. Baltimore: Johns Hopkins University Press, 1979.
Koch, Tom. *Cartographies of Disease: Maps, Mapping, and Medicine*. Redlands, CA: ESRI Press, 2005.
Langmuir, A. D. "Epidemiology of Airborne Infection." *Bacteriological Review* 25 (1961): 173–181.
Rosen, George. *A History of Public Health*. Expanded Edition. Baltimore: Johns Hopkins University Press, 1993.

TOM KOCH

FERNEL, JEAN (1497–1558). Born at Montdidier near Amiens, Fernel entered medical training quite late because of uncertainty as to where his true talents lay. After publishing three promising mathematical works, he turned to medicine and received his M.D. in 1530. Dissatisfied with the institutionalized version of medicine he had been taught, he pursued his own course of study. This led him to write a work that pointed the way to the reform of medical theory, *On the Hidden Causes of Things*, in about 1538. Aware of its radical nature, Fernel suppressed this book while he prepared the first major summary of the anatomy and physiology of the ancient medical authority, **Galen**, which formed the basis of all **medical education** (and from which Fernel wanted to depart). This was published in 1542 as *On the Natural Part of Medicine*, but later appeared as the *Physiologia*, accompanied by the *Pathologia*, and the unfinished *Therapeutice*, in his *Medicina* (1554). *On the Hidden Causes of Things* was published in 1548. Fernel also rose to become one of the best practitioners in France and spent the last two years of his life as the royal **physician**. He should be recognized as one of only three would-be reformers of medicine in the sixteenth century, alongside **Paracelsus** and **Girolamo Fracastoro**.

On the Hidden Causes of Things is concerned with three sorts of diseases with "hidden causes": poisonous, contagious, and pestilent. All three present the standard physiological concept of disease of the Galenic tradition with severe difficulties. The unvarying pattern of such diseases, such that all patients irrespective of body type or temperament respond in essentially the same way, seemed to belie the physiological view of disease based **humoral theory**. Consequently, Fernel offered his own alternative account. Diseases of these types were held to act not on the humors, but on the substantial form or "total substance" of the body. Furthermore, they acted by means of some occult (hidden) power. A substance entering the body from outside, either through a bite or a wound, or by ingestion or inhalation, could wreak havoc in a healthy body, and so quickly that corruption of the humors—the traditional explanation—could hardly have taken place. If nothing else, Fernel pointed the way to a concept of diseases as entities in their own right, not merely collection of symptoms caused by humoral imbalances. He tried to provide details of the occult powers that could cause such rapid deterioration (drawing chiefly on **astrology** and alchemy). His considerable influence was eclipsed, however, when the advent of new mechanical philosophies of the seventeenth century rejected explanations that relied upon occult powers. *See also* Contagion Theory of Disease, Premodern; Paracelsianism; Scientific Revolution and Epidemic Disease.

Further Reading

Fernel, Jean. *Physiologia (1567)*. Translated by John M. Forrester. *Transactions of the American Philosophical Society* 93 (2003). Philadelphia: American Philosophical Society.

Forrester, John M., trans., and John Henry, ed. *Jean Fernel's On the Hidden Causes of Things: Forms, Souls and Occult Diseases in Renaissance Medicine*. Leiden: Brill, 2005.

Sherrington, Sir Charles. *The Endeavour of Jean Fernel*. New York: Cambridge University Press, 1946.

JOHN HENRY

FILM.   *See* Cinema and Epidemic Disease.

FIRST PLAGUE PANDEMIC.   *See* Plague of Justinian.

FLAGELLANTS.   *See* Black Death, Flagellants, and Jews.

FLIGHT.   Since the earliest times, flight has been one of the most commonly practiced individual responses to **epidemic** disease throughout history. People have resorted to flight as a means to protect themselves from outbreaks of disease and the horrors that sometimes accompany them. Even before the etiology of epidemic diseases and the exact nature of **contagion** were accurately understood, popular wisdom suggested that physical proximity could induce disease **transmission**; changing places was therefore considered a means for protection. Early theories of **miasma** that posited "corrupted air" as the cause of disease also recommended flight from affected areas.

Ancient medical systems had varying degrees of awareness regarding disease transmission and a variety of attitudes toward flight. In traditional **Chinese disease theory**, it was common understanding that people could transmit their sickness to others, and flight was therefore seen as useful. Similarly, ancient Indian **Ayurvedic** medicine vaguely recognized the transmissibility of epidemic diseases like plague and warned against the danger of remaining in an area where such a disease broke out, therefore encouraging flight. In the same way, ancient Greco-Roman medical theories that held that disease could either be transmitted by interpersonal contact or through fetid air considered flight a legitimate means to avoid disease.

Islamic teaching, on the other hand, prohibited flight from plague-stricken areas based on a tradition of the Prophet Muhammad (570–632), who advised: *"If you hear that plague has broken out in a country, do not go there; if it breaks out in a country where you are staying, do not leave it."* This principle was further confirmed by Muslim scholars who warned that traveling would cause fatigue and make one more vulnerable to disease. Islamic plague literature, mostly written by legal scholars during and after the **Black Death** (1347–1352) legitimized this prohibition by maintaining that the plague was a blessing or mercy of God and a means of martyrdom for the believer. Therefore, Muslims were to be patient in times of plague and not flee: first because they believed that there is no way of escaping death that is sent by God and second because by fleeing plague, a Muslim would lose the status of martyr and thus the eternal reward of heaven. In practice, however, flight in search of a place free from the disease was common throughout the Islamic world during plague episodes. Sultans in the Islamic world would move their courts and entire households from plague-infested cities like Cairo to disease-free areas, staying away until the disease abated in the city.

During the recurrent outbreaks of plague following the Black Death, flight gradually became more of a routine practice for urban communities in the Islamic world, who would move to their countryside residences in times of outbreaks. This is also reflected in the changing attitudes of Islamic legal scholars to the issue. Although the major works concerning the topic of plague written by Islamic scholars during the fourteenth century did not authorize leaving plague-infested cities, works written in the Ottoman Empire from the fifteenth century onward have a dramatically different legal viewpoint on proper conduct during times of plague. Sixteenth-century Ottoman plague literature granted legitimacy to the need to exit a plague-infested city in search of clean air and legally authorized it.

Flight was also common practice in Europe, especially during and after the Black Death. European plague literature, both popular and medical, enthusiastically recommended flight as a first resort. Popular wisdom decreed that one should flee early, go far, and come back late. However, in practice, flight was not an option for all. Often only the affluent had the means to leave plague-stricken cities for the countryside. Especially after the initial wave of the Black Death, when recurrent outbreaks became more or less routine, the affluent urban dwellers would move to their permanent countryside residences where they would stay until the end of the outbreak. During violent plague outbreaks, city officials, doctors, and clergy left, whereas lower class individuals who could not afford to leave were bound to stay in cities. As a result of deaths and flight, deserted cities offered reduced taxes to attract newcomers from the countryside as laborers.

Although the European medical literature recommended flight as the foremost prophylaxis, Christian teaching denounced this practice, and instead preached repentance, patience, and prayer for protection from divine wrath. Those who fled were heavily condemned for further increasing God's wrath and anger. Poet Giovanni Boccaccio (1313–1375) used the theme of flight as a moral critique of the fourteenth-century Florentine society in his *Decameron*, a literary treatment of flight from disease wherein ten young Florentines leave for the countryside to escape the plague in the city and entertain themselves by telling each other stories for 10 days. Throughout the Second Pandemic, preachers and moralists slammed **physicians**, community officials, and clergy who fled plague-stricken towns for their own safety when their services were needed most. Some cities fined absent civic officials, and King Charles II (1630–1685)—who had fled with his court—rewarded those who stayed put during London's Great Plague in 1665.

One major problem with flight was that it could and did spread disease from its source. By the seventeenth century country folk shunned and even drove away refugees from plague-wracked cities, sometimes leaving the sick to die along the roadside. From the time of the Black Death, refugees were stopped at city gates and refused entry, and many states and locales required **quarantine** to guarantee the healthiness of those admitted. Immigration quarantine facilities at Grosse Île in Canada and in eastern port cities like New York and Boston were swamped with the disease-ridden **Irish** who fled the potato famine and epidemics in the later 1840s. Governments developed increasingly sophisticated *cordons sanitaires* to block the entrance of suspect travelers and those who were fleeing from infected areas into their own territories, or to keep their own victims isolated within a limited zone.

In the modern era, although there are national and international laws for declaring and enforcing public health measures like quarantine and isolation, flight is still extensively practiced. During the **Pneumonic Plague in Surat, Gujarat, India, 1994,** hundreds of thousands of people fled the city and further spread the disease to a wider geographic area. Similarly, in China, when Beijing was hit by **Severe Acute Respiratory Syndrome (SARS),** over a million migrant workers left the city for their hometowns in rural areas in 2003, considerably extending the areas affected by the disease. Likewise, in Africa, thousands of people fled their homes in Congo-Brazzaville in 2003, in fear of the Ebola virus. More recently, in 2007, tens of thousands of Iraqis left their homes fearing the further spread of **cholera** in northern Iraq.

Flight has been and still is a factor for the spread of epidemic diseases around the globe. With the advanced travel technologies of the modern world, flight presents an extraordinary risk for disease transmission on both national and international levels. The recent implementation of the International Health Regulations (2005) by the **World Health Organization** (WHO) is an effort for international cooperation against the global risks of pandemics. *See also* Geopolitics, International Relations, and Epidemic Disease; Historical Epidemiology; International Health Agencies and Conventions; Medical Ethics and Epidemic Disease; Personal Liberties and Epidemic Disease; Poverty, Wealth, and Epidemic Disease; Public Health in the Islamic World, 1000–1600; Trade, Travel, and Epidemic Disease; War, the Military, and Epidemic Disease.

Further Reading

Boccaccio, Giovanni. *The Decameron.* New York: Norton, 1982.
Byrne, Joseph P. *Daily Life during the Black Death.* Westport, CT: Greenwood Press, 2006.
Dols, Michael W. *The Black Death in the Middle East.* Princeton: Princeton University Press, 1977.

NÜKHET VARLIK

FLU.   *See* Influenza.

FOLK MEDICINE.   Folk medicine may be considered the oldest form of medical practice because its roots can be traced to the earliest forms of human culture. Practitioners of folk or "traditional" medicine use locally available plants; animals (alive and as ingredients); and rituals, charms, and magic ("passing through" ceremonies, the spiritual healing system known as *curanderismo* in Latin America, faith healing) to cure their patients.

Historically practiced within isolated agrarian communities and among the peasant class, it continues to be used today by groups geographically or economically isolated from the medical mainstream. Whereas professional medicine generally entails a course of formal training in prevailing mainstream medical models, folk medicine has traditionally been transmitted orally among community members, and practitioners are accorded authority based on their accumulation of knowledge or on tradition (in some traditions the seventh son of a seventh son was supposed to have powerful healing talents). In Europe many folk practitioners were women, often called "root wives," "cunning women" (from *kennen*, to know), or "healers." Any given system of folk medicine is founded on the values, beliefs, and customs of the community that uses it. Although some folk medical practices have been partially accepted by professional medicine today, many are considered unscientific at best, or at worst, potentially harmful. Mainstream cultures have often perceived folk medicine practitioners as witches.

Folk medical responses to **epidemic** disease tend to be preventative (prophylactic), palliative (reducing symptoms), or curative. An African American method for preventing **tuberculosis** involved letting a cat sleep at the foot of one's bed. Palliative treatments included salves made with animal fat and used to minimize the scars caused by **smallpox**. Lady Frances Catchmay (fl. 1615–1630), a practitioner in early seventeenth-century England, claimed that she had cured over 300 victims of **syphilis** with an herbal drink and a special diet.

Some folk remedies mirrored major breakthroughs in mainstream medicine. It has been shown that long before Lady Mary Wortley Montagu (1689–1762) imported the practice of **inoculation** for smallpox from Turkey to Britain in the early eighteenth century, the practice of placing smallpox pus under the skin of a healthy person was used in ancient China and India. However, there is also evidence of its use by folk practitioners in Africa, as well as evidence that slaves brought knowledge of it to Boston before local physicians practiced inoculation.

Elements of the folk herbarium have found their way into the modern pharmacopoeia as biochemical researchers discover the healing properties of traditional medicinal herbs and other plants. Today, recognizing that traditional medicine is often the only source of medical attention for many of their citizens, some African governments have taken steps to foster collaboration between traditional practitioners and mainstream medical workers. The **World Health Organization** (WHO) notes that certain plants used in traditional African medicine are being tested as treatments for symptoms of **HIV/AIDS**. Groups such as the Consortium of Academic Health Centers for Integrative Medicine (CAHCIM) seek to systematize the integration of traditional ideas into mainstream medicine, but, as folklorist Wayland D. Hand (1907–1986) argued, some of the magical aspects of folk medicine may be ultimately incompatible with mainstream medical practice. *See also* AIDS in Africa; Apothecary/Pharmacist; Black Death (1347–1352); Disinfection and Fumigation; Empiric; Flight; Magic and

Healing; Medical Ethics and Epidemic Disease; Physician; Quacks, Charlatans, and Their Remedies.

Further Reading

Davies, Owen. *Cunning-Folk*. London: Hambledon and London, 2003.

Hand, Wayland D. "Magical Medicine: An Alternative to 'Alternative Medicine'." *Western Folklore* 44.3 (1985): 240–251.

Imperato, Pascal. *African Folk Medicine: Practices and Beliefs of the Bambara and Other Peoples*. Baltimore: York Press, 1977.

Jones, Michael Owen, dir. *Online Archive of American Folk Medicine*. University of California Los Angeles. http://www.folkmed.ucla.edu/index.html.

Kliger, Benjamin, Rita Benn, and Gwen Alexander, eds. *Curriculum in Integrative Medicine: A Guide for Medical Educators*. Working Group on Education, Consortium of Academic Health Centers for Integrative Medicine (CAHCIM), 2004. http://www.imconsortium.org/img/assets/20825/CURRICULUM_final.pdf.

Loux, Françoise. "Folk Medicine." In *Companion Encyclopedia of the History of Medicine*, edited by W. F. Bynum and Roy Porter, pp. 661–676. New York: Routledge, 1993.

Trotter, Robert T., and Juan Antonio Chavira. *Curanderismo: Mexican American Folk Healing*. Athens: University of Georgia Press, 1997.

World Health Organization. *Traditional Medicine*. World Health Organization Media Center. http://www.who.int/mediacentre/factsheets/fs134/en/

MELISSA SMITH

FRACASTORO, GIROLAMO (ca. 1478–1553).   Girolamo Fracastoro was an Italian humanist physician and poet who offered a new explanation of **contagion** for the transmission of diseases like **syphilis, typhus,** and the **Black Death**. He was born in the city of Verona in the Republic of Venice and studied mathematics, philosophy, and medicine at the University of Padua, receiving a B.A. degree there in 1502. Thereafter, he served as poet and physician to a number of leading Venetians until he was summoned to serve as physician to the members of the Council of Trent (1545–1563) under Pope Paul III (1468–1549). His two best-known works, *On Contagion and Contagious Diseases and Their Cure* (1546) and the poem, *Syphilis or the French Disease* (1530), from which the name of the venereal disease derived, were both concerned with the causes of infectious diseases and their treatment.

In the second century, **Galen** had mentioned the possibility that "seeds of disease" were responsible for the spread of contagious diseases, but he had given precedence to the theory that disease was spread by noxious airs or miasmas, rather than by human-to-human contact. According to miasmatic theory, putrefied airs act like poisons and cause a **humoral** imbalance and illness in those who inhale them and are constitutionally predisposed for the disease. In *On Contagion*, Fracastoro proposed a new explanation of contagion, arguing that imperceptible particles or "seeds" spread contagious diseases. He contended that these seeds were passed from an infected person to a new victim in three ways: directly by touch, indirectly by seeds called "fomites" which were carried by an intermediary object like clothing, or at a distance through the **air**. Furthermore, Fracastoro maintained that each disease was caused by a different kind of seed which was normally generated inside a sick person, but which could also originate as a result of an unfavorable planetary alignment.

Fracastoro's concept of disease-causing seeds coincided with efforts during the Renaissance to explain natural phenomena that occurred without direct physical contact (like the attraction of iron shavings to a magnet) without postulating "occult" (hidden or spiritual) causes. In this case "seeds" provided a physical, *material* cause that explained human-to-human contagion via direct and indirect contact or at a distance. Although Fracastoro's theory might appear to prefigure modern **germ theory**, it was not incompatible with miasmatic theory, nor did his contemporaries perceive it as revolutionary. Indeed, Fracastoro's **contagion theory** was easily reconciled with the theory of bad airs, and many physicians even suggested that the seeds were responsible for putrefying the air. See also Astrology and Medicine; Medical Education in the West, 1500–1900; Plague in Europe, 1500–1770s; Syphilis in Sixteenth-Century Europe.

Further Reading

Fracastoro, Girolamo. *Hieronymi Fracastorii De contagione et contagiosis morbis et eorum curatione: libri III* [Girolamo Fracastoro's Three Books on Contagion and Contagious Diseases and Their Cures]. Translated by Wilmer Cave Wright. New York: G. P. Putnam's Sons, 1930.

———. *The Sinister Shepherd: A Translation of Girolamo Fracastoro's Syphilidis sive de morbo gallico libri tres.* Translated by William van Wyck. Whitefish, MT: Kessinger Publishing, 2007.

Nutton, Vivian. "The Reception of Fracastoro's Theory of Contagion: The Seed that Fell among Thorns?" *Osiris*, 2nd series 6 (1990): 196–234.

Pantin, Isabelle. "Fracastoro's *De Contagione* and Medieval Reflection on 'Action at a Distance': Old and New Trends in Renaissance Discourse on the Plague." In *Imagining Contagion in Early Modern Europe*, edited by Claire L. Carlin, pp. 3–15. New York: Palgrave Macmillan, 2005.

WILLIAM H. YORK

FRENCH DISEASE.   *See* Syphilis.

FROST, WADE HAMPTON (1880–1938).   Wade Hampton Frost was a critical figure in the transformation of nineteenth-century "sanitary science" into the twentieth-century discipline of public health. As a **physician**, researcher, and teacher, he exemplified the increasingly specialized skills of public health experts in the first half of the twentieth century. Born to a country doctor, Frost received his medical degree from the Medical College of Virginia in 1903. The following year he passed the examination for the Public Health and Marine Hospital Service—later the Public Health Service (PHS)—where he began more than 20 years of service beginning in 1905.

Frost was involved as an investigator in a range of studies, including works regarding issues of **water** quality and its effect on disease. In 1905, for example, Frost was a critical federal investigator of a virulent New Orleans **yellow fever** epidemic, and in 1909 he was instrumental in the analysis of a waterborne **typhoid fever** outbreak in Williamson, Virginia. Across his public health career, he was principal in the research into a series of **epidemic** and **pandemic** outbreaks. In these studies his careful examination contributed to an understanding of diseases whose etiology was then unknown, including **poliomyelitis** in 1910–1912 and the **1918–1919 influenza** outbreak in the United States.

After his work on the 1918–1919 influenza outbreak, in which he and an economist determined the effect of the epidemic on U.S. cities, he was hired by the new School of Hygiene and Public Health then being established at Johns Hopkins University in Baltimore. He was hired originally as a "guest lecturer," and he remained a commissioned officer in the PHS, albeit on detached service, through the 1920s. During this period his first duties at Johns Hopkins were to teach **epidemiology** and disease studies through the case study method. He encouraged the adoption of epidemiology as a scientific study, as was the case with medical research, and his clear, precise methods of study laid the foundation for the future of epidemiology. He also introduced biostatistics as an important tool for judging confidence in data. In 1927 Frost published a "state of the art" text that defined the evolving science of the epidemiologist and focused on disease studies, along with public health promotion from the perspective of the public health practitioner. *See also* Influenza Pandemic, 1918–1919; Poliomyelitis, Campaign Against; Public Health Agencies, U.S. Federal; Typhoid Fever in the West since 1800; Yellow Fever Commission, U.S.; Yellow Fever in the American South, 1810–1905.

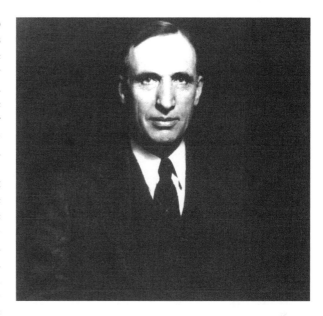

Wade Hampton Frost. Courtesy of the National Library of Medicine.

Further Reading

Daniel, Thomas M. *Wade Hampton Frost, Pioneer Epidemiologist 1880–1938: Up to the Mountain.* Rochester, NY: University of Rochester Press, 2004.

Maxcy, Kenneth F., ed. *Papers of Wade Hampton Frost, M.D.: A Contribution to Epidemiological Method.* New York: The Commonwealth Fund, 1936.

TOM KOCH

FUMIGATION.   *See* Disinfection and Fumigation.

G

GALEN (129–ca. 217). Claudius Galenus of Pergamum, or Galen, one of medicine's most influential figures, was a **physician** who lived through the devastating **Antonine Plague** of the Roman Empire. Prolific, pedantic, and ruthlessly self-promoting, Galen authored about 350 works and created the framework of medical ideas and ideals dominant in the West until the eighteenth century.

Galen was from a prominent family of Pergamum (Bergamo, Turkey). His father Nicon, a cultured architect, immersed Galen practically from birth in the finest education available and, because of a dream, directed Galen at 16 toward medicine. When Nicon died three years later, he left Galen ample means to continue a lavish and lengthy education, traveling and studying a wide range of subjects with experts at Smyrna (Izmir, Turkey) and Alexandria (Egypt). After a prolonged stay in Alexandria, he returned home in 157 to take a prestigious job as **surgeon** for a troop of gladiators. Galen's ambitions, however, outgrew Pergamum, and he moved to Rome in 162. His connections, education, and flair served him well in the theatrical and highly competitive practice of treating Rome's affluent class and brought him to the attention of the imperial court. Emperor Marcus Aurelius (121–180), on campaign in the east, summoned Galen (who was in Pergamum at the time) to his service in 166. After returning to Rome, another opportune dream kept Galen from accompanying the emperor on campaign; he was, instead, assigned to safeguard the health of the emperor's son, the future infamous emperor Commodus (161–192). Except for one other trip to Pergamum, Galen remained in Rome and associated with Rome's imperial elite past the turn of the century.

Galen encountered an epidemic in Rome while he was with Marcus Aurelius in Aequilia in 168–169. Although he wrote late in life that he had left Rome in 166 to avoid the pestilence, he earlier had claimed that he had left for fear of his rivals. His comments on the epidemic are thus secondhand, scattered throughout his works, and they focus more on individuals' symptoms than on overall generalizations (except with regard to fever). They appear to indicate **smallpox**, although **measles** has also been suggested. Galen thought, according to his own theories of the role of *pneuma* (breath), that treatment entailed purifying poisoned **air** within the body. In *Theriac to Piso* he suggests *gelenê* (a multi-ingredient antidote and tonic) as a prophylactic and remedy, making an analogy with the famous story of **Hippocrates** burning agents to purify the air during the **Plague of Athens**; in *Method of Healing* Galen observes that "drying drugs" were effective for a young man, perhaps reflecting the common theory that plague existed in overly dense and wet air. Galen's observations and theories on epidemic plagues long remained authoritative. His copious writings shaped **Islamic disease theory and medicine**, as well as that of the Christian West so powerfully that "Galenic" defined Western medicine until the **Scientific Revolution** and the development of **germ theory** overthrew his authority. *See also* Greco-Roman Medical Theory and Practice; Humoral Theory; Medical Education in the West, 1100–1500; Medical Education in the West, 1500–1900; Paracelsianism; Paracelsus; Smallpox in the Ancient World.

Further Reading

Arrizabalaga, Jon, et al., eds. *Galen and Galenism: Theory and Medical Practice from Antiquity to the European Renaissance.* Burlington, VT: Ashgate, 2002.

Cruse, Audrey. *Roman Medicine.* Stroud, UK: Tempus, 2004.

Littman, R., "Galen and the Antonine Plague," *American Journal of Philology* 94 (1973): 243–55.

Mattern, Susan P. *Galen and the Rhetoric of Healing.* Baltimore: Johns Hopkins University Press, 2008.

Nutton, Vivian. *Ancient Medicine.* New York: Routledge, 2004.

Prioreschi, Plinio. *Roman Medicine.* Lewiston, NY: Mellen, 1998.

ERIC D. NELSON

GEOPOLITICS, INTERNATIONAL RELATIONS, AND EPIDEMIC DISEASE.

History is replete with examples of **epidemic** diseases that have shaped, and in turn been shaped by, geopolitics—the intertwining of geography, political, and economic relations. The **Black Death** of the Middle Ages spread from Central Asia to Europe via **trade** routes, killing so many that Europe's social and political structures were irrevocably altered. European conquest of the "New World" was enabled by raging epidemics of **measles, smallpox**, and other infectious diseases, which—combined with **warfare**, forced labor, and displacement—killed between one-third and one-half of the indigenous population. Proliferation of international commerce and migration was again fundamental to the global pandemics of **cholera** that occurred through the 1800s, facilitated by rapid transport via steamships and the opening of the Suez Canal.

Cholera outbreaks, together with **yellow fever** and the reemergence of the **bubonic plague**, motivated the first international health meetings, treaties, and organizations in the late nineteenth and early twentieth centuries in Europe and the Americas. These efforts called for mutual notification of epidemic diseases and inspection and **quarantine** of both humans and goods, with the aim of safeguarding international **trade** and protecting home populations.

On another front, military action also spurred epidemics and their control: partly spread via troop movements, the **influenza pandemic of 1918–1919** killed upwards of

50 million people, far more than World War I (1914–1918), and was itself a deciding factor in several battles. As these various examples show, the emergence and transmission of epidemic disease is interconnected with global trade, migration, militarism, and international relations.

Geopolitical matters also shaped the first international disease campaigns. In addition to fears that disease outbreaks would interrupt the profitable transfer of goods and resources, Europe's imperial powers were concerned that disease problems could threaten colonists, provoke unrest, and reduce worker productivity in profitable plantations, mines, and other industries. Britain's colonial office, for example, sought to control **tuberculosis** among African miners and **malaria** among Asian agricultural workers. U.S. geopolitical interests in Latin America also shaped disease control efforts. The U.S. spearheaded the creation of the world's first international health agency, now known as the Pan American Health Organization, in 1902: for decades the organization was focused almost exclusively on stopping the spread of epidemics through commercial routes.

Precursor to today's **World Health Organization** (WHO), founded in 1948, the League of Nations Health Organization (LNHO), established after World War I, was launched by a commission to forestall the threat to Western Europe of **typhus** and other epidemics in Eastern Europe. The LNHO also became involved in cooperative efforts to address epidemics, such as infant mortality, that were rooted in poor social conditions. Following World War II (1939–1945), the WHO pursued a series of technical disease campaigns framed by Cold War politics. The WHO's Global Malaria Eradication Campaign, started in 1955, sprayed DDT against malaria-bearing mosquitoes but also used it as a strategy in the Cold War. The campaign's funders, primarily the United States and other Western countries, believed that malaria-free populations would be less attracted to communism. Subsequent campaigns against vaccine-preventable diseases, first smallpox, then **polio** and measles, followed.

Today, as in the past, international economic, political, and social relations and structures facilitate the (re)emergence and spread of both old and new pathogens and shape the ways in which epidemics are addressed by multinational entities, including public, private, and civil society agencies. Two intertwined sets of factors, both of which have intensified over the past decade, are central: globalization and renewed attention to global health governance, including the prominence of health on the foreign policy agendas of many countries.

Epidemic Disease and Globalization. Globalization refers to the growing political, economic, social, and cultural connections among individuals, communities, and countries that occur as business interests, people, goods, ideas, and values travel around the globe. In many respects, today's epidemic disease threats stem from the increased pace and intensity of global trade, financial transactions, travel, communication, and economic integration that have occurred over the past two decades. Economic globalization—the development of an increasingly integrated global economy via the removal of barriers to free trade and capital flow—is particularly important in explaining current patterns of epidemic disease.

Although international exchange and interdependence have occurred as long as global trade has existed, today's globalization is exceptional because of the unprecedented worldwide integration of markets and the increased role of transnational corporations and international financial institutions in social policy making. The World Bank (WB), International Monetary Fund (IMF), and World Trade Organization (WTO)—together with corporate interests writ large—have enormous influence over global and domestic social and economic policymaking; international health policy is, in turn, dominated by a market-led paradigm that fosters privatization and overlooks the underlying determinants of disease.

For much of the post–World War II period, it was assumed that economic development and technical progress would eliminate the problem of infectious disease; global life expectancy has indeed increased, and there have been some key advances in disease control (most notably, the **eradication of smallpox**) as a result of international cooperation. However, not all attempts at disease control have been so successful. Many diseases once thought to be in retreat, including malaria, cholera, and tuberculosis (TB), have reemerged in recent decades, partly as a consequence of current global economic patterns and policies. New diseases, such as **HIV/AIDS** and **Severe Acute Respiratory Syndrome** (SARS), are also linked to economic conditions and global interrelations.

For both new and reemerging diseases, the privatization and dismantling of government-funded social protections and programs that have accompanied economic globalization—in many developing countries via the Structural Adjustment Programs (SAPs) of the World Bank and IMF—have increased vulnerability to disease for marginalized groups.

As an example, the resurgence of cholera in South America in the early 1990s began with a freighter ship's discharge of cholera-infected ballast water from China off the coast of Peru. The cholera *Vibrae* infected local shellfish and entered the food supply, reaching the Peruvian population. Thereafter, the **bacteria** spread rapidly through overcrowded slums (economic conditions having forced many to migrate to urban areas in order to find work). Government cutbacks in public health, sanitation, and infrastructure—imposed by IMF and World Bank loan conditionalities starting in the 1980s (following the Latin American debt crisis, yet another feature of geopolitics)—enabled the disease to spread unchecked, killing thousands in Peru and neighboring countries.

Political and economic upheaval is a key factor in today's disease epidemics. Following the breakup of the Soviet Union in 1991, Russia has experienced increased unemployment, **poverty**, and inequity, which, together with the collapse of public health and social security systems, has resulted in escalating TB rates, particularly among the homeless, migrant workers, and prisoners. Russia's severely overcrowded and underfunded prison system has become a breeding ground for multidrug-resistant (MDR) TB, which is now spreading to the general population, with the poorest and most vulnerable least able to access treatment.

Like mass refugee movements in war-torn African nations, the trade, travel, and economic development accompanying contemporary globalization have exposed new disease reservoirs and expanded opportunities for exposure between pathogens and people. Today's mass movements of people and goods increase the chances of disease vectors being introduced into areas where they previously did not exist. The large-scale exploitation of natural resources leads to human encroachment on previously uninhabited areas where they may be exposed to pathogens to which they have no immunity. In central Africa, for example, logging, and consequent road construction, has brought people into contact with the **Ebola virus** via an increase in bush meat consumption. In many other areas of the world, clear-cutting, farming, and urban sprawl have enabled diseases such as **Dengue** fever, malaria, yellow fever, and **West Nile virus** (all spread via mosquito vector) to spread into human settlements. Climate change, also linked to **industrialization**, has also contributed to the transmission of **insect**-borne diseases, as warmer temperatures have expanded vector habitats.

Perhaps the most visible link between globalization and the spread of disease is the increased speed and volume of global travel. As demonstrated by the SARS outbreak of 2003, an infectious agent appearing anywhere in the world can circulate around the globe in a matter of days, with health and economic consequences for both individuals and countries. SARS also illustrated the ability of globalization to help contain disease; the speed of global communication enabled accurate surveillance, reporting, quarantine, and eventual containment, especially because the threat appeared imminent to the well-off.

Globalization has also affected nutritional patterns, interpersonal violence, medical practices and personnel, and environmental health problems such as pollution. In some cases, rapidly diffused information helps to address disease, for example through the sharing of medical information and techniques via open source journals and international training programs. But in other ways, the work and living patterns of a "globalized world" increase people's susceptibility to disease as a result of work stress, consumption of unhealthy food, and exposure to pollutants in the home, workplace, and surroundings.

Under-nutrition remains a major issue in much of the developing world, but obesity is also a growing concern. Diabetes and cardiovascular disease, conditions previously associated with affluent societies, have become global epidemics, posing great challenges to countries with weak health infrastructures (7 of the 10 countries with the largest numbers of diabetics are in the developing world). These chronic disease epidemics are attributed to globalization, in that trade liberalization has brought processed food and drinks and sedentary lifestyles to the developing world. Yet the relationship between globalization and chronic disease epidemics is more complex than the simple transmission of lifestyle and individual nutrition "choice."

Although many societies—and even public health authorities—blame poor diets on individual choices and lack of education, these problems are rooted in the mass production and marketing of food products. Dietary patterns derive from tradition, culture, and household resources, but are also increasingly influenced by the industrialization of food production. Despite its complex production, marketing, and distribution chain, processed food has become far cheaper per calorie than fresh produce and basic foodstuffs in most cities—and even rural areas—around the world.

Along with increasing exposure and susceptibility to disease, globalization has also limited governmental capacity to address ill health. The migration of doctors and nurses from developing to wealthier countries—the "brain drain"—is a key factor here. Drawn by higher wages, improved working conditions, and better supported health care systems, thousands of health-care workers trained in developing countries (usually with public resources) have emigrated to wealthier nations, worsening the human health-care resources deficit in their home countries and widening health-care inequities worldwide.

The supremacy of trade liberalization has also limited governments' abilities to address epidemic disease, as international trade agreements promote profits over human wellbeing. The WTO's agreement on Trade Related Intellectual Property Rights (TRIPS), negotiated in 1994, has exacerbated the impact of diseases such as HIV/AIDS in low-income countries by protecting profit-making, patented pharmaceuticals, effectively blocking treatment for millions of people. The WTO's 2001 "Doha Declaration" affirms the rights of states to protect public health in emergency situations, transcending TRIPS requirements. Many developing countries, however, lack the capacity to adopt the Doha provisions of compulsory licensing (local manufacture of drugs) and parallel importing of patented pharmaceuticals. Moreover, many developing countries are pressured to avoid adopting measures to protect public health in order to safeguard trade interests.

Marginalized populations—the poor, migrant workers, refugees—bear the brunt of (re)emerging epidemic disease, but in a globalized world everyone feels threatened. This perception of threat—often fuelled by overblown media coverage of remote risks such as "mad cow disease"—has led to the intensification of health diplomacy and the formalization of foreign health policy on the part of many nations in both the developed and developing world.

Epidemic Disease and Foreign Policy.   Because epidemic disease does not respect borders, it has long been a focus of diplomatic concern. Health cooperation—the provision of funding, materials, and/or human resources to address health needs—has occurred as long as international relations have existed. But efforts to address epidemic disease are motivated by goals beyond improving health conditions. Since the 2001 terrorist attacks on the United States, the ubiquitous concern with national security has extended to epidemic disease. The potential intentional spread of infectious disease, such as the use of anthrax or smallpox as a bioweapon by terrorists, is considered a national security concern. Disease is also understood as a contributing factor to conflict around the world because disease and premature death are a potential cause of economic and social instability. War and social disorder in turn foster the conditions in which further epidemic disease can flourish.

In order to protect domestic health and national security, an increasing number of governments, in particular those of the United States and the United Kingdom, are providing aid to prevent the emergence and spread of epidemic disease. Within this larger foreign policy context, health aid is understood to confer a number of advantages on donor countries, including protecting the health of their own citizens; promoting political stability, economic productivity, and a vibrant civil society; and encouraging research, debt relief, and primary care. The pursuit of such goals results in donor priorities dominating aid agendas and, often, in a failure to address questions of social conditions and resource distribution in development assistance strategies.

A growing number of developing and emerging countries are also engaged in government-to-government health cooperation, including Taiwan, the Czech Republic, Iceland, Korea, Latvia, Lithuania, and the Slovak Republic. Various countries, such as China, Turkey, Saudi Arabia, and Brazil, are both aid donors and recipients. Perhaps most notably, since the early 1960s, dictator Fidel Castro's Cuba has sent medical missions to over 100 countries in Asia, Africa, and Latin America providing disaster relief, medical personnel and training, and health systems policy advice, as well as training thousands of foreign doctors in Cuba as a way of enhancing its international image.

Other kinds of cooperation among nations of the southern hemisphere (South-to-South cooperation) are also materializing. South Africa provides aid to Mali and the Democratic Republic of the Congo, and in turn receives aid in the form of ophthalmologists from Tunisia to eliminate its cataract backlog. The "Bolivaran Alternative for the Americas" is a regional group that includes Bolivia, Venezuela, Cuba, and Nicaragua. Member states contribute funds, goods, and services to be used by other members. The India–Brazil–South Africa (IBSA) trilateral agreement, which promotes South-South dialogue, cooperation, and common positions on issues of international importance, includes a working group on health focused on epidemiological surveillance; sanitary regulations; traditional medicines; and Intellectual Property Rights.

Geopolitics and the Fight Against Epidemic Disease.   The rapid spread of diseases across national boundaries underscores the need for global collaboration in fighting epidemics beginning with international systems of disease surveillance and reporting. International agreements to monitor and prevent the spread of disease have existed since the 1892 adoption of the International Sanitary Conventions that evolved into the World Health Organization's International Health Regulations (IHR) in 1969. Updated in 2005, the new IHR was implemented in 2007; 192 countries are currently party to the regulations, which require member governments to inform the WHO of any reportable diseases within a specific timeframe, but do not require further action.

Today, much global health funding and activity is led by interested parties beyond traditional state players and the WHO, including private foundations, **non-governmental organizations**, international financial institutions, multilateral organizations, and business groups. Private funding, led by the Bill & Melinda Gates Foundation, now accounts for one-fourth of all development funding targeted at health. Combined with an overall rise in health-related development assistance funds in the majority of donor nations since 2000, this means that more money is currently directed at global health challenges than ever before.

The adoption of the United Nations' Millennium Development Goals (MDGs) in 2000 has been a key impetus behind the increased funding for global health. Although not legally binding, the 189 signatory nations agreed to work toward the achievement of eight development goals, three of which are directly health related (reducing child mortality; improving maternal health; and combating HIV/AIDS, malaria, and other diseases), by 2015—a deadline that most experts agree is unlikely to be met.

Whereas the MDGs embody broad development objectives, most of the initiatives implemented to meet them have very narrow targets. For example, reducing epidemic disease is approached on a disease-by-disease basis, a strategy that obscures the contributions of the global political economy and related poverty and inequity.

In sum, global public health efforts, reflecting geopolitical power, are not democratic. Priorities to address epidemic disease are almost inevitably set by donors, be they foundations, multilaterals, or governments. Diseases that receive media attention in rich countries garner the most funding (e.g., the Global Fund to fight AIDS, Tuberculosis, and Malaria); currently, HIV/AIDS drives most global health spending. Although all killers are undoubtedly worthy of attention, high-profile diseases draw resources away from competing health concerns.

Recent increases in both public and private funding for global health, along with new attention to disease on foreign policy agendas, suggest that the political will to address epidemic disease exists. Success requires greater coordination among donors, meaningful involvement of aid recipients, and, above all, attention to the underlying environmental factors of disease. Increasing aid alone will never solve global epidemic disease problems. Vanquishing epidemic disease must be understood not simply as a goal in it itself, but as an essential component of improving global health. *See also* Capitalism and Epidemic Disease; International Health Agencies and Conventions.

Further Reading

Bashford, Alison, ed. *Medicine at the Border: Disease, Globalization and Security 1850 to the Present.* Basingstoke, NY: Palgrave Macmillan, 2006.

Fort, Meredith, et al., eds. *Sickness and Wealth: The Corporate Assault on Global Health.* Cambridge, MA: South End Press, 2004.

Garret, Laurie. *Betrayal of Trust: The Collapse of Global Public Health.* New York: Hyperion, 2000.

Globalization and Health [online journal]. www.globalizationandhealth.com

International Relations (Special Issue on Global Health) 19, 4 (2005).

Peterson, Susan. "Epidemic Disease and National Security." *Security Studies* 12 (2006): 43–81.

KLAUDIA DMITRIENKO AND ANNE-EMANUELLE BIRN

GERM THEORY OF DISEASE.   The germ theory of disease, also known as the pathogenic theory of medicine, proposes that microorganisms too small to be seen by the naked eye are the cause of many diseases. After decades of research and observation suggested that living organisms could be responsible for disease, the theory became generally accepted in the scientific community by the end of the nineteenth century, with profound effects on medical treatment and our cultural response to illness. Highly controversial when first proposed, germ theory is now the fundamental basis for clinical microbiology and, indeed, for all of modern medicine. Our understanding of the role of microscopic organisms in human suffering and death has led to the extensive use of **antibiotics**, immunity-producing **vaccinations**, and disinfectants; a much greater investment in sanitation; and an increased concern for **personal hygienic** practices almost everywhere. As a result, germ theory is perhaps the most important contribution to the improvement of health and the extension of life expectancy among people around the world.

Early Explanations for Disease.   The significance of the germ theory of disease is best understood when compared to earlier explanations. Although previous accounts turned out to be inadequate, they each foreshadowed the direction medical science would later take in its search for the cause of human illness. For example, **humoral theory**, the leading Western concept for over two millennia, suggested that diseases were caused by substance imbalances within the body of the patient. This theory identified such crucial substances, or "humors," as blood, phlegm, yellow bile, and black bile, and each of these was in turn associated with a major organ in the body, such as the heart, brain, liver, and spleen. Its adherents emphasized diet, exercise, and rest for retention of good health. A second theory explained the suffering and death created by epidemics, focusing largely on the presence of "miasmas," or poisonous **airs**, as the proximate cause of the spread of disease. Although addressing what appeared mysterious at the time, miasmatic arguments emphasized what we would today think of as **environmental** factors in disease causation. It led people to drain swamps, burn refuse and human waste, and otherwise dispose of or neutralize these sources of unseen "miasmas." Finally, there were hypotheses that suggested that diseases might be spread by "contagia"—agents that could be passed from one person to another through air, water, clothing, bedding, or cooking utensils. Although the precise cause of disease was clearly not understood, it was apparent that many diseases followed a course of **contagion** from one individual to another, and this thinking found its best expression later in the germ theory of disease.

Developing the Germ Theory.   Although earlier theories of the cause of human and animal diseases may seem quaint and primitive today, some suggested that living organisms like tiny seeds or spores could be related to disease. During the second half of the nineteenth century, observers came to exactly that conclusion. The French chemist and microbiologist **Louis Pasteur** led the way when he determined the cause of rabies, cholera, anthrax, and silkworm disease. In the 1860s Pasteur's work also led to the development of several effective vaccines, and his efforts set the stage for modern biology and biochemistry. Central to Pasteur's work was his discovery that microorganisms are present in the air but are not created by the air—a critical challenge to earlier theories of the spontaneous generation of disease. He did this by proving that broth became contaminated when exposed to the air but, once sanitized by boiling, the same broth did not reveal the contaminants. He also discovered that fermentation, for example turning grape juice to wine, was a biological process carried out by microorganisms and concluded that if germs could cause fermentation, they might just as well cause diseases; if so, then the laboratory manipulation of the germs that caused diseases could be used to immunize people and animals.

In the 1870s the German **physician Robert Koch** firmly established the practice of bacteriology when he purified the anthrax bacillus and demonstrated that it created endospores that, once caught in the soil, could cause "spontaneous" outbreaks of the disease. Koch also showed that the organisms could be seen in every instance of the disease, that the germ could be produced in a pure culture, that the disease could be reproduced in experimental animals, and that the organism could be retrieved from the inoculated animal and grown again in another culture. Koch also created a series of techniques still used today, including the staining and purification of samples, the development of bacterial growth media, and the use of the Petri dish and agar plates for specimen samples. Using these methods, he later demonstrated the bacterial roots of the devastating disease **tuberculosis**, and identified the *Vibrio* bacterium that caused cholera. For these discoveries, Koch later received the Nobel Prize in Medicine.

Joseph Lister (1827–1912), a British physician and Professor of Surgery at Glasgow University, noticed that many people survived the trauma of surgery but then died later from "ward fever." Lister believed that microbes in the air of the **hospital** caused the disease to spread in the recovery wards, and that people who had been operated on were especially susceptible to illness, as surgery had left them weak, and their open wounds provided an entry point for the germs. His experiments included the careful cleaning of the wounds of patients who had suffered compound fractures and risked the onset of gangrene. He dressed the wounds with thin layers of lint covered in carbolic acid, and enjoyed an immediate increase in the survival rate of these patients. Lister established beyond doubt the relationship between poor sanitation and the spread of disease, especially in the hospital setting, and he established careful procedures for sanitizing surgical and other treatment equipment. Among other honors received in his lifetime, modern-day mouthwash Listerine offers tribute to Lister's contributions to sanitation and health.

By the end of the nineteenth century it was clear that earlier theories explaining the cause and spread of disease were either incomplete or wrong, and the germ theory of disease came to play a crucial role in our understanding of human suffering and death. Once the presence of pathogenic agents had been established, researchers armed with increasingly sensitive **microscopes**, dyes to stain biological samples, and other tools launched a series of discoveries that continue to determine our understanding of medicine today. In the 1890s **Alexandre Yersin**, a student of Pasteur, and **Shibasaburo Kitasato**, one of Koch's protégés, simultaneously discovered the bacterium that caused the dreaded plague, and Yersin worked to develop a serum to combat it. Scientists, physicians, and the general public rightly celebrated these developments, and the evidence is indisputable that each new discovery marked an increase in the quality of human life. The germ theory of disease led to the theoretical foundations of the modern science of **epidemiology**, inspired the development of newer and more effective antibiotic drugs, established principles for hygienic practices in hospitals and other medical care facilities, and informed our understanding of public sanitation, wastewater treatment, and a host of other practices.

Once controversial, germ theory is now accepted by virtually everyone associated with modern medicine, although we are well advised to recall that a complex network of factors also play a significant role in the rise and spread of disease. For example, environmental exposure to materials such as asbestos, benzene, tobacco, and lead has also produced human suffering on an unprecedented scale. *See also* Contagion Theory of Disease, Premodern; Fracastoro, Girolamo; Human Immunity and Resistance to Disease; Immunology; Protozoon, –zoa.

Further Reading

Ewald, Paul. *Plague Time: The New Germ Theory of Disease*. New York: Anchor Books, 1977.
Harvard University Library. *Contagion*. http://ocp.hul.harvard.edu/contagion/germtheory.html
Karlen, Arno. *Man and Microbes: Disease and Plague in History and Modern Times*. New York: Simon and Schuster, 1996.
Pasteur, Louis, and Joseph Lister. *Germ Theory and Its Applications to Medicine & On the Antiseptic Principle of the Practice of Surgery* (Great Minds Series). New York: Prometheus Books, 1996.
Stephen Abedon Lecture at Ohio State University [online]. http://www.mansfield.ohio-state.edu/~sabedon/biol2007.htm
Waller, John. *The Discovery of the Germ: Twenty Years that Transformed the Way We Think about Disease*. New York: Columbia University Press, 2003.
Worboys, Michael. *Spreading Germs: Disease Theories and Medical Practice in Britain, 1865–1900*. New York: Cambridge University Press, 2000.
Zimmerman, Barry E., and David J. Zimmerman. *Killer Germs: Microbes and Disease that Threaten Humanity*. New York: McGraw-Hill, 2002.

BART DREDGE

GONORRHEA AND CHLAMYDIA.   Gonorrhea is an infectious inflammatory disease that primarily affects the urethra but may involve the genitalia, joints (arthritis), skin, eyes, and occasionally other organs. It is caused by a specific **bacterium**, the gonococcus. This Greek term literally means "discharge of seed"; its earlier designation, "*blennorhea*," means discharge of mucus. Involuntary urethral discharges were referred to in ancient writings, but because of the absence of associated pain, it is unlikely that gonorrhea was being described. London **physician** Andrew Boorde (1490–1549) cited a painful condition that resulted from "meddling with a harlot" and could be transmitted to another woman. Uro-genital symptoms in women are generally less severe, and diagnosis was not recognized in women for another 200 years. Furthermore, gonorrhea was considered to be a symptom of **syphilis**, rather than a discrete disease. The differentiation made by Benjamin Bell (1749–1806), a Scots **surgeon**, in 1793 was accepted only gradually.

The Gonococcus.   In 1879, when Albert L. Neisser (1855–1916) was a 24-year-old trainee in the dermatology department of the University of Breslau (Prussia), he made microscopic examinations of secretions from typical cases of gonorrheal urethritis (inflammation of the urethra), neonatal infections, and ophthalmia (eye inflammation) of adults.

He stained the microscopic slides with methyl violet dye and in each case observed structures having a similar appearance. At the time only two diseases had a proven bacterial cause; hence, even Neisser was uncertain of the significance of his observation. He was unsuccessful in finding a medium on which to grow these presumed bacteria. In 1882 he described these structures in more detail and called them "gonococcus," even though he remained uncertain about whether they were the actual cause of the inflammation at the various locations. Two problems impeded research on this question. No animal was found that could be infected with this germ, and it was difficult to grow in an artificial medium. Culturing first succeeded in 1885, and research into how to grow this bacterium reliably continued for the next 70 years.

The genus of bacteria to which the gonococcus belongs is called Neisseria that includes not only the meningococcus that causes spinal meningitis, but also nonpathogenic bacteria that occur in the human mouth. The simplest way to identify the gonococcus is to apply the Gram stain to secretions that have been dried on a microscope slide and to find stained round bacteria, usually in pairs, within leukocytes (white blood cells). If no gonococci can be detected, but symptoms are suspicious of gonococcal disease, then fresh secretions must be placed on a specialized culture medium, preferably with added carbon dioxide. After at least two days of incubation, any growth is examined. Growth requirements of gonococci are more complex than those of meningococci.

Symptoms of Gonococcal Infection.   All extra-genital complications of gonorrhea were recognized before their etiologic relationship with gonococcal infection, or the discovery of the gonococcus itself. In the early nineteenth century, gonococcal **conjunctivitis** was confused with trachoma, and the possibility that they were separate diseases hinged on giving credence to trachoma patients who stated that they had not been sexually active. Although any joint may be involved, arthritis usually affects only one or two joints, particularly the knee and ankle. Because joint pain is such a common symptom, it appeared likely that its occurrence in a person with gonorrhea was a coincidence. Proof of the causative relationship was obtained by injecting synovial fluid from an inflamed joint of men who had gonorrhea into the urethra of healthy men. The development of typical gonorrhea proved the identity of the cause. Before there were **antibiotics**, the vast majority of gonococcal arthritis cases were men, but since the 1960s most have been women. The probable explanation is that because silent, untreated gonococcal infection is more common in women, their risk of an eruption of symptoms is more persistent.

Uro-genital symptoms in men usually begin two to five days after having become infected. If a woman becomes symptomatic, this begins about 10 days after having been infected. Between 10 and 20 percent of infected women develop pelvic inflammatory disease, which may cause sterility as a result of scarring of the fallopian tubes. Once the body harbors gonococci, various extra-genital manifestations may occur, either from direct contact or from dissemination through the blood. Since the advent of antibiotic therapy, these events have become less frequent and occur mainly in persons who lack recognized symptoms of the genital infection. Manifestations as a result of direct contact are pharyngitis from fellatio ("oral sex"), proctitis from anal intercourse, and conjunctivitis from inadvertently touching the eye with a contaminated substance or finger. The most frequent manifestations of gonococci disseminated through the blood are arthritis and dermatitis; involvement of the liver or heart is rare. Pain may be limited to a tendon, but more often a few joints become inflamed. Arthritis tends to occur during the latter half of pregnancy. The most typical skin eruption consists of tiny red spots, some with blistering, mainly on the hands and feet. Skin and joint symptoms often occur simultaneously.

Treatment.   The first successful treatment that pertained to gonococcal infection was aimed at preventing the blinding of the eyes of newborns who had been infected in the birth canal. In 1880 Carl S. Credé (1819–1892), a German obstetrician, introduced placement of a 2 percent solution of silver nitrate into the eyes of newborns. This practice gradually became routine, and by 1910 the ocular manifestation of gonorrhea had virtually been eliminated from newborns.

Injection of silver nitrate or potassium permanganate into the urethra of symptomatic men became the main treatment among many that were tried. Vaccines prepared from gonococci had no effect on the disease. Arthritis was treated by inducing fever or by locally heating affected joints. However, the first reliable eradication of gonococcal infection occurred in 1938 with sulfanilamide. This required 4 grams of pills per day for at least three weeks and cured about 80 percent of cases. The bacteria soon became resistant to sulfanilamide, but the infection would temporarily respond to one related sulfa drug after another. The real breakthrough occurred in 1943 when it was found that one injection of a small dose of **penicillin** would be curative, even in patients whose **sulfa drug** treatment had been unsuccessful. However, strains of gonococci that required increasingly large doses of penicillin for cure became more frequent. In about 25 years, the curative dose of penicillin increased some 60-fold to 4.8 million units. Tetracycline taken by mouth was shown to be effective, and between 1962 and 1972 it was replacing penicillin in the treatment of gonorrhea. Resistance to tetracyclines developed more rapidly than it had to penicillin. Consequently, new chemically unrelated antibiotics have been introduced every few years. Cephalosporin was the favorite antibiotic in 1990, and since then drugs in the fluoro-quinolone group have in part replaced it. It has been found that after a once-effective antibiotic has fallen into disuse for some years, the prevalence of resistant strains of gonococci diminishes, so that it again becomes possible to treat initially with the least expensive antibiotic, penicillin. If this is not rapidly successful, other agents are available.

The problem of antibiotic resistance in the United States has two causes: adaptation of local strains to various antibiotics and importation of resistant strains, mainly from Southeast Asia and Africa, by infected people who are returning from these areas.

Differential Diagnosis: Chlamydia Trachomatis.   The most frequent microbe in the differential diagnosis of gonococcal infections is *Chlamydia trachomatis.* This is a peculiar bacterium that survives only within cells of certain species. Dr. Julius Schachter, of the University of California San Francisco, discovered it in humans in 1966. Identification is ordinarily made by immunologic methods performed on urine, rather than by culture. Chlamydia is present most frequently in sexually active young women.

This infection may be cured by several antibiotics. Azithromycin in a single oral dose or doxycycline for one week are currently favored in most circumstances. Erythromycin is preferred for neonates. The development of resistance to initially effective antibiotics has been less of a problem with Chlamydia than with gonococci.

Epidemiology of Gonococcal and Chlamydial Infection.   With recognition of the importance of infection with Chlamydia, gonorrhea has fallen to become the second most prevalent venereal disease in the United States. The actual prevalence of both infections can only be estimated because as many as half of the cases of gonorrhea and even more with Chlamydia are not reported to health departments. According to a report from 2003, a peak prevalence of gonorrhea occurred in 1978, with a steady decline until 1995, when this disease leveled off. In 2005 more than 330,000 cases of gonorrhea and more than 900,000 cases of infection with Chlamydia were reported to U.S. health departments. According to a population survey, rather than health department data collection, of the 14–39 year age group, conducted during 1999–2002, these events have become less frequent: the mean prevalence of gonorrhea was 0.16 percent in males and 0.33 percent in females; Chlamydia was found at a rate of 2 percent in males, 2.5 percent in females. Of those with Chlamydia, 2.7 percent of males and 6.8 percent of females also had gonorrhea. In a larger national survey conducted in 2001–2002, 70 percent of individuals with gonorrhea were also infected with Chlamydia. Both infections have been detected substantially more frequently in African American than in other racial cohorts. The availability of effective treatment has reduced the occurrence of complications.

Persistence of Symptoms.   The symptoms that used to be called post-gonococcal urethritis usually reveal a Chlamydial infection that was masked until the gonococcal infection had been cured. Chlamydial infection has a longer incubation period than gonorrhea and may require a different antibiotic for treatment.

Reactive arthritis (formerly called Reiter's disease) is believed to result from an immunologic reaction to various bacteria, but predominantly Chlamydia. The typical patient develops urethritis, followed by conjunctivitis and arthritis or tendonitis, thus closely mimicking symptoms of disseminated gonococcal infection. This syndrome occurs predominantly in men and does not respond reliably to antibiotics. *See also* Drug Resistance in Microorganisms.

Further Reading

Bavoil, Patrick, and Priscilla Wyrick. *Chlamydia: Genomics and Pathogenesis.* New York: Taylor and Francis, 2007.

Centers for Disease Control and Prevention. *Gonorrhea.* http://www.cdc.gov/std/Gonorrhea/default.htm

Hook, E. W., and H. H. Handsfield. "Gonococcus"; "Chlamydia." In *Sexually Transmitted Diseases,* 3rd edition, edited by K. K. Holmes, et al. pp. 391–422, 451–466. New York, Mc-Graw Hill, 1999.

Kollar, Linda, and Brian Schmaefsky. *Gonorrhea.* Philadelphia: Chelsea House, 2005.

Mayo Clinic. *Gonorrhea.* http://www.mayoclinic.com/health/gonorrhea/DS00180

Stamm, W. E., R. B. Jones, and B. E. Batteiger. "Gonococcus"; "Chlamydia." In *Principles and Practice of Infectious Diseases,* 6th edition, edited by G. L. Mandell, J. E. Bennett, and R. Dolin, pp. 2236–2268, 2514–2529. New York: Elsevier, 2006.

World Health Organization. *Sexually Transmitted Diseases.* http://www.who.int/vaccine_research/diseases/soa_std/en/index2.html

THOMAS BENEDEK

GORGAS, WILLIAM CRAWFORD (1854–1920).   William Gorgas, whose use of sanitation techniques to rid Panama of mosquito-borne **malaria** and **yellow fever** resulted in the successful completion of the Panama Canal in 1914, "found himself leading the most costly, concentrated health campaign the world had yet seen," as historian David McCullough (b. 1933) expressed it.

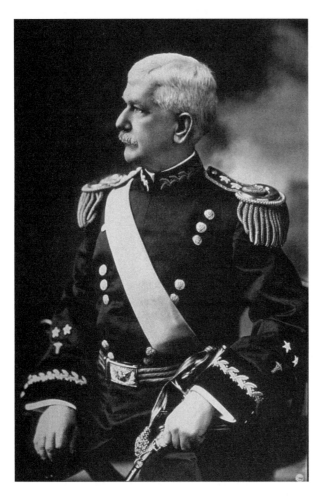

William Crawford Gorgas. Courtesy of the National Library of Medicine.

Gorgas was born near Mobile, Alabama, and though he was unable to realize his dream of attending West Point military academy, the medical degree that he received from Bellevue Medical College in New York City allowed him to enter the military as a **physician**. After being sickened by yellow fever and developing immunity, he was posted to Havana, Cuba, as chief sanitary officer. He arrived at the close of the Spanish-American War of 1898, which had placed Cuba under American control. Many diseases, including **dysentery** and **typhoid**, were raging. At that time, Gorgas believed that unsanitary conditions caused yellow fever, and though Havana was thoroughly cleaned, yellow fever persisted.

In 1884 French physician **Alphonse Laveran**, working in Algeria, suggested that malaria was a mosquito-borne disease, and around the same time, Cuban physician Carlos J. Finlay (1833–1915) theorized that the mosquito transmitted yellow fever. In 1899 British tropical medicine specialist **Ronald Ross** discovered that the parasite that causes malaria is transmitted by the bite of the *Anopheles* mosquito, and the following year, American physician **Walter Reed's** experiments showed the involvement of the mosquito now known as *Aedes aegypti* in yellow fever transmission, confirming the theory that Finlay had been unable to prove. Gorgas was then able to bring the diseases under control within 18 months by hiring a large staff of inspectors to locate and cover or eliminate all mosquito breeding grounds, enforce fines for harboring mosquitoes or mosquito larvae, fumigate homes, enforce the use of netting, **quarantine** the sick, and deal with city residents' resentment and suspicion.

Desiring a quicker sea route from the Atlantic to the Pacific Ocean, a French engineering company had begun to build a canal across the Isthmus of Panama in the 1880s. Mainly because of the high death rate from malaria and yellow fever, they were unable to continue and sold the unfinished canal to the United States. The digging resulted in unfinished sewage drains and shallow trenches that collected water and were breeding grounds, but government officials did not believe that the **insects** were the cause of these diseases. When Gorgas was made Panama's chief sanitary officer, he was able to turn to President Theodore Roosevelt (1858–1919) for support, and, using measures similar to those proven in Cuba, the diseases were entirely eradicated within eight months.

Gorgas was made Surgeon General of the U.S. Army and, after he retired, served as a consultant on the control of malaria and yellow fever in Brazil and South Africa. He died suddenly in England, however, before he could carry out his plan to study outbreaks of yellow fever in West Africa. *See also* Malaria in Africa; Sanitation Movement of the Nineteenth Century; War, the Military, and Epidemic Disease; Water and Epidemic Diseases; Yellow Fever in Latin America and the Caribbean, 1830–1940.

Further Reading

Gibson, John M. *Physician to the World: The Life of General William C. Gorgas*. Durham, NC: Duke University Press, 1950.

Harvard University Library: *Contagion*. http://ocp.hul.harvard.edu/contagion/gorgas.html

McCullough, David. *The Path between the Seas: The Creation of the Panama Canal, 1870–1914*. New York: Simon and Schuster, 1977.

Noble, Robert E. "William Crawford Gorgas." *American Journal of Public Health* 11, 3 (1921): 250–256; online at: http://pubmedcentral.gov.

MARTHA STONE

GREAT PLAGUE OF LONDON.   *See* London, Great Plague of (1665–1666).

GREAT POX.   *See* Syphilis.

GRECO-ROMAN MEDICAL THEORY AND PRACTICE.   The medicine of classical antiquity, though not a single intellectual tradition, formed the medical knowledge of the medieval West, the Islamic world, and some modern medicine into the Enlightenment. The Greek medical tradition arose around the same time as the Pre-Socratic natural philosophers in Attica and the Aegean Islands: the fifth century BCE. The earliest extant Greek medical texts are called the "Hippocratic corpus" in reference to **Hippocrates**, the (probably legendary) author and **physician**, who was considered the founder of the school that produced these texts. Although many folk medical traditions already existed, such as the cult of the healing god Aesclepios, the Hippocratic texts provide the earliest evidence of a medical system organized around observation and analysis. Hippocratic medicine claimed that explicable natural phenomena underlay illness, and physicians seeking to heal diseases must understand their natural causes.

Greek **humoral theory**, derived from the Hippocratic corpus, viewed health as the equilibrium of fluids in the **human body** called humors; it was believed that if these became imbalanced, illness resulted. The humors—blood, yellow bile, phlegm, and black bile—were often associated with particular organ systems and used for their classification. Whereas medieval physicians fixed the number of humors at four, the Hippocratic authors give no set number. These early theories developed from the observation of sick patients, but little dissection or anatomical study occurred. Hippocratic medicine emphasized the role of the environment in the development of plagues and asthma. Greek physicians correlated both meteorological and astrological influences with the epidemic diseases of populations. Plagues were viewed as the consequence of many natural factors converging on a location; thus, epidemics were believed to result from temporary conditions acting on specific places.

Ancient physicians were aware of the limitations of their art. They could observe the course of a disease, predict its worst moments (crisis), and estimate the point beyond which recovery was unlikely or impossible, but rarely could they effect an immediate cure. Fevers and the healing of wounds modeled the course of illness generally. Prediction was vitally important to ancient physicians because their ability to attract clients depended on their skill in predicting an accurate outcome to illnesses. Diagnosis was based on systematic observation of the patient, the taking of the pulse in various locations, and the examination of urine (uroscopy) and of the complexion. Once a doctor decided that a patient's condition had a remedy, he would design treatment for that specific patient. Treatment regimens often included carefully chosen **diets**, because diet was believed to affect the humors. Most drugs were derived from herbs, though some were mineral or animal products. Following humoral theory, the goal of a treatment regimen was the restoration of humoral balance. To this end, purges, controlled bleeding, baths, and similar cures were prescribed. Although the Hippocratic Oath delineated surgery as separate from medicine, many physicians performed surgical procedures, along with cleansing wounds with wine and wrapping them, setting fractures, and making braces to correct the posture. Healers who were not physicians, known as **empirics**, also performed many of these procedures. The efficacy of Greek practice varied greatly, with better results for chronic than acute diseases. Because there was no precise pharmaceutical knowledge, categories of drug therapy were often vague, and whenever possible, physicians adjusted their care to the changing needs and illnesses of the patient. The wealthy were treated in either the home of the physician or that of the patient, whereas the poor often traveled to healing shrines. Although the knowledge of **quarantine** existed to some extent, ancient medicine encouraged those suffering from plague to flee the location where they were stricken, and thus escape to places with better "**air**."

Aristotle's biological and psychological writings significantly affected medicine and physiology in the Greek world. Aristotle's detailed zoological writings contributed anatomical detail to the often-hazy anatomy of the Hippocratics, and his hierarchy of functions for the heart, brain, lungs, and liver became part of standard Greek physiology. Though rival schools held different hierarchies for organ function (Plato's followers believed the brain was the central organism against Aristotle's claims for the heart), none of them approached Aristotle's level of systematic study. The rise of Alexandria, Egypt, as a center of Greek culture and learning during the Hellenistic Age led to new advances in medicine. Ptolemaic Egypt produced innovative physiologists, particularly the fourth-century anatomist Hierophilus and early-third-century Erisistratus. Systematic human dissections were performed for the first time in this city in the third century BCE, and the wide cultural exchanges in the city led to many new treatments being added to the Greek pharmacopoeia.

During the Hellenistic Age, Greek medicine was introduced into the Roman Republic. The Latinization of Greek medicine is the principal cause of its survival as the bedrock of Western medical thought into modernity. As Rome expanded and came to dominate the Mediterranean, Greek culture became a large influence in Roman intellectual and social life. Wealthy Romans consulted medically trained Greek slaves and freedmen, and Hippocratic-Alexandrian medicine began to replace traditional Roman healing methods in urban centers, if not in rural regions. Also, the Roman army routinely employed Greek surgeons by the first century CE. The great army doctor

Dioscorides (c. 40–90), for instance, wrote influential guides to pharmacology. Whereas some traditional Romans were bothered by the alien nature of Greek natural philosophy, most physicians who criticized Greek medicine followed basic humoral theory in their own texts.

Galen was the greatest physician of the classical world. His theories changed Greco-Roman medicine immensely. Innate bodily heat was one of his key concepts. Galen thought it was the difference between living and nonliving matter, maintained by the heart, which received blood from the liver and *pneuma* (air and "spirit") from the lungs. He believed, in opposition to Aristotle, that there was no "chief" organ, but that the brain controlled behavior, the liver digestion, and the heart the innate heat. Galen's work on the nervous system introduced the relationship between nerves and muscular movement into Greco-Roman medicine. The medieval inheritance of classical medicine was largely shaped by Galenic language and concepts, especially the doctrine of innate heat. *See also* Apothecary/Pharmacist; Avicenna (Ibn Sina); Ayurvedic Disease Theory and Medicine; Black Death (1347–1352); Chinese Disease Theory and Medicine; Contagion Theory of Disease, Premodern; Environment, Ecology, and Epidemic Disease; Epidemiology, History of; Islamic Disease Theory and Medicine; Magic and Healing; Malaria in the Ancient World; Medical Ethics and Epidemic Disease; Plague of Athens; Plagues of the Roman Empire; Plagues of the Roman Republic; Rhazes; Smallpox in the Ancient World; Surgeon.

Further Reading

Cruse, Audrey. *Roman Medicine*. Stroud, UK: Tempus, 2004.

Grmek, Mirko. *Western Medical Thought from Antiquity to the Middle Ages*. Cambridge, MA: Harvard University Press, 1999.

Jackson, Ralph. *Doctors and Disease in the Roman Empire*. Stillwater: University of Oklahoma Press, 1988.

Longrigg, James. *Greek Rational Medicine: Philosophy and Medicine from Alcmaeon to the Alexandrians*. New York: Routledge, 1973.

Nutton, Vivian. *Ancient Medicine*. New York: Routledge, 2005.

DENNIS GREGORY CARAMENICO

H

HAFFKINE, WALDEMAR MORDECHAI (1860–1930). Waldemar Haffkine, who began his career as a zoologist, developed the first vaccine for **bubonic plague** and one of the first vaccines for **cholera**. He understood how to translate laboratory findings into effective means of disease control in humans.

Haffkine was born in Odessa, Russia, where he received his doctoral degree in natural sciences and became involved in anti-Czarist revolutionary causes. He studied under Russian zoologist and microbiologist Elie Metchnikoff (1845–1916), who assisted him at critical times in his career. He was invited to Paris where he became bacteriologist **Louis Pasteur's** assistant, began to study **typhoid fever** and **cholera**, and experimented with inoculation against cholera using attenuated (weakened) **virus**. In 1883 German bacteriologist **Robert Koch** had identified the **bacterium** that causes cholera, but scientists dismissed the idea of an anticholera vaccine after Catalan bacteriologist Jaime Ferran y Clua (1852–1929) refused to cooperate with various scientific organizations that were investigating his cholera vaccination program, and his results were dismissed as invalid.

Haffkine studied cholera in laboratory animals and inoculated himself and three of his friends before reporting his findings and declaring that his vaccine was safe for humans. In 1893 he was invited by the Indian government, at Pasteur's recommendation, to help control a cholera outbreak there. He faced problems ranging from dosage variations to fatal attacks of cholera after inoculation. Though Haffkine's vaccine was weak and only moderately effective, statistics indicated that it lowered the death rate significantly.

In 1896 India announced an outbreak of plague, and Haffkine was asked to develop a vaccine, following the discovery of its cause by French Swiss bacteriologist **Alexandre Yersin** and Japanese bacteriologist **Shibasaburo Kitasato**. Haffkine's vaccinations were carried out in many stricken Indian cities, but he was often thwarted by the government's sanitarian approach to the illness, which involved the removal of patients from their homes and forced admission into hospitals, as well as many residents' resistance to **vaccinations**.

Haffkine had to battle complicated political intrigue for many years, when a laboratory accident resulted in the death, from tetanus, of 19 people who were being immunized against the plague. After an enquiry, Haffkine was eventually exonerated, thanks in part to the efforts of tropical medicine specialists **William Simpson**, from Scotland, and **Ronald Ross**, from England. His career, however, did not recover, and some believed that he had not used correct scientific methods, though, as scholar Ilana Lowy wrote, "Haffkine tirelessly asserted his right be recognized as the true pioneer of scientific vaccination."

Though Haffkine was unable to regain his influence, the laboratory where he had worked in Bombay (now Mumbai), India, was renamed the Haffkine Institute in 1926, 11 years after he retired, and is still in existence. *See also* Cholera: Fourth through Sixth Pandemics, 1862–1947.

Further Reading

Lowy, Ilana. "From Guinea Pigs to Man: The Development of Haffkine's Anticholera Vaccine." *Journal of the History of Medicine and Allied Sciences* 47 (1992): 270–309.

Lutzker, Edythe, and Carol Jochnowitz. "Waldemar Haffkine: Pioneer of Cholera Vaccine." *ASM News* 53, 7 (1987): 366–339; available online at http://www.asm.org/

Waksman, Selman A. *The Brilliant and Tragic Life of W. M. W. Haffkine, Bacteriologist.* New Brunswick, NJ: Rutgers University Press, 1964.

Waller, John. *The Discovery of the Germ: Twenty Years that Transformed the Way We Think about Disease.* New York: Columbia University Press, 2002.

MARTHA STONE

HANSEN, GERHARD ARMAUER (1841–1912). In 1873 Norwegian **physician** and researcher Gerhard Armauer Hansen discovered the bacillus that causes **leprosy**, which would become known as Hansen's disease. Through clinical observation and epidemiologic study, he had developed the conviction that leprosy was an infectious disease with a specific causal agent, rather than the product of **heredity** or **environmental** factors, the conclusion of most experts at the time. The bacilli Hansen observed in the diseased cells of leprosy sufferers demonstrated for the first time that a microorganism could cause a chronic disease.

Born in Bergen, Norway, Hansen trained in medicine at the University of Christiana in Oslo. In 1868 he returned to Bergen, Europe's center for the study of leprosy, to study the disease under Daniel C. Danielssen (1815–1894).

Hansen's research soon departed radically from his mentor's, which was premised upon leprosy's hereditary transmission. Early studies in which Hansen observed yellowish, granular masses within leprous nodules, along with his clinical observations, suggested to him a different etiology. In 1871 Hansen began conducting epidemiologic studies in western Norwegian districts where leprosy affected many, and in 1872 he published a report asserting that the disease was infectious. Referring in detail to the observations he had made among lepers and their families, he systematically dismantled the arguments in support of heredity, constructed his argument for contagion, and pointed toward his microbiological findings. In 1873, using a primitive staining process, Hansen revealed the rod-shaped bacilli that came to be known as the cause of leprosy. In 1875 he was appointed Norway's Chief Medical Officer for Leprosy.

Controversy arose when Albert Neisser (1855–1916), a German researcher, used a more sophisticated technique to demonstrate the microorganism's existence even more clearly and claimed primacy for his discovery. Ultimately, however, the overwhelming majority of Hansen's professional peers credited him with the discovery.

Having identified the bacillus, Hansen worked to prove that it was the etiologic agent for leprosy and to dispel persistent skepticism about communicability. He traveled to the United States to conduct studies among leprous Norwegian emigrants, a population uniquely useful for epidemiologic observation, as the disease had not previously existed in the area. He also unsuccessfully sought to cultivate the bacillus and transfer it to animals or people in order to demonstrate pathogenesis. In 1879 he inoculated a patient ocularly with leprous material against her will and was found guilty of the act in a court of law. The court stripped him of his position as resident physician at the Bergen Leprosy Hospital, but he remained Chief Medical Officer for Leprosy until his death in 1912. As such, he served as the president of the Second International Congress on Leprosy held in Bergen in his honor in 1909.

Hansen convinced Norwegian authorities to enforce mandatory isolation of the most contagious leprosy patients. Previously, admission to hospitals had been voluntary for leprosy sufferers, and usually only the most debilitated presented themselves. Hansen used data from the National Leprosy Registry to demonstrate that incidence of the disease had diminished most appreciably in regions with strictly enforced hospitalization. Hansen's work ultimately resulted in widespread recognition that leprosy was a contagious disease, if not a highly contagious one, the transmission of which could be controlled by aggressive public health measures. *See also* Demographic Data Collection and Analysis, History of; Leprosarium; Leprosy in the Premodern World; Leprosy in the United States; Leprosy, Societal Reactions to.

Further Reading

Hansen, G. A., trans. *The Memories and Reflections of Dr. G. Armauer Hansen*. Würzburg: German Leprosy Relief Association, 1976.

Irgens, Lorentz M. "Leprosy in Norway: An Interplay of Research and Public Health Work." *International Journal of Leprosy* 41 (1973): 189–198.

Vogelsang, Thomas. M. "Gerhard Henrik Armauer Hansen, 1841–1912: The Discoverer of the Leprosy Bacillus, His Life and Work." *International Journal of Leprosy* 46 (1978): 257–332.

AVA ALKON

HANSEN'S DISEASE.   *See* Leprosy.

HANTAVIRUS.   *See* Hemorrhagic Fevers; Hemorrhagic Fevers in Modern Africa.

HEMORRHAGIC FEVERS.   The term hemorrhagic fevers describes a broad group of human illnesses caused by **viruses** from four families: Arenaviridae (including Lassa and New World Arenaviruses), Bunyaviridae (including Hantavirus), Filoviridae (including Ebola and Marburg viruses), and Flaviviridae (including the viruses responsible for **Yellow Fever** and Dengue fever). All hemorrhagic fever viruses (HFVs) have RNA for their genetic material, and all are enveloped in a fatty (lipid) covering. Although there is significant variation from virus to virus, in general they can cause a severe, potentially fatal illness affecting several different organ systems. The severity of the illness depends on several factors, including the type of virus, the size of the dose, and the route of infection.

After exposure, the virus incubates for 2 to 21 days and then attacks cells in the bloodstream, typically white blood cells (macrophages) and their predecessor cells (monocytes), leading to general fever and aches in the early stages of illness. From the blood, the infection can spread to a number of different organs including the kidneys, liver, and lungs. In many cases, as the disease progresses it damages the smallest blood vessels, the capillaries, causing fluid leakage into the surrounding tissues. It may also cause significant internal and external bleeding (hemorrhage), from which viral hemorrhagic fevers take their collective name. In severe cases, patients may bleed from the skin and eyes and may excrete copious amounts of blood through vomiting and diarrhea. Death can result from several causes, including heart or kidney failure, blood loss, pulmonary distress, seizure, or shock.

All viral hemorrhagic fevers are of animal origin (zoonotic). Ordinarily the virus replicates in a host species, typically a rodent or arthropod, which suffers few if any ill effects from the infection. Hemorrhagic fever viruses are therefore geographically restricted to the areas inhabited by their host species. Infection of the **human body** results from close contact with the host species. HFVs can be spread to humans via bites, as is commonly the case when arthropods such as ticks or mosquitoes are the host species. When rodents are the host, the virus is usually secreted in saliva, droppings, or urine, which can then dry and become airborne as dust particles. In some cases, the primary host may spread the virus to other animals such as livestock, which then pass the virus on to the humans who care for or slaughter them. Because HFVs exist normally in an animal reservoir, human outbreaks are sporadic and very difficult to predict.

Transmission.   The jump from host species to human is called primary **transmission**. Many hemorrhagic fever viruses are incapable of spreading from person to person, and their outbreaks are caused entirely by primary transmission. However, some HFVs can be spread from person to person in a process called secondary transmission. Secondary transmission occurs via direct contact with infected blood or other bodily fluids. There is little evidence that HFVs are normally transmitted via coughing or sneezing, although such a means of spread cannot be ruled out entirely. Secondary transmission can occur through the skin if infected fluid contacts a cut or other break in the surface. Puncturing the skin via a needle stick allows the virus direct access to the bloodstream and is therefore a particularly dangerous mode of transmission. In numerous documented cases, the repeated use of syringes under conditions of poor hygiene has served to amplify naturally occurring outbreaks of HFVs, contributing to both the spread and the lethality of the illness. HFVs are probably not transmissible from person to person before major symptoms have manifested themselves.

Because poor public health practices have contributed so significantly to the emergence of viral hemorrhagic fevers, it follows that good public health has been the most effective way to halt outbreaks. In cases of secondary transmission, quick identification, followed by **quarantine** of suspects and isolation of infected individuals has been successful. For some such outbreaks, the introduction of basics for **personal hygiene** such as clean water, soap, gloves, and appropriate clothing has been sufficient to halt secondary transmission of the illness via contact with infected fluids. Proper use and disposal of equipment such as needles and thermometers is essential. In cases of primary transmission via rodents, controlling the host population through trapping or poisoning has been effective, as have efforts to eliminate rodents from human dwellings and food sources where their urine and feces readily come into contact with people. When arthropods serve as the host, measures such as **fumigation**, wearing of proper clothing, and use of nets, screens, and other barriers are effective.

Treatment.   There has been little opportunity to observe most hemorrhagic fevers in a clinical setting, so evidence regarding individual treatment is sketchy at best. For all hemorrhagic fevers, treatment consists of supportive therapy—the administering of fluids and electrolytes to ensure that blood pressure and circulatory volume remain high enough to allow the body's defenses to deal with the infection. Careful observation must accompany fluid treatment, as damage to blood vessels can permit the leakage of added fluids from the circulatory system into surrounding tissues causing complications such as pulmonary edema, the swelling of lung tissue leading to suffocation. In the case of Lassa fever, the use of antiserum derived from the blood of previously infected patients has been effective in early stages of the disease, but this necessitates prompt and accurate diagnosis, which often is not available in early stages of hemorrhagic fever outbreaks. Trials have shown that treatment with the drug ribavirin after infection may reduce the mortality rates of several hemorrhagic fever viruses. There are no known treatments for illnesses caused by the Filoviridae and Flaviviridae families. With the exception of yellow fever, there are no licensed vaccines for any hemorrhagic fever viruses.

HFVs as Biological Weapons.   Since the 1990s hemorrhagic fever viruses have received considerable public attention as potential weapons in **biological warfare** or **bioterrorism**. There is some justification for this concern. Outbreaks of the Ebola virus in 1976 killed between 53 percent and 88 percent of infected persons, and in Angola, an outbreak of the closely related Marburg virus killed 235 of 257 infected individuals in 2005 (a 91.4 percent mortality rate). In addition, both the Soviet Union and the United States worked on weaponizing various HFVs during the Cold War, and the Soviet Union is known to have worked with Ebola and Marburg. Studies carried out in former Soviet bioweapons facilities have demonstrated that high concentrations of these agents in aerosolized form can cause illness in guinea pigs and nonhuman primates. In addition, a nonvirulent strain of the Ebola virus, dubbed Ebola Reston, may be somewhat transmissible in aerosol form. This evidence suggests that although HFVs such as Ebola and Marburg are not ordinarily very infectious, they are a short evolutionary leap away from high infectivity. The lethality of these viruses coupled with the lack of any effective therapy would make such a modified form a devastating weapon. Accordingly, in 1999 the **Centers for Disease Control and Prevention** (CDC) in Atlanta classified hemorrhagic fever viruses as Category A bioweapon agents.

Families of Hemorrhagic Fever Viruses

Arenaviridae.   Arenaviruses are spherical and have a grainy appearance under the electron microscope. The host species for arenaviruses are rodents. There are four strains of arenavirus in the Western Hemisphere, which cause Argentine, Bolivian, Venezuelan, and Brazilian hemorrhagic fevers. All four of these hemorrhagic fevers tend to occur in limited, sporadic outbreaks. The best-known arenavirus causes Lassa fever, which is endemic in several countries of western Africa. In approximately 80 percent of patients, Lassa fever shows few if any observable symptoms. In the remaining 20 percent, the virus causes a severe disease that may affect the liver, spleen, and kidneys. For approximately 1 percent of all infected individuals, death occurs within 14 days of infection. Approximately 300,000 to 500,000 cases of Lassa fever occur each year in West Africa, with about 5,000 fatalities. Lassa may be spread from person to person via direct contact with infected fluids, but there is no definitive evidence to support direct airborne transmission of the virus. The animal reservoir for the Lassa virus consists of several closely related species of rat; because these rats have a wide geographic distribution, the Lassa virus may have a wider range than is currently believed. Treatment with ribavirin in the early stages of infection may reduce the mortality rate in Lassa fever outbreaks.

Bunyaviridae. Bunyaviridae is a large family of viruses including five genera, each with many different serotypes. Bunyavirus diseases have been documented throughout much of the world, including Africa, Asia, and most recently North America. In Africa, the primary Bunyavirus diseases are Rift Valley Fever (RVF; genus Phlebovirus) and Crimean-Congo Hemorrhagic Fever (CCHF; genus Nairovirus). In both cases the animal host of the virus is an arthropod—mosquitoes in the case of RVF and ticks for CCHF. RVF is confined to Sub-Saharan Africa. Mosquitoes transmit the virus to both people and livestock, which then pass it on to humans. In most people RVF causes a mild illness with few if any symptoms, but in some patients the disease can progress to hemorrhagic fever accompanied by **encephalitis** and eye damage, including **conjunctivitis**. Approximately 1 percent of infected humans die of the disease. In late 2006 and early 2007, the **World Health Organization** (WHO) reported outbreaks of Rift Valley Fever in the United Republic of Tanzania, Kenya, and Somalia, all of which had extremely high mortality rates ranging between 23 percent and 45 percent, but this is at least partially attributable to the fact that surveillance was only able to detect severe cases of the disease. In contrast, CCHF is endemic throughout Africa, Asia, the Middle East, and Eastern Europe. Ticks transmit the virus for CCHF to humans and many other species of mammal. CCHF often causes death from liver, kidney, or lung failure, with a mortality rate of approximately 30 percent. The use of ribavirin in the early stages of infection may reduce the mortality of both illnesses.

The third genus of Bunyaviruses that cause hemorrhagic fever in humans are the Hantaviruses. In Asia, Hantavirus infections often lead to kidney failure and are thus referred to as hemorrhagic fevers with renal syndrome. These illnesses have been known in China and Russia for centuries; they received international attention during the Korean War, when thousands of UN troops became ill with Hantavirus infections. The virus was not identified until 1976, followed by identification of the main host species, the striped field mouse, several years later. Recently a new form of Hantavirus endemic to the southwestern United States has been discovered, one that causes an immune reaction producing very fine damage in the capillaries, which allows fluid but not cells to leak out. Consequently the lungs of victims fill with liquid while the blood congeals, leading to rapid death from pulmonary edema. By 1995, 115 cases of this new Hantavirus disease had been confirmed, most in the four corners region of the southwestern United States; the mortality was a very high 51.3 percent. The host animals for this virus are also mice. There is evidence that Asian Hantaviruses respond to treatment with ribavirin, but there seems to be no treatment other than supportive therapy with careful observation for the American Hantavirus.

Filoviridae. Filoviruses are the most recently discovered family of hemorrhagic fever viruses, having first been observed in 1967. The name means threadlike or filamentous, describing the threadlike structure of the viral particles. There are two genera of filoviruses, Marburg and Ebola, and Ebola has four sub-types, three of which cause severe hemorrhagic fevers in humans. Marburg virus was discovered in 1967 when workers in Marburg, Germany, were exposed to the virus via a shipment of green monkeys from Uganda. In this initial outbreak, there were 31 confirmed cases in Germany and Yugoslavia, of which 7 (23 percent) were fatal. Ebola first became known through two unrelated but simultaneous outbreaks in Zaire (now Democratic Republic of Congo) and Sudan in 1976. Each outbreak resulted in approximately 300 confirmed illnesses. The mortality rate for the Sudan epidemic was 53 percent; that of Zaire was 88 percent. There was another major Ebola epidemic in Congo in 1995, leading to 316 illnesses and a 77 percent mortality rate. The most recent epidemic, as noted above, was an outbreak of Marburg in Angola in early 2005, which killed a staggering 235 of 257 known cases (91.4 percent mortality).

The courses of all filovirus infections are similar. After an incubation period of 2 to 21 days, in which the virus infects the macrophages and monocytes, the illness spreads to other tissues such as the kidneys and spleen. Victims suffer high fevers and excruciating pain. In later stages the viruses cause capillary damage resulting in massive internal and external hemorrhaging. The cause of death is typically described as terminal shock. Filoviruses are spread via direct contact with infected fluids. Airborne spread has not been observed among people, but laboratory research suggests it might be possible. Poor public health has been a significant factor contributing to the secondary transmission of filovirus infections. In all three major Ebola outbreaks, hospitals have served to amplify rather than reduce the incidence of the disease by reusing syringes, needles, and other medical equipment without sterilization. There is no known treatment for filovirus infections other than supportive therapy. The natural range for most filovirus strains appears to be Africa, but some strains (such as the Reston strain) occur naturally in Asia and the Philippines. The animal host of filoviruses is currently unknown, but evidence is increasingly pointing toward bats as the host species. The mode of primary transmission from host to human remains unknown.

Flaviviridae. Viruses of the Flaviviridae family cause four hemorrhagic fevers in human beings: **yellow fever**, Omsk Hemorrhagic Fever, Kyasanur Forest Disease, and Dengue fever. Omsk Hemorrhagic Fever and Kyasanur Forest Disease have ticks as their host species and have a limited impact on human health. Of the four, Dengue fever poses the greatest public health threat. Dengue may be caused by one of four closely related types of flavivirus. In most cases it causes a severe flu-like illness, but in a minority of cases the fever leads to symptoms consistent with other HFVs—high fever, liver damage, internal and external bleeding, and death as a result of general shock. Dengue is a very widespread disease, endemic in more than 100 countries, particularly in Southeast Asia and the western Pacific. The incidence of Dengue has increased dramatically in the past two decades. Currently, WHO estimates that there may be 50 million cases of Dengue infection worldwide every year, with approximately 500,000 cases requiring hospitalization. Dengue is most prevalent in urban and semi-urban environments, affects children under the age of 15 preferentially, and is the leading cause of hospitalization and death among children in several countries. Dengue viruses are transmitted via the bites of infected female mosquitoes. There is no treatment for Dengue fever, but proper supportive therapy can reduce mortality to 1 percent or lower. There is no vaccine, and the only current method for controlling the spread of Dengue is to combat the mosquitoes that transmit the virus.

Future Research.   Currently, far more is unknown than known about hemorrhagic fever viruses, leaving all major areas of research open. Much more needs to be done in the identification of host species and determination of ranges of the viruses. The same is true for modes of transmission, primary and especially secondary. Greater opportunity for clinical observation is necessary for improving our understanding of the course of the diseases. Finally, the overall lack of drug therapies and effective vaccines indicates that these areas also await extensive further investigation. *See also* Air and Epidemic Diseases;

Animal Diseases (Zoonoses) and Epidemic Disease; Diagnosis and Diagnostic Tools; Diet, Nutrition, and Epidemic Disease; Environment, Ecology, and Epidemic Disease; Epidemiology; Hemorrhagic Fevers in Modern Africa; Human Immunity and Resistance to Disease; Insects, Other Arthropods, and Epidemic Disease; International Health Agencies and Conventions; Pesticides; Pharmaceutical Industry; Poverty, Wealth, and Epidemic Disease.

Further Reading

Crawford, Dorothy H. *The Invisible Enemy: A Natural History of Viruses.* New York: Oxford University Press, 2000.

Ergonul, Onder. *Crimean-Congo Hemorrhagic Fever: A Global Perspective.* New York: Springer, 2007.

Garrett, Laurie. *Betrayal of Trust: The Collapse of Global Public Health.* New York: Hyperion, 2000.

Gubler, Duane J. "Dengue and Dengue Hemorrhagic Fever." *Clinical Microbiology Review* 11 (1998): 480–496.

Leuenroth, Stephanie J. *Hantavirus Pulmonary Syndrome.* Philadelphia: Chelsea House, 2006.

Oldstone, Michael B. A. *Viruses, Plagues, and History.* New York: Oxford University Press, 1998.

Raymond, J. Kay, and Deborah J. Baglole. "Lassa Fever: Epidemiology, Clinical Features, and Social Consequences." *British Medical Journal* 327 (2003): 1271–1275.

Ryabchikova, Elena I., and Barbara B. S. Price. *Ebola and Marburg Viruses: A View of Infection Using Electron Microscopy.* Columbus, OH: Battelle Press, 2004.

Ryan, Frank. *Virus X: Tracking the New Killer Plagues.* New York: Little, Brown, and Company, 1997.

Smith, Tara C. *Ebola.* Philadelphia: Chelsea House, 2005.

JEFFREY LEWIS

HEMORRHAGIC FEVERS IN MODERN AFRICA. **Hemorrhagic fevers** are human illnesses caused by **viruses** that result in damage to the blood vessels, making them more permeable and potentially resulting in internal bleeding. Hemorrhagic fevers are distributed throughout the world, but those that are found in Africa include Ebola, Marburg, Lassa, Crimean-Congo, Dengue, and Hantavirus. Outbreaks of Ebola and Marburg have primarily taken place in Central Africa, including the Democratic Republic of Congo (Congo Kinshasa), the Republic of Congo (Congo Brazzaville), Uganda, and Sudan, whereas outbreaks of Dengue have taken place not only in Africa but in other tropical regions of the world, including Asia, the Pacific, Australia, and the Americas.

Although the occurrence of Marburg and Ebola hemorrhagic fevers are considered rare when compared to illnesses caused by other viruses such as **Human Immunodeficiency Virus** (HIV), they are important illnesses because when they do strike, the consequences are devastating. Furthermore, there is evidence that outbreaks of Ebola, for example, have been occurring with increasing frequency since the mid-1990s. In the case of Marburg hemorrhagic fever, whereas in earlier years there were only a few documented outbreaks, in 1998 a large outbreak occurred in the Democratic Republic of Congo (DRC) resulting in a case fatality of 83 percent. The deadliest outbreak of Marburg to be recorded occurred in Angola in 2005 where it claimed at least 300 lives.

Indeed, Marburg and Ebola hemorrhagic fevers have arguably caused the most terror and are considered the most severe of the hemorrhagic fevers because of their ability to spread through large populations in a short period of time if not contained, and also possibly because our knowledge of the viruses that cause these illnesses is limited. Our knowledge of viral hemorrhagic fevers is indeed small when compared to our knowledge of other viral infections such as HIV.

Dengue hemorrhagic fever, although having a good prognosis if treated early, can also be fatal. It is also one of the most common viral illnesses spread by mosquitoes, with hundreds of thousands of people becoming ill every year. In the early 2000s, there have been more frequent **epidemics** of Dengue hemorrhagic fever occurring in major cities in the tropics, causing this illness to become a major public health concern.

Outbreaks of Ebola have been common in Central African countries such as the DRC and the Republic of Congo, claiming the lives of scores of people. Examples of prominent outbreaks of Ebola hemorrhagic fever included the outbreak in Yambuku, Northern Zaire in 1976, which later spread to Southern Sudan. This was the first outbreak of Ebola to be well documented.

Outbreaks of these hemorrhagic fevers are unfortunately not history. Since the 1976 outbreak of Ebola Hemorrhagic fever, there have been scores of epidemics in various countries in Africa. In October 2007, the **World Health Organization** (WHO) reported an ongoing outbreak of Ebola confirmed in the previous month, in which there was a total of 25 out of 76 suspected cases from a province in the DRC.

Since the 1976 Ebola outbreak in Zaire (DRC), researchers, health-care providers, public health experts from agencies such as the World Health Organization and the American **Centers for Disease Control and Prevention** (CDC), and government officials have made great strides in ensuring the accurate and systematic documentation of outbreaks. Wherever outbreaks of these three hemorrhagic fevers have occurred, there has been efficient communication among various international bodies and important parties. Necessary personnel have been deployed to the areas not only to assist in containing the virus causing the hemorrhagic fever but also to document relevant information pertaining to how the outbreak began and how it spread, in an effort to gain a better understanding of these deadly diseases and to prevent future outbreaks.

These diseases are especially dangerous when they reach epidemic levels on the African continent, given the many challenges faced by the African countries where these hemorrhagic fevers tend to occur. To give an example, the likelihood of death resulting from Ebola in Africa is 50 to 90 percent, with health-care providers directly involved in caring for those infected being at great risk of contracting the virus. Indeed, the mortality rate for medical workers who contract Ebola is 50 percent. While the likelihood of death from Marburg is lower than that of Ebola—about 25 percent—both diseases may spawn complications, a few of which include liver inflammation, inflammation of the spinal cord with possible permanent paralysis, and, in men, inflammation of the testicles.

The prognosis of a patient suffering from Dengue fever is better than that of Marburg and Ebola, with most patients recovering from Dengue fever if health care is provided promptly and in an aggressive manner. Nevertheless, half of the patients suffering from Dengue fever who are not treated go into shock and die.

To date, there is neither a cure nor a vaccine for these easily transmittable deadly hemorrhagic fevers, with exposure occurring through contact with body fluids. Infected persons are isolated and provided with supportive treatment and care, which means that they receive fluids and electrolytes to maintain hydration and medications to help relieve the symptoms of the disease and treat resulting complications. Furthermore, little is known about how the animal host transmits the virus to the human host. As such, the need for further research that would yield information critical to the development of a cure or even a vaccine is essential.

With the world becoming more and more of a global village and with people traveling with ease from one part of the globe to another, there is need for the understanding of such diseases that have the potential to spread among scores of people within a very short time frame. Diseases that once only occurred in a remote African village can now be easily transported through a human host traveling from Central Africa to the Americas to be transmitted to someone else in that part of the world. It is therefore critical that any outbreaks of hemorrhagic fevers on the African continent be speedily curbed as a way of not only protecting the health of Africans but also that of citizens of other countries in the world.

Challenges for African Countries. The African countries that have experienced epidemics of hemorrhagic fevers are also some of the very poorest countries in the world. Many lack the infrastructure, as well as the health and social services personnel, to care adequately for those who are infected. Take, for example, the DRC, which has a gross domestic product (the total market value of all final goods and services produced within a country in a year) per capita of $123, compared to that of the United States, which is $11,004. The poor economy of the DRC has undoubtedly limited domestic funding for the establishment of health-care infrastructure, as well as for the education, training, and adequate compensation of health-care personnel necessary for the containment of outbreaks of deadly diseases.

Limited Medical Supplies. In resource poor countries, containing epidemics resulting from hemorrhagic fevers can indeed be challenging. Because the diseases are transmitted through contact with bodily fluids, including contact with equipment such as needles that have been used on or handled by an infected person, it is important to take strict precautions when handling anything that has come into contact with the infected person. As such, it is recommended that those coming into contact with the infected person's body fluids or anything else that the person has been in contact with put on gloves, gowns, goggles, and masks, items that are often not readily available in hospitals or clinics in the African countries affected by these epidemics. It is also recommended that needles that have been used on infected persons be sterilized or disposed of appropriately using standard protocols. In the 1976 epidemic of Ebola hemorrhagic fever in Yambuku mission hospital in Northern Zaire, it is clear that inability to contain the virus effectively through proper sterilization of needles and syringes contributed to the rapid spread of the virus, which eventually claimed the lives of 280 of the 318 people infected. It is documented that at the time of the outbreak, the routine was for five needles and syringes to be issued to the nursing staff every morning for their use on the hospital units. These needles and syringes were rinsed between patients with warm water and sometimes boiled at the end of the day.

Today, we know that because these viruses are spread through direct contact with infected body fluids, nondisposable protective equipment such as gowns or masks must not be reused unless they have been properly disinfected. Moreover, needles and syringes that have been used on the infected person are definitely not to be reused. The Centers for Disease Control and Prevention report that contaminated needles and syringes have played a significant role in spreading infection where outbreaks of Ebola hemorrhagic fever have occurred. Clearly, even today, poor African countries such as the DRC can ill afford adequate disposable needles and the equipment necessary to ensure proper and continuous sterilization of needles. Neither can they afford to dispose of important protective gear.

Lack of available medications also complicates the delivery of efficient and much needed health care to victims of epidemics of hemorrhagic fevers. Basic medications that are sorely lacking in hospitals when there is no outbreak, such as fever-reducing medications, become all the more needed when there is one.

Limited **diagnostic tools** that would allow for the prompt identification and isolation of cases are also in short supply, making it difficult to contain the virus following prompt identification, thus resulting in amplification of the virus leading to outbreaks. Early detection and containment of the viruses causing hemorrhagic fevers are further made difficult because the signs and symptoms of hemorrhagic fevers, such as headache, fever, and vomiting, are very similar to those of other diseases such as **malaria, dysentery**, and **influenza** commonly present in Central Africa. During the Ebola epidemic in Kikwit in the DRC in 1995, laboratory tests were unavailable, and patients exhibiting fevers were empirically treated with antimalarials and **antibiotics** rather than the medications indicated for Ebola.

Infrastructure.   Isolation of infected persons, required to ensure the effective containment of the viruses causing hemorrhagic fevers, is a challenge when there is limited infrastructure to house those infected. During the Ebola outbreak of 2003 in the Republic of Congo, one of the rural hospitals had only two rooms available for use as isolation rooms. These two rooms had a metal cot with no mattress, a bucket, broken windows, and no running water or toilets.

Health-Care Personnel.   In addition to the need for infrastructure, in order to save the lives of those already infected, aggressive treatment is essential. As mentioned earlier, treatment involves fluid replacement therapy and administration of medications that will help treat the signs and symptoms of the disease as well as the complications resulting from the disease. In cases of an outbreak, there is therefore an urgent need for health-care personnel who will not only provide such aggressive treatment but also ensure strict monitoring of patients for prompt identification of complications and rapid ensuing medical response. Yet in African countries that experience outbreaks of hemorrhagic fevers, there is routinely a dire need for health-care personnel. To give an example, according to the **World Health Organization**, the DRC had an average of 0.53 **nurses** and 0.11 **physicians** per 1,000 population in the year 2004. This need naturally intensifies when there is an outbreak of a hemorrhagic fever.

The short supply of health-care personnel engaged in the treatment and the containment of outbreaks of hemorrhagic fevers such as Ebola and Marburg face not only the risk of acquiring the viruses themselves as they tend to patients with limited supplies but also the stigmatization by other members of the community and from their own families. Further complicating the situation faced by health-care providers when such epidemics occur in African countries are the two very divergent sociocultural models used to curb the spread of hemorrhagic fever epidemics: On one hand, there is the Western biomedical model in which Westerners respond to the epidemic with the provision of important resources, assistance in isolating and providing treatment to the sick, and conducting of hygienic rituals such as bagging infected **corpses** for appropriate handling. Such actions of Westerners in response to epidemics of hemorrhagic fevers on the African continent are viewed from a different perspective by the observing Africans who may have a limited understanding of Western infection control procedures. On the other hand, for the

Africans, there is the traditional model in which African peoples in the midst of an epidemic offer their own explanations for what is taking place in their communities, based on their own frame of reference and their traditional medical and religious beliefs.

African health-care providers find themselves caught in the middle of these two different and sometimes conflicting models. Often they do not reveal what occurs in the African context to the Western health-care providers for fear of being labeled backwards and ignorant. At the same time, they are mistrusted by their fellow Africans who associate them with the Westerners whom they do not understand and perhaps also do not trust. One important issue to note is that although some of the indigenous practices used by Africans in an effort to contain the spread of a hemorrhagic fever epidemic may serve to amplify the outbreak, other practices complement those instituted by Western health-care professionals. The two cultures, although different, can negotiate, and a common ground, more collegial in nature, can be discovered to strengthen the response to fever epidemics on the African continent.

Although much has been said about the challenges faced by resource-poor African countries in which outbreaks of these deadly diseases occur, there is also much to be said about the unity, cooperation, and resilience of human beings when epidemics such as Marburg and Ebola occur. For instance, on August 31, 2007, the World Health Organization reported an outbreak of an unknown illness in the province of Kasai Occidental in the DRC, with 50 percent of the cases identified as children less than 10 years of age. An investigation team that included officials from the ministry of health in the DRC, WHO officials, and those from other agencies took important measures, such as obtaining clinical samples for laboratory testing, mobilizing support for epidemiological investigation and logistics, ensuring the provision of supplies and safe **water**, promoting safe burial practices, and strengthening infection control. Clinical samples were also sent to the CDC in Atlanta, Georgia. Less than two weeks later, the Ministry of Health of the DRC confirmed that laboratory analysis performed at the Centre International de Recherches Médicales de Franceville in Gabon and at the CDC in the United States indicated that the unknown illness in the province of Kasai Occidental was an outbreak of Ebola hemorrhagic fever. The prompt response of both national and international officials to the needs of an African nation with limited resources in the midst of such a crisis is a testimony to the results yielded by human cooperation and unity. This is only one example that indicates that with each subsequent outbreak of hemorrhagic fever and with the acquisition of more knowledge and experience, national and international teams of health-care experts and social scientists become better organized in their clinical management and documentation of cases, and the mortality rates resulting from the epidemics are consequently lower.

The commitment of local nurses during the outbreaks occurring in the DRC in 1995, in Uganda in 2001–2002, and in the Republic of Congo in 2003 also speaks to the resilience and commitment of health-care providers who often place their own lives at risk while prioritizing the lives of others in the midst of a deadly outbreak.

On the Frontiers.   Over the past decade, significant progress has been made through various studies that have increased scientists' understanding of the molecular mechanisms that are involved in the **transmission** of viruses from the host cells and the processes that lead to hemorrhagic fevers themselves. One of the most important advances in combating these viruses through research is evidenced through the extraordinary successes of two vaccine platforms that have proven to be capable of completely protecting nonhuman primates against some strains of the Ebola and Marburg viruses.

Swift measures in the detection and treatment of the viruses causing Marburg, Ebola, and Dengue hemorrhagic fevers and continued investigation into the disease source and the disease process through research speak to the international unity and cooperation among organizations and countries that is necessary for not only the containment but ultimately the elimination of these deadly hemorrhagic fevers. *See also* AIDS in Africa; Animal Diseases (Zoonoses) and Epidemic Disease; Folk Medicine; Geopolitics, International Relations, and Epidemic Disease; Non-Governmental Organizations (NGOs) and Epidemic Disease; Pharmaceutical Industry; Trade, Travel, and Epidemic Disease.

Further Reading

Berger, Stephen A. *Exotic Viral Diseases: A Global Guide.* Hamilton, ON: B.C. Decker, 2005.

Gear, J. H. S. *Handbook of Viral and Rickettsial Hemorrhagic Fevers.* Boca Raton, FL: CRC Press, 1988.

Guimard, Y, et.al. "Organization of Patient Care during the Ebola Hemorrhagic Fever Epidemic in Kikwit, Democratic Republic of Congo, 1995." *The Journal of Infectious Diseases* 179 (1999): 268–273.

Hensley, L. E., et al. "Ebola and Marburg Viruses: Pathogenesis and Development of Countermeasures." *Current Molecular Medicine* 5 (2005): 761–772.

Hewlett, B. S., and Amola, R. P. "Cultural Contexts of Ebola in Northern Uganda." *Emerging Infectious Diseases* 9 (2003): 1242–1248.

Hewlett, B., and Hewlett, B. S. "Providing Care and Facing Death: Nursing during Ebola Outbreaks in Central Africa." *Journal of Transcultural Nursing* 16 (2005): 289–297.

Howard, Colin R. *Viral Haemorrhagic Fevers.* New York: Elsevier, 2006.

Pattyn, S. R., ed. *Ebola Virus Hemorrhagic Fever.* New York: Elsevier, 1978.

LUCY MKANDAWIRE-VALHMU

HENDERSON, DONALD AINSLIE (1928–).   As head of the **World Health Organization's** (WHO) worldwide **smallpox eradication** program from 1966–1977, Dr. Donald A. Henderson led the only successful disease eradication program to date. This unprecedented triumph marked the containment of a **virus** that had plagued humankind for millennia (killing 300 million people in the twentieth century alone) and established Henderson as a key figure in the history of global public health.

Born to Canadian parents in Lakewood, Ohio, Henderson earned his Masters in Public Health degree from Johns Hopkins University in 1960. Initially employed by the **Centers for Disease Control** (CDC) in Atlanta (first as chief of the **epidemic** intelligence service from 1955–1957, then as chief of the surveillance section from 1960–1966), he was recruited as WHO's chief medical officer for the smallpox eradication campaign in 1966.

As head of the program, Henderson oversaw the thousands of public health workers who carried out the massive **vaccination** campaign. Using a combined approach of mass vaccination and surveillance and containment (or "ring vaccination"), Henderson and the national eradication teams that made up the worldwide campaign were able to prevent the spread of—and eventually vanquish—the disease. Such a successful outcome had eluded eradication efforts against hookworm, yellow fever, and malaria earlier in the century.

In speaking about eradication initiatives, Henderson cited several advantages in the case of smallpox: there was an effective, easily administered, and inexpensive vaccine available for a disease with no animal reservoir, and the political will existed to achieve the goal. Henderson's own determination and initiative were also key factors in the victory. For example, he befriended Emperor Haile Salassie's personal physician in order to ensure Ethiopia's participation in the face of fiscal concerns and traveled to Moscow (against orders) personally to demand improved quality of vaccine donated from the USSR. In recounting the campaign, Henderson describes smallpox eradication as a "Cold War victory" noting that the atmosphere of international competition helped to drive the success of the program. Nonetheless, Henderson was also critical of the neglect and under-funding of other pressing health issues beyond smallpox that occurred as a result of the eradication campaign, leading him to argue against future disease eradication attempts in later years.

Knowing that the eradication program was almost complete, Henderson left the WHO to become Dean of the Johns Hopkins School of Public Health (1977–1990), just prior to the report of the last natural case of smallpox in Somalia in 1977. Following his role in the smallpox eradication campaign, Henderson has continued to be involved in public health and disease eradication/control issues in both academic and government settings, serving as White House science advisor (1991–1993) and deputy assistant secretary for health and science for the federal Department of Health and Human Services (1993–1995). Henderson is the recipient of numerous international awards and honorary degrees, including the Presidential Medal of Freedom (received in 2002), the highest civilian honor in the United States.

Although smallpox was officially declared eradicated in 1980, Henderson continues to be troubled by the virus and its potential role in **biological warfare**, a concern that resulted in his appointment as founding director of the Center for Civilian Biodefence Strategies at the Johns Hopkins School of Public Health in 1997. His work on bioterror-ism and public health security has continued via his 2001 appointment as head of the federal Office of Public Health Preparedness and 2003 transfer to the Center for Biosecurity at the University of Pittsburgh Medical Center. Rather ironically, Henderson currently spends much of his time making public health contingency plans in the unlikely event of intentional reintroduction of the very disease that he helped to wipe out.

Further Reading

Henderson, D. A. "Eradication: Lessons from the Past (Smallpox Eradication)." *Bulletin of the World Health Organization* 76, 2 (1998): S17.

Henderson D. A . "Smallpox Eradication—A Cold War Victory." *World Health Forum* 19 (1999): 113–119.

Henig, Robin Marantz. "D. A. Henderson: Eradicating One of History's Deadliest Diseases was Just the Beginning." *Smithsonian* 35, 8 (2005): 70–71. Also online at http://www.smithsonianmag.com/issue/November_2005.html.

Reed, J. D. "Virus Vanquisher: D. A. Henderson led the global campaign to eradicate smallpox; now he's working against its return." *Smithsonian*, 32, 11 (2002): 28–29.

KLAUDIA DMITRIENKO AND ANNE-EMANUELLE BIRN

HEPATITIS. The word hepatitis is a catchall term that refers to any inflammation (*–itis*) of the liver (*hepar*) and does not imply a specific cause or connote contagiousness. Inflammation of the liver is defined as an irritation or swelling of liver cells. Hepatitis is a term that encompasses many different causes. Only hepatitis caused by a **virus** (viral hepatitis) is potentially infectious to others. Consequently, hepatitis from causes other than viruses, such as alcohol (alcoholic hepatitis) or fat (fatty liver hepatitis), cannot be spread through food or by interpersonal or sexual contact.

Hepatitis is generally described using two broad categories. One category refers to how long a person has hepatitis, and the other category refers to what factor caused the hepatitis. Inflammation of the liver that lasts less than six months is known as acute hepatitis. Within six months, people with acute hepatitis are completely healed. The liver typically self-repairs any short-term damage it may have suffered, and no long-term consequences are suffered. Viral hepatitis A is an example of acute hepatitis.

Inflammation of the liver that lasts longer than six months is known as chronic hepatitis. People who progress from acute hepatitis to chronic hepatitis are at risk of developing cirrhosis (severe scarring of the liver that is typically irreversible) and the complications of cirrhosis, such as liver cancer, internal bleeding, and liver failure. Viral hepatitis B and viral hepatitis C can lead to chronic hepatitis.

Hepatitis is also described by its cause. Although hepatitis is most frequently caused by viruses, other stimuli may cause forms of the disease. These include autoimmune liver disease (autoimmune hepatitis), obesity (nonalcoholic fatty liver hepatitis), alcohol (alcoholic hepatitis), and some medications and herbs (toxin-induced hepatitis). This entry only discusses potentially infectious viral hepatitis. A virus is a tiny microorganism that is much smaller than **bacteria**. Its main activity and goal consists of reproducing more viruses and causing damage. A virus is capable of growth and multiplication only once it has entered a living cell. The main goal of the hepatitis virus is to enter a liver cell, reproduce more hepatitis viruses, destroy the cell, and move on to attack the next liver cell.

The History of Viral Hepatitis.   Viral hepatitis can be traced back to ancient times, when it was believed by scientists that some type of virus existed that attacked the liver, resulting in a yellow discoloration of the skin and eyes, now known as jaundice. From the late 1800s to the early 1900s, scientists believed that there were only two forms of viral hepatitis: infectious hepatitis and serum hepatitis.

In 1963 a major breakthrough in research occurred—the cause of serum hepatitis was identified, and the virus was given the name hepatitis B virus (HBV). It took an additional 10 years for scientists to isolate the cause of infectious hepatitis. This virus was given the name hepatitis A virus (HAV). Around this time, medical researchers realized that other forms of viral hepatitis must exist that were not caused by either HAV or HBV because there were still so many cases of hepatitis that were not the result of one of these two viruses. These cases of unknown viral origin were lumped into the category of non-A non-B (NANB) hepatitis. In 1989 the virus that caused the majority of NANB hepatitis was identified through cloning experiments and was named the hepatitis C virus (HCV).

Although the three most common viruses causing hepatitis are hepatitis A, B, and C, other hepatitis viruses also exist. The hepatitis delta virus (HDV), first isolated in the mid-1970s, was shown to exist only in the presence of HBV. The existence of another hepatitis virus, which is similar to HAV, was suggested throughout the 1980s but was not successfully cloned until 1990, at which point it was named the hepatitis E virus (HEV). Evidence of the existence of a hepatitis F virus (HFV) is, at present, only anecdotal. Hepatitis viruses that do not appear to be significant causes of liver disease are the hepatitis G virus (HGV), discovered in 1995; the transfusion-transmitted virus (TTV), identified in 1997; and the SEN-V, identified in 1999. Other viruses, such as herpes simplex virus and Epstein-Barr virus, can also attack the liver. However, since the liver is not the principal organ damaged by these viruses, they are considered not to be a significant cause of viral hepatitis. Because approximately 10 percent of hepatitis cases still do not have an identified cause, researchers suspect that one or more as yet unidentified hepatitis viruses may exist.

Incidence and Prevalence.   In the United States, HAV is the most common cause of acute viral hepatitis. Each year, approximately 134,000 Americans are infected with HAV. In fact, around 33 percent of all Americans have at some point been infected with HAV. Almost 100 percent of people who live in U.S. communities with substandard **water** and sewage sanitation systems, in addition to people living in economically developing countries such as Africa, Asia, and Latin America, have been infected during **childhood**.

Approximately 2 billion people worldwide have been infected by hepatitis B, and almost 400 million people worldwide, including 1.25 million people in the United States, are chronic carriers of this virus. Approximately 65 million of those chronically infected will die of the disease. HBV is the single most common cause of cirrhosis and liver cancer worldwide. Hepatitis B is endemic in Southeast Asia, China, and Africa. In these areas of the world, more than 50 percent of the population has been exposed to HBV at some point in their lives. The virus has a relatively low prevalence in North America, Western Europe, and Australia, and accounts for only 5 to 10 percent of all chronic liver diseases in these areas.

HCV is the most common cause of chronic liver disease in the United States. It is estimated that almost 5 million Americans (over 2 percent of the U.S. population) and more than 1 percent of the world's population are infected with HCV. Although the incidence of people becoming acutely infected with HCV is decreasing, approximately 8,000 to 12,000 deaths are attributed to hepatitis C each year.

How Hepatitis Viruses Are Transmitted.   Hepatitis A virus is transmitted by the enteric or fecal-oral route. Enteric transmission consists of introduction of a virus into the body by way of the digestive tract. It occurs when a virus is present in the feces (fecal) of an infected person, and is then transmitted to another person via ingesting (oral) a small amount of infected stools. HBV, HDV, and HCV are transmitted via the parenteral route, meaning that these viruses are introduced into the body by any way other than via the intestinal tract. HBV is transmitted either through contaminated blood, during sexual contact, or from mother to child during childbirth. HDV only occurs in individuals who already have hepatitis B. HCV is transmitted only by blood-to-blood contact. This includes intravenous drug use, blood or blood product transfusions prior to 1992, and possibly tattoos and body-piercings. Sexual **transmission** of HCV is very rare, and transmission from mother to child at childbirth occurs in only 3 to 5 percent of cases.

The Symptoms and Physical Signs of Hepatitis.   These may vary greatly. At one extreme, some people are very ill, with jaundice, fever, decreased appetite, abdominal pain, nausea, vomiting, and fatigue. At the other extreme, and more commonly, people with hepatitis may be totally asymptomatic—meaning that they have no symptoms—or may have vague, nonspecific symptoms, such as mild fatigue or flu-like symptoms. The severity of symptoms that a person is experiencing often bears no correlation to the amount of damage done to the liver.

Diagnosing Hepatitis.   The only way to determine the type of hepatitis one has, what caused it, and how much damage has been done to the liver, is through a combination of tests. These include blood tests, such as liver function tests (LFTs) and hepatitis-specific blood tests (such as antibody and antigen tests); imaging studies done by a radiologist, such as a sonogram; and a liver biopsy (removal of a tiny piece of liver tissue using a special needle).

Treatment and Prevention.   Medications used to treat viruses are known as antivirals. Treatment of acute hepatitis, such as hepatitis A, is mostly supportive. This means that treatment is based upon the symptoms being experienced, and no antiviral medication is typically needed.

Treatment of chronic hepatitis, such as chronic hepatitis B or C, is more complicated and depends on numerous factors. Treatment of hepatitis B may include an injectable medication known as interferon, or one or more oral medications either alone or in combination, known as nucleoside and/or nucleotide analogues. Typically, hepatitis B cannot be cured, and treatment is life-long. Treatment of chronic hepatitis C involves the use of pegylated interferon (a once-a-week injectable medication), in combination with an oral medication known as ribavirin, which is taken daily. Treatment lasts for 24 to 48 weeks. Hepatitis C is the only virus that can potentially be cured, with recovery rates greater than 55 percent.

Prevention is, of course, the best treatment for any disease, and fortunately, hepatitis A and B **vaccinations** are available. The development of the hepatitis B vaccine represents one of the most important advances in medicine. This is the first and only vaccine in history that can simultaneously prevent liver cancer, cirrhosis, and a sexually transmitted disease. This vaccine has been incorporated into the immunization programs of more than 80 countries, and routine hepatitis B vaccination of all newborns in the United States has been in mandatory since 1999. The hepatitis A vaccine has been available since 1995. There is currently no vaccination for hepatitis C. *See also* Human Body.

Further Reading

Boyer, Thomas, et al. *Zakim and Boyer's Hepatology.* New York: Malcolm Saunders, 2006.
Centers for Disease Control. *Viral Hepatitis.* http://www.cdc.gov/ncidod/diseases/hepatitis/
Palmer, Melissa. *Dr. Melissa Palmer's Guide to Hepatitis and Liver Disease.* New York: Penguin Putnam Avery Press, 2004.
Schiff, Eugene, et al. *Schiff's Diseases of the Liver,* 10th edition. New York: Lippincott Williams & Wilkins, 2006.
Thomas, Howard C., et al. *Viral Hepatitis.* New York: Wiley-Blackwell, 2005.
World Health Organization. *Hepatitis.* http://www.who.int/topics/hepatitis/en/

MELISSA PALMER

HEREDITY AND EPIDEMIC DISEASE.   Humans differ significantly in their susceptibility to **epidemic** diseases. These disparities are the result of a wide range of biological, developmental, geographical, social, economic, cultural, behavioral, and psychological factors. Recent studies have confirmed what **physicians** and patients, ancient and modern, have generally believed: that hereditary variations can play a key role in determining who does or does not succumb to a given disease. Long before the advent of gene studies of twins and adoptees, for example, medical writers used such terms as diathesis, constitution, or hereditary predisposition to denote the way in which certain kinds of illness seemed to "go by blood." Not until the mid-1700s, when Pierre-Louis Moreau de Maupertuis (1698–1759) studied the **transmission** of polydactyly (extra fingers or toes) in a German family, did the role of heredity in the onset of disease or abnormality start to emerge as a field of scientific inquiry. And it took the twentieth century's development of improved statistical techniques, advances in our understanding of twinning and genetic relatedness, and the advent of genomic analysis for robust data to emerge. As genotyping becomes quicker and easier, more and more genes are being identified that can reduce or enhance an individual's infectivity and her chances of overcoming infection.

The high level of polymorphisms among genes involved in immune function, not least the human leukocyte antigen (HLA) genes, reveals the intense selective pressure humans have been exposed to from disease. Often as a result of genetic variations, some individuals and groups have a heightened resistance to infection. Members of the Fulani tribe of West Africa, for instance, seem to have a high frequency of genes conferring a degree of resistance to the *Plasmodium* parasite that causes **malaria**. Members of African populations with hemoglobin C also appear to enjoy a raised level of protection against severe cerebral malaria. And those who lack the Duffy blood group on their red blood cells may have complete resistance to *vivax* malaria.

Genetic linkage studies, including some genome-wide scans, have recently identified a number of chromosomal regions bearing genes that are likely to confer enhanced disease resistance. Certain HLA alleles have been shown to correlate with the rapid clearance of **hepatitis** B infections in the Gambia, Europe, and Korea. Non-HLA genes have been implicated in protection against **leprosy** and **tuberculosis**; in the latter case, the Vitamin D receptor gene may play an important role. And it has been established that between 5 and 21 percent of Caucasians carry a mutation, CCR5Δ32 (Δ=delta), which means that their macrophages and lymphocytes lack a coreceptor that certain HIV strains require for entering them. This can give homozygotes protection against HIV infection and can afford heterozygotes a delay in the onset of full-blown AIDS.

In addition, selection for certain blood types may have been related to infectious disease. The occurrence of Blood Group O, for example, is especially high among those suffering from severe forms of **cholera**, indicating that other blood groups might have evolved to confer resistance to such deadly infections. Yet epidemic diseases typically exert less intense selective pressures than endemic infections like malaria, leprosy, or tuberculosis. Specific outbreaks can, of course, be devastating—for instance, bubonic plague during the Middle Ages in Europe. Nevertheless, the cumulative death toll from infections like plague, **typhoid**, and cholera tends to be far less than that from endemic infections that kill persistently over successive centuries. Even so, some investigators associate the high frequency of certain mutations with past epidemics. It has been suggested, for example, that the CCR5Δ32 mutation was selected for as a result of the bubonic plague outbreaks of the Middle Ages. There is, however, some dispute as to whether the selective pressures would have been adequate to produce the observed frequency of the gene among modern Caucasians. Other researchers have argued that CCR5Δ32 was an adaptation for combating **smallpox**, a disease that was undoubtedly a potent selective force, killing countless people before reproductive age. Such debates are difficult to resolve partly because other factors might also account for the frequency of the genes in question.

Less benign genetic mutations certainly confer selective advantages against disease. The benefits for people in malarial regions of carrying single recessive genes for sickle-shaped hemoglobin, α-thalassemia, or β-thalassemia are well known. Mutations that are highly deleterious in homozygote form may also have evolved to help combat epidemic diseases. The high rates of the recessive gene for cystic fibrosis (CF) in western Europe suggest that heterozygote carriers once enjoyed some level of **immunity** against one or more major killers. The frequency of the main CF gene does not in itself prove that it conferred a survival advantage. But there is evidence that CF genes could have provided protection against typhoid: the mutation causing CF appears to make it harder for the bacteria responsible, *Salmonella typhi*, to enter the body's cells. Other groups of researchers have suggested that CF genes gave a heterozygote advantage against cholera, diarrhea, or tuberculosis.

Conversely, certain alleles are associated with increased susceptibility to infectious disease and/or a lowered ability to fight against an existing infection. Twin studies have demonstrated high levels of concordance in cause of death between parents and children for such infections as tuberculosis, leprosy, and **poliomyelitis**. More recently, researchers in many countries have identified genes that are disproportionately common among those suffering from various, though typically endemic, infections. For example, the study of HLA alleles has revealed an association between specific mutations and susceptibility to tuberculosis and leprosy in Indian populations. Moreover, separate studies among Brazilian and West African families indicate the presence of a mutation on chromosome 5, in a region associated with immune response, which may lessen resistance to **schistosomiasis**.

The identification of genes or gene complexes involved in disease susceptibility has vastly improved in recent years. In particular, the ease of genotyping has now made genome-wide linkage studies more viable. Researchers in the field are confident that in the coming years a far more complete picture will emerge of the links between human genetics and the incidence of disease. It is also hoped that a fuller understanding of the genetics of susceptibility will contribute to the development of more effective therapies and vaccines. *See also* Human Subjects Research.

Further Reading

Cooke, Graham S., and Adrian V. S. Hill. "Genetics of Susceptibility to Human Infectious Disease." *Nature Genetics* 2 (2001): 967–977.

Hill, Adrian V. S. "The Genomics and Genetics of Human Infectious Disease Susceptibility." *Annual Review of Genomics and Human Genetics* 2 (2001): 373–400.

JOHN WALLER

HIPPOCRATES (ca. 460–375/350 BCE) AND THE HIPPOCRATIC CORPUS. Although Hippocrates is widely regarded as the father of western medicine and is famous for treating a plague in antiquity, we actually know very little about him or this incident. Plato (428–348 BCE; *Protagoras* 311b–c) and Aristotle (384–322 BCE; *Politics* 1326a14), in the fourth century BCE, recognized him as a **physician** of some renown, but by the first century BCE, he had become a heroic figure associated with many deeds, beliefs, and texts. **Galen**, physicians of the Renaissance and Enlightenment (such as **Paracelsus** and **Thomas Sydenham**), and even contemporary medicine have looked back to Hippocrates as a foundational hero in their own image. In short, Hippocrates became, from very early on and through a process that we do not fully understand, an iconic figure onto whom people throughout the ages have projected their own ideas of the best of medical knowledge, practice, and ethics. He has gained the status of the principal figure in the fifth-century rationalization of Greek medical theory and practice. Hippocratic medicine attributed disease to purely natural, rather than religious or magical, causes and sought natural preventive measures and therapies.

Hippocrates was born on Cos, a Greek island just off the present-day coast of Turkey. He was a member of the Asclepiadai ("Sons of Asclepius"), a clan that claimed descent from both Asclepius (the god of healing) and Heracles (Hercules). He seems to have been active as a physician and teacher primarily in northern Greece in the last half of the fifth and early fourth centuries BCE. His son Thessalus, a son-in-law Polybus, and grandson Hippocrates (physician to Alexander the Great [356–323 BCE]) also reportedly became famous physicians. However, specific traditions about Hippocrates' life are mostly later fictions, and what he actually believed is disputed even by ancient authorities. Plato (*Phaedrus* 270c) says that Hippocrates thought it important to consider "the whole" (although what this means has been of debate since antiquity), whereas Aristotle (according to the Anonymus Londinensis papyrus, whose source appears to go back to Aristotle's pupil Meno) and Galen present differing versions of Hippocrates' core beliefs.

Similar uncertainty attends the "Hippocratic Question," namely which—if any—of the works of the "Hippocratic" Corpus (a group of about 65 medical texts assembled in Alexandria in the third and second centuries BCE) Hippocrates actually wrote. These works cover many different subjects and come from a variety of sources and authors with differing medical beliefs. The seven books entitled *Epidemics* are not about **epidemics** in the modern sense of a widespread occurrence of a common disease, but contain individual case studies and generalized observations concerning patients and locations mostly in northern Greece. Among these, however, a plague at Thasos near Lemnos appears in *Epidemics* 3.3–4, and cases and observations concerning **malaria**, and possibly **influenza**, occur in *Epidemics* 1 and 2.

Hippocrates' earliest extant association with epidemic plague (or *loimos* in Greek) comes from two works of the pseudepigrapha (texts written to appear to be something else, such as letters or speeches composed as if they were written by a famous person) found at the end of the corpus: the "Presbeutikos," a fictitious oration composed between 350–250 BCE, and the "Decree," a fictitious Athenian honorary decree composed shortly thereafter. They credit Hippocrates with diagnosing a plague in the late fifth century BCE and with saving Greece by circulating an effective therapy. In this early version, envoys from the Barbarian kings of Illyria and Paeonia (roughly modern Albania and Kosovo) arrive at Hippocrates' residence in Thessaly (northern Greece) and promise him great riches if he comes to help them. Hippocrates questions the envoys and, once he has learned enough of the disease, pretends to be unable to travel and sends the envoys away. But he then composes a therapy, distributes it throughout Greece, and sends his sons and pupils to take it to various areas (it is unspecified, however, just what this therapy entailed). When he finally arrives in Athens, the Assembly honors him and his son Thessalus.

By the first century BCE, this episode had become widely associated with the famous Athenian plague of 428–427 BCE deemed incurable by the historian Thucydides (460–400 BCE; *The Peloponnesian War* 2.47–54). The Roman historian Varro (116–27 BCE; *On Rural Farming* 1.4.5) credits him with saving "many cities," and Pliny the Elder (23–79 CE; *Nat-*

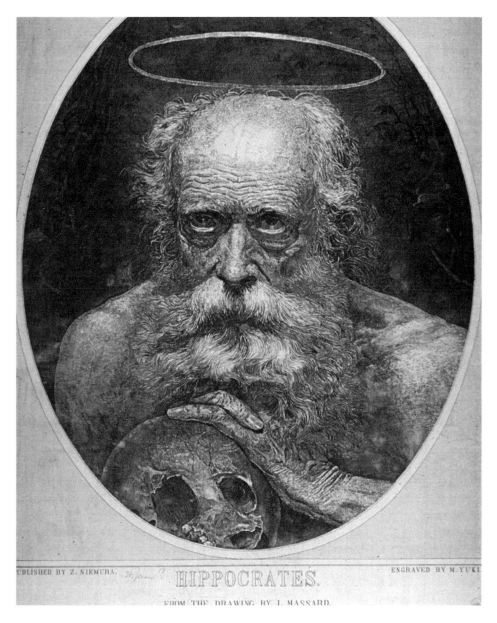

UBLISHED BY Z. NIEMURA.   HIPPOCRATES.   ENGRAVED BY M. YUKI

FROM THE DRAWING BY L. MASSARD.

Hippocrates. Engraved by M. Yuki. From the drawing by L. Massard. Courtesy of the National Library of Medicine.

ural History 29) repeats the assertion, found in the "Presbeutikos" and "Decree," that he was honored for this service. In these and some other versions of the story, such as those by Galen ("Theriac to Piso" 16), Plutarch (46–127; "Isis and Osiris" 383c) and Aetius Amidenus (6th century CE; *Tetrabibloi* 5.95), Hippocrates used a bonfire composed of various materials to dry and correct the imbalances in the **air** thought to cause plague according to the prevailing theories of the time. This tale survived through the Renaissance in medical literature and art, and is featured on the cover of the famous 1588 Venice edition of the corpus.

Another famous story, found first in the pseudepigrapha (Letters 1–9) and in several later accounts ("Vita Hippocratis Secunda Soranum," Suda, Johannes Tzetzes [1110–1180]), involves a request made to Cos by the Persian king Artaxerxes II (c. 436–358 BCE). With a plague ravaging his army, the king sends for Hippocrates, promising him riches and honors. Hippocrates, supported by Cos, refuses to aid an enemy of the Greeks. Although Greek writers (and others) saw this as an example of Hippocrates' patriotism, courage, and character, the Roman Cato (95–46 BCE; Pliny, *Natural History* 29.13–14; Plutarch, "Cato" 23) may have had this story in mind when he criticized Greek doctors and warned his son that "they have sworn to kill all barbarians with medicine, and to charge a fee for it as well." *See also* Avicenna (Ibn Sina); Environment, Ecology, and Epidemic Disease; Greco-Roman Medical Theory and Practice; Islamic Disease Theory and Medicine; Medical Education in the West, 1100–1500; Medical Education in the West, 1500–1900; Medical Ethics and Epidemic Disease.

Further Reading

Note: Works of the Hippocratic Corpus in Greek with modern English translations have been published in the Loeb Classical Library (Harvard University Press).

Jouanna, Jacques. *Hippocrates*. Translated by Malcolm DeBevoise. Baltimore: Johns Hopkins University Press, 1999.

Lloyd, G. E. R., ed. *Hippocratic Writings*. New York: Penguin, 1984.

Nutton, Vivian. *Ancient Medicine*. London: Routledge, 2004.

Pinault, Jody. *Hippocratic Lives and Legends*. Leiden: Brill, 1992.

Smith, Wesley D. *The Hippocratic Tradition*. Ithaca: Cornell University Press, 1979.

ERIC D. NELSON

HIPPOCRATIC CORPUS.   *See* Hippocrates.

HISTORICAL EPIDEMIOLOGY.   As one of the sciences of public health, **epidemiology** is concerned with the descriptions and explanations of the origins, etiologies, and **transmission** of diseases in populations. Historical epidemiology is the description, analysis, and explanation of patterns of epidemic diseases and their consequences in historical populations. A rather new field of study, historical epidemiology is interdisciplinary: it uses the traditional tools of social history, as well as the techniques of modern epidemiology, medical demography, medical geography, evolutionary biology, and genetics. Historical epidemiology can help researchers form a more complete understanding of the current trends in infectious, chronic, and reemergent diseases facing the world today.

The origins of the discipline of epidemiology help to explain the scope of historical epidemiology. Although the field has older roots, as a branch of medical science, epidemiology can be dated to the founding of the London Epidemiological Society in 1850. The founding members of this public health–minded group included William Budd (1811–80), Richard Bright (1789–1858), **John Snow**, and **William Farr**, the Statistical Superintendent at the Registrar General. From its inception, the aim of the society was, "to endeavor, by the light of modern science, to review all those causes which result in the manifestation and spread of epidemic diseases . . . to collect together facts, on which scientific researches may be securely based." Although epidemiologists and historical epidemiologists still investigate the major infectious diseases, the domain of the discipline has shifted to respond to recent trends in the changing relationship between human hosts, disease pathogens, and the environment.

Historical epidemiology plays a vital role in public health and the history of disease. By analyzing changing disease patterns over time and the impacts of public health responses on the health of populations, historical epidemiology helps to develop a more complete picture of the long term impacts of modern medicine and public health policies. The most important focus has been the impact of social reforms, environmental interventions, technological changes, and advances in medical knowledge on the development of the modern world. The study of the history of public health has also been widely influenced by historical epidemiology. For example, decreases in mortality and morbidity have increasingly been related to triumphs of public health in the late nineteenth and early twentieth centuries, as well as to the modern transition to preventive medicine in western societies. In this way, historical epidemiology's focus on changes in the health of populations can better delineate the impact of modern medicine on infectious and chronic diseases, changes in the environment, diet, and nutrition.

The Demographic Transition.   Historical epidemiologists recognize that epidemics help define social relationships, cultural norms, and political practices. Thus, the study of changing demographic patterns has occupied a central role in this field of study. One of the most interesting questions that has vexed historical epidemiologists is the occurrence of what has been called the "demographic transition"—the transition from the high birth rates and death rates of preindustrial societies to the low birth rates and death rates of industrial and postindustrial societies. The outcome of this demographic change has been a dramatic and continuing increase in world population. The demographic transition has left many questions unanswered: what is the relationship between economic modernization and the demographic transition? How did rising living standards affect this change? What were the effects of technological, scientific, and curative or preventative medicine? These are the types of questions that historical epidemiologists have sought to answer.

Understanding the demographic transition has both important historical implications and current applications. By the early twentieth century, in most European and North American countries, the collective population had begun to experience health and disease on terms dramatically different from those of previous centuries. As many epidemic diseases such as cholera, typhoid, and scarlet fever entered a period of relative stagnation and ultimate decline, adults started to live longer, and infant and child mortality rates steadily declined. Historically human population had grown very slowly, but this pattern was disrupted in the last two centuries by exponential human population growth. In 2007 the world population exceeded 6.5 billion and is projected to continue to grow throughout this century. Historical epidemiologists have been at the center of answering the complex questions of why this transition occurred.

Of the many historical epidemiologists to examine the modern rise of populations, the Irish-born physician and professor of Social Medicine at the University of Birmingham, Thomas McKeown (1912–1988), is perhaps the most important. In a body of research developed from the 1950s to the 1980s, McKeown argued that the growth in modern populations from the eighteenth century was the result of broad improvements in overall standards of living, particularly improved diet and nutrition. Using historical data on changes in death rates, McKeown noted that population growth was primarily affected by a decline in mortality from infectious disease. The basis for this decline, according to McKeown, was improved economic conditions that followed as a result of the Industrial Revolution. These changes led to rising standards of living that enhanced nutrition and strengthened human resistance to disease. Although the above formulation was the crux of his argument, McKeown also noted that other developments also contributed to the demographic transition, such as public health reforms, the enlargement of preventative and curative medicine, and the decline in virulence of infectious organisms. These last three factors were seen as minor contributors to the demographic transition particularly before the twentieth century.

The essential question that McKeown's research has raised is whether human agency, in the forms of medicine and public health or changes in economic growth, stimulated the rise of modern populations. The implications for this research are immense: should public health be directed at specific interventions or broader measures to reorganize the socioeconomic determinants of health? McKeown's stress on broad social and economic changes, as opposed to specific public health and medical interventions, has remained highly controversial and largely unresolved. Although his methodology has been called into question, the main complaint that has been generated against McKeown is the little weight given to medical science in contributing to the mortality decline before the twentieth century. Recent research has suggested that inoculation, vaccination, local public health efforts, and improvements in medical prevention perhaps played a much larger role in the mortality decline than has been suggested. An important instance is the experience of Britain. John Snow's epidemiological research on the mode and transmission of cholera in mid-nineteenth-century London, the growth of state medicine under the public health officer John Simon (1816–1904), and the numerous Parliamentary public health acts all facilitated the improvement of water supplies and methods of sewage disposal. By the beginning of the twentieth century, public health in Britain occupied a central role in British government and society, and directly influenced the control of epidemic disease.

Although a great deal of work in this field still remains, new epidemiological methods and disease ecology modeling are promising for the future. Although numerous scholars have since discredited McKeown's findings, his ideas have shaped the direction of subsequent research both in Western countries and in the developing world.

The Epidemiological Transition.   Epidemic disease has played a key role in the demographic development of all societies. Throughout history, frequent mortality crises caused by epidemics of plague, cholera, typhoid fever, and smallpox have been the determining factor in demographic growth and decline. Related to the demographic transition, one of the other chief areas of focus for historical epidemiologists has been the "epidemiological transition," which can be defined as the general shift from acute infectious pandemics and deficiency diseases to chronic noncommunicable and degenerative diseases. Examination of this phenomenon lies at heart of the interests of historical epidemiologists: specifically, the interactions between disease patterns and their demographic, social, and economic consequences.

Historical epidemiologists have identified three stages of the epidemiological transition. The first is called "The Age of Pestilence and Famine." This stage describes most preindustrialized societies and is characterized by high mortality rates and low life expectancy, somewhere between 20 and 40 years. The major causes of death in this stage were epidemics, famines, and wars. A good example is the epidemiological work of the seventeenth-century London statistician and pioneer epidemiologist John Graunt (1620–1674). By analyzing London's Bills of Mortality (lists of the numbers who died by cause of death printed weekly by the Company of Parish Clerks), Graunt demonstrated that nearly three-fourths of all deaths were attributed to infectious diseases, malnutrition, and maternity complications. Other more chronic conditions such as cancer were responsible for less than 6 percent.

"The Age of Receding Pandemics" is the second stage of the epidemiological transition. During this stage, mortality rates began to decline progressively in relation to the decreased frequency and virulence of epidemics. The average life expectancy increased to somewhere between 30 and 50 years. This stage characterized most western countries in the late nineteenth and early twentieth centuries. Better nutritional standards, increased economic prosperity, and more vital and sustained public health activities all contributed to the changes during this phase. Nonetheless, rapid **industrialization** and **urbanization** also took their toll in the forms of increased crowding, and air and water pollution. By the end of the nineteenth century, however, increased public health efforts in most Western countries led to improved sewer systems, drainage, and the provision of clean, filtered water. In countries of the developing world where public health reforms have been delayed, mortality rates remain high, particularly from waterborne and deficiency diseases.

"The Age of Degenerative and Human-Made Diseases" is the third stage, in which mortality rates stabilized at a fairly low level and the average life expectancy increased to beyond 50 years. Sustained economic improvements coupled with massive industrialization and urbanization during this stage led to an increase in chronic diseases. As behavioral changes such as increased caloric diet and lower daily caloric expenditure occurred and were accompanied by an increase in activities such as smoking, the kind of diseases experienced dramatically changed. Some researchers have recently added a fourth stage, in which major technological advances in medicine lead to a delay of death from chronic cardiovascular diseases and cancer.

The demographic transition and the epidemiological transition are subject to regional variation because of differing social, economic, demographic, and environmental forces. They occur at different times in different places. The factors that influence the changes broadly described by these transitions are complicated. They involve the ecological and biological determinants of mortality, namely the complex balance among disease agents, fluctuating levels of host resistance, and the ever-changing environment.

The historical relationship between demographic changes and patterns of disease is complex. It involves a dynamic, continuously changing process whereby some diseases disappear and others appear for the first time, reemerge, or mutate from existing species. Recent projects in the genome sequencing of both humans and diseases indicate that this process is not unidirectional. The emergence of new infectious diseases like AIDS is one prime example. Recent work in historical epidemiology has suggested the need for a change in the global approach to the emerging problems of changing patterns of disease. *See also* Demographic Data Collection and Analysis, History of; Diagnosis of Historical Diseases; Epidemiology, History of; Paleopathology.

Further Reading

Hardy, Anne. *The Epidemic Streets: Infectious Disease and the Rise of Preventive Medicine: 1856–1900.* Oxford: Oxford University Press, 1993.

Landers, John. *Death and the Metropolis: Studies in the Demographic History of London 1670–1830.* Cambridge: Cambridge University Press, 1993.

McKeown, Thomas. *The Modern Rise of Population.* London: Edward Arnold Press, 1976.

Mooney, Graham, and William Luckin. "Urban History and Historical Epidemiology: The Case of London, 1860–1920." *Urban History* 24 (1997): 37–54.

Omran, Abdel. "The Epidemiologic Transition: A Theory of the Epidemiology of Population Change." *Milbank Memorial Fund Quarterly* 49 (1971): 509–538.

Rosen, George. *A History of Public Health,* expanded edition. Baltimore: The Johns Hopkins University Press, 1993.

Winslow, Charles-Edward Amory. *The Conquest of Epidemic Disease: A Chapter in the History of Ideas.* Madison: The University of Wisconsin Press, 1980.

JACOB STEERE-WILLIAMS

HIV/AIDS. *See* Human Immunodeficiency Virus/Acquired Immune Deficiency Syndrome (HIV/AIDS).

HOSPITALS AND MEDICAL EDUCATION IN BRITAIN AND THE UNITED STATES.

According to European hospital historians, the role of hospitals in medical education seemed assured as early as the 1770s. Medical education, formerly conducted in medical school classrooms or on a one-to-one basis between master and apprentice, was literally brought into hospitals in the mid-eighteenth century. Links between the two institutions only grew stronger over the next hundred years. Although appearing both inseparable and essential to the education of medical practitioners, the combination of medical education and hospital instruction was not yet a reality on both sides of the Atlantic. Though clinical clerking had become a common experience, even a right, at many European medical schools, American schools, like their German counterparts, rarely provided such extensive hands-on ward instruction. Instruction continued to be provided by part-time teachers, whereas preclinical courses more quickly came under the influence of scientific ideas than did clinical training. As a result, by the late nineteenth century, the hospital school of medicine lost ground to the university as the favored site of medical instruction. Reformers tackled these and other disparities in the first decades of the twentieth century. By the end of the century, clinical instruction in a hospital setting was firmly embedded in the medical curriculum in both England and America.

Significant progress in clinical teaching had been made at American medical schools since the Civil War (1861–1865). The period devoted to clinical subjects had grown to two years, and section teaching had brought students into the hospital wards. As in the United Kingdom, specialization only increased in pace during this period, with the proliferation of both specialist hospitals and specialist clinics in general hospitals. However, teaching remained largely demonstrative. Few students learned practically by carrying out tasks in hospitals. Patients were cared for in the presence of students, but they were not cared for *by* students. Reformers aimed to rectify this through the introduction of clinical residencies (clerkships in Britain), requiring students to spend significant periods of the day addressing their patients' needs, rather than collectively walking the wards for an hour. According to William Osler (1849–1919), who was engaged in and understood both the North American and English systems of medical education, all other forms of clinical instruction were "bastard substitutes" for the residency. Though common practice at Johns Hopkins, where Osler had been based between 1889 and 1905, and moderately successful at other schools, such as Western Reserve University, Jefferson Medical

DURING THE FRENCH REVOLUTION, FRENCH MEDICAL EDUCATION REFORMER PHILIPPE PINEL ENCOURAGES "THE CLINICAL TRAINING OF DOCTORS" (1793)

Medicine must be taught in the hospitals—The healing art should only be taught in hospitals: this assertion needs no proof. Only in the hospital can one follow the evolution and progress of several illnesses at the same time and study variations of the same disease in a number of patients. This is the only way to understand the true history of diseases. In these shelters for suffering humanity, young students can analyze the influence of the seasons and of each year's medical constitution. And only in a hospital can the physician be certain that patients receive the specific diet and medication he prescribes, and that nascent symptoms are carefully observed.

Need for an appropriate teaching hospital—. . . all modern medical schools have emphasized observation as a characteristic aspect of medicine when it is viewed as a major branch of the natural sciences. Leyden [The Netherlands], Edinburgh [Scotland], Vienna [Austria], Pavia [Italy], etc, have stressed the need of selecting a small number of patients for didactic purposes and grouping them on teaching wards. This offers the advantage of focusing the students' attention on a small number of well-defined cases, without neglecting any aspect of cleanliness or health.

Project for a teaching hospital: Proposal by the Society of Medicine—At a time when education is being restored in France and public instruction organized, the Society of Medicine turns its attention to a matter of supreme importance, the creation of teaching hospitals. Only clinical teaching can spread knowledge of the healing art in a uniform manner and restore the rigorous, oft-neglected principles of observation. All other public teaching of medicine by the lecture method is pointless and unproductive.

From *The Clinical Training of Doctors: An Essay of 1793*, edited and translated by Dora P. Weiner (Baltimore: Johns Hopkins University Press, 1980).

College, and the universities of Pennsylvania and Michigan, the practice of residency was struggling for survival when Abraham Flexner's (1866–1959) report on medical education appeared in 1910. As a result, the famed survey of 155 North American medical schools indicted clinical teaching more severely than all other branches of American medical education. Even where residencies existed, usually only a fraction of medical students could be accommodated by limited ward places. Most attended outpatient clinics where opportunities for observing acute patients were limited. Equally limited were possibilities of following the daily course of diseases and therapies. Further progress required providing students direct participation in the management of patients.

Residency continued to struggle until American medical schools attained some control over affiliated teaching hospitals. Although most schools were associated with such clinical facilities, they often had very little control over hospitals. Johns Hopkins was one of few schools that exercised control over its teaching hospital, a point recognized by Flexner. Though bedside instruction in hospitals has been traced to fifteenth-century Europe, many hospital governors continued to tolerate teaching in the wards as long as it was strictly regulated and did not interfere with daily hospital activities. Unlike in London, where hospitals gradually developed their own schools during the eighteenth and nineteenth centuries, American medical schools and hospitals developed separately from one another. By the late-nineteenth century, it had become clear that hospitals in the United States would have to become more closely associated with medical schools, especially during the clinical years of training. For many schools, the answer lay in building their own hospitals.

Although the English system allowed for the appointment of clerks and dressers in the wards, as became common at St Bartholomew's for example in 1865, the need for further progress in clinical education was recognized. The Haldane Commission, the British equivalent of the Flexner report, highlighted the key deficiencies in the British context. Established in 1909 and published in 1912, the Commission found fault with clinical medicine carried out by physicians and surgeons whose main interest lay in private practice. Given the length of the inquiry, by the time of its publication, the commissioners had become greatly influenced by Flexner's report. Equally influential was William Osler, Regius Professor of Medicine at Oxford from 1905 to 1919, who called for a full-scale invasion of hospitals by the universities. In their report, the Commissioners advised the establishment of professorial units in clinical medicine and surgery. Quoting Osler, the report suggested that only such units would allow a professor to carry out the three-fold duty of curing the sick, studying the problems of disease, and giving students a university education in the science of their profession. The advent of the British University Grants Committee after the First World War transformed some of these ideas into reality. Academic units with professors at the head became the general rule for the preclinical subjects, and some teaching hospitals experimented with full-time professorial units in medicine and surgery. Nevertheless, the bulk of clinical teaching remained, as it does today, in the hands of part-time visiting staff, and only 13 full-time clinical chairs were established in Britain's medical schools before World War II. As a result, experimental science was more often encountered in laboratories than in hospital wards, where staff employed traditional methods of observation and undertook little clinical research.

Rectification of the key deficiency in American medical education involved building hospitals and would cost schools considerably more than professorial units. Washington University contemplated building a teaching hospital in 1903, until it was estimated that it would cost $1 million. Yale abandoned plans to build a hospital in 1910 when its projected cost reached $3 million. Even a well-endowed university like Harvard abandoned plans to build a teaching hospital years earlier on the grounds of cost. Instead, many schools decided to form links with existing community hospitals. Before 1910 only Western Reserve University and Dartmouth College managed such affiliations. Other hospital boards, though managing vast clinical resources, permitted only demonstrative teaching. Most resisted the efforts of medical school staff to improve clinical teaching before 1910.

In the next decade, however, these difficulties were largely overcome. Most American medical schools managed to improve relationships with nearby voluntary hospitals. In 1910 alone, three significant unions occurred. These involved Columbia and Presbyterian Hospital in New York, Harvard Medical School and Peter Bent Brigham Hospital in Boston, and Washington University Medical School and Barnes Hospital and St Louis Children's Hospital in St Louis. In some instances, teaching hospitals had to be constructed at the taxpayers' expense. In each case, Johns Hopkins remained the model of best practice. In the case of Washington University Medical School, Flexner's report was particularly influential in provoking cooperation, though not at other institutions, where overlapping boards of trustees facilitated union.

Formerly hostile to clinical residencies, most American hospital trustees had become convinced that their institutions would benefit from association with a medical school. Besides better patient care, close association promised state-of-the-art care, including laboratories and the latest medical equipment, and enhanced their potential research output. The division of labor was also mutually advantageous. Like business corporations, unions between medical institutions promised to make medical schools and hospitals more efficient administrative units. Failure to acquire a teaching hospital, on the other hand, often resulted in the closure of a school. The difficulties facing rural schools were occasionally insurmountable. As a result, medical education became ever more urban as great numbers of rural schools disappeared. By 1921 every surviving American medical school had affiliated with a hospital that it either controlled or owned. In 1926 the American Medical Colleges announced that residencies had been introduced at all medical schools. With student numbers in decline during this period, schools found it easier to offer pupils residencies. Though a uniform system of residency remained to be created at the 76 medical schools in existence in 1930, subsequent changes were of degree, not kind.

Though the modern system of medical education in the United States had emerged by the 1920s, the relationship between medical schools and hospitals in the United Kingdom continued to be debated in the 1940s with the introduction of a National Health Service. The fullest expression of these discussions is in the report of the Special Commission on Medical Education, known as the Goodenough Report (1944), which was charged with a review of medical schools in the knowledge of impending government health legislation. Among other things, the committee found that accommodation for teaching and research fell below ordinary requirements at most teaching hospitals. Among its many recommendations was that students no longer be taught simply about sick people in hospital beds, but of the social and industrial causes of ill health. As a result, in contrast to American schools where education became ever more standardized, English medical schools began to offer an increasing number of electives. Recognizing the additional reality of specialization, the Goodenough Report also proposed a comprehensive system of postgraduate education, rather than leaving qualified practitioners to self-educate. Based less on examinations and professional associations than in the American case, this involved the establishment of a national system of specialized postgraduate institutes, organized around specialist hospitals. The four Scottish medical schools set up a joint body to organize postgraduate training, which in England was organized regionally. The British Postgraduate Medical Federation of the University of London was established in 1945 and integrated more than a dozen hospital-affiliated specialist units in the capital, including the British Postgraduate Hospital and Medical School at Hammersmith, which was established in 1935.

With the introduction of a National Health Service (NHS), the institutions of medical education in England were significantly reorganized. Instead of being under one of the fourteen regional hospital boards under the jurisdiction of the Ministry of Health, English teaching hospitals were placed under independent boards of governors responsible to the Ministry of Health from whom they were financed. Medical school, staff, and university were all represented on these boards. Rather than being handed to the universities, medical schools were also put under independent boards of governors responsible to the university from which they received their funding but on which the governing board of its teaching hospital was represented. In this way, each school was ensured some control in the selection of staff and hospital policy, and each teaching hospital was guaranteed a voice in the election of staff and in control of the school's policies. The hospital provided the school with the necessary facilities for the business of medical instruction in return for the numerous services rendered by the high-powered scientific departments that the schools now maintained, subsidized by the university. The autonomy of teaching hospitals was removed in 1974 when the boards of governors were abolished and the hospitals placed under new Area Health Authorities. In the 1990s, trust status promised British teaching hospitals a return to the independence they lost in 1974.

Besides organizational issues, the advent of the National Health Service has had an impact on medical education and has accelerated changes in clinical teaching methods. Given the slow rate of hospital construction since the introduction of the NHS, facilities for clinical instruction began to fall short of the recommended bed numbers. Though the Goodenough Committee suggested 1,000 beds for each annual intake of 100 first-year, clinical students, the Ministry of Health limited hospitals to 800 beds for several years. As a result, students had to travel more extensively in the post-war period in order to obtain sufficient clinical experience, especially in obstetrics. Changes in the distribution of the population have further prevented teaching hospitals from offering the clinical work necessary for the education of students, whose numbers have only increased. Selective and controlled admission to suit teaching interests remains unrealistic. This has encouraged additional training in nonhospital environments, but reform has been limited. More often students enter nonteaching hospitals to escape the artificial atmosphere of a teaching hospital. In the 1960s, teaching hospitals more regularly appointed full-time staff in general medicine, surgery, and obstetrics, and not only in pathology, radiology, and anesthesiology. Funds for medical research more often came from private foundations than from research councils, and they increased exponentially in this decade.

Like the NHS, medical schools in the second half of the twentieth century grew dramatically in size and bureaucracy. English schools were also unusually concentrated in London. In 1965 there were 12 schools within five miles of Charing Cross, leading the Todd Report (1968) to suggest that schools be combined. Cuts in funding in the 1980s encouraged further mergers, and new provincial schools were created. In both the U.K. and U.S. contexts, the close union of medical schools and teaching hospitals brought science and medicine closer together, though students in Britain's two dozen medical schools often remained less aware of research undertaken in clinical departments. Many more had become aware of the fact that medical facilities of British universities were lagging far behind those in America. Instead of American medical students traveling to Europe to receive the best training, after World War I many more Europeans were choosing to attend North American medical schools. In Britain, the decline in medical facilities at universities was emphasized in the Porritt report (1963). Although much clinical research is still funded by notable individual benefactors, hospital policy now tends to be determined by medical boards, whose decisions trustees generally follow. The traditional conflicts between hospitals and medical schools continue to exist, but the reputations of both rely on affiliation. The tensions between education and patient needs have also been resolved in favor of education, which the public generally accepts. The patient, on the other hand, is no longer simply central to hospitals' teaching functions. With federal educational subsidies in decline since the 1980s, American teaching hospitals more often resort to aggressive marketing in order to attract patient revenue. Consequently, the language of clinical instruction in the teaching hospitals of the nation's 125 medical schools more often signals the triumph of marketplace rhetoric and values than of prevention and the relief of suffering. Whereas the number of cases treated in hospitals only increases, the average length of stay has fallen, once again making it difficult for students to see patients. These changes encourage further rethinking of clinical education and generate additional critiques of hospital-based learning. *See also* Hospitals in the West to 1900; Hospitals since 1900; Medical Education in the West, 1500–1900; Medical Ethics and Epidemic Disease; Nurses and Nursing; Public Health Agencies in Britain since 1800; Public Health Agencies, U.S. Federal.

Further Reading

Bonner, Thomas Neville. *Becoming a Physician: Medical Education in Britain, France, Germany, and the United States, 1750–1945*. Baltimore: Johns Hopkins University Press, 1995.

Ludmerer, Kenneth M. *Learning to Heal: The Development of American Medical Education*. New York: Basic Books, 1985.

———. *Time to Heal: American Medical Education from the Turn of the Century to the Era of Managed Care*. New York: Oxford University Press, 1999.

Poynter, F. N. L., ed. *The Evolution of Medical Education in Britain*. London: Pitman Medical Publishing Company Ltd., 1966.

Stevens, Rosemary. *In Sickness and in Wealth: American Hospitals in the Twentieth Century*. Baltimore: Johns Hopkins University Press, 1999.

Waddington, Keir. *Medical Education at St Bartholomew's Hospital, 1123–1995*. Woodbridge, Suffolk: Boydell Press, 2003.

Walker, R. Miles. *Medical Education in Britain*. London: Nuffield Provincial Hospitals Trust, 1965.

JONATHAN REINARZ

HOSPITALS IN THE WEST TO 1900.   The earliest known hospitals were examples of Christian charity. They were not exclusively meant to heal the sick but also to house the poor; they were "guesthouses" rather than hospitals in a modern sense, an idea that is expressed in the Latin term *hospitium*. Travelers, pilgrims, the disabled and injured, the infirm elderly, and those such as poor widows who lacked resources found shelter and sustenance. Over time the hospital evolved first into the social institution dedicated to the care of the chronically ill, and then into a more multipurpose care-providing facility.

Ecclesiastical authorities created shelters to house the needy and the sick in response to famine, **war**, and **epidemics**. Because of this close link with Christianity, prayer, religious rituals, and reflection were important therapies alongside rest, nutrition, and medication. The earliest such shelters were established in Byzantium (Constantinople) between the fourth and sixth centuries; the Gallo-Roman *hôtels-dieu* of the same period also fall in this category.

Non-Christian roots of the hospital include ancient Greek temples to the god of healing, Asclepius, which also served as healing places. In the Roman Empire, *valetudinaria* were shelters for injured or exhausted slaves. Islamic societies created "places for the sick," the **bimaristan**; one of the earliest of which was established in Damascus, Syria, in 707.

Paralleling the development of hospitals were **leprosaria**, where chronic sufferers of **Hansen's Disease** and related maladies found shelter and care and isolation from the stigmatization of wider society. With the Black Death and subsequent plagues from the fourteenth through eighteenth centuries, many leprosaria and hospitals were transformed into short-term pest houses where victims of plague either recovered or died. Larger hospitals set aside special wings or wards for infectious disease cases or appended outbuildings during local epidemics. In the sixteenth and seventeenth centuries, new or previously rare infectious diseases emerged: syphilis, influenza, typhus, and smallpox, among others. Hospitals wrestled with their obligations to their communities: the elderly and chronically ill who resided in most hospitals were threatened by the acutely diseased, though the mechanisms of disease transmission were but dimly understood. With the Renaissance in the sixteenth century and the **Scientific Revolution** in the seventeenth, hospitals became more closely related to medical education and primitive research. The ideas of philosophers of the Enlightenment made rulers and their medical doctors realize that healing could not exclusively be achieved on the basis of speculations. Hence, by the early nineteenth century, a new concept of the (poor) citizen-patient with a right to hospital care was emerging. The patient became an object of medical observation, **diagnosis**, and treatment. This new "rational" medicine was based on an empirical method that combined observation of the sick with systematic examinations of the deceased.

Large hospitals were an excellent place to put these ideas into practice. They acquired importance as clinical research centers, as they provided medical doctors and students with numerous cases of diseases to study, such as **tuberculosis**. In the United Kingdom, a hospital system had emerged in the eighteenth century that extended throughout the country. The Royal Infirmary in Edinburgh was established in the 1720s and became one of the foremost institutions for medical instruction in Europe. In France hospitals were reformed after 1789, in the course of the French Revolution. The General Hospital (*Allgemeines Krankenhaus*) in Vienna was a 2,000-bed facility inspired by Paris's late eighteenth-century *hôtel-dieu*.

Yet unexplained in the period before the advent of **germ theory**, these large hospitals were feared by patients for their high mortality rates. These were often the result of inadequate hygienic and sanitary conditions—for example, in connection with autopsies and subsequent patient examinations that contributed to spreading of infectious diseases, a connection that was not yet understood.

In the nineteenth century medical innovations occurred in a transatlantic setting. For example, in the early 1800s medical students from all over Europe and America flocked to the huge hospitals in Paris and Vienna, whereas those of the late nineteenth century turned to Germany. Americans also contributed to the changing outlook of the hospital.

Moreover, **nursing** emerged as a skilled profession particularly for women, a development in which the British nurse Florence Nightingale (1820–1910) played a leading role. In contrast, in 1687 Elizabeth Cellier (d. c. 1688) had unsuccessfully petitioned English King James II (r. 1685–1688) for a College of Midwives. The professional nurse became a feature of the modern nineteenth-century hospital.

Hospitals were the sites of numerous new inventions that would ultimately serve the goal of diagnosing and fighting infectious diseases. In 1816 the French **physician** René Théophile Hyacinthe Laënnec (1781–1826) developed the stethoscope; a great help in diagnosing pulmonary complaints such as tuberculosis. In 1846 ether was first successfully used as anesthesia during surgeries in the Massachusetts General Hospital in Boston. The news soon spread to England. With the elimination of pain, longer surgeries on, for example, infected internal organs became possible.

Also in the 1840s the relationship between the performance of autopsies and high mortality rates in hospitals was discovered: when doctors and medical students proceeded from the dissection table to examining patients, they failed to scrub all "death matter" off their hands. This endangered, among others, women who had just given birth. Puerperal fever was known as early as in ancient Greece, yet staring in the eighteenth century it became a major problem in maternity hospitals. In a way, the creation of big hospitals thus highlighted problems in transmitting infectious diseases that could subsequently be solved. Physicians Oliver Wendell Holmes Sr. (1809–1894) in New England and **Ignaz Semmelweis** in Vienna both understood the connection between childbed fever and autopsies; yet they were little successful in effecting changes.

Only with the birth of bacteriology did practices begin to change. In 1867 the British surgeon Joseph Lister (1827–1912) published his observations with regard to the antiseptic method. Lister had been inspired by **Louis Pasteur's** findings on fermentation. He concluded that microorganisms might be responsible for surgical infections and began using carbolic acid to disinfect wounds. Nonetheless, two or three patients occasionally shared a bed even in his day—a practice that disregarded the potential dangers of possible infections spreading among those convalescing from surgery. Ironically, at about the same time, physicians realized that it was most important to prevent germs from entering a surgical site. This could be achieved through the aseptic method, such as the sterilization of instruments with heat. Pasteur's English collaborator Charles Chamberland (1851–1908) developed this method. Hence, even though many revolutionary discoveries were made in the second half of the nineteenth century, implications for preventing the spread of contagious diseases were not always immediately recognized.

The late nineteenth century witnessed the establishment of new hospitals with research laboratories in addition to facilities for patient care, such as at the medical school of the Johns Hopkins University in Baltimore, Maryland, which was launched in 1889 and which, in the 1890s, first introduced rubber gloves as a means to increase hygiene. Further discoveries changed the routine at hospitals: German physicist Wilhelm Konrad Röntgen's (1845–1923) work on X-rays (1895) became an important means for diagnosis of diseases like tuberculosis. On the basis of the findings of Pasteur and **Robert Koch**, the 1880s marked the beginning of immunization as we know it today, to which **Emil Adolf von Behring** contributed when he developed an antitoxin for **diphtheria** in the 1890s. Hospitals could provide cures and therapies that could rehabilitate, and they were slowly losing their stigmata as warehouses for the poor and terminally ill.

With the prevention of the spread of infectious diseases and the advent of widespread **vaccination**, hospitals in the future would no longer serve primarily to receive hundreds of victims during the outbreak of an infectious disease, such as the **cholera** epidemic in Hamburg as late as in 1892. An awareness of germ theory and subsequent development of treatments, as well as improvement of living and hospital conditions, marked the beginning of a new area in the history of hospitals on the eve of the twentieth century. *See also* Disinfection and Fumigation; Hospitals since 1900; Medical Education in the West, 1500–1900.

Further Reading

Bowers, Barbara. *The Medieval Hospital and Medical Practice*. Aldershot: Ashgate, 2007.

Carruthers, G. Barry, and Lesley A. Carruthers. *A History of Britain's Hospitals*. New York: Book Guild, 2005.

Foucault, Michel. *The Birth of the Clinic: An Archaeology of Medical Perception*. Translated by A. M. Sheridan Smith. New York: Pantheon Books, 1973.

Frangos, John. *From Housing the Poor to Healing the Sick: The Changing Institution of Paris Hospitals under the Old Regime and Revolution*. London: Associated University Press, 1997.

Granshaw, Lindsay, and Roy Porter, eds. *The Hospital in History*. London: Routledge, 1989.

Henderson, John. *The Renaissance Hospital*. New Haven: Yale University Press, 2006.

Hickey, Daniel. *Local Hospitals in Ancien Regime France: Rationalization, Resistance and Renewal, 1530–1789*. Montreal: McGill University Press, 1997.

Horden, Peregrine. "The Earliest Hospitals in Byzantium, Western Europe and Islam." *Journal of Interdisciplinary History* 35 (2005): 361–389.

Miller, Timothy. *The Birth of the Hospital in the Byzantine Empire*. Baltimore: Johns Hopkins University Press, 1997.

Park, Katherine. "Healing the Poor: Hospitals and Medical Assistance in Renaissance Florence." In *Medicine and Charity before the Welfare State*, edited by Jonathan Barry and Colin Jones, pp. 26–45. New York: Routledge, 1991.

Risse, Guenter B. *Mending Bodies, Saving Souls: A History of Hospitals*. New York: Oxford University Press, 1999.

Tuchman, Arleen M. *Science, Medicine, and the State in Germany: The Case of Baden, 1815–1871*. New York: Oxford University Press, 1993.

Anja Becker

HOSPITALS SINCE 1900.   Over the past hundred years or so, hospitals have evolved from providing care (often long term) for the indigent patient with chronic infectious disease and the infirm elderly. With America in the forefront, hospitals have concentrated health-care functions and services as the medical profession has become increasingly specialized and reliant on technology. The revolution in prophylaxis and treatment of traditional epidemic diseases, with vaccines and antibiotics for example, has meant that hospitals in developed countries have acquired a new clientele. In developing countries, however, hospitals treat a wide range of complex conditions that often combine one or more infectious diseases with complications stemming from such factors as malnutrition, birth defects, and violence.

Western Hospitals.   The current structure and function of hospitals are those of either a modern high-tech palace that focuses on short-term high intensity intervention, or a hospital for specialized care or long-term care of chronic conditions. Hospitals can be categorized by size (number of beds), teaching (university affiliated) versus nonteaching functions, privately owned versus government-owned status, general care versus specialized care (hospice, psychiatric care) provision, or length of care (acute care, long-term care) provision. Private hospitals can be either for-profit or nonprofit. Nonprofit hospitals are often associated with religious institutions. In the United States, most psychiatric hospitals are owned and operated by the state, whereas the federal government owns and operates military and veterans hospitals. Most **tuberculosis** (TB) hospitals were state-operated. In developed countries other than the United States and Canada, the government owns and controls the majority of hospitals. Most hospitals in the United States have up to 800 beds, those in Sweden up to 1,000 beds, and those in Russia up to 1,250 beds.

In the early 1900s, TB, pneumonia, bronchitis, **diphtheria**, and enteritis were major causes of death. For the first half of the twentieth century, infectious diseases were the most common cause for hospital admissions. TB hospitals (**sanatoriums**), in use up to 1960, often hosted patients for two years or more. Some hospitals had whole wards for treating **typhoid fever, smallpox**, or scarlet fever. In the early 1900s, **syphilis** was also common, until an effective treatment was discovered in 1909. General hospitals played a major role in patient care. For example, in 1943, general hospitals admitted over 90 percent of all U.S. patients, even though they had only 40 percent of the total number of hospital beds.

Group hospitalization insurance was introduced by Baylor University Hospital in the United States in 1929 and was soon widely adopted. Prior to health insurance, patients paid for their care with their own resources or worked for the hospital after they recovered from their illness. Insurance induces demand for health care services, since the payer is a third party. As a result, hospital utilization grew. In 1945 about 30 million people in the United States had hospital insurance, and their rate of hospitalization was 50 percent higher than that of the population as a whole. The average cost per day per patient in 1910 was less than $2, whereas in 2006 it was between $900 and $1800 depending on the level of care provided.

The Hill-Burton Hospital Construction Act of 1946 provided federal funds to build new hospitals, expand existing hospitals, and add new technology to hospitals. Medicare and Medicaid programs began in the 1960s. The number of hospital beds in the United States peaked in the 1960s, a time that was considered the golden era for hospitals. Between 1946 and 1976, as a result of specialization and technology, hospitals were at the center of American health care.

In 1973 the U.S. Congress passed the Health Maintenance Organization (HMO) Act to help finance the development of HMOs, and thus to control costs. In 1983 Congress introduced the diagnosis-related group (DRG) as a means to cut Medicare spending. This greatly reduced reimbursement payments of Medicare part A, the hospitalization portion of Medicare. In the 1990s, there were many hospital mergers and conversions of nonprofit to for-profit status. Many hospitals closed during this time. Also in the 1980s and 1990s, malpractice concerns forced many **physicians** to use more (often unnecessary) laboratory tests in practicing defensive medicine. Worldwide, beginning in the 1980s, health-care administrators focused on cutting costs, improving efficiency, and preventing the occurrence and spread of disease. In the United States, the average number of days (length of stay) for patients in the acute care hospital went from about 21 in 1910, to 9 in 1960, to 6 in 1994.

In most hospitals, nursing is the largest department, followed by dietary services, and then housekeeping. Other departments include laundry, medical records, pharmacy, laboratory, social services, respiratory therapy, patient education, and nutrition counseling. Identification and treatment of infectious agents, improved sanitation, infection control, and improved nutritional status of the patients all help to decrease the incidence and spread of infectious disease.

Hospitals and Epidemic Disease.   Epidemic **typhus** was a major problem in World War I (1914–1918) and in World War II (1939–1945). **Measles**, mumps, and **meningitis** were also common in WWI, but overall improved hospital sanitation significantly reduced deaths from infectious disease. After WWI, the **Spanish influenza pandemic** (1918–1920) hit and killed more people than the war itself. During the pandemic, temporary hospitals were established to meet the sudden increase in need. One such hospital was the Emergency Influenza Hospital in Kirksville, Missouri, which was the Theta Psi Fraternity House at Southeast Missouri State College before being converted to the temporary hospital. Worldwide, nearly 20 million people died from this catastrophic pandemic. In 1957 the Asian flu pandemic hit many areas of the world, and a second wave occurred in early 1958. In 1968 the Hong Kong flu pandemic occurred, returning in 1970 and 1972. Regional epidemics of the flu occurred in 1976 with the swine flu, in 1977 with the Russian flu, and in 1997 and 2003 with the avian flu. Since 2000 influenza has resulted in about 226,000 annual U.S. hospitalizations. Since the 1990s, multiple-drug-resistant TB has been spreading rapidly. In 1993 the **World Health Organization** (WHO) declared war on TB and initiated programs for TB identification, treatment, and control. Accordingly, hospitals are required to have isolation policies and procedures in place to deal with TB.

A major challenge facing hospitals in the later decades of the twentieth century is infections that are acquired in the hospital. In the United States, according to the **Centers for Disease Control and Prevention** (CDC), there are about 1.7 million cases and 99,000 deaths each year as a result of infectious diseases acquired while in the hospital.

About 32 percent of these infections are urinary tract infections (UTI), 22 percent are infections of surgical sites, 15 percent are pneumonias, and about 14 percent are bloodstream infections. Whereas the number of admissions, the average length of stay, the number of inpatient surgical procedures, and the total number of hospital-acquired infections have all decreased, the incidence of hospital-acquired infections in the United States has increased over recent decades.

In 1983 the CDC advised all health-care workers to use universal precautions to help decrease the spread of infectious disease and in 2007 recommended hospital infection-control report cards. Process measures such as timely administration of perioperative **antibiotic** prophylaxis, insertion practices of vascular catheters, and hand hygiene practices could be measured. Outcome practices such as intensive care unit infection rates associated with central vascular catheters and complications as a result of surgical-site infections could be measured and reported.

Hospital Quality. Technology dominates many hospitals today. Health-care consumerism in the community, a focus on costs from the health-care administration, and a lack of personal attention to patients are current challenges facing many hospitals. But issues of quality are far from new. Richard C. Cabot (1868–1939), the "father of medical social work," wrote *Diagnostic Pitfalls Identified during a Study of Three Thousand Autopsies* in 1912, and five years later hospital reformer Ernest A. Codman (1869–1940) published *A Study in Hospital Efficiency*. These two men helped initiate quality control in hospitals by bringing to the attention of hospital trustees and medical professionals the identification and measurement of hospital treatment outcomes. In this vein, in 1918, the American College of Surgeons started a survey program to establish hospital standards. Also in the early 1900s, American registrars started using the International List of Causes of Death, which had been designed by the French statistician Jacques Bertillon (1851–1922).

U.S. hospitals are rated according to Avedis Donabedian's (1919–2000) three-element model of health-care quality: structure, process, and outcome. Since 1990, *U.S. News & World Report* has annually published the list of "America's Best Hospitals." HealthGrades is a different, relatively new, grading system for U.S. hospitals. As a result of cost-containment strategies, health-care systems in developed countries seem to be moving toward increased delivery of services via clinics and other outpatient care settings. Because the greatest proportion of health-care spending is on hospital costs, the shifts in hospital marketing and management are geared toward cost reductions. The Joint Commission on the Accreditation of Healthcare Organizations (JCAHO) and the Institute for Healthcare Improvement (IHI) support quality improvement by enhancing organizational learning, sharing lessons learned, benchmarking, and using the continuous quality improvement process to improve hospital quality.

Hospitals in Developing Countries.   During the twentieth century, hospitals played a major role in the globalization of Western medicine. Charitable, mission-based hospitals in particular have introduced Western medicine and provided training to populations in developing colonial and postcolonial countries. Health care in these regions is predominantly curative rather than preventive, and centralized hospitals are usually in competition with primary care clinics for scarce health-care resources. From the 1970s the **World Health Organization** (WHO) has advocated a decentralized system focused on primary care in zonal and regional facilities. Urban political elites, however, tend to support the larger centralized systems. When reliant on local personnel, clinics tend to have minimally educated and prepared caregivers because those with options easily find work in larger cities or abroad. Yet even larger urban health centers have problems with sexism, low morale, and lack of adequate training, funding, supplies, and the confidence of the community. African traditional medicine, for example, still has sway among large segments of the population, and one of the challenges is to blend it with Western medical approaches to healing.

Care for children and responses to epidemic diseases such as polio, tuberculosis, plague, yaws, and cholera, as well as more recent pestilences such as HIV/AIDS and Ebola are serious issues for African hospitals. Initiatives tend to be reactive rather than pro-active, with few (but increasing) resources devoted to health education, public health initiatives, and preventive medicine. In 2000 and 2005, WHO published clinical guidelines for pediatric (children's) health care in areas and facilities with limited resources. Follow-up reports and studies from Asian, African, and Oceanic countries have shown that hospitals in developing countries have shown clear decreases in case fatality rates when guidelines like these are applied, along with greater attention to personnel training and resource management. *See also* Contagion and Transmission; Diagnosis and Diagnostic Tools; Drug Resistance in Microorganisms; Hospitals and Medical Education in Britain and the

---

EBOLA EMERGES ON WESTERN MEDICINE'S FRONTIER, 1976

The hospital conditions in Abumombazi were not as deplorable as in other parts of the country. A prominent Zairian general came from the region. He had the clout to attract a white doctor to the village, and there, with Belgian nuns, [Danish physician] Grethe [Rask] worked with what she could beg and borrow. This was central Africa, after all, and even a favored clinic would never have such basics as sterile rubber gloves or disposable needles. You just used needles again and again until they wore out; once gloves had worn through, you risked dipping your hands in your patient's blood because that was what needed to be done. The lack of rudimentary supplies meant that a surgeon's work had risks that doctors in the developed world could not imagine, particularly because the undeveloped part, specifically Central Africa, seemed to sire new diseases with nightmarish regularity. Earlier that year, not far from Abumombazi, in a village along the Ebola River on the Zaire-Sudan border, a virulent outbreak of a horrifying new disease had demonstrated the dangers of primitive medicine and new viruses. A trader from the village of Enzara, suffering from fevers and profuse, uncontrollable bleeding, had come to the teaching hospital for nurses in Maridi. The man had apparently picked up the disease sexually. Within days, however, 40 percent of the nurses in Maridi were stricken with the fever, transmitted by contact with the patient's infected blood either through standard care procedures or through accidental needle sticks.

Frightened African health officials swallowed their pride and called the World Health Organization, who came with a staff from the American Centers for Disease Control. By the time the young American doctors arrived, 39 nurses and two doctors were dead.

From Randy Schilts's *And the Band Played On: Politics, People, and the AIDS Epidemic* (New York: Stonewall Inn Editions, 2000) p. 4.

United States; Hospitals in the West to 1900; Nurses and Nursing; Pharmaceutical Industry; Sanatorium.

Further Reading

Bynum, W. F., et al. *The Western Medical Tradition, 1800 to 2000*. New York: Cambridge University Press, 2006.

Risse, Guenter B. *Mending Bodies, Saving Souls: A History of Hospitals*. New York: Oxford University Press, 1999.

Siegel, J. D., et al. *Guideline for Isolation Precautions: Preventing Transmission of Infectious Agents in Healthcare Settings 2007*. June 2007. http://www.cdc.gov/ncidod/dhqp/pdf/isolation2007.pdf

World Health Organization. "Hospital Care for Children: Guidelines for the Management of Common Illnesses with Limited Resources." Geneva: WHO, 2005. http://www.who.int/child-adolescent-health/publications/CHILD_HEALTH/PB.htm

MARK A. BEST

HUMAN BODY.   This section will present the major systems of the body in a way that links the names of each individual part (or the anatomy of the system) to the way that they work together (or the physiology of the system). It is important to understand these details in order to appreciate how and why they can become diseased (the pathology of the system).

The Integumentary System.   The largest organ in the body, the skin forms a protective layer between the body and the harsh world around it. One way it does this is by regulating the body's fluids and temperature. If hot, the skin has pores that open to release sweat and cool off the body as the sweat evaporates; if cold, blood vessels in the skin constrict, thereby diverting blood to the core of the body where it is most needed. In addition to sweat glands, oil glands next to the hair roots keep the skin supple and the hair lubricated. Different types of nerve receptors in the skin offer perhaps the greatest protection to the body: the abilities to touch, sense temperature, and feel pain. The skin has two different layers: the epidermis is the outermost section of skin made of piled up layers of cells, and the dermis, made up of thicker fibrous material, lies beneath it.

Unlike armadillos, which have a hard shell of skin protecting them, humans are incredibly soft and vulnerable to trauma. Because the skin barrier is so easy to breach, many serious infections can enter the body via this route. A simple cut, for example, can allow **bacteria** to enter and cause infections, such as a *cellulitis* (a superficial infection of the skin) or an abscess (a deeper, walled-off infection). **Insects** that bite the skin can introduce into the blood parasites that cause serious diseases such as **malaria** or Lyme disease. On the other hand, the so-called viral exanthems, diseases such as **measles** and rubeola, are caused by **viruses** that infect the entire body but make themselves present with a rash or "eruption" on the skin.

The Respiratory System.   The lung can be thought of as a giant balloon that inflates and deflates more than 20,000 times a day. Unlike a hollow party toy, however, it is made up of millions of microscopic balloons called alveoli. These alveoli are like spring buds at the end of the branches of the respiratory tree, which starts at the trachea (windpipe) and branches out in the lungs into ever smaller bronchi, and then into bronchioles. Inhaled air is composed of a number of gases, but most importantly oxygen (O_2), which is the elixir that the body's cells need to burn energy, and carbon dioxide (CO_2), which is one of the byproducts created by the body in return. The alveoli absorb O_2 and expel CO_2 from the bloodstream through a net of thin-walled blood vessels that surround them, called capillaries. This exchange maintains the acid-base balance, or metabolic equilibrium, of all the body's processes. The proper passage of air through the lungs, and the effective transfer of gases, is therefore absolutely essential to life.

If the lungs become diseased, however, the essential process of gas exchange could be jeopardized. If the alveoli fill up with infection or fluid, such as with pneumonia or **Severe Acute Respiratory Syndrome** infection, oxygen cannot be absorbed, and carbon dioxide cannot be exhaled, putting the body at risk of complete respiratory failure. In **tuberculosis**, the lung architecture can be so severely damaged that those who survive the disease are sometimes left with considerably less lung function.

The Circulatory System.   The main function of the heart is to squeeze bright red blood full of O_2 to different parts of the body. Blood makes this journey through different types of tubes that vary in composition and caliber. Starting from the most powerful chamber of the heart, the left ventricle, blood leaves through the largest artery in the body, the aorta. It then flows through smaller arteries, and then into even smaller arterioles. All these arterial blood vessels are relatively muscular and can contract or relax, depending on factors such as the blood pressure and temperature of the body. Following the arterioles, a network of capillaries penetrate deep into the tissues and organs of the body and allow for the easy transfer of O_2 as well as CO_2 and other toxins. Dark blue blood, full of these metabolic by-products, then travels back to the heart in the thin walled veins and venoules of the venous system. From here, the blood collects in the right atrium, passes into the right ventricle, and is ejected into the lungs. Another vascular system in the lungs delivers blood to the single-cell-walled capillaries that line the alveoli so that effective gas exchange can once again occur. Upon leaving the lungs, the blood will collect in the *left* atria before entering into the left ventricle to begin the journey anew. Between the atria and the ventricles, and between the ventricles and the large arteries that take blood away from the heart to either the body or the lungs, there are four leathery valves that contain the blood in the proper heart chamber before it moves on. It is their opening and closing that produces the *lub-dub* sound of the heart beating. The heart beats because its rhythmic contractions are controlled by an electrical system that periodically produces a signal that travels from the sinus node in the right atrium down to the ventricles.

The Lymphatic System.   Any fluid that squeezes out from the blood vessels is brought back to the venous circulation through a separate series of thin-walled conduits called the lymphatic system. This system is also important in the immune function of the body. It is composed of the lymph glands, which serve as docking stations for activated white blood cells; the thymus and tonsils, which also work with the immune system's white blood cells; and the spleen, which filters and purifies the blood. Each patch of lymph nodes has its own name, depending on where it is located and what area of the body it drains.

Swollen lymph nodes and an enlarged spleen usually suggest that the body is fighting off an infection. If most of the nodes that one finds are swollen and the spleen is enlarged, then the infection is likely a total body infection, such as **Human Immunodeficiency Virus** or mononucleosis. If only a small patch of lymph nodes are swollen, such as those under the neck, under the arm, or in the groin, a localized infection can usually be found by tracking back to where these lymphatic channels drain. In **bubonic plague**, the presence of a large lymph node exuding pus, called a bubo, suggests that a flea carrying plague bacteria has bitten the skin that is drained by that lymph node.

The Hematologic and Immunologic Systems.   Flowing through the arteries, veins, and capillaries of the body, the blood is full of specialized cells that perform different functions: red cells transport oxygen, white cells fight off infections, and platelets clog up ruptures that cause bleeding. All these are created deep within a latticework of dividing cells inside the bones, called the bone marrow. Many pathogens live or travel inside the bloodstream, and some parasites such as malaria's actually live inside the red blood cells. The importance of white blood cells in preventing infection is especially evident when they are compromised: the Human Immunodeficiency Virus (HIV) is a retrovirus that eliminates one of the most important white blood cells, the CD4+ T-cell, thereby putting the body at risk for countless infections. It usually is not HIV, per se, that kills the infected person, but the many other germs that the compromised immune system cannot control, a syndrome of diseases called **Acquired Immune Deficiency Syndrome**.

In addition, blood is full of many other proteins and dissolved molecules that help the body function correctly: there are proteins that fight off infections, called antibodies; proteins that work with platelets to stop bleeding, called coagulation factors; and excreted toxins that are by-products of metabolic processes. Diseases such as the **hemorrhagic fevers** Ebola and Dengue alter the coagulation factors such that the body cannot stop bleeding once it begins, often leading to the infected person's death.

The Endocrine System.   Various organs throughout the body that form the Endocrine system secrete biologically active proteins called hormones into the blood so that their effect can be carried throughout the body. The main organs considered part of this system are the pituitary gland, the hypothalamus, the thyroid gland, the parathyroid glands, the insulin-producing cells of the pancreas, the adrenal glands, the ovaries, and the testicles. Each hormone produced has its own set of actions and helps to regulate processes as complex as menstruation and puberty. Even small alterations in any of these organs or hormones can have dramatic effects on the growth, development, and health of a human being.

The Digestive System.   Once food is swallowed, a wavelike motion called peristalsis will pulsate through the esophagus, the tube of muscle that brings the food from the mouth to the stomach. Before entering the stomach, the food will meet a band of muscle that contracts or relaxes to control the flow of food, called the lower esophageal sphincter (LES). This pattern essentially mirrors the form of the entire gastrointestinal (GI) tract: a succession of tubes and sphincters that regulate the transport of food, altering it at each stage so that the body can absorb necessary nutrients. Once in the stomach, acid and enzymes dissolve and digest the chewed up food, especially proteins, but stop short of digesting the stomach organ itself because of a protective lining of mucous along the stomach wall. The stomach muscle simultaneously contracts powerfully so as further to mash the chewed up food mechanically. The stomach gets ulcers when the protective layer is damaged, usually by an infection, allowing the acid to burn the stomach wall. Once fine enough to move through the tight opening of the pyloric sphincter at the end of the stomach, the chewed up food, now called chime, enters the small intestine, which has three parts. First, in the duodenum, carbohydrates are processed with a stew of digestive enzymes and anti-acidic solutions that pour out from a gland called the pancreas, and fats are processed with bile that comes from a collecting sack that sits just under the liver called the gallbladder. The other two parts of the small intestine, called the jejunum and ileum, work with the duodenum to absorb nutrients into the blood through tiny finger-like projections, called villi, on their inner walls. As digestion progresses, carbohydrates are reduced to simple sugars, fats break down into fatty acids, and proteins are divided into their amino acids. All the blood of the intestines collects in what is called the portal venous system that passes through the liver so that the nutrients can be further processed, and toxins may be neutralized. Any medicines absorbed into the blood may also be altered as they pass through the liver. Once past the large intestine, the ingested food, now stool (feces), sits in the rectum until it can pass through the final sphincter, the anus.

When the process of digestion up to the point of the small intestine malfunctions, terrible consequences can happen to the body. For example, in many developing countries, parasitic worms, such as tapeworms, infect the small intestine and intercept the nutrients from consumed food before they are absorbed by the body. Sometimes worms such as roundworm grow and divide, becoming such masses that the entire small intestine plugs up and stops working.

Many diseases that cause infectious diarrheas work at the level of the large intestine by either breaking down the inner lining (the mucosa), thereby preventing it from absorbing water correctly, or by poisoning the cells themselves so that they secrete water. **Dysentery** is sometimes called a "bloody diarrhea" because the damage to the mucosa, or the inner lining of the intestine, caused by the toxins produced by the pathogenic bacteria cause it to bleed. **Cholera**, on the other hand, is one type of "secretory diarrhea" which does not destroy the mucosa, but yet can kill a human in only a few days because the amount of fluid lost through the poisoned and malfunctioning cells can fatally dehydrate the body. Oral Rehydration Therapy (ORT) is a simple but effective treatment that works to replace lost vital fluids by using both salt and sugar dissolved in water to help pull hydration back into the body. Its wide use has saved millions of lives to date and forms the cornerstone of any effective diarrhea treatment.

The Reproductive System.   Despite being a source of embarrassment in many cultures, the human genitals play the most important role in the survival of our species: sex and reproduction. When a fetus is first forming, the tissues that change to become either male or female sex organs originate from the same dividing cells, and therefore, the female genitalia and male genitalia are very much alike. The most sensitive parts of the genitals are the tip of the penis, or the glans, and the front of the vagina near the pubic bone, or the clitoris. The shaft of the penis and the lips, or labia, of the vagina develop from the same folds of tissue, as do the scrotum and the mounds of skin next to the labia called the mons venus. A key difference though, is that the female gonads, or the ovaries, are internal, whereas the male gonads, or testes, are outside the abdominal cavity. During intercourse, once a man ejaculates semen into a woman's vagina, the sperm from his testicles may combine with her egg, or *ovum*, that has come from the ovary down the *fallopian tubes*. The fertilized egg will usually implant in the woman's *uterus* and, if successful, the fetus will grow, producing the same genitals that will someday start the process anew.

Sexual intercourse involves the exchange of fluids through these organs, so if one partner is infected with a sexually transmitted disease (STD), his or her sexual partner is also at risk of becoming infected. Different diseases infect people differently. **Syphilis** forms a painless ulcer on the external genitals, making infected people unaware that they are infecting their partners. Chlamydia and **gonorrhea** inhabit the sexual fluids, making

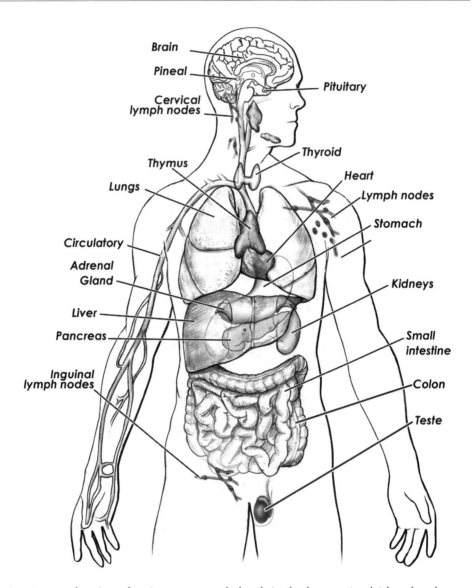

A cut-away drawing of major organs and glands in the human (male) head and torso.
Courtesy of Megan Rojas.

them pus-like and contagious. HIV infects the blood and can enter the sexual fluids, but
it can also infect someone through the exchange of blood, as can happen with blood
transfusions or the sharing of needles during intravenous (IV) drug abuse.

The Muscular and Skeletal System.   The human skeleton can be thought of as a
puppet: the bones are like the sticks that play the arms and legs, and the muscles are like
the strings that pull the sticks. Bones are connected to one another at the joints in different ways. The shoulder and hip joints, for example, have a ball-in-socket type joint that

allows for a full range of circular motion. The knee, on the other hand, is like a hinge and can move in only one path. Muscles are connected to bones by tendons, and bones are connected to other bones by ligaments. Each bone has a name, as does each muscle, ligament, and tendon.

The Urinary System.   The kidney is made up of a complex network of cells, called nephrons, which concentrate salt and toxins in urine. By doing this, the kidney filters the blood, rids it of many impurities, and helps maintain the metabolic equilibrium of the body. Once the urine is produced, it flows out through the ureters into the bladder. The urethral sphincter will hold it back until it can flow out through the urethera. **Schistosomiasis** is a parasite that lives some of its lifecycle in the urinary system and is therefore passed onto other people who swim in fresh water in which an infected human host has urinated.

The Nervous System.   The very design of the central nervous system works to resist damage. Protected by the thick skull bone of the head, called the cranium, the brain is composed of the cerebrum (the part that processes most thinking, from controlling speech to doing math calculations) and the cerebellum (the part that controls the body's coordination and balance). Both sit on top of the brain stem, which controls basic bodily functions like breathing and defecation. Entering at this level, the spinal cord is the long highway of nerves that brings messages back and forth from all parts of the body. Covering all of these parts is a bath of cerebrospinal fluid and a series of protective layers called the meninges. Entry into the brain space is therefore incredibly difficult; even the substances in the blood itself have to cross the so-called blood–brain barrier. If bacteria do happen to breech this barrier, they can cause a profound inflammation in the meningeal space, called **meningitis**. If the infection enters into the brain itself, it is called **encephalitis**. Depending on where it does damage, dramatic changes in bodily function and personality can occur. Indeed, there is a tremendous amount of specialization in each part of the nervous system, with different types of nerves bringing messages to different types of tissues in the body. Some nerves bring messages for skeletal muscle movement whereas others may bring messages for digestion. Similarly, the diverse lobes and folds of the brain work to control different aspects of various thoughts or actions. *See also* Antibiotics; Ayurvedic Disease Theory and Medicine; Chinese Disease Theory and Medicine; Contagion and Transmission; Corpses and Epidemic Disease; Diet, Nutrition, and Epidemic Disease; Germ Theory of Disease; Greco-Roman Medical Theory and Practice; Heredity and Epidemic Disease; Human Immunity and Resistance to Disease; Immunology; Islamic Disease Theory and Medicine; Personal Hygiene and Epidemic Disease.

Further Reading

Blakemore, Colin, and Sheila Jennett. *The Oxford Companion to the Body*. New York: Oxford University Press, 2002.

Cotran, Ramzi S., et al. *Robbins and Cotran Pathologic Basis of Disease*, 7th edition. Philadelphia: W. B. Saunders Company, 2004.

The Encyclopedic Atlas of the Human Body. North Charleston, SC: Global Book Publishing, 2004.

Martini, Ric, and Ed Bartholomew. *Essentials of Anatomy and Physiology*. Upper Saddle River, NJ: Prentice Hall, 2006.

Netter, Frank H. *Atlas of Human Anatomy*, with netteranatomy.com. East Hanover, NJ: Novartis, 2006.

Nuland, Sherwin B. *How We Die: Reflections on Life's Final Chapter.* New York: Vintage, 1995.

Sacks, Oliver. *The Man Who Mistook His Wife for a Hat: And Other Clinical Tales.* New York: Harper-Collins, 1985.

DANIEL PALAZUELOS

HUMAN IMMUNITY AND RESISTANCE TO DISEASE.   A continual interplay occurs between microbes and our immune systems. Our immune systems have evolved to provide us with resistance to most microbes encountered throughout life. Yet pathogenic microbes evolve increasingly elaborate strategies to exploit weaknesses in our immune responses and cause disease. Defects in either innate or adaptive components of the human immune system can profoundly reduce a host's resistance to infection. Consequently, infectious microbes often suppress or evade aspects of the immune system in order to cause disease, for example during **bubonic plague, influenza**, and **tuberculosis**. The ability of the immune system to resist infection is also reduced in **AIDS** and is a major cause of morbidity and mortality in human immunodeficiency virus (HIV)–infected individuals.

Barriers to Infection.   The initial barriers to infection are the epithelial surfaces of the body. These include skin and the mucous layers of the eyes, lungs, gut, and other body surfaces. The importance and strengths of these barriers are attested by the fact that billions of nonpathogenic microbes inhabit these epithelial surfaces every day of our lives without causing disease. Those few microbes that do manage to cross an epithelial barrier soon encounter immune cells—such as macrophages, dendritic cells, and neutrophils—that can eat (phagocytose) microbes or debris from damaged tissues. The immune cells also produce a variety of toxic products that directly damage or destroy invading microbes, as well as numerous secreted hormone-like products (cytokines) that recruit and activate other components of the immune system. Those few nonpathogenic microbes that happen to cross epithelial barriers are thus rapidly eliminated by our innate immune system.

In some cases, dendritic cells will transport invading microbes or their products to lymph nodes that drain the infected tissue. This enables the dendritic cells to present antigens that activate antigen-specific antibody-producing B lymphocytes and T cell receptor–producing T lymphocytes within the lymph node. Once activated, T cells contribute to the increased activation of macrophages and other immune cells through their ability to produce cytokines such as interferon gamma (IFNγ). IFNγ is also produced by natural killer (NK) cells in response to hormone-like cytokines produced by infected cells. NK cells can also respond to stress-induced changes in expression of molecules at the surface of infected cells. T cells and NK cells can also directly lyse (kill) infected target cells, thereby preventing the growth of viruses and other intracellular pathogens. B cells produce antibodies that recognize the pathogen or its antigens.

In contrast to harmless, nonpathogenic microbes, pathogenic organisms have evolved strategies to subvert or evade destruction by the innate immune system. One common mechanism used is to avoid destruction by phagocytes. For example, *Streptococcus pneumoniae* **bacteria** produce slippery polysaccharide capsules that interfere with the ability of phagocytic cells to internalize the bacterium. **Viruses** and some other bacteria do not prevent phagocytosis itself, but rather avoid destruction by a phagocyte once phagocytosed. For example, *Mycobacterium tuberculosis* is readily engulfed by macrophages, but in most cases it continues to live inside these cells without being killed. Other viruses and bacteria have evolved strategies to prevent antigen presentation by cells they infect, so that T cell responses are not efficiently activated.

A common feature associated with a variety of antimicrobial immune responses is the formation of a structure called the *granuloma*. The granuloma is a collection of immune cells that forms to surround and wall off sites of infection within the body. Small cytokine-like molecules known as chemokines are crucial for recruiting the immune cells to sites of infection. These chemokines form a path leading out from the site of infection and bind to receptors on the surface of nearby immune cells. The immune cells then move along the path to the site of infection. Although granulomas can help to limit the dissemination of pathogenic microbes through the body, the collection of activated immune cells also causes localized tissue damage that may contribute to disease symptoms or severity.

Detection of Invading Microbes.   In order to contribute to resistance against infection, phagocytes and other immune cells must be able to detect the presence of the invader. To do this, immune cells express a variety of "innate" receptors that play important and complex roles in the immune response.

One class of receptors is specific for the "Fc region" of antibody molecules. The Fc region is a conserved region found on the opposite end from the antibody antigen binding site. Because of this separation of the two regions, each antibody molecule can bind simultaneously both a microbial protein or particle and a host "Fc receptor." In the case of cells that phagocytose microbes, binding of Fc receptors to antibodies bound to a microbe's surface can enhance the ability of the leukocyte to eat that microbe. This process is called *opsonization*. The immune cells that are most capable of phagocytosis are macrophages, dendritic cells, and neutrophils. On other, nonphagocytic, immune cells Fc receptors can alter the function of the cell or cause the cell to release toxic products. For example, when an antigen and antibody triggers the Fc receptors present on a natural killer (NK) cell, this cell is triggered to kill infected cells. Conversely, Fc receptors on mast cells (that contain histamines) trigger the release of products that cause allergic-type reactions.

A second class of innate immune receptors detects microbes independently of antibodies. Rather, conserved components of pathogens are detected. These include components of the cell wall of bacteria, elements in virus particles, or material produced by **protozoon** pathogens. Examples of this class of receptors include scavenger receptors, Toll-like receptors (TLRs), and the related Nod-like receptors (NLRs). These receptors typically cause the release of cytokines, which regulate immune responses and enhance the ability of cells to kill phagocytosed microbes.

In addition to cells, conserved blood proteins also have a role in preventing the dissemination of invading microbes and/or in killing these microbes. Proteins involved in blood clotting are activated by microbes and can cause blood clots to form at sites of infection. These clots then physically wall off invading pathogens. Proteins of the "complement system" also recognize pathogens. "Complement" proteins bind to the pathogen and can cause death of the pathogen by breaking down the cell wall. Similar to antibodies and Fc receptors, complement can also cause opsonization of microbes, which are then more readily eaten and killed by phagocytic cells.

Impact of Immune Deficiency on Host Resistance.   Animal models of infection have been crucial in defining components of the immune system that promote resistance to infection. Rendering mice deficient for specific immune cell populations, cytokines, or other killing mechanisms has enabled immunologists to make several generalizations with regard to which immune responses are most important for resistance to a specific pathogen or class of pathogen. T cells are usually important for eliminating infections with intracellular pathogens, either through direct lysis of infected cells or production of cytokines that regulate innate immune cell functions. For example, animals rendered genetically deficient for IFNγ or tumor necrosis factor (TNF)-γ are highly susceptible to infections by intracellular bacteria such as *Mycobacterium tuberculosis* and *Listeria monocytogenes*, as well as viruses like murine cytomegalovirus (MCMV). B cells and antibodies play a more substantial role in immune resistance to extracellular pathogens and toxins, such as **diphtheria** toxin, but can also contribute to resistance against viruses such as *influenza*.

Cytokines produced by T cells, NK cells, and other cell types also have diverse effects during antimicrobial immunity. For instance, in addition to activating antimicrobial killing mechanisms of macrophages, IFNγ and TNFγ are thought to contribute to immunity by promoting granuloma formation and maintenance. Cytokines such as IL-12, IL-18, and IL-1 regulate the production of these cells and also influence more general host responses to infection such as fever. It is important to note that cytokines have numerous effects and sometimes can have opposite effects on infection with different microbes. For instance, type I IFNs can regulate the survival of infected cells as well as the ability of such cells to produce proteins that degrade nucleic acids in viruses. Mice deficient for type I IFNs are thus more susceptible to infections with several viruses, including MCMV. Yet, these same mice are considerably more resistant to infection with certain intracellular bacteria, such as *L. monocytogenes*.

With regard to humans, mutations in several genes have been shown to predispose one toward specific pathogens or classes of pathogens. For example, humans who lack expression of the receptor for IFNγ or for IL-12 show increased susceptibility to infections with intracellular bacteria such as *Mycobacteria* and *Salmonella*. Mutations in the chemokine receptor CCR5 are associated with a reduced risk of **human immunodeficiency virus (HIV)** infection in otherwise high-risk individuals. This is at least partially because HIV exploits CCR5 for entry into infected cells. *See also* Contagion and Transmission; Drug Resistance in Microorganisms; Heredity and Epidemic Disease; Human Body; Immunology; Vaccination and Inoculation.

Further Reading

DeFranco, Anthony. *Immunity: The Immune Response to Infectious and Inflammatory Disease*. New York: Oxford University Press, 2007.

Playfair, J. H. L., and Benjamin Chain. *Immunology at a Glance*. New York: Wiley-Blackwell, 2005.

LAUREL LENZ

HUMAN IMMUNODEFICIENCY VIRUS/ACQUIRED IMMUNE DEFICIENCY SYNDROME (HIV/AIDS).   AIDS is a new infectious disease whose symptoms are the end result of infection with the Human Immunodeficiency **Virus** (HIV). In June 1981, AIDS was first recognized in the medical literature, but at that time, the causative agent of AIDS was unknown, so the disease was given several names describing either symptoms exhibited by patients or social characteristics of those patients. "Wasting disease," "slim disease," "opportunistic infections," and "Kaposi's sarcoma (KS)," were used singly or together to describe the symptoms. Because the disease was first recognized in the homosexual communities of large U.S. cities, "Gay-Related Immune Deficiency (GRID)" and

"Gay cancer" described a salient identity of patients. By 1984 medical researchers had identified a retrovirus as the causative agent in the disease. In 1986 this virus was named Human Immunodeficiency Virus (HIV), and in 1987 the disease AIDS was defined by the U.S. **Centers for Disease Control and Prevention** (CDC) and the **World Health Organization** (WHO) as the end stage of infection with this virus—hence the name HIV/AIDS. HIV is transmitted by intimate contact between bodily fluids. Over 2 to 10 years, the virus kills key controlling cells of the body's immune system until an infected person has no immunological defenses against many different opportunistic infections and cancers. Because infected and contagious people appear healthy for many years, HIV has spread rapidly in geographic locations where individuals engage in sexual relations with many partners, infected women become pregnant and transmit the virus unknowingly to their babies, and injecting drug abusers share needles. In areas of the world with large populations and few medical resources, the rapid spread of HIV and subsequent epidemic of AIDS has destabilized societies by killing the young adults most likely to become infected and thus leaving children without parents and communities without leadership.

The Virus and its Effect on the Human Body.   HIV is a retrovirus, composed of ribonucleic acid (RNA). The term *retro* originates from the property of these viruses to transcribe themselves, via an enzyme called reverse transcriptase, into a DNA form that is then integrated into the invaded cell's genome. The creation of new viruses then becomes a part of the cell's own genetic instructions. In the early decades of the twentieth century, the AIDS virus mutated in West Africa from a form that infected only chimpanzees to one that could infect humans.

Retroviruses had been known to cause disease in animals since 1911, when Peyton Rous (1879–1970), a scientist at the Rockefeller Institute for Medical Research in New York City, discovered that a particular type of cancer in chickens could be transmitted by grinding up a tumor and injecting it into another chicken. By the 1970s, the molecular structure of retroviruses was known, but none had ever been identified as causing disease in humans. In 1980 Robert C. Gallo (b. 1937) and his colleagues at the National Cancer Institute, National Institutes of Health, in Bethesda, Maryland, demonstrated the existence of retroviruses that caused cancer in humans by triggering unchecked replication of T cells.

In contrast, HIV, the retrovirus that causes AIDS, kills the helper T cells that regulate the immune system, thus destroying the body's natural defenses against opportunistic infections and cancers. When the initial infection takes place, HIV causes fever, headache, malaise, and enlarged lymph nodes—symptoms similar to those of many other virus infections. These symptoms disappear within a week or two, but the infected individual is highly contagious at this point, with HIV present in large quantities in genital fluids. For the next 10 years in adults (and approximately 2 years in infants infected at birth), there may be no disease symptoms at all. During this period, however, HIV is destroying the T cells that are the body's key infection fighters, and this decline is measurable. Once the immune system has reached a certain level of disruption, the infected person begins to experience symptoms. Lymph nodes may enlarge again, energy may decline, and weight may be lost. Fevers and sweats may become frequent. Yeast infections may become frequent or persistent, and pelvic inflammatory disease in women may not respond to treatment. Short-term memory loss may be observed. Infected children may grow slowly or have many bouts of sickness.

The CDC defines the advent of full-blown AIDS as the moment when an individual infected with HIV experiences a T cell count below 200 per cubic millimeter of blood (healthy adults have T cell counts of 1,000 or more). This is the point at which the immune system is so ravaged that it cannot fight off **bacteria**, viruses, fungi, parasites, and other microbes normally kept in check by the immune system. Symptoms of people with AIDS may include coughing and shortness of breath, seizures, painful swallowing, confusion and forgetfulness, severe and persistent diarrhea, fevers, loss of vision, nausea and vomiting, extreme fatigue, severe headaches, and even coma. Children with AIDS may experience these same symptoms plus very severe forms of common childhood bacterial diseases such as **conjunctivitis**, ear infections, and tonsillitis. People who develop AIDS also may develop cancers caused by viruses, such as Kaposi's sarcoma and **cervical cancer**, or cancers of the immune system known as lymphomas. Eventually, the person with AIDS is overwhelmed by the opportunistic infections and cancers and dies. Antiviral drugs are able to suppress the damage to the immune system but not to eradicate the virus. People living with AIDS must take antiviral drugs, which have many side effects, for the rest of their lives.

Transmission. HIV is not easily transmitted. It is *not* transmitted by hugging, kissing, coughing, using public toilets or swimming in public pools, or sharing eating utensils or towels in the bathroom. Transmission of HIV requires close contact between an infected person's bodily fluids and the blood or other bodily fluids of a noninfected person. The principal way in which AIDS is transmitted is through sexual intercourse—genital, anal, or oral. It is also transmitted easily when injecting drug users share needles, or when needles used in tattooing or body piercing are reused without being sterilized. HIV may be transmitted from mother to child before, during, or after birth, and it may be transmitted in breast milk. Before 1985, when a test for HIV was released, the AIDS virus was also transmitted through contaminated blood and blood products used in surgery or to treat hemophilia.

Education about the routes of transmission, programs to encourage abstinence from sex or faithfulness to one partner, the distribution of condoms and clean needles, and free testing so that people may learn their HIV status have been the major methods by which the transmission of AIDS has been slowed, when such methods have been utilized. Religious taboos against the use of condoms during sex and political views that oppose the distribution of clean needles to drug abusers have inhibited prevention efforts. Cultural resistance to permitting women to refuse unsafe sex and the existence of informal multipartner sexual networks in which individuals do not think of themselves as promiscuous because they have sex with only a few people whom they know well have also hindered the interruption of transmission of HIV.

Epidemiology. As a new disease, AIDS was literally "constructed" by epidemiologists in the years after it was first identified in the medical literature. Between 1981 and 1984, epidemiologists had to answer many questions: What did it mean to have AIDS? How was the disease transmitted? What did the epidemiological data suggest about possible etiological agents? How much morbidity and mortality did the disease exact and over what time periods? How was the disease dispersed geographically? Which populations were most at risk for contracting the syndrome?

The first on-the-ground investigations of the new syndrome were done as collaborations between the CDC and state or local health agencies. Public health officials followed up every case they could find of KS and *Pneumocystis carinii* pneumonia (PCP). A 30-page, detailed questionnaire was developed that produced a picture of AIDS in the United States. By early 1982, statistics showed that the average age of patients was 35. All of the patients were gay men, and they were living in the strong gay communities of San Francisco, New York, and Los Angeles, all areas of high opportunity for gay men. They had a large number of sexual partners. They all went to the same nightclubs and most used the drugs known as poppers (isobutyl nitrite or amyl nitrite).

By June 1982, however, information about cases of AIDS outside the gay communities had been collected, and the understanding of AIDS was broadened. AIDS was identified in injecting drug users and their sexual partners, in newborn babies, and in heterosexual patients who had undergone surgery. These new observations suggested a blood-borne pathogen. The discovery of cases in hemophiliacs reinforced the evidence for transmission via blood, like **hepatitis** B.

HIV infection and AIDS are concentrated in places where the methods of transmission are most prolific and where prevention methods are not employed. It was first identified in the United States, for example, in the gay communities of large cities, where frequent and unprotected sexual encounters took place, enabling rapid spread of the virus. Injecting drug users, communities of whom are often concentrated in large cities, spread the virus to one another through shared needles and to their sexual partners during sex. In much of Sub-Saharan Africa, in contrast, AIDS is more often transmitted heterosexually. HIV transmission is concentrated along highways traveled by men working far from home and seeking sex with female sex workers. Once infected, the men may unknowingly infect their wives. When the wives become pregnant, their unborn children may become infected as well. Cultural practices that discourage the discussion of sex may lead men to deny infection. Because women in many African cultures have no recognized right to demand that their husbands wear condoms during sex, they have almost no options to protect themselves from infection. A popular superstition that a man will be cured of his HIV infection by having sex with a virgin may lead men to have forcible intercourse with young girls, thus spreading the infection further. In Southeast Asia and in India, the sex trade in large cities has been a principal locus of HIV transmission.

Sociocultural Construction of the Disease.   As a mental picture of AIDS was constructed by epidemiologists from the medical evidence they observed, the meaning of the disease was also constructed in the social, political, cultural, and religious contexts of the societies in which it existed. "Having AIDS" meant much more in all societies than mere infection with a virus and the physical consequences of that infection. Because HIV was transmissible sexually, views about marriage, homosexuality, adultery, and premarital sex all colored the perception of someone with AIDS. In cultures that had strong prohibitions against homosexuality, AIDS became a symbol of how God punished gay people. In cultures that held religious beliefs against the use of condoms during sex, that method of AIDS prevention was discounted as being of no importance. In cultures in which political leaders implemented pragmatic rather than ideological policies, strong prevention efforts such as education, condom distribution, and programs to distribute clean needles to addicts reduced the incidence of new infections.

History of Research on and Control of HIV/AIDS.   As soon as epidemiologists understood that AIDS attacked the helper T cells that controlled the immune system, they urged virologists to search for a hitherto unknown virus that fit this description. The only viruses known to attack human T cells were the retroviruses identified by the Gallo laboratory at the National Cancer Institute (NCI) in Bethesda, Maryland. These viruses were known as Human T-Cell Lymphotrophic Virus, Types I and II (HTLV-I and HTLV-II), which caused cancer in humans. Three groups of investigators began searching for retroviruses as possible causative agents of AIDS. In addition to Gallo's group, there were virologist Luc Montagnier's (b. 1932) group at the Pasteur Institute in Paris and medical researcher Jay Levy's (b. 1938) group at the University of California San Francisco (UCSF). In 1984 Gallo's group published four papers in the journal *Science* that demonstrated a retrovirus as the cause of AIDS. They initially believed that it was in the same family as the other two HTLV viruses; hence, they named it HTLV-III. Montagnier's group at the Pasteur Institute and Jay Levy's at UCSF also identified the causative retrovirus of AIDS at about the same time. They named their viruses, respectively, lymphadenopathy associated virus (LAV) and AIDS related virus (ARV). Within a year, these viruses were shown to be identical. Because the AIDS virus caused destruction of infected T cells instead of the uncontrolled reproduction that occurred in cancer, it was deemed separate from the HTLV family. In 1986 an international group of scientists proposed that the name of the retrovirus that caused AIDS be changed to *Human Immunodeficiency Virus* (HIV).

The first medical intervention developed for the control of AIDS was a diagnostic test adapted from the laboratory assay that confirmed the presence of antibodies to HIV in cell cultures. This enzyme-linked immunosorbancy assay (ELISA) can have false positives, however, so a second test, known as the Western blot, which assays for specific viral proteins, was used to confirm a positive ELISA test. In 1987 the U.S. Food and Drug Administration (FDA) required that both tests be used before someone would be told that he or she was infected with AIDS. Twenty-five years into the epidemic, these diagnostic tests arguably remain medicine's most useful interventions for addressing the AIDS epidemic because they provide a measurable, replicable means to identify infected individuals.

During the two years of intensive laboratory research during which HIV was identified and characterized genetically, information also emerged about the virus that helped suggest which preventive interventions by political and public health leaders might be possible. Within just a few months after HIV was identified, molecular biologists understood that it mutated far too rapidly—up to 1,000 times as fast as **influenza** virus—for a traditional vaccine to be made against it. Instead of being able to vaccinate against AIDS, political and public health leaders needed to use educational methods aimed at curbing high-risk behavior to slow transmission, a much harder task.

Molecular and genetic studies also identified the key points in the virus's life cycle, which, if interrupted, would halt the spread of the virus. The first was the CD-4+ receptor on the cell wall of the host cell to which the virus attached. Second was the point at which the enzyme reverse transcriptase caused the single-strand RNA virus to make a complementary copy that transformed it into double-stranded DNA. Third, the enzyme integrase caused the viral DNA to be spliced into the genome of the host cell. Finally came the point at which the enzyme protease cut newly constructed polypeptides into viral proteins in the final assembly of new virus particles. By 1986 intellectual strategies were in place to intervene in each of these four steps, but scientists were not technologically capable of implementing most of them, and a great deal of molecular information about HIV, such as the existence of necessary co-receptors in step 1, was not yet known.

In 1984 some drugs were known to inhibit reverse transcriptase, so this is where the work on an AIDS therapy began. Scientists utilized an anti-cancer drug-screening program at the NCI to identify potential drugs for use against AIDS. One of these that showed promise *in vitro* was azidothymidine, commonly called AZT. After truncated clinical trials in which AIDS patients showed a clear response to AZT, it was approved for use by the FDA in record time and sold under the brand name Retrovir or the generic name zidovudine. Within a few more years, two additional reverse transcriptase inhibitors, known in chemical shorthand as ddI and ddC, were approved by the FDA for treating AIDS. The reverse transcriptase inhibitors improved the condition of AIDS patients but had a number of toxic side effects and were subject to the development of resistance by HIV.

Other than these antiretroviral drugs, treatments for AIDS focused on existing drugs for treating the opportunistic infections and cancer that people with AIDS developed. In 1995 the first of a new class of antiretroviral drugs was introduced.

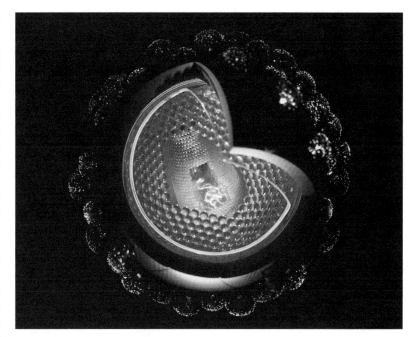

Cut-away model of the human immunodeficiency virus (HIV), the cause of AIDS. John Wildgoose.

Known as protease inhibitors, these drugs interfered with the final enzymatic step in the viral assembly process. For a brief period, there was optimism that the protease inhibitors would "cure" AIDS because viral loads—the number of virus particles in a quantity of blood—disappeared. It soon became apparent, however, that HIV was only suppressed and that it rapidly rebounded if the drugs were withdrawn. These drugs, too, caused unpleasant side effects. The combination of reverse transcriptase inhibitors and protease inhibitors known as Highly Active Antiretroviral Therapy, or HAART, is nevertheless the most effective "cocktail" of drugs for long-term therapy against AIDS. Pharmaceutical research still works toward a rationally designed, molecularly based drug with minimal toxicity as a therapy for AIDS, but at present, that goal has not been attained.

Current Situation of AIDS. In November 2006, WHO reported that 2.9 million people had died of AIDS-related illnesses and estimated that 39.5 million people were living with HIV/AIDS. WHO also reported that there were 4.3 million new infections in 2006, 65 percent of which occurred in Sub-Saharan Africa. There were also important increases in Eastern Europe and Central Asia.

Research continues on a preventive vaccine and on new antiviral drugs. The most effective means for controlling the epidemic, however, still remains diagnosis of individuals infected with HIV, education about how the virus is spread, and public health efforts to change behavior to minimize the risk of infection. *See also* all AIDS-related entries; Animal Research; Capitalism and Epidemic Disease; Cinema and Epidemic Disease; Disease, Social Construction of; Human Body; Human Immunity and Resistance to

Disease; Literature, Disease in Modern; Medical Ethics and Epidemic Disease; Personal Hygiene and Epidemic Disease; Personal Liberties and Epidemic Disease; Pharmaceutical Industry; Popular Media and Epidemic Disease: Recent Trends; Poverty, Wealth, and Epidemic Disease; Religion and Epidemic Disease; Sexual Revolution.

Further Reading

Barnett, Tony, and Alan Whiteside. *AIDS in the Twenty-First Century: Disease and Globalization*, 2nd revised edition. New York: Palgrave Macmillan, 2006.

Campbell, Catherine. *Letting Them Die: Why HIV/Aids Prevention Programs Fail*. Bloomington: Indiana University Press, 2003.

Centers for Disease Control and Prevention. *HIV/AIDS*. http://www.cdc.gov/hiv/

Engel, Jonathan. *The Epidemic: A Global History of AIDS*. New York: Smithsonian/ HarperCollins, 2006.

Fan, Hung. *AIDS: Science and Society*, 5th edition. Boston: Jones and Bartlett, 2007.

Frontline [PBS]. *25 Years of AIDS: The Age of AIDS*. http://www.pbs.org/wgbh/pages/frontline/aids/cron/

Grmek, Mirko. *History of AIDS: Emergence and Origin of a Modern Pandemic*, translated by Russell C. Maulitz and Jacalyn Duffin. Princeton: Princeton University Press, 1990.

Hunter, Susan. *AIDS in America*. New York: Palgrave Macmillan, 2006.

———. *AIDS in Asia: A Continent in Peril*. New York: Palgrave Macmillan, 2005.

———. *Black Death: AIDS in Africa*. New York: Palgrave Macmillan, 2003.

Levy, Jay A. *HIV and the Pathogenesis of AIDS*, 3rd edition. New York: ASM Press, 2007.

Mayo Clinic. *HIV/AIDS*. http://www.mayoclinic.com/health/hiv-aids/DS00005

National Institute of Allergy and Infectious Diseases. *AIDS*. http://www.niaid.nih.gov/publications/aids.htm

New York Times. The AIDS Epidemic: AIDS at 20. http://www.nytimes.com/library/national/science/aids/timeline

San Francisco AIDS Foundation. *Milestones in the Battle Against AIDS: 25 Years of an Epidemic*. http://www.sfaf.org/aidstimeline/

World Health Organization. *HIV Infections*. http://www.who.int/topics/hiv_infections/en/

VICTORIA A. HARDEN

HUMAN PAPILLOMA VIRUS AND CERVICAL CANCER.   Many people consider **epidemic** diseases to be those that affect populations suddenly, accompanied by severe symptoms like diarrhea and rashes that are dramatic and strike quickly. A corollary might be that if an epidemic struck slowly, modern medicine could catch up to it and wipe it out. Cervical cancer is an epidemic disease that progresses gradually and can be detected and even cured if found early. But despite the opportunity to stop this epidemic, it continues to be a leading cause of cancer death among women in many developing countries.

It may seem unusual to think of cancer as an epidemic, but the remarkable distinction of cervical cancer is that it is caused by a **virus**, just like **influenza** or the common cold. The Human Papilloma Virus (HPV) in some forms causes simple warts, like those commonly found on hands or feet. The virus comes into contact with the cells in the topmost, or epidermis, layer of human skin, and causes the skin cells to divide and grow more than normal. On the hands, a little bump with a crown like a cauliflower will form; on the cervix of a woman, cancer can develop.

The cervix is a round lip at the end of a woman's uterus, which separates it from the vaginal canal. It is covered with skin very much like the skin anywhere else on the body. When cervical skin cells are infected with an HPV that is potentially cancerous, visible changes occur in how these cells look under a microscope. Normally, the cells look like clear bags with a stained circle in the middle of each cell. This dot is the *nucleus*, where the DNA of the cell is located. This DNA holds all the information on how the cell functions, divides, and dies. Once infected with HPV, the DNA changes; the nucleus may become larger in comparison to the rest of the cell, look darker, or look more irregularly shaped—all changes that are easily spotted under the microscope. There are many different types of HPV, and the most dangerous are four subtypes (numbered 16, 18, 31, 45) that hold oncogenes, the genes that affect the DNA and cause cancer.

In the United States and the rest of the developed world, cervical cancer used to be one of the leading causes of cancer death among women. All this changed when Dr. George Papanicolaou (1883–1962) developed a test in the 1920s that allowed healthcare providers to look for the very changes mentioned. First, a small sample of cells from a woman's cervix is collected. Then, these cells are placed on a glass slide, stained with various dyes, and viewed under a microscope. If changes are found, then the infected cells on the cervix can be either cut out or burned off with a super-cold probe. The cervix does not have any pain nerves so this does not cause the patient pain. After many years of implementation, this procedure all but eradicated cervical cancer among the women with access to a Papanicolaou (Pap) smear test. If left alone to continue changing, however, the infected cells of the cervix can grow into cancer. They may continue to develop until they have invaded organs nearby; cancerous cells can even travel throughout the body to implant and grow in places far away from the cervix. This is called metastatic cervical cancer, and it is usually fatal.

A study of American women in 2003–2004, published in the *Journal of the American Medical Association* in February 2007, found that at any given moment 26.8 percent have some form of the virus. Other studies indicate that 80 percent of women will acquire the virus at some point, that 14,000 will develop cervical cancer each year, and that almost 4,000 American women will die of it each year. Worldwide estimates in 2004 were 493,000 new cases annually and 274,000 annual deaths.

The reason so many women continue to die of a disease that is entirely preventable has more to do with politics and economics than with science and medicine. Although it is a simple test that does not require much equipment, the Pap smear has some critical shortcomings. First, many women are unaware of the causes and dangers of cervical cancer and have never heard of it or have never been offered an explanation of it. Second, getting a sample is sometimes embarrassing or uncomfortable for women. It entails inserting a speculum into the vaginal canal, which spreads the vaginal lips so that the cervix can be seen and then sampled. Although most trained health-care practitioners can perform this exam while avoiding discomfort, the patient has to know and trust that all this is actually worth the trouble. Some traditional and modern societies highly value modesty, and a stranger, particularly a man, is not trusted to perform such a sensitive procedure. In addition, even if women want the test, in cultures in which men have control over their wives' and daughters' activities, women are not allowed to decide this issue for themselves. Third, Pap smear analysis and follow-up can be extremely difficult in developing countries. The slides from the Pap smear must be transported to another doctor, who will examine the sample to see whether it is abnormal. If abnormal cells are seen, the patient must then be notified to return to the clinic for further care. In many developing countries, some women have to walk or ride for hours to get to the nearest clinic. The process of obtaining the results can take months if a good system of transport and analysis of the sample does not exist. Similarly, some countries have not been able to develop reliable laboratory systems that can provide accurate results in a reasonable amount of time. For example, some studies from Latin America show that a result may return as long as six months after the sampling date, and may have a false-negative rate of up to 50 percent, meaning that the abnormal cells were missed by the pathologist in up to half of the patients who actually had cellular changes. With a system that entails multiple visits to screen, receive results, and treat, cervical cancer prevention has not reached places that lack good roads, dependable lines of communication, and governments that choose to invest in these procedures.

In order to address this epidemic, some groups are trying different approaches. The HPV that causes cervical cancer is transmitted sexually, but studies show that condoms alone do not prevent the **transmission** of the virus from one person to another. Multiple new screening strategies have been developed. The goals of a good screening test are to catch all the people who have the disease and to minimize falsely diagnosing those who do not have the disease. The most promising alternatives have been Visual Inspection with Acetic Acid (VIA) and HPV testing. In VIA the cervix is coated with a vinegar-like solution and if there are areas that have been infected by the HPV, they turn white. In HPV testing, samples of vaginal fluids are taken and tested for the worst types of HPV.

To utilize these methods most efficiently, some groups are developing a system called the "one visit screen and treat" approach. In one technique, VIA is performed, and if positive many of the abnormal cells are treated by burning them off at the same visit. The benefit of this approach is that the women do not have to travel to the clinic more than once. Similarly, other groups have explored having patients self-collect vaginal samples to test for HPV. Some women have considered this preferable to a Pap smear because it may be less embarrassing and more comfortable. But if her test returns positive, a woman will still have to undergo a vaginal exam to have the precancerous cells removed. The one visit screen and treat approach has not yet proven to be as effective as the Pap smear in reducing the incidence of cervical cancer, although there is great potential.

The discovery of HPV as the cause of cervical cancer has led to a number of important advances, including the recent release of a vaccine that is able to prevent infection with the most dangerous types of HPV. Even this vaccine, however, is not a perfect cure: it is relatively expensive, lasts only a number of years, and is only helpful in women who are not yet infected with HPV. It is most promising for young women who are not yet sexually active, but it does not address the millions already infected.

Cervical cancer, a deadly disease affecting women, has a cure. This cure, however, is not available to everyone in the world, especially those women who are most commonly affected by this slow moving epidemic. New methods have been developed that may help these women access the screening process and subsequent treatment. The critical next step, however, is securing the health-care practitioners to perform the tests, along with the support necessary from their governments, to ensure that this process begins.

Further Reading

Centers for Disease Control and Prevention. *Human Papillomavirus (HPV) Infection.* http://www.cdc.gov/std/hpv/default.htm

Goldie, S. J., L. Gaffikin, et al. "Cost-effectiveness of Cervical-cancer Screening in Five Developing Countries." *New England Journal of Medicine* 353 (Nov 17, 2000): 2158–2168.

Mayo Clinic. *HPV Infection.* http://www.mayoclinic.com/health/hpv-infection/DS00906

Shah, Keerti V., and Thomas E. Rohan. *Cervical Cancer: From Etiology to Prevention.* New York: Springer, 2004.

Sompayrac, Lauren. *How Cancer Works.* Boston: Jones and Bartlett Publishers, 2004.

World Health Organization. *Human Papillomavirus.* http://www.who.int/immunization/topics/hpv/en/

DANIEL PALAZUELOS WITH LINDSAY BROOCKMAN

HUMAN SUBJECTS RESEARCH.   Scientists have included humans as the focus of both basic and applied research ranging from biomedical to behavioral studies, and despite the specific focus of a project, the general purpose of the research has been to extend human understanding beyond what is already known. As they gathered observable, empirical, and measurable evidence, scientists subjected their analysis to rigorous standards of reasoning and technical method, and new medical products, improved clinical procedures, and more sophisticated knowledge of physiology, pharmacology, biochemistry, and human behavior followed.

From the start, the scientific method distinguished itself from other means of establishing knowledge, and researchers developed specific hypotheses to explain natural phenomena as they designed experimental studies to test these predictions for accuracy and consistency. Today, the systematic observation, description, and measurement of data—as well as the exposure of experimental results to the critical scrutiny of other scientists—provide the fundamental bases of the modern sciences such as chemistry, biology, and psychology.

A human subject is typically a living individual who participates in scientific research by interacting directly with the investigator. For example, a human subject may surrender bodily materials such as cells, blood, or other tissues if required by the research design. In other cases, he or she may disclose personal medical, family, or psychological information to the scientist, or perform exacting tasks such as undergoing rigorous physical exercise or completing batteries of psychological tests. In larger epidemiological studies, scientists are concerned with the health and welfare of whole populations as they systematically collect and analyze data related to the frequency, distribution, and causes of human disease. No matter its specific focus, the application of the scientific method provides a variety of potential benefits such as the testing of new drugs, the discovery of new health products and technologies, the development of better diagnostic methods, and the improvement in comfort and quality of life. Though the causes of some epidemic diseases, such as bubonic plague, were discovered by studying dead victims, many more discoveries were the result of studying living victims. This is especially important for understanding the transmission, course, and other patterns of a given disease.

A good example of very early human subjects research was **Edward Jenner's** trials of cowpox vaccine in the late eighteenth century. Jenner kept careful and detailed notes on those he vaccinated, the doses he used, and their reactions to the injections. This provided important information to later physicians. Later in the century, Dr. Eduard Arning (1855–1936) offered Hawaiian death row inmates the choice of execution or inoculation with potentially deadly leprous material. He wanted to study the contagious nature of **Hansen's Disease**. Some early researchers used themselves as test subjects, as with members of **Walter Reed's yellow fever** team in 1900. In a second phase of his study Reed coupled inducements—including money—with early informed consent contracts that laid out the risks involved. These are at the heart of modern research approval processes.

The testing of the antibiotic streptomycin for use against pulmonary tuberculosis began in England in 1946. Researchers pioneered the double blind, randomized control clinical trial. One group of subjects received the drug, whereas a control group got the standard drug of the day. Patients were randomly assigned to groups, with neither the doctor nor the patient aware of who received which drug (double blind). This model has become one of the standards for pharmaceutical testing. In 1953 the U.S. National Institutes of Health (NIH) opened a 540-bed research hospital in Bethesda, Maryland, for subjects of their studies.

The inhumane "medical experiments" carried out by Nazi German and Imperial Japanese doctors in the 1930s and 1940s led to the establishment of **medical ethics** standards for researchers. In 1979 the NIH established written guidelines for ethical project design and conduct, a development followed by western European countries by the 1990s. The Council of International Organizations of Medical Science and World Medical Association ethics standards require that before any research may be conducted on human subjects, including vaccine trials, a research ethics committee (REC) or an institutional review board (IRB) must approve a formal proposal that outlines the proposed research and the protections offered to human subjects. The review committee is charged with determining whether the research is scientifically valid, whether the benefits to medical knowledge outweigh the risks to the subjects, and whether people participating in an experiment, or their surrogates, have been adequately informed of the risks and whether, knowing these risks, they have given their informed consent to participating as subjects. *See also* Epidemiology; Epidemiology, History of; Heredity and Epidemic Disease; Hospitals and Medical Education in Britain and the United States; Leprosy in the United States; Personal Liberties and Epidemic Disease; Pharmaceutical Industry; Poliomyelitis, Campaign Against; Public Health Agencies, U.S. Federal; Scientific Revolution and Epidemic Disease.

Further Reading

Achinstein, Peter. *Science Rules: A Historical Introduction to Scientific Methods.* Baltimore: Johns Hopkins University Press, 2004.

Eckart, Wolfgang U. *Man, Medicine and the State: The Human Body as an Agent of Government Sponsored Research in the Twentieth Century.* Stuttgart: Franz Steiner Verlag, 2006.

Goliszek, Andrew. *In the Name of Science: A History of Secret Programs, Medical Research, and Human Experimentation.* New York: St. Martin's Press, 2003.

Goodman, Jordan, et al., eds. *Useful Bodies: Humans in the Service of Medical Science in the Twentieth Century.* Baltimore: Johns Hopkins University Press, 2003.

Grodin, Michael A., and Leonard H. Glantz, eds. *Children as Research Subjects: Science, Ethics, and Law.* New York: Oxford University Press, 2006.

Guerini, Anita. *Experimenting with Humans and Animals: From Galen to Animal Rights*. Baltimore: Johns Hopkins University Press, 2003.

Lederer, Susan E. *Subjected to Science: Human Experimentation in America before the Second World War*. Baltimore: Johns Hopkins University Press, 1994.

Washington, Harriet A. *Medical Apartheid: The Dark History of Medical Experimentation on Black Americans from Colonial Times to the Present*. New York: Doubleday, 2006.

BART DREDGE WITH ROBERT BAKER

HUMORAL THEORY.   Developed in Classical Greece, humoral theory provided the basis for Western medicine from the fifth century BCE to the nineteenth century. According to humoral theory, the body contains four principle substances, or humors—blood, phlegm, yellow bile, and black bile—and good health requires a balance among them. This was first articulated in the writings of fifth-century BCE Greek physician **Hippocrates** and his followers, and then accepted by later intellectuals, including the Greek philosopher Aristotle (384–322 BCE) and the Roman **physician Galen**. The writings of these two men expanded upon the original theory and helped ensure it would become the standard explanation of health and disease in both European and Islamic civilizations until the nineteenth century.

The humors, like their corresponding elements of the natural world (earth, **air**, fire, **water**), combine the four principle qualities of hot, cold, dry, and wet: blood (air) is hot and wet, phlegm (water) is cold and wet, yellow bile (fire) is hot and dry, and black bile (earth) is cold and dry. Humoral theory held that all human bodies contain these four substances, though each person maintains a particular ratio among them. Each body's humoral balance is affected daily by external factors commonly known as the six nonnaturals: air, food and drink, sleep and waking, exercise and rest, evacuation and repletion, and passions. Thus, illness is a result of imbalance in the humors, which can be restored to balance through manipulations of diet and lifestyle. In addition, balance may be restored through the removal of excess humors, principally through bleeding. One result of this theory was the perception of illness as a continuum of "nonhealth" rather than as a result of a discrete disease with a unique causative agent. **Diagnosis** of problems was therefore subjective, and physicians tailored therapy to each individual.

While humoral theory worked well to explain individual ailments such as fever or congestion, **epidemic** disease required a more intricate explanation to account for widespread (but not universal) experiences of similar symptoms. Of primary use for explaining epidemics was the first of the non-naturals—air. Corrupt or unhealthy air (miasmas) could spread a similar set of symptoms within a large population, particularly affecting those whose natural humoral balance left them susceptible to such contaminations. In this way, the ability of some in the population to escape an epidemic could be explained through either lack of sufficient exposure to the miasma or through lack of predisposition to the miasma.

Whereas popular ideas of **contagion** began to emerge in response to plague in the fourteenth century, coherent medical theories of contagion did not emerge until the sixteenth century with Italian physician **Girolamo Fracastoro**. These offered alternative explanations for some diseases, but did not seriously undermine the widespread acceptance of humoral theory in general. Challenged by **Paracelsianism** in the sixteenth and seventeenth centuries, humoralism was finally supplanted by **germ theory** in the nineteenth century. *See also* Greco-Roman Medical Theory and Practice; Islamic Disease Theory and Medicine; Medical Education in the West, 1100–1500; Plague and Developments in Public Health, 1348–1600.

Further Readings

Arikha, Noga. *Passions and Tempers: A History of the Humours*. New York: Ecco, 2007.

Harvard University Library. *Contagion*. http://ocp.hul.harvard.edu/contagion/humoraltheory.html

Lindberg, David. *The Beginnings of Western Science*. Chicago: University of Chicago Press, 1992.

Nutton, Vivian. *Ancient Medicine*. New York: Routledge, 2004.

KRISTY WILSON BOWERS

I

IMMUNITY. *See* Human Immunity and Resistance to Disease.

IMMUNIZATION. *See* Vaccination and Inoculation.

IMMUNOLOGY. Immunology is the scientific discipline that seeks to explain the human host immune system and its many roles in health and disease. The immune system has important roles in maintaining health and in fighting diseases such as cancer, autoimmunity, and infections.

At least as early as ancient Greece, it was recognized that humans who recover from some specific infectious diseases are resistant to a second attack of the same disease. We now know this is true because the immune system can recognize infectious agents or products of these agents (called antigens). This recognition leads to activation of an immune response and, frequently, to the elimination of these antigens or pathogens. The reason we avoid getting sick a second time is that our immune system "learns" from the first encounter and "remembers" how to eliminate the infectious agent before it can again cause disease symptoms. Importantly, this "immunological memory" is highly specific and is shaped by and adapted to the immunological experiences of each individual.

Beginning in the late 1800s, scientists discovered that the ability of our immune system to remember antigenic challenges is dependent on specific types of white blood cells and by one of their secreted protein products called antibodies. Antibodies are made by B lymphocytes (B cells). Antibodies recognize and bind with very specific sites ("epitopes") on a pathogen or antigen. This binding can reduce the ability of the pathogen to cause disease by blocking the function of the antigen or causing destruction of the pathogen. Pathogen destruction occurs either directly, by a process called complement fixation, or indirectly by a process called opsonization. Opsonization occurs when an antibody coats a pathogen so that it can be detected and eaten by phagocytic cells. When eaten, the microbe is usually killed and digested.

Each antibody recognizes a distinct epitope with high affinity and exquisite specificity, as conferred by the antibody's unique antigen binding site. Because there is an enormous number of potential pathogens and antigens that might be encountered by each human or animal, the immune system has evolved a mechanism to generate millions of different antibody molecules. DNA rearrangements occur during the development of each B lymphocyte clone. These DNA rearrangements join together three individual DNA regions (V, D, and J) to form a single antibody-encoding gene. Because of imperfect joining and a large number of different V, D, and J regions in the genome, up to approximately 10^{10} distinct antibody molecules can theoretically be made within a given individual. A similar process of gene rearrangement occurs within T lymphocytes (T cells) in order to create a diverse array of cell-surface T cell receptors (TCRs). Whereas antibodies recognize the three-dimensional structure of an antigen, individual TCRs recognize peptide fragments of protein antigens that are displayed on the surface of infected cells. Some T cells can directly kill infected cells. They do this by recognizing host-derived surface proteins that are components of the major histocompatibility complex (MHC), which are able to bind and present small peptides that are processed from pathogen-derived antigens.

Because V, D, and J gene rearrangements occur separately within individual T cells and B cells that develop in the body, each cell produces a unique antibody or TCR. When an individual T or B cell senses an antigen that binds its TCR or antibody, it is activated to proliferate and mature into a more developed stage. A single T or B cell can thus quickly expand into a clonal population containing thousands of cells. These cells then produce antibodies or kill infected cells. After eliminating the antigen or infection, many of the responding T and B lymphocytes will die, but the remaining cells persist at a frequency 10 to 1,000 times greater than in the previously uninfected "naïve" individual. These cells also differ from their parents in that they respond more rapidly and efficiently to a second encounter with a given antigen. Thus, the ability of the immune system to prevent re-infection is the result of the persisting "memory" T and B cell populations that rapidly eliminate any reencountered antigen or pathogen.

The ability of the immune system to remember previously encountered antigens is the basis for vaccines and **vaccination**. The development of an effective vaccine by **Edward Jenner** ended a worldwide **epidemic** caused by **smallpox virus** and ultimately enabled humankind to eradicate this deadly disease. Similarly, vaccines developed against poliovirus by **Jonas Salk** and **Albert Sabin** have reduced the worldwide incidence of **poliomyelitis** to a point where this infection may also someday be completely eradicated. It is hoped that vaccines can be developed that will help eradicate other epidemic pathogens, such as **AIDS** and **tuberculosis**.

Immunologists often categorize the immune response into two phases: *adaptive* (acquired) and *innate* immunity. T lymphocytes, B lymphocytes, and the antibodies they produce are considered to participate in *adaptive* immunity. By contrast, *innate* immunity is comprised of other white blood cells; as well as the ermline- (genetically) encoded products of cells that promote immunity. Innate immune responses are not specific to a particular pathogen or antigen and do not undergo DNA rearrangements. Rather, they are more generic for broad classes of pathogens (e.g., Gram-negative **bacteria**) and are largely identical among different individual humans or animals of a given species.

In the absence of infection, most T and B lymphocytes circulate through the bloodstream and the lymphatics. The lymphatics are vessels that drain the fluid (*lymph*) that collects in tissues of the body. The lymph passes through a series of lymph nodes, which are collections of immune cells that act to filter out microbes or antigens from the lymph. Antigens collected by dendritic cells or macrophages can trigger the activation of naïve T and B cells that transiently pass through the lymph node draining a site of infection. These activated immune cells then proceed to direct the adaptive and innate components of the immune response against the antigen or pathogen. The activation of an immune response can also cause the lymph node to swell. Swelling of lymph nodes is a common symptom of infection but is more pronounced during some specific diseases, such as **bubonic plague**.

Although our understanding of the immune system and its roles in health and disease is far from complete, studies of innate and adaptive immunity have enabled immunologists to understand how our bodies resist infection and re-infection. It is also clear that defects in one or more components of the immune system can strongly contribute to plagues, pestilence, and pandemics. *See also* Contagion and Transmission; Drug Resistance in Microorganisms; Heredity and Epidemic Disease; Human Body; Human Immunity and Resistance to Disease.

Further Reading

Sompayrac, Lauren. *How the Immune System Works.* New York: Wiley-Blackwell, 2008.

LAUREL LENZ

INDUSTRIALIZATION AND EPIDEMIC DISEASE. The shift from hunter-gatherer living to early **Neolithic** farming and domestication of **animals**, which began around 10,000 years ago, created the first "big bang" opportunity for novel infectious disease agents to enter the human species. The settled and denser agrarian way of life allowed sustained and closer contacts with animals and their microbes, the proliferation of pest species (rodents, flies, etc.) as vectors of infectious agents, and, in due course for some infectious agents as towns and early cities formed, the opportunity for continuous circulation and survival in populations of sufficient size to sustain a supply of susceptible (non-immune) persons.

The second era of great new opportunity for microbes came with industrialization, initially in late eighteenth-century England; then in Europe, North America, Australia, and beyond; and now in many lower-income countries that have been undergoing industrialization in the late twentieth and early twenty-first centuries. Prior to the advent of industrialization, the human population was mostly rural, with fewer than 1 in 20 persons living in either town or city. When factories arose, and mechanized manufacturing, agriculture, and transport spread for the first time, there were large populations of densely crowded, impoverished, malnourished factory and sweat-shop laboring classes. This, of course, was an ideal "culture medium" for many potentially **epidemic** and endemic infectious diseases: hence the public health scourges of **tuberculosis, smallpox, measles, diphtheria**, pertussis **(whooping cough), cholera**, and others.

Tuberculosis (TB) has long been predominantly a disease of the poor and crowded segments of urban-industrial populations. It persists as a scourge in crowded shantytowns and slums around the world. In the early **Industrial Revolution** tuberculosis was rife, and in the nineteenth century it was known as "the white plague." This disease, which was no respecter of persons and was readily transmitted by coughing, has also provided the stuff of much romance in the history and stories of nineteenth-century Europe.

Miasmas, Germs, and People.   The biological nature of the often rampant "crowd diseases" of industrialization was not understood before the advent of the **germ theory** in the 1880s. The prevailing view in the earlier decades of industrialization was that epidemic diseases were spread by "**miasmas**," foul airborne emanations from dank and dirty soil and rotting organic matter such as **corpses**. Highly visible air pollution from soft coal–burning homes and early factories, which were rarely far apart, seemed to substantiate the notion that "corrupted air" had deleterious effects on the human body. The miasma theory could also explain, for example, why cholera and other such diseases were epidemic in places where the **water** was undrained and foul-smelling.

The record of infectious disease impacts and societal responses is particularly well documented in England. There, miasma theory motivated the epoch-defining sanitary revolution beginning in the mid-nineteenth century. **Edwin Chadwick**, sanitary engineer and utilitarian, looms large in this story with his hugely influential 1842 *Report on the Sanitary Conditions of the Labouring Population of Great Britain.* Chadwick argued that the local miasmatic atmospheric conditions arising from putrefaction and excreta caused the "endemic and contagious diseases" that afflicted the populace, particularly in the poor and crowded sections of London. Disposal of sewage and wastes via public sanitation would rid society of this economically draining miasmatic scourge.

Late in the nineteenth century, germ theory was propounded, drawing on the work of **Louis Pasteur** in France and then **Robert Koch** in Germany. "Contagious" diseases came to be understood as being caused by "germs" via the process of person-to-person "infection"; they did not arise by themselves from miasmatic emanations. The retreat of cholera in England in the later decades of the nineteenth century, as both public sanitation and domestic hygiene improved, gave good corroboration to this ground-breaking theory—a theory that, during the twentieth century, would reshape much thinking, research, and practice within a new "biomedical" frame that would bring more reductionistic insights and perspectives to the study of causation and prevention of infectious diseases.

Food Production and Processing.   As the twentieth century unfolded, other aspects of industrialization also began to affect patterns of infectious diseases. In particular, there have been many, and continuing, unexpected consequences of the intensification of food production methods.

The commercialization of poultry production in much of Southeast Asia appears to have contributed to the amplification of the spread, during 2004–2007, of the highly pathogenic H5N1 strain of **avian flu** ("bird flu"). This strain has killed, or prompted owners or authorities to kill, many millions of birds, both wild and domestic. By 2007 it had also infected more than 300 humans, with approximately 200 fatal cases, two-thirds of which were in Vietnam and Indonesia. The actual origin of the new strains of influenza is thought to lie in the small-hold farming practices of southern China and adjoining countries, but the opportunities for wider spread and for zoonotic transmission to humans are multiplied via the industrial-scale production of poultry for urban food markets.

The most notorious and exotic of zoonotic diseases occurred late in the twentieth century in the United Kingdom, when the nation's "mad cow disease" disaster spilled over into the human population. This disastrous episode arose from the unnatural practice (introduced to accelerate productivity of dairy cattle and growth of beef cattle) of feeding cattle with industrially-treated proteinaceous and energy dense "bovine offal"—scraps of recycled meat, fat, gristle, and offal from slaughtered cattle. This resulted in the surprise occurrence of a "prion" disease that affected the bovine brain. The prion molecule, a type of rogue protein molecule, has the unusual capacity to "multiply" by inducing normal protein molecules in the brain to undergo copy-cat molecular deformation. This caused cow "madness"—bovine spongiform encephalopathy (BSE)—by rendering the brain tissue spongy. Subsequently, and somewhat against expectations, prions were transmitted to human consumers of beef products in the United Kingdom and caused over 150 fatal cases of a degenerative brain disease called variant Creutzfeldt-Jakob disease (vCJD).

Less exotically, the reported rates of infectious food poisoning have increased markedly in Western countries during the past two decades. Several outbreaks of the potentially lethal toxin-producing *Escherichia coli* 0157 in North America and Europe in the mid-1990s originated in contaminated beef imported from infected cattle in Latin America. Inevitably, in an industrial era, in light of the modern scale of food production and the length of commercial supply lines from source to consumer, there are frequent outbreaks of gastroenteritis (food poisoning) as a result of faults or mishaps in the production and distribution of processed foods.

Concomitants of Industrialization: Infectious Disease Risks from Urbanization; Medical Technologies; Antimicrobial Resistance.   The industrial age has entailed the rapid growth of cities as the engines of the modern economy, along with the evolution of a range of new technologies—for transport, workplace automation, health-care facilities, and other purposes. Cities have been described as "highways for microbial traffic." The relevant features extend beyond the obvious influences of large numbers and crowding upon risks of infection. Urban living also typically entails a loosening of traditional family and social structures, and it allows a greater personal mobility with extended social networks. These features, along with access to modern contraception, have facilitated a diversification of sexual contacts and practices and, hence, the spread of sexually-transmitted infectious diseases (STDs). Around the world, the familiar STDs, **gonorrhea** and **syphilis**, persist widely. In many cities they are increasingly supplemented by chlamydia, herpes viral infections, and now **HIV/AIDS**. Sadly, the growth in sex tourism in today's increasingly interconnected and mobile world—a form of tourism that capitalizes in an exploitative fashion on the desperation of migration and **poverty**—amplifies the risk of STD **transmission** in many of today's developing countries. Cities are also the epicenters of the international drug trade and of illicit drug use. Intravenous drug injection has become a major source of spread of infection, including HIV/AIDS and **hepatitis** B.

The discovery of natural **antibiotic** substances in the mid-twentieth century spawned a new era of infectious disease control and a rapidly growing enterprise for the **pharmaceutical industry**. Some evidence of the evolution of bacterial resistance to **penicillin** appeared within a decade of its generalized use in health care. Nevertheless, the range and use of antimicrobials increased rapidly over the next few decades, not just to treat infectious diseases in humans, but also for enhancing the growth of livestock (including, more recently, aquaculture). This increasingly widespread use of antimicrobials has resulted in a serious spread of antimicrobial resistance, entailing threats of localized outbreaks of **hospital**-based "epidemics" of resistant strains of bacterial infections. Over two-thirds of the bacteria that cause hospital-acquired infections are now resistant to one or more of the usual antibiotics used to treat them.

Other modern medical technologies have also facilitated the spread of infectious disease agents. The unhygienic use of hypodermic needles for therapeutic injection can be one vehicle for transmission. Indeed, within the past decade there has been a tragic episode of widespread hepatitis C dissemination in Egypt as a result of the unhygienic use of needles used for a campaign to control of bilharzia (**schistosomiasis**). Blood transfusion and organ transplantation also pose risks of infectious agent transmission. This furthermore raises the worrying prospect of the possible future entry into humans of occult (hidden) **viruses** via xenotransplantation—that is, organ transplants for humans from genetically bred pigs that naturally harbor a range of viruses.

Meanwhile, industrialization has conferred various benefits for the reduction of infectious disease risks in the health-care setting. Modern autoclaves and sterilizing procedures provide a far higher level of cleanliness in hospitals and clinical settings. Industrial production of medical instruments, diagnostic tools, and other hardware has provided practitioners around the world the highest quality of equipment in history. Likewise, reliance on handcrafted pharmaceuticals has been superseded by their production under standardized and quality-controlled conditions, making them more affordable, safer, and longer lasting. The provision of drugs and the means of administering them in large and reliable quantities made the **eradication** of smallpox and the elimination of **polio** in the United States possible, and they hold the promise of reducing and perhaps eradicating other infectious diseases. *See also* Animal Diseases (Zoonoses) and Epidemic Disease; Capitalism and Epidemic Disease; Colonialism and Epidemic Disease; Drug Resistance in Microorganisms; Pesticides; Poliomyelitis, Campaign Against; Public Health Agencies, U.S. Federal; Sanitation Movement of the Nineteenth Century; Smallpox Eradication; Tuberculosis and Romanticism; Vaccination and Inoculation; Venereal Disease and Social Reform in Progressive-Era America.

Further Reading

Dubos, Rene, and Jeanne Dubos. *The White Plague*. Boston: Little Brown and Company, 1952.

Johnson, Steven. *The Ghost Map: The Story of London's Most Terrifying Epidemic—and How it Changed Science, Cities and the Modern World*. New York: Riverhead Books, 2006.

McMichael, Anthony. *Human Frontiers, Environments and Disease: Past Patterns, Uncertain Futures*. New York: Cambridge University Press, 2001.

Porter, Dorothy. *Health, Civilization and the State: A History of Public Health from Ancient to Modern Times*. New York: Routledge, 1999.

Schwartz, Maxime. *How the Cows Turned Mad: Unlocking the Mysteries of Mad Cow Disease*. Translated by Edward Schneider. Berkeley: University of California Press, 2004.

Walters, Mark J. *Six Modern Plagues, and How We Are Causing Them*. Washington, DC: Island Press, 2003.

ANTHONY MCMICHAEL

INDUSTRIAL REVOLUTION.   Industrial revolution is the transformation from agrarian societies to industrialized market economies geared towards **capitalism** and profit making, which implies large-scale production in factories on the basis of new technologies. The origins of the modern Industrial Revolution can be traced back to seventeenth-century Europe, but major modifications of many aspects of life were not felt until the late eighteenth century.

Industrialization is an ongoing process rather than a singular event that triggered subsequent changes. In the Western world three waves of **industrialization** that constituted the Industrial Revolution may be identified: A first wave started with mechanization of eighteenth-century British textile manufacture. It spread to continental Europe and North America. Innovations in that early period included the invention of the steam engine in 1690 and improvements to the weaver's loom with the result that more linen or cotton cloths could be produced with less human power. A second wave occurred in the mid-nineteenth century with the advent of large-scale steel production, railroads, steamboats, and steamships, which also promoted a transportation revolution. The introduction of the Bessemer process for steel making in the1850s and new furnaces in the 1870s allowed the inexpensive and efficient production of a previously rare and precious product. A third wave of industrialization set in after World War II (1939–1945), spreading older and innovative industrial organization and processes that affected the whole world. Yet the Industrial Revolution had been an international phenomenon from the beginning, as the mechanized production process depended on functioning trade relations with countries all over the world from which raw materials were procured and to which products were sold.

From the beginning there existed an awareness of health hazards for human beings in the new production processes. In 1700 the Italian professor of medicine, Bernardino Ramazzini (1633–1714), published a book on the influences of particular trades on health, which was quickly translated into English. England pioneered in showing early concern about the "Sanitary Condition of the Laboring Classes," as indicated by **Edwin Chadwick's** 1842 report with that title. A few years earlier, the English **physician** Charles Turner Thackrah (1795–1833) had examined death rates in certain trades in Leeds. In the nineteenth century, a general concern with health problems as a consequence of **environmental** and living conditions—including **air** pollution, inadequate sewage disposal, tainted **water** supplies, poor ventilation, and crowded quarters—particularly in urban areas, also led to a growing interest in occupational diseases.

The combination of demand for labor in the new factories and improved infrastructure resulted in the migration of people from smaller communities to industrial centers. It also meant increasing emigration from Europe to America. The new means of transportation sometimes had positive effects. For example, the replacement in the mid-nineteenth century of sailing vessels with steamships not only shortened transatlantic crossings, but it also meant that travelers no longer had to wait for a suitable wind in unhygienic conditions that might expose them to new diseases. Then again, the increasing mobility also brought the danger of importing diseases: when immigrants arrived at U.S. ports such as Ellis Island in New York they were subjected to health examinations, and a considerable percentage were returned to their home countries.

Because industrial production was geared towards making profit, the health and safety of workers were of minor concern to factory owners, particularly because the causes of infectious diseases were unknown until the late nineteenth century. Workers labored in steel plants under harsh conditions twelve hours a day. Heat, fumes, and physically exhausting work provided numerous health hazards that resulted in greater susceptibility to disease and short life expectancies. Often urban families took boarders into their already crowded living quarters to supplement their income. Hence, in the industrial centers, overcrowded, ill-ventilated, and unsanitary living and working conditions favored the spreading of infectious diseases such as **tuberculosis, typhoid,** and **cholera**, which in early modern times had replaced the **epidemic** scourges of the Middle Ages.

Industrial or occupational medicine developed in the context of **industrialization** and discoveries in medical science in the late nineteenth century. For instance, the awareness of microorganisms that caused and spread disease led a new generation of middle-class people to educate the working class about sanitary living conditions and healthy nutrition.

Starting with Toynbee Hall in a slum in East London in 1884, college and university graduates initiated the settlement house movement. It soon became an opportunity for women to enter the professional sphere as social workers. The best-known institution in the United States was Hull House in Chicago. One of the residents was Alice Hamilton (1869–1970), a physician and pioneer of industrial medicine. Studying typhoid fever in Chicago around 1900, Hamilton pointed out the connection between disease and sanitation and called for public health reforms. In 1919 she became the first woman to earn professor rank at Harvard University.

However, with the development of bacteriology in the late nineteenth century, the focus of attention shifted to **germ theory of disease** and its implications for public health. For example, researchers studied pulmonary ailments that were caused and transmitted by germs in dusty air. Other causes for occupational diseases were regarded as less significant in the general excitement over the discovery of microorganisms. Still, infectious diseases such as cholera had declined in the Western world by the middle of the twentieth century. This decline was the result of new realizations, for example, that water containing germs caused the disease, and thus proper sewage would prevent spreading of the disease. Yet in the new and more hygienic surroundings, in which mild, routine childhood exposure to certain germs was greatly reduced, "cleanliness diseases" such as epidemic **poliomyelitis** emerged. *See also* Hospitals in the West to 1900; Pesticides; Pharmaceutical Industry; Poverty, Wealth, and Epidemic Disease; Trade, Travel, and Epidemic Disease; Urbanization and Epidemic Disease.

Further Reading

Grob, Gerald N. *The Deadly Truth: A History of Disease in America*. Cambridge, MA: Harvard University Press, 2002.

Hillstrom, Kevin, and Laurie Collier. *The Industrial Revolution in America*, 9 vols. Santa Barbara: ABC-CLIO, 2005.

Stearns, Peter. *The Industrial Revolution in World History*, 2nd edition. Boulder, CO: Westview Press, 1998.

ANJA BECKER

INFANTILE PARALYSIS.   *See* Poliomyelitis.

INFLUENZA.   In humans, influenza is a potentially lethal respiratory illness caused by a large number of closely related **viruses** of the family Orthomyxoviridae, whose genetic material is RNA (ribonucleic acid). Influenza viruses can infect birds as well as humans and other mammals. Influenza viruses evolve rapidly, resulting in new outbreaks of disease on a regular basis. Depending on the strain of the virus and the host species, influenza infections range from the benign to the highly communicable and pathogenic. There are three major categories of influenza viruses: A, B, and C. In humans, all three viruses can cause respiratory illness. Type C influenza can infect humans and swine; type B infects only humans; and type A can infect humans, swine, and other mammals, but is endemic in both domestic and wild birds. Type A influenza viruses also mutate much more rapidly than do types B and C. Because they evolve rapidly and are capable of cross-infecting different species, type A influenza viruses are responsible for new and highly contagious forms of the disease and are therefore of great significance from the perspective of public health and **epidemic** disease.

In birds, influenza ordinarily infects the gastrointestinal system, but in humans and other mammals it infects the respiratory system, making it very transmissible via coughing and sneezing. The disease incubates for approximately one to five days after exposure and may be transmitted before recognizable symptoms are apparent, making it one of the most contagious human diseases known. In this form, influenza often resembles a very severe cold. Symptoms include fever, sore throat, coughing/sneezing, and muscle aches but can also include headache, dizziness, vomiting, and diarrhea. It is therefore very difficult to diagnose influenza by symptoms alone.

Influenza often is not a direct cause of death but instead tends to encourage secondary **bacterial** infections by destroying the cells that line the nose, throat, and lungs and by weakening the immune system. These bacterial infections can lead to pneumonia, which is very often the direct cause of death during influenza outbreaks. Influenza death via secondary bacterial infection is most common in those in poor health or with weak immune systems; thus, the victims in most flu epidemics tend to be the very young and the elderly. In rarer cases, the virus can trigger an excessive immune system response, comparable to an allergic response, which causes massive damage to the lungs. Known as acute respiratory distress syndrome (ARDS), this condition can very quickly lead to death. In contrast to bacterial pneumonia, this condition occurs most often in relatively young people with strong immune systems. Influenza is seasonal, affecting the greatest number of people during the winter months. According to the **Centers for Disease Control and Prevention**, a typical flu season in the United States results in the hospitalization of approximately 200,000 people, of whom about 38,000 die. Between 1 and 1.5 million people worldwide die of the disease on an annual basis.

Structure.   Viewed under very high magnification, the influenza virus resembles a spike-covered ball. The ball contains the viral RNA, which occurs in eight segments that are analogous to chromosomes in higher organisms. These eight segments produce a total of nine proteins, some of which structure the virus and some of which copy the viral RNA once in a host cell. The most common "spikes" on the surface of the virus are made of a protein called hemagglutinin (H). This protein allows the virus to attach itself to, and then enter, cells of the host organism. The other protein "spike" on the surface of the virus is neuraminidase (N). This protein is responsible for allowing newly created viral particles to break free from the surface of their host cells. These two proteins serve as the primary antigens by which the immune system of the host organism recognizes the virus. Currently 16 different strains of hemagglutinin proteins and 9 different strains of neuraminidase proteins have been identified.

The number of these two surface proteins provides a general naming system for flu viruses. For example, the virus that caused the devastating **influenza pandemic of 1918–1919** was covered with hemagglutinin 1 and neuraminidase 1 proteins, and is therefore known as H1N1. Avian influenza, which is currently a major public health concern, has the hemagglutinin 5 protein and is therefore H5N1. Historically, humans have been most susceptible to viruses with the H1, H2, and H3 antigens, whereas all 16 types are capable of infecting birds. There can also be significant variation within each type of viral surface protein, so in addition to the 144 major strains of influenza (16 H types x 9 N types yields 144 possible different HN combinations) there are hundreds of sub-strains. For example, a recent survey of influenza types among domestic birds in Guangdong province of China revealed more than 500 different strains of the virus, including 53 subtypes of the H9 strain. Among research and medical professionals, a more precise naming system is used to account for these sub-strains.

Mutability and Variation.   The enormous number of influenza strains and sub-strains results from the extraordinary mutability of the virus, which ensures that novel forms and combinations of the HN surface proteins (antigens) emerge year after year. Two properties of the influenza virus account for this variation. The first is "antigenic drift," which results from imperfect copying of the virus's RNA genome. Influenza RNA is a single-stranded molecule, unlike DNA, which has two complementary strands, and therefore two copies of the information contained with the genetic sequence. This allows the cellular machinery to check one copy against the other and make corrections where necessary, resulting in very accurate copying of the genetic message. Organisms with single-stranded RNA genomes have no such mechanism for correction, and consequently the copying of their genetic messages during replication is much more error prone. In fact, relatively few of the copies made of an influenza virus will have the exact same genetic sequence, which has led researchers to think not in terms of populations of identical viruses, but instead in terms of swarms of closely related, but different, viral copies. Any of these copying errors has the potential to lead to a viable mutant sub-strain of virus slightly different from the parent strain. When such changes occur in the surface proteins of the virus, the immune system of the host organism may have a difficult time recognizing the new antigens, and the process of antigenic drift has taken place. This genetic variation drives influenza virus evolution at an extraordinarily accelerated rate—the virus evolves approximately 1 million times faster than the DNA-based life forms it infects.

Genetic reassortment is the second process that drives influenza mutation by splicing together genes from different influenza viruses, leading to the phenomenon known as "antigenic shift." Genetic reassortment results from the coinfection of a host cell by more than one strain of influenza virus. During the process of copying and assembly of the viral components, there is sometimes an intermingling or reassortment of the eight RNA segments from the different viruses. When this happens, a new strain of hybrid virus can result. Such hybrids possess features of both "parent" viruses, but in a novel combination. Since viruses from different species can coinfect the same cell, reassortment offers the possibility for new strains of virus to cross the biological barrier between species. Reassortment is therefore capable of producing dramatically new populations of viruses in a short time. Thus, for many years researchers believed that reassortment/antigenic shift was responsible for all new epidemic forms of the disease, but recent research has shown that this is not accurate. In 2005 researchers working on the virus responsible for the global influenza pandemic of 1918–1919 demonstrated that it gained its virulence via simple genetic mutations (antigenic drift) instead of reassortment and recombination of human and bird influenza genes (antigenic shift).

History.   The rapid emergence of new strains of influenza virus enables the disease to reoccur on a yearly basis. In most years, the new strains of virus that infect human populations are not especially virulent, making the annual flu season somewhat manageable and predictable. However, extremely lethal strains also emerge regularly, albeit unpredictably. These strains result in global pandemics whose consequences dwarf those of the regular flu season. The most devastating pandemic in history was the 1918–1919 flu pandemic that probably killed 50 million or more people in about a year, 675,000 of them in the United States. Inaccurately remembered as the Spanish flu, the origins of this strain are not yet certain, although recent research suggests that it may have emerged at Army bases in the United States. It spread rapidly thanks to its own infectivity as well as the movement of soldiers and populations accompanying the end of World War I (1914–1918). The virus was a strain of the H1N1 type and was unique in that it killed a large percentage of its victims directly via ARDS. Public health services in developed countries, which to that point had been making dramatic progress in the reduction of infectious disease, were helpless. They did not have the technical ability to isolate and identify viral pathogens, and the presence of secondary bacterial infections in the lungs of some (but not all) of the victims confounded the efforts of physicians to attribute the pandemic to a single causal agent. The virus was not identified until the early 1930s, and it was not until the post–World War II era that the mechanism of viral infection began to be unraveled. There have been two major global pandemics since 1918: the "Asian" or "Chinese Flu" (H2N2) of 1957–1958, which killed approximately 2 million people globally, and the "Hong Kong Flu" (H3N2) of 1968–1969, which killed about 1 million people.

In early 1976, David Lewis, a healthy 18-year-old private in the U.S. Army, died of influenza after an all-night training hike through winter weather. By February, public health officials were convinced that the strain that killed Lewis was very similar to the 1918 strain. Fearing a repeat of that pandemic, they convinced President Gerald Ford (1913–2006) to launch a costly and much-publicized program to vaccinate all Americans against this strain. Because new strains of influenza typically originate in their bird hosts and cross the species barrier to humans using pigs as intermediaries, the strain was identified in pigs and became popularly known as "Swine Flu." The vaccine program was delayed by the reluctance of the insurance industry to underwrite it. By the time that trials of the new vaccine began in late summer, no new cases of the disease had been reported. The trials demonstrated that the vaccine was effective in adults but less so in children, raising concerns about its overall effectiveness. By the end of the year no further cases of the flu had emerged, but in a small number of patients the vaccine had contributed to the development of Guillain-Barré syndrome, a neurological condition that is potentially fatal. That December the **vaccination** program was ended, having become a public relations catastrophe for the presidency as well as for leading public health officials.

Treatment.   As with all viral diseases, there is no effective **antibiotic** treatment for influenza, although there is currently an effective class of antiviral agents called neuraminidase inhibitors that can reduce influenza symptoms if taken after infection and may reduce likelihood of infection if taken as a preventative measure. The most commonly available is oseltamivir, available commercially as Tamiflu. The most effective route for combating influenza remains vaccination. Each year researchers must gauge which new influenza strains are most likely to infect humans; to do this they analyze strains that have already moved into swine populations, as these are the most likely to make the jump to humans. It takes several months to develop, test, and market a new vaccine. To ensure maximum efficiency, the annual flu vaccine is designed to confer **immunity** against the three most likely flu strains.

Avian Influenza.   In 1997 the H5N1 strain of influenza began to receive widespread attention when it led to an unusually destructive disease in its bird hosts. It quickly became known as avian influenza, or "bird flu" for short. The virus was able to spread to humans where it also was very lethal—in this first outbreak, 18 human cases were documented, of which 6 led to death. Several sub-strains of the virus have caused subsequent outbreaks among birds and humans. As of August 2006, over 220 million birds had been either killed by the virus or deliberately slaughtered by people to end localized outbreaks. As of April 2007, there had been 291 laboratory-documented cases of H5N1 in human beings in 12 different countries; 172 of these cases (59 percent) have been fatal. This is an

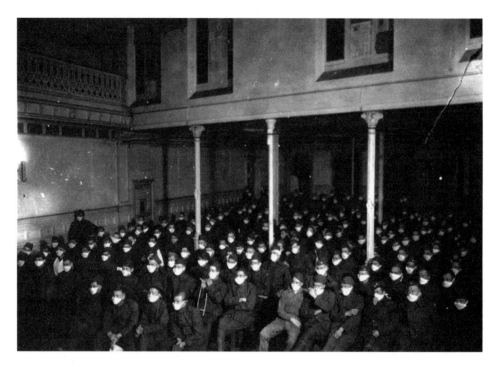

U.S. Army Hospital Number 30, Royat, France. Patients at moving-picture show wear masks because of an influenza epidemic, 1918. Courtesy of the National Library of Medicine.

exceptionally high mortality rate for human influenza, exceeding by far that of the 1918 pandemic strain. The virus has not yet demonstrated the ability to be transmitted easily from person to person, although one case has been documented. Should the virus evolve in such a manner that it becomes easily communicable among people, it would become a public health threat of the highest order. Currently, it is impossible to predict when or if such a change in the virus might take place.

Future Research.   There are many questions about influenza waiting to be answered. Understanding the relationship between the surface antigens and human disease, especially their role in transmission, is of great importance, as it may allow us to better anticipate the emergence of dangerous sub-strains. There is also a great deal of current research on new types of anti-viral drugs. Relying on one class of anti-viral drugs, the neuraminidase inhibitors, is risky as it is very likely that resistant forms of the virus will emerge. Finally, much attention is being paid to vaccine research. Here research is split between developing new vaccines and new processes for manufacturing vaccines. The goal is ultimately to develop vaccines that can be produced very quickly and can confer immunity against a range of potential viral sub-strains. *See also* Drug Resistance in Microorganisms; Influenza Pandemic, 1889–1890; Influenza Pandemic, 1918–1919; Severe Acute Respiratory Syndrome (SARS).

Further Reading

Barry, John. *The Great Influenza: The Story of the Greatest Pandemic in History*. New York: Viking, 2004.

Crosby, Alfred. *America's Forgotten Pandemic: The Influenza of 1918*, Revised First Edition. New York: Cambridge University Press, 2003.

Davies, Pete. *The Devil's Flu: The World's Deadliest Influenza Epidemic and the Scientific Hunt for the Virus That Caused It*. New York: Henry Holt, 2000.

Davis, Mike. *The Monster at Our Door: The Global Threat of Avian Flu*. First Edition, Revised and Expanded. New York: Owl Books, 2006.

Emmeluth, Donald. *Influenza*. Philadelphia: Chelsea House, 2003.

Kolata, Gina. *Flu: The Story of the Great Infuenza Pandemic of 1918 and the Search for the Virus that Caused It*. New York: Touchstone, 1999.

Monto, Arnold S. *Contemporary Diagnosis, Prevention, and Management of Influenza*. Newtown, PA: Associates in Medical Marketing Company, 2002.

Morse, Stephen, ed. *Emerging Viruses*. New York: Oxford University Press, 1993.

Potter, C. W. *Influenza*. Amsterdam: Elsevier, 2002.

Radetsky, Peter. *The Invisible Invaders: The Story of the Emerging Age of Viruses*. Boston: Little, Brown, 1991.

Silverstein, Arthur. *Pure Politics and Impure Science: The Swine Flu Affair*. Baltimore: Johns Hopkins University Press, 1981.

JEFFREY LEWIS

INFLUENZA PANDEMIC, 1889–1890.   During the summer of 1889, a severe **influenza epidemic** was reported in the Russian Empire's impoverished central Asian city of Bukhara (in modern Uzbekistan), to which destination Russia had just completed 900 miles of the Trans-Caspian Railroad. The associated high mortality of 5 to 8.75 percent (the norm is around 2 percent) suggests that if flu was involved, there may have been a coexisting disease such as **malaria**. Other sources give the **pandemic**'s origin as western Siberia and northern Kazakhstan. By October the illness had traveled to Moscow and St Petersburg and thence into Poland, as well as along the highways, railroads, and rivers into Finland, Hungary, southern Russia, Germany, and Austria. In Western Europe it was named "Russian flu," but the Russians believed it was a **miasma** that had been wafted on pestilential breezes into the Empire from China, following the flooding, in 1888, of the Yellow River (Huang He), in which up to 2 million humans and animals were drowned. They called it the "Chinese cold." A popular French theory maintained that the Chinese cold was transformed into influenza by Russian peasants living in filth and squalor.

The citizens of Paris, London, and Edinburgh were laid low with flu by the end of October and into March the following year. Steamship traffic carried influenza across the Atlantic to the United States where, by mid-December 1889, it was reported in New York and Boston. By January it had crossed the Midwest and entered Canada. Simultaneously, it passed through the Mediterranean into North Africa, and via Atlantic and Pacific seaports (dock workers were often its first victims) into South Africa, South America, Japan, the west coast of the United States (January), China via Hong Kong, Singapore (February), India, Australia, New Zealand, and Indonesia (March). The secretary of the Illinois State Board of Health observed that in just three months influenza had encompassed the globe, whereas in 1843, just prior to the railroad and steamship age, its journey to and through the United States had taken six months. There were exceptions. Remote Kashmir was not affected until December 1890. Similarly, influenza's progress along the circuitous **trade** routes of central Africa was slow, and it eventually reached British Nyasaland (Malawi) in September 1890. To black Africans, who claimed never to have experienced influenza, it was a disease of white colonization. Indeed, **colonialism** and globalizing trade links increased the volume and speed of international communications and therefore its spread. Throughout the world, the pattern of transmission was generally from large cities to small towns and thence into rural districts.

Most reports suggest that the largest group affected by influenza were those aged 15 to 40 years, followed by the elderly, who had perhaps gained some immunity from the pandemics of the 1840s but were in any case less socially active, and then children and infants. Most deaths, however, were among the elderly.

In Europe, the 1889–1890 influenza was the greatest single killer epidemic of the nineteenth century, claiming 270,000 to 360,000 lives, although the overall mortality rate was only 1 percent. In Britain, influenza interrupted the decline in adult deaths from infectious diseases that had for a generation accompanied rising living standards and sanitation reform. Deaths in London from **whooping cough**, pulmonary **tuberculosis**, bronchitis, **diphtheria, typhoid**, and **measles** were higher during 1889–1890 than the previous ten-year average, suggesting that influenza lowered resistance to other infections. Nevertheless, influenza killed by far a smaller percentage of Londoners (0.5 per 1,000) than Parisians (2.5 per 1,000) or the people of Lisbon (1.6 per 1,000). Influenza was also considered to be a major cause of nervous and **psychological** disorders by acting as a "devitalizing agent." Descriptions of influenza sequelae included "depression," "shattered nerves," "neurasthenia," and "despondency." During 1890, for example, an unprecedented 140 melancholics afflicted with influenza "poison" were admitted to Scotland's Royal Edinburgh Asylum. Coroners also cited influenza as a reason for "temporary insanity" in cases of suicide. Across Europe, rates of suicide (mostly male) and attempted suicide (mostly female) rose during the 1890s. In England and Wales, there was a 25 percent increase in suicides between 1889 and 1893. Paris witnessed a 23 percent rise during 1889–1890 compared with the average, and there were also increased rates in Germany and Switzerland.

The pandemic disrupted manufacturing, public services, and transport as workers fell sick simultaneously (the incubation period is one to four days). In Massachusetts, about 27 percent of the workforce in affected establishments was absent for an average of five days per employee. In London, during the Christmas mail rush, 1,346 post office workers (about 15 percent) went sick for an average of 15 days each. Two died. Next door to the city's main post office was St. Bartholomew's Hospital, which treated about 25 flu victims during the outpatient hour every working day throughout January and February. Winter sickness rates among the London Metropolitan Police were four times higher than usual, with 1,660 out of 14,000 (12 percent) succumbing to influenza in January alone. Even British Prime Minister Lord Salisbury (1830–1903) took to his bed. Among the eminent individuals who died of flu were the poets Robert Browning (1812–1889) and Alfred Lord Tennyson (1809–1892), and Queen Victoria's (1819–1901) grandson, the Duke of Clarence (1864–1892). Post-influenza lassitude left many people unfit for work, and in an unprecedented move, Pope Leo XIII (1810–1903) granted a dispensation in the matter of abstinence to people suffering from flu during the Church's penitential season of Lent. Sick pay for British workers was not universal, and those who were not covered or who were inadequately covered by insurance were often unable to pay their doctors' fees. Indeed, local benefits clubs sometimes collapsed under the payouts for influenza and associated illnesses. Financial problems were enough to induce feelings of despair in poor and middling workers even if suicide was not actually contemplated.

Physicians used the word "**virus**" to explain the immediate cause of influenza, although only in the sense of its being a hypothetical pathogenic microorganism. Many combined the new Pasteurian **germ theory** with traditional ideas about **contagion**, miasmas, constitutional disturbance, atmospheric influences, and local **environmental** conditions. A typical viewpoint, suggested by the physician to the Edinburgh Royal Infirmary, was that the influenza microorganism existed in all parts of the world but only under certain conditions did it become sufficiently active to cause severe symptoms in humans and animals. Like other doctors in the northern hemisphere, he commented on the unseasonably warm winter of 1889–1890, although influenza prevailed independently of season, climate, and weather, appearing in the cold of Russia and the heat of India. Others invoked high and low pressure atmospheric gradients, varying ozone levels, electrical storms, recent earthquakes, and volcanic eruptions across Europe, the United States, and the Pacific as material energizers of dormant germs, spores, or atmospheric "fomites." Once the germs had been activated, according to these theories, they turned contagious and infectious and were able to pass from host to host in the usual way. Less plausible ideas about comets and meteors carrying poisonous gases from outer space nevertheless appeared in medical literature as well as the popular media.

Some military and naval surgeons believed that influenza was the tropical disease called **Dengue** or breakbone fever, modified by climate. The symptoms of aching joints and limbs were similar, and those who had suffered Dengue in the past believed they were experiencing relapses. The concept of vector-borne transmission, influenced by the recent work of **Patrick Manson** on mosquitoes, nematode worms, and elephantiasis, was proven immaterial in areas where higher than normal levels of **insects** were observed or where crop yields were poor, indicating infestation. Migrating birds were also proposed as carriers of the influenza agent, and in some locales there were excess deaths among fowls, cage birds, cats, dogs, and particularly horses. Epidemics of equine ("horse"; type A) influenza or "pink-eye," a frequently fatal respiratory disease in horses, were observed during the early 1890s in Glasgow, Lisbon, and Warsaw, and there was a severe outbreak in St Petersburg in 1889, preceding the influenza. A century later, in 1989–1990, horses in northeast China were stricken with a similar respiratory disease. Mortality in some herds reached 20 percent. The causative virus was classified as an influenza H3N8 subtype that originated in birds.

Medical opinion, in general, was converted during the course of the 1889–1890 pandemic from a belief in the miasmatic origin of influenza to its being a communicable disease. The German bacteriologist Richard Pfeiffer (1858–1945; **Robert Koch**'s son-in-law) announced in 1890 his discovery of the influenza organism although attempts at replicating flu symptoms with "Pfeiffer's bacillus," and at producing an anti-flu serum, proved unsatisfactory. Nevertheless, "Pfeiffer's bacillus" was still being discussed in the bacteriology literature of the 1920s. It subsequently proved to be *Haemophilus influenzae*, a bacterium implicated in some of influenza's secondary infections. Proof of the viral nature of influenza did not occur until the development of the electron microscope in the 1930s.

Most physicians understood that the pandemic influenza of 1889–1890 was more virulent than ordinary sporadic influenza but that there were no specific treatments to shorten its duration. Bed rest, antipyretics, purgatives, and bland food were the usual recommendations. A plethora of patent remedies, preventives, and fortifying tonics appeared

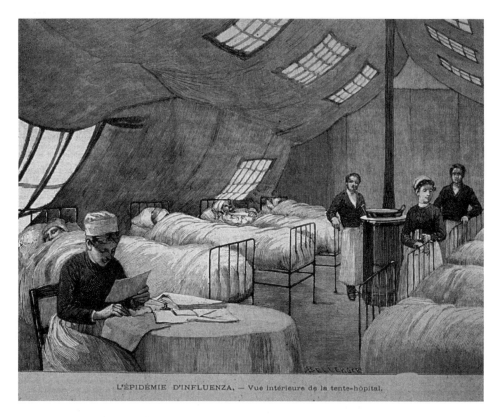

L'ÉPIDÉMIE D'INFLUENZA. — Vue intérieure de la tente-hôpital.

Interior view of a supplemental tent hospital during the 1889 influenza pandemic, showing a nurse sitting at a table, several beds with patients, and nurses standing near a stove. Illustration from *L'Illustration,* January 4, 1890. Courtesy of the National Library of Medicine.

on grocery and pharmacy shelves, and it is likely that many sufferers resorted to these rather than consulting a doctor. Public opinion was against enforced **quarantine**, which was seen as official meddling with everyday business to contain what most regarded as a minor illness. In Edinburgh, where an isolation hospital *was* provided, not a single patient was admitted throughout the epidemic. Edinburgh physicians were disappointed at being denied an opportunity to study the disease, particularly because a scientific committee appointed by the Royal College of Physicians had been established for this purpose. The pandemic was extremely well documented worldwide, with many countries publishing detailed studies of their experiences. Maps and statistical tables were compiled, and this reflected the growing preoccupation of nations with their own vital statistics. Moreover, the growth of scientific medicine had resulted in the increasing publication of medical journals, which encouraged the reporting and international dissemination of such studies.

Influenza epidemics occurred in many countries during much of the decade following the 1889–1890 pandemic and were often associated with higher mortality than the initial pandemic. For example, the Irish death rate at 19.4 per 1,000 during the 1892 wave was the highest since registration began in 1864. Excess mortality in Chicago rose from

1,200 in 1890 to 2,000 the following year. In the northern English town of Sheffield, fewer than 5 people died of flu during one week in March 1890 compared with over 100 during the same week in 1891. This suggests that minor viral mutations ("drift") of the pandemic strain continued to circulate around the world. *See also* Animal Diseases (Zoonoses) and Epidemic Disease; Demographic Data Collection and Analysis, History of; Human Immunity and Resistance to Disease; Influenza Pandemic, 1918–1919; Public Health Boards in the West before 1900.

Further Reading

Crosby, Alfred W. *America's Forgotten Pandemic: The Influenza of 1918.* Cambridge: Cambridge University Press, 2003.

Patterson, David K. *Pandemic Influenza, 1700–1900: A Study in Historical Epidemiology.* Totowa, NJ: Rowman & Littlefield, 1986.

Smith, F. B. "The Russian Influenza in the United Kingdom, 1889–94." *Social History of Medicine* 8 (1995): 55–73.

Wolfe, Robert J. "Alaska's Great Sickness, 1900: An Epidemic of Measles and Influenza in a Virgin Soil's Population." *Proceedings of the American Philosophical Society* 126 (1982): 91–121.

CAROLE REEVES

INFLUENZA PANDEMIC, 1918–1919.   Influenza is a viral disease with a very high morbidity rate. Virulence varies from outbreak to outbreak because of the constantly shifting nature of the **virus**. Like all viruses, it reproduces itself by penetrating the cell of a host and using the host's genetic material. The influenza virus, like other RNA viruses, is particularly adept at mixing its own genetic material with the host's, reconstructing its own so that when the invaded cell bursts (the cause of being ill), large numbers of new variations are released. Most are not viable, but a few not only are but also have new biological characteristics. The result is that eventually, sometimes quickly, the human immune system no longer recognizes the virus, and the illness again gains the potential to become a pandemic. It also has the potential to be more deadly than previous variations. All the dangerous possibilities merged in 1918. The pandemic that began in the spring and produced two subsequent waves—fall 1918 and spring 1919—spread quite literally over the entire planet and, although records are at best incomplete, killed at least 40 million people.

The Influenza Pandemic of 1918 to early 1919 was a global event and cannot be accurately understood in any other context. To isolate it geographically for study is to understate its presence and impact. There was nowhere on earth that boasted even a small collection of human residents who did not suffer from influenza in 1918–1919. Although there are good local studies, there is, as yet, no satisfactory global history of the pandemic.

The death count is also less than satisfactory. The longtime common assertion of about 20 million deaths over the 46 week period of the pandemic is significantly low. That figure was usually credited to Edwin O. Jordan's 1927 study *Epidemic Influenza*, one of the first scholarly studies of the pandemic. As more was learned, it became increasingly clear that Jordan had no solid statistics for what might today be called the Third World. The illness was everywhere—explorers at the pole isolated for six months got sick. In fact, one pathologist suggests that fully half of the human race was infected. Although it is sometimes still seen, Jordan's estimate has been revised upward to the point that many now regard doubling it to be appropriate.

Even doubling the number may not be enough—though we will never actually know with any certainty. Unfortunately, records were not kept very consistently even in developed states. The Atlanta city fathers, for instance, were very concerned about the healthful image of their city. Furthermore the annual Southeastern Fair was held in October. The fair was both a money-maker and an important public relations event. Local businessmen were concerned about precautionary measures that closed places of amusement or required gauze masks (a common but actually worthless precaution) in public places. Neither they nor the city government's leaders wanted either the fair closed or attendance—normally drawn from all over the region—to be reduced by health concerns. They dealt with the situation by underreporting. Perhaps this was not as cynical and self-serving as it seems. In Atlanta the summer wave of the disease had been mild (almost nonexistent) and Grady Hospital—the Atlanta public facility—was closed to influenza patients during the fall wave as a result of the impact of the disease on its staff. Thus information about the local situation may have been obscured. Wishful thinking could have done the rest. On the other hand, the international horrors of the disease were known, and soldiers at Atlanta's Fort Gordon were suffering badly. By the first week in October, local civic groups had made 100,000 masks for the men at the fort. By the second week of the month, cases at the base had risen to 2,941. Although some precautionary closings were ordered, the fair was exempted, and city health officials, including Dr. J. P. Kennedy, founder of the Atlanta City Health Department, insisted there was no **epidemic** in Atlanta. By the middle of the month they had acknowledged only 2,500 cases and 81 deaths. Falling back on the **race** card, they also implied that the worst of what little problem there was could be found in the parts of the city populated by African Americans. Actually, African Americans did not suffer a disproportionate number of cases. By the end of the month, the City Council on the advice of Dr. Kennedy overruled the Board of Health and canceled the closing orders. The fair went on with historic success—setting an attendance record. The city failed to submit the required annual health report for 1918 to the state. A comparison of the actual official reports to an apology from the telephone company in which poor service is attributed to the number of sick operators seems to indicate that telephone operators were far and away the worst hit group in Atlanta. A different conclusion might be reached from one Atlantan's recollection that people "were dying like leaves falling off the trees."

The story of Atlanta illustrates the unreliability of records. It is safe to say that the pandemic killed more Americans than World Wars I and II, Korea, and Vietnam combined, but it is much less safe to say exactly how many more—and this confusion reigned in a relatively well-developed society with, for the day, good communications and health care and little disruption as a result of the **war**. In Europe, particularly eastern Europe, the impact of the war was enormous. In many parts of the rest of the world, there was little health care and little infrastructure for meaningful reporting of mortality let alone morbidity.

Typically influenza causes high fever, body aches, and malaise with respiratory distress in only a minority of victims. It is a relatively minor disease. The first wave—there are typically three—became obvious in June 1918. It was mild, though quite infectious, and was not much noticed until it swept through Spain, when it gained the tag "Spanish Influenza." It probably started in Central Asia with infections in swine or fowl—another typical element of influenza—though the mildness meant that it had spread too far to be very effectively tracked before it was noticed. Other theories have abounded since 1918. As noted above, some recent scholarship suggests that the key mutation and the first outbreak were at Fort Riley, Kansas, in March 1918. It appears the disease was spread by military personnel, who did, in fact, move around the country and world that spring. There are, however, also records of scattered pockets of an unusually virulent "flu" in 1917. A 1918 article in the British medical journal *The Practitioner* went so far as to blame the Germans by attributing the disease to **corpses** rotting at the bottom of the sea poisoning seafood or causing some miasma to bubble up and poison the ether. However improbable this miasmic theory is, it is not unusual for the era of the pandemic. Whatever the origin, the infection was clearly spread by wartime transport. The first wave caused some disruption. Absenteeism at defense plants rose and battle plans had to be adjusted. Both sides were hit at once, however, so neither in June 1918 nor later could any army take much advantage of the other's disability. By the end of the summer, the malady seemed to be gone.

The second wave came in the mid- to late fall. It too was highly infectious (and the degree of resistance from June attacks did not seem to be as high as might be expected), but it was much more deadly. In the fall and subsequent late winter waves, the virus had a tendency to cause lesions in sufferers' lungs, which tended to produce pneumonia. The worst cases soon showed signs of cyanosis, which almost always meant death. With the complication of pneumonia, the death rate may have reached 20 percent. Again available statistics may be inaccurate. A block study conducted by the British Ministry of Health right after the war ended showed that fewer than half of the mortal cases in England were attended by a health-care worker—even a **nurse**. Thus questions about diagnoses, symptoms, and mortality are going to remain. And how much less likely was a very sick person to see a **doctor** or nurse in Nigeria or Indochina, for instance, than even in wartime England? The third wave, early in 1919, was more like the second than the first, though it was neither as infectious nor as deadly (there appears to have been more resistance from second to third than from first to second). For most people, of course, "flu" meant 10 days of misery and then recovery, commonly with some attendant depression. The latter symptom, historian Alfred Crosby asserts, afflicted U.S. President Woodrow Wilson (1856–1924) as he tried to cope with the wily David Lloyd George (1863–1945) and Georges Clemenceau (1841–1929) at the climatic point of negotiating the Paris Peace Settlement that ended World War I.

There was another oddity about the 1918 influenza mortality. A graph of a pandemic's mortality according to age usually looks roughly like a fishhook. There is a relatively high rate of death among the very young. This declines steadily with age through about 50 and then steadily increases, peaking among the very old. Such a graph for 1918–1919 is almost exactly turned over. It shows a relatively high death rate among the very young and then a steady increase with age peaking in the mid-30s and then decreasing with age. The very elderly were surprisingly safe. In fact, the Ministry of Health's statistics indicate that an 80-year-old Englishman was less

---

A DITTY ON THE FLU (1919)

If we but knew
The cause of flu
And whence it comes and what to do,
I think that you
And we folks too
Would hardly get in such a stew
Do you?

Printed in *Indiana State Board of Health, Monthly Bulletin*, v. 22:1, January 1919, p. 5.

likely to die of influenza in 1918 than in a normal year. This pattern held throughout the world. There was some variation in the age of peak death rate, but it was always in mid-adulthood. Thus, the demographic impact of the pandemic was maximized, for the worst cases and most deaths were among those in their most productive span of years. It was complementary to the trenches, though much worse of course because the war only took about 10 million lives.

Today there is some explanation for this unusual virulence and odd age pattern of mortality. The unusual virulence of the virus caused the immune systems of youthful, strong victims to overreact. This defensive reaction caused the lungs to fill with fluid and froth, leading to death. In 1918, however, isolation of viruses was more than a decade away, and although some doctors speculated about a filter-passing organism, the disease was commonly but mistakenly blamed on Pieffer's bacillus, which was quite frequently found in those afflicted. By the time viruses could be meaningfully studied, the influenza virus had evolved to a point that the unusual symptoms were no longer found in the infected. More recently it was realized that bodies from 1918 buried in the permafrost might harbor viable examples of that era's version of the virus. In the 1980s it was felt that finding and culturing the virus was more dangerous than it was worth.

In the twenty-first century, with the ability to delineate DNA and RNA sequences, the fear of the virus has taken a backseat to the possible gains from studying it. Expeditions have been mounted to exhume bodies, isolate the virus, and study it. In 1998 scientists at the Armed Forces Institute of Pathology mapped the genetic makeup of the 1918 virus.

The people facing influenza in 1918 had little to improve their morale. Most of those infected had aches and fever that worsened, peaking in three to five days and abating in eight to ten. Patients were then urged to stay home for several extra days because of a pattern of relapses observed among those who returned to normal routines too quickly. But more dramatic cases frequently appeared. In Chicago a class of school children seemed healthy, put their heads on their desks, and were prostrate by lunch. Shoppers collapsed on the street and were dead before they reached the hospital. Fear, even terror, was the result, but there was little an individual could do.

Public health authorities took precautionary measures in many places. Authorities or owners closed gathering places—theaters, cinemas, schools, places of entertainment, and public transport systems. Masks—actually useless—were distributed. Although the disease continued to spread to every part of the planet, surely keeping people apart reduced the level of infection—if such isolation could be sustained. As in Atlanta, many local authorities did not sustain it; more commonly, people found that they had to go to work, and public transportation was their only means of doing so. Employers were not necessarily sympathetic to weeks—even unpaid weeks—off the job.

The impact of the pandemic was enormous. During the 46 weeks of its ravages, 47 percent of deaths in the United States were caused by influenza or its complications. At the Cook County Hospital in Chicago, the death rate for influenza during the pandemic was 39.8 percent. The rate for hospitalized cases in Frankfurt, Germany, was 27.3 percent. Reports from Africa indicated whole villages had been depopulated. Eskimos in Alaska also saw whole communities die. Recent estimates of deaths in India approach 20 million—long the total given for the entire planet. Although it is probable that the Black Plague of the fourteenth century killed a greater proportion of the human species, more people died in the influenza pandemic of 1918–1919 than from any other single outbreak of disease in history. **AIDS** seems virtually certain to surpass the total, but the AIDS epidemic has taken more years to do so than there were months in the 1918–1919 pandemic. *See also* Contagion and Transmission; Influenza Pandemic, 1889–1890.

Further Reading

American Experience—Influenza, 1918 [film]. PBS Home Video, 2005.

Barry, John M. *The Great Influenza: The Epic Story of the Deadliest Plague in History.* New York: Viking, 2004.

Byerly, Carol R. *Fever of War: The Influenza Epidemic in the U.S. Army during World War I.* New York: New York University Press, 2005.

Collier, Richard. *The Plague of the Spanish Lady: The Influenza Pandemic of 1918–1918.* New York: Atheneum, 1974.

Crosby, Alfred W. *America's Forgotten Pandemic: The Influenza of 1918.* New York: Cambridge University Press, 1989.

Davies, Pete. *The Devil's Flu: The World's Deadliest Influenza Epidemic and the Scientific Hunt for the Virus that Caused It.* New York: Henry Holt, 2000.

Harvard University Library. *Contagion.* http://ocp.hul.harvard.edu/contagion/influenza.html

Heaton, Matthew M. "Global Explanations versus Local Interpretations: The Historiography of the Influenza Pandemic of 1918–19 in Africa." *History in Africa* 33 (2006): 205–230.

Johnson, Niall. *Britain and the 1918–19 Pandemic: A Dark Epilogue.* London: Routledge, 2006.

Kolata, Gina. *Flu: The Story of the Great Influenza Pandemic of 1918 and the Search for the Virus that Caused It.* New York: Farrar, Straus, and Giroux, 1999.

National Museum of Health and Medicine. http://nmhm.washingtondc.museum/collections/archives/agalleries/1918flu/1918flu.html

Patterson, K. David. *Pandemic Influenza, 1700–1900: A Study in Historical Epidemiology.* Totowa, NJ: Rowman and Littlefield, 1986.

van Hartesveldt, Fred R., ed. *The 1918–1919 Pandemic of Influenza: The Urban Impact in the Western World.* Lewiston, NY: Edwin Mellin Press, 1992.

FRED R. VAN HARTESVELDT

INOCULATION.   *See* Vaccination and Inoculation.

INSECT INFESTATIONS.   Since long before historical accounts recorded them, insect infestations have had a major impact on the success of agriculture, food storage, and the human psyche. In this context the term "infestation" refers to a far higher than normal number of **insects** occurring over a wide geographic area. Examples of insect species whose infestations have severely limited food and fiber production include the flightless Mormon cricket of western North America and the desert locust of Sub-Saharan Africa, the Near East, and Southwest Asia. Some insects that appear in great numbers have a more significant impact on the human psyche than upon agriculture. Periodical cicadas, often mistakenly referred to as "locusts," emerge in eastern North America in 13- or 17-year cycles and can elicit fear and despair though they pose no threat to humans and cause little damage to native trees. Even wingless insects that also lack the ability to disperse by walking, such as bed bugs, can become significant pests. Insect species that are purposely or accidentally introduced to geographic areas to which they are not native can also reach infestation levels because they are no longer limited by their natural predators and parasites.

Desert locust (*Schistocerca gregaria*) swarms in Sub-Saharan Africa average 60 million individuals per square kilometer, often reaching as many as 10 billion individuals in a single swarm. Constituting the eighth **biblical plague** of Egypt described in Exodus 10, such swarms can cover 75 miles (120 km) per day. These insects directly compete with humans for food, often devastating crops such as peas, beans, tomatoes, and grains, and thus causing famine in their wake. The presence of locusts has also driven human migration to areas free of these insect pests. Locusts can exist in more than one form, depending on their environment. When these insects mature in areas where they have little contact with other individuals, they become "solitarius" adults, are not very restless, and have longer lives. However, when immatures grow up in an area crowded with other locusts and when other conditions such as rainfall are present, they mature into more restless, "gregarious" adults that display aggregate behavior, even when flying. This migratory, gregarious phase has the greatest impact upon human agriculture, with the bugs often stripping all vegetation in their path. Amazingly, some swarms have been carried by winds from Africa to the Caribbean and northern South America, a distance of about 3,750 miles (6,000 km). All of the transitional stages between the solitarious and gregarious phases can be seen in nature. Phase changes can occur in other species of locusts that can also reach plague proportions in many parts of the world. Among these are the Migratory locust, the Moroccan locust, the Red locust, the Australian plague locust, the Bombay locust, the Central American locust, and the South American locust.

In the United States the Mormon cricket (*Anabrus simplex*)—not a true cricket but rather a short-winged, long-horned grasshopper—can be devastating to agricultural crops. Mormon crickets do not fly like migratory locusts but move over land in vast numbers and are known to feed on at least 250 plant species. The Mormon cricket received its name in the spring of 1848 when swarms of this insect descended upon the crops of the first Mormon settlers of the Valley of the Great Salt Lake in Utah. As the story goes, great flocks of sea gulls appeared after three days of fasting and prayer and began gorging themselves on the crickets. A prominent statue commemorating the gulls is mounted in Salt Lake City's Temple Square.

The periodical cicadas (*Magicicada* spp.) of the eastern United States are among the longest-lived insects, living as nymphs underground for 13 or 17 years before emerging en masse to breed and overwhelming their predators in the process. The brightly colored, conspicuous, and noisy adults may emerge with as many as 1.5 million individuals per acre. Periodical cicadas occur in different broods with different distributions. Each brood contains three species, with the males of each brood producing a distinctive call. Rarely, a 13-year brood and a 17-year brood will emerge in the same year (in one area every 221 years) resulting in prodigious numbers of these insects. The mated females cut into tree branches to lay eggs, but this rarely damages native trees. Though they do not consume the foliage of plants, periodical cicadas are often called locusts because they occur in tremendous numbers. European settlers along the eastern coast of the United States saw their emergence as a bad omen and interpreted the dark "W" on their wings to mean that there would be an Indian war.

An example of an annoyance/nuisance insect that has reached infestation proportions is the bazaar fly of the Eastern Hemisphere. This fly prefers to rest on the heads of humans and returns immediately after being brushed away. Its increase in numbers and geographic range is thought to be the result of increases in the fly's larval habitat, dog feces, which is related to human population growth in particular areas. Another fly species that can occur in great numbers and can be annoying at times in Florida is the Lovebug (*Plecia nearctica*). The common name refers to the fact that males and females remain attached for up to three days during mating. The adult flies are a nuisance to motorists because they are attracted to highways where they splatter on the hoods and windshields of automobiles. Large numbers of lovebugs can cause overheating of liquid-cooled engines, reduce visibility, and damage automobile paint. Strangely, lovebugs were not even known to science until 1940, and it has been proposed that the ever-mounting amount of organic waste produced by the increasing human population in Florida has provided still more habitats for this fly's immature stages. The presence of wings or powerful walking legs is not essential for insects to reach infestation levels. Bed bugs possess neither, relying on humans to transport them from place to place. These human-loving, blood-feeding insects have recently reemerged as a pest in North America.

Over 200 species of insects have been introduced to the United States through **trade and travel**. Examples of insect species that have reached infestation levels since their introduction into the United States include the multicolored Asian lady beetle, the Asian tiger mosquito, the Japanese beetle, and the gypsy moth. Though a beneficial predator of aphids, adults of the multicolored Asian lady beetle (*Harmonia axyridis*) tend to aggregate in the fall on doors, windows, walls, and porches of buildings. These beetles then overwinter in wall voids from which they can emerge to invade the interior of homes in great numbers during the winter. A native of Southeast Asia, the Asian tiger mosquito (*Aedes albopictus*), was introduced to the United States in 1985 and has since spread to 26 southeastern states. It has been more successful than native container-breeding mosquitoes and is easily transported in its immature stages by the transport of discarded automobile tires. Unlike native container-breeding species, the Asian tiger mosquito aggressively bites in the daytime and can reach landing counts greater than 50 per five minute interval. The fact that this mosquito species readily utilizes human-made water-filled containers has also increased its numbers in the United States.

First discovered in the United States in 1916, Japanese beetle (*Popillia japonica*) adults are known to feed on more than 300 species of plants and are now well established in all states east of the Mississippi River except Florida. Adult Japanese beetles feed on foliage, flowers, and fruits. Leaves are typically skeletonized or left with only a tough network of veins. Japanese beetles can apparently live anywhere that there is sufficient foliage on which to feed, including the gardens of homeowners. Japanese beetles have wings and travel and feed in groups. A swarm of these beetles has been known to strip the foliage of a peach tree in as few as 15 minutes. The larvae or grubs, feeding in the soil, damage the roots of turf and pasture grasses, vegetables, nursery seedlings, and field crops. The gypsy moth (*Lymantria dispar*) is perhaps North America's most devastating forest pest. Originally introduced from France to an area near Boston, Massachusetts, in 1869, it has been spreading slowly south and west ever since. This insect gets some assistance by humans, who inadvertently transport its egg masses to previously uninfested areas. The larvae or caterpillars of the gypsy moth are known to feed on the foliage of hundreds of species of plants and can cause tree mortality (e.g., in oaks) after several successive years of defoliation. With the help of a strand of silk they produce, the larvae can "balloon" for miles to establish new infestations. Within the range of the gypsy moth, fall color enthusiasts are often disappointed because many of their favorite trees have been defoliated by this pest species.

Though many millions of dollars continue to be spent on **pesticide** research, biological control methods, and integrated pest management strategies, the infestations of insects described above will be with us for the foreseeable future.

Further Reading

Evans, Howard E. *The Pleasures of Entomology: Portraits of Insects and the People Who Study Them.* Washington, DC: Smithsonian Institution, 1985.

Kritsky, Gene. *In Ohio's Backyard: Periodical Cicadas.* Columbus: Ohio Biological Survey, 1999.

Lockwood, Jeffrey A. *Locust: The Devastating Rise and Mysterious Disappearance of the Insect That Shaped the American Frontier.* New York: Basic, 2004.

Peters, T. Michael. *Insects and Human Society.* New York: Van Nostrand Reinhold, 1988.

STEVE MURPHREE

INSECTICIDE.   *See* Pesticides.

INSECTS, OTHER ARTHROPODS, AND EPIDEMIC DISEASE.   Human beings have had to engage and interact with the world of insects from time immemorial. Insects have been held responsible for destroying food crops. They have been seen as harbingers of famine and economic disaster. In almost every part of the world, human beings have had to devote considerable energy and skill in trying to protect themselves from insects. Insects have also benefited humanity. They have often been used as sources of food and drink in certain cultures. Over time, insects have sustained a wide variety of industries: silk, wax, cochineal, shellac, and so forth.

Insects have also been considered detrimental to human life, however. They have been attributed with causing human diseases. The work of **travel** writers and natural historians has reflected such concerns for centuries. However, it was in the late nineteenth century, with the advent of medical entomology as a distinct branch of scientific knowledge, that the relationship between human diseases and insects became an area of sustained and organized academic research.

Robert Koch of Germany and **Louis Pasteur** of France, along with a host of other scientists in the nineteenth century, propounded the "**germ theory** of disease causation." This theory suggested that living microorganisms in the blood caused an extensive range of human diseases. Following this theory, scientists eventually suggested the role of insects in transmitting diseases. It was argued that insects acted as vectors in transmitting harmful microorganisms from one **human body** to another. Henceforth, the role of insects in causing epidemic diseases has been studied in great detail. Anthrax was the first disease to have come under experimental scrutiny. These initial experiments, however, failed to affirm definitively whether insects caused the **transmission** of anthrax.

Research conducted by **Patrick Manson** in Amoy (China) and published in 1878 and 1884 confirmed that mosquitoes caused elephantiasis in humans. His works suggested that mosquitoes transmitted the filarial worm from one body to another. Manson showed that the larvae of the filarial parasite entered the body of the mosquito once it had sucked the blood of an infected person. After the mosquito died, the filarial parasite inherent in its body was released in **water**. Human beings who drank that water acquired the disease. Manson's work was eventually modified. It was later shown that filarial infection did not result from drinking infected water. Instead, it followed the bite of an infected mosquito. Despite this, his research firmly confirmed the long held hypothesis that insects play a crucial role in causing human diseases.

Following Manson's lead, many scientists set out to discover the causes behind the propagation of many epidemic diseases. Manson inspired similar research not only on human diseases but also on veterinary diseases. In the late 1860s a fever epidemic among the cattle in Texas threatened to devastate the existing livestock economy. This "Texas cattle fever" was also referred as Spanish fever, red-water fever, and dry murrain. In 1893 Theobald Smith (1859–1934) and Fred Lucius Kilborne (1858–1936) showed that that the disease was caused by **protozoa** that were spread by cattle ticks. After sucking blood from an infected animal, a tick would drop off into the grass and lay eggs from which would hatch young ticks already harboring the protozoa. Weeks after the original tick dropped from its longhorn host, its progeny were still capable of infecting other cattle. This finding was later followed by the discovery of vectors of the "Rocky Mountain spotted fever" of humans, tularaemia, and other similar diseases.

Several other forms of cattle diseases in other parts of the world were later found to be transmitted by insects. In 1895 it was shown that the fatal Nagana cattle disease in Africa was conveyed from sick to healthy animals by bloodsucking tsetse flies. This discovery paved the way for the demonstration of the cause and method of spread of the deadly human African **sleeping sickness**.

Alphonse Laveran had shown in 1880 that a parasitic protozoon caused **malaria**. Patrick Manson had hinted that mosquitoes could transmit malaria. Combining these understandings, **Ronald Ross** demonstrated how female *Anopheles* mosquitoes carried malarial parasites from one human body to another. This was soon followed by the discovery of the mode of the transmission of **yellow fever** by mosquitoes. A United States Army Commission (1900) headed by **Walter Reed**, who was assisted by James Carroll (1854–1907), Jesse Lazear (1866–1900), and Aristides Agramonte (1868–1931) supplied proof toward this discovery. Malaria and yellow fever were both considered a bane to the entire colonial world as they killed thousands of European soldiers, traders, and missionaries. Such knowledge inspired extensive projects of mosquito extermination in Africa, different parts of India, Hong Kong, the Philippine Islands, Cuba, and Panama, along with several other regions.

Dengue, or breakbone, fever is another febrile disease that was found to be caused by mosquitoes. Dengue is rarely fatal, is accompanied by rash, and can cause severe debilitating effects. The *Aedes aegypti* and *Aedes albopictus* species of mosquitoes most frequently transmit Dengue. During the World War II, an epidemic of Dengue broke out in Hawaii in 1943 and on various Pacific Islands in 1944, having an adverse effect on the military operations of the U.S. army and navy.

The sand fly fever caused by the bite of sand flies continues to be an acute and debilitating, though not fatal, disease. It is widely distributed across southern Europe, Latin America, Asia, and Africa. Attacks of large swarms of black flies classified under the species *Simulium*, apart from destroying poultry and domesticated animals, cause Onchocerciasis among **children** in various parts of tropical Africa and Latin America.

Bubonic plague is an acute infectious disease that affects both humans and rodents. Plague is primarily a disease of rodents: rats, mice, ground squirrels, and many other species are affected. The rat-flea *Xenopsylla cheopis* has been found to be the most effective vector of bubonic plague. This knowledge has been effectively employed in attempts to eradicate plague. Extermination of rats and their fleas has been an important feature of plague control. It has often been feared that bubonic plague might be carried to different parts of the world by rats through ships. As a routine practice, ships from infected ports are **fumigated** to kill the rats and their fleas.

Lice are the agents for the transmission of **typhus**. It has been shown that *Rickettsia quintana*, a microorganism found consistently in the stomach of infected lice, causes trench

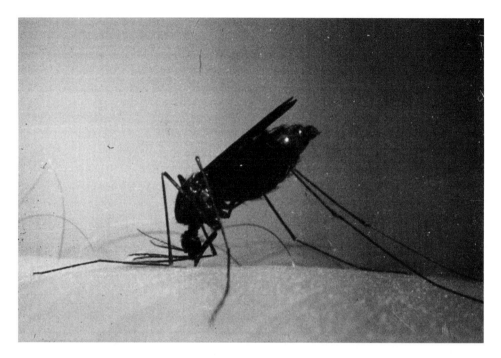

A common malaria mosquito (anopheles quadrimaculatus) in biting position. It is full of blood down to the last three segments. Courtesy of the National Library of Medicine.

fever. The housefly, in addition to being a vector of **typhoid fever**, has been incriminated along with closely related species as a vector of a number of other **animal diseases**. *See also* Ectoparasites; Environment, Ecology, and Epidemic Disease; Insect Infestations; Pesticides.

Further Reading

Gratz, Norman G. *Vector- and Rodent-Borne Diseases in Europe and North America: Distribution, Public Health Burden, and Control*. New York: Cambridge University Press, 2006.

Hays, J. N. *The Burdens of Disease: Epidemics and Human Response in Western History*. New Brunswick, NJ: Rutgers University Press, 1998.

Marquardt, William H. *Biology of Disease Vectors*, 2nd edition. New York: Academic Press, 2004.

ROHAN DEB-ROY

INTERNATIONAL HEALTH AGENCIES AND CONVENTIONS. Neither diseases nor the organisms that cause them recognize the political boundaries that separate human populations into nations. The natural boundaries that long isolated islands and continents—and their unique biological populations—have been crossed with increasing frequency and effectiveness. Today we live in a truly globalized society, sharing pathogens with the world. Never has international cooperation in monitoring, planning for, and confronting infectious diseases been more important. The medieval plague prompted Italian city-states to surveille their neighbors for signs of an outbreak and to recognize each other's health passes, guaranteeing a traveler's lack of disease. Early modern maritime nations at least tacitly recognized each others' **quarantine** and isolation procedures, and *cordons sanitaires* along national borders were generally respected because no one had an interest in spreading pestilential disease. Yet the earliest multistate effort to confront **epidemic** disease began only in the mid-nineteenth century as cholera raged across European countries and their colonies.

By the 1850s Europe was rapidly undergoing **industrialization** and **urbanization** and was beginning to experience the closer ties created by such innovations as steamships, railroads, and the telegraph. Imperialism linked a lengthening list of European states to far-flung colonies, many of which served as reservoirs for infectious tropical diseases. At the same time, the medical profession in Europe was gaining increasing popular respect, raising the prospect that diseases might soon be understood and conquered. In 1830 an outbreak of epidemic **cholera** prompted the Ottoman Empire to initiate a program of international monitoring of sea and land routes between Asia and Western nations directed by the Conseil Supérieur de Santé de Constantinople (Istanbul). Two decades later, in the midst of another cholera pandemic, diplomats, **physicians**, and scientists from 12 nations participated in the First Sanitary Conference, which opened on July 23, 1851. A lack of consensus on causation led to a lack of consensus on action, but the first step had been taken. In 1859 the Second Conference convened again in Paris, but with only the diplomats present. Even so, no agreement on measures to combat cholera was ratified. The medical men rejoined the diplomats for the Third in Istanbul in 1866, and **yellow fever** was added to the agenda, but no real headway resulted. Though the agendas broadened somewhat, the same must be said for the Fourth Conference (Vienna, 1874), the Fifth (Washington, D.C., 1881; with a greater emphasis on yellow fever), and the Sixth (Rome, 1885).

During this period other developments reinforced international collaboration on matters of health and disease. The International Statistical Congresses, beginning in 1853, helped disseminate the emerging ideas and tools of the new science of **epidemiology**; the International Congress of Medicine held 11 sessions between 1867 and 1900; and the U.S. Surgeon-General began publication of the *Index Medicus*, an up-to-date international catalogue of books and articles of medical relevance. The German **Robert Koch** and Frenchman **Louis Pasteur** made their respective microbiological discoveries that confirmed modern **germ theory** of disease, while **Rudolf Virchow** in Germany and **John Snow** and **William Farr** in England paved the way for modern epidemiology.

The Seventh International Sanitary Conference, held in Rome in 1892, was a breakthrough, as it unanimously ratified the First International Sanitary Convention (agreement). Though limited to establishing quarantine protocols for ships passing into the Mediterranean through the new Suez Canal, it opened the door to a series of conventions drafted and approved by the subsequent conferences. The Eighth Conference met in Dresden, Germany, in 1893 and agreed on certain prophylactic measures and required notification during future cholera outbreaks. In 1894 the Ninth Conference convened in Paris and established guidelines for reducing the spread of cholera during the annual Islamic pilgrimage to Mecca. By 1897 **bubonic plague** had reemerged in the form of the Third Plague Pandemic and was appropriately the focus of the Tenth Conference, held in Venice. Its Fourth Convention dealt with international notification and quarantining to contain the spread of plague. Six years later, the Eleventh Conference met in Paris. Delegates agreed to work toward controlling rat populations, which had only recently been linked to the plague; toward codifying the quarantine and other procedures established at previous conferences; and toward establishing a new organization, the Office International d'Hygiène Publique (International Office of Public Hygiene [OHIP]), which would have a largely European scope. The OHIP was founded by 12 countries—including the United States and Brazil—and met for the first time in Paris in 1908. It tackled the issue of monitoring **leprosy, tuberculosis, typhoid,** sexually transmitted diseases, and **water** quality (for cholera). Only three more conferences of this series would be held, the last in Paris in 1938.

The Eighth International Sanitary Conference, held in Washington, D.C., in 1881, laid the foundation for the First International Conference of American States, held in Washington in 1890. From this meeting emerged the International Union of American Republics, which later became the Organization of American States. Representatives at the Second International Conference of American States (Mexico City, 1901) organized the First General International Sanitary Convention of the American Republics (Washington, D.C., 1902). As a permanent executive board for executive oversight, the convention created the International Sanitary Bureau (ISB; later the Pan American Health Organization or PAHO), which remains the world's oldest international health agency. Based in Washington, the ISB was directed by the U.S. Surgeon-General and often collaborated with the **Rockefeller Foundation's** International Health Division and the U.S. Institute for Inter-American Affairs. As with the OHIP, the chief function of the ISB was to monitor and report on levels or outbreaks of infectious disease in the Western Hemisphere and to supervise its quarantine procedures.

World War I (1914–1918) not only killed millions of combatants and countless civilians in Europe but also spawned terrible outbreaks of cholera and **typhus** in its wake. More deadly than the **war** itself was the worldwide **influenza pandemic of 1918–1919.** The failures of international diplomacy that sparked the war led to the founding of the League of Nations (1919), and the medical emergencies to the League of Nations Health Organization (LNHO, 1923). Because the United States was not a member of the League, it could not participate in LNHO activities, so the OHIP and ISB (now the Pan American Sanitary Bureau) remained independent and active as monitors and quarantine supervisors that worked with the LNHO. Complementarily, the LNHO took a much more proactive role in supporting practical measures to prevent the outbreak and spread of disease. Aided by Rockefeller Foundation funds, the Organization disseminated the latest information, strategies, and techniques, and published a monthly report on medical situations worldwide. Unlike earlier international efforts, the LNHO covered East Asia, from an office in Singapore. It collaborated with the International Red Cross and the International Labor Office in providing public education, sending experts to trouble spots, and sponsoring committees and conferences. It sponsored research and development of treatments, public hygiene, and worldwide standardization of epidemiological matters from cause of death reporting to medical products.

The LNHO recorded many successes, but the Great Depression and weaknesses of the League of Nations helped limit the organization's effectiveness. World War II (1939–1945) severely curtailed its activities. The Allied-sponsored United Nations Relief and Rehabilitation Administration (UNRRA) emerged in 1943 amid fears of pandemics like those that followed World War I. In the wake of the war, the United Nations Conference on International Organization established a new World Health Organization (WHO) that would absorb the LNHO, OHIP, PASB, and UNRRA. On April 7, 1948,

POINTS [FOR PUBLIC HEALTH OFFICIALS] TO CONSIDER AT THE START OF AN OUTBREAK OF MEASLES (1999)

POPULATION DATA	Obtain most recent population size and age distribution.
WHAT'S BEEN DONE	List any actions already taken.
CASE REVIEW	List reports of cases in area during previous six months.
COVERAGE RATES	Obtain existing coverage data and include unofficial estimates.
SPOT MAP	Use pins or a pen to mark the location(s) of case(s) and areas targeted for immunizations on a map.
RESOURCES	Determine what resources are available at all levels for outbreak control (transportation, vaccine, cold chain materials, promotional materials, etc.). Human resources should include filed staff to assist in the outbreak, including staff from other programs, district staff, medical and nursing students, interpreters, and drivers. Arrange for transport and for travel advances.
ARRIVALS	Inform appropriate health/community authorities when/where any special teams will be arriving, and ensure that specific health staff/community representatives will be present.
SUPPLIES	Organize necessary supplies:

1. Adequate vaccine based on estimated target population.
2. Cold chain materials: ice packs, cold boxes, vaccine carriers, thermometers, refrigeration capacity (locally available or must be brought in), possibility of purchasing ice locally.
3. Adequate supply of forms
   - Line Listings of Suspected Cases
   - Case Investigation Forms
   - Outbreak Control Summary
   - Mop-up Work Sheets
4. Promotional materials: pamphlets, posters, etc.

From *Measles Eradication Field Guide* (Technical Paper #41), published by the Pan American Health Organization, Pan American Sanitary Bureau, Regional Office of the World Health Organization (Washington, D.C., 1999).

the required 26 nations ratified its constitution, and it assembled for the first time in June. The International Sanitary Conventions evolved into the World Health Organization's International Health Regulations (IHR), adopted in 1969. Updated in 2005, the new IHR was implemented in 2007; 192 countries are currently party to the regulations. These require cooperating governments to inform the WHO of any reportable diseases in a timely way but do not require further action.

Since 1948 the WHO has been in the forefront as an organizer of international efforts to maintain high levels of general health, prevent the emergence or spread of disease, treat victims, and, in some cases, eradicate diseases. Controlling and eventually eradicating infectious diseases are among the highest of WHO's priorities, and success with **smallpox eradication** in 1977 set the tone for current efforts against **measles**, TB, **malaria**,

SOME WHO-AFFILIATED INFECTIOUS
DISEASE-FIGHTING ORGANIZATIONS (2008)

FOR SPECIFIC DISEASES
International AIDS Vaccine Initiative (1996):
    http://www.iavi.org/
Pediatric Dengue Vaccine Initiative (2003):
    http://www.pdvi.org/PdviMain.htm
Medicines for Malaria Venture (1999):
    http://www.mmv.org/rubrique.php3?id_rubrique=15
Malaria Vaccine Initiative (1999):
    http://www.malariavaccine.org/
TB Alliance: Global Alliance for TB Drug Development
    (2000): http://www.tballiance.org/home/home.php
Aeras: Aeras Global TB Vaccine Foundation (1997):
    http://aeras.org/

GENERAL HEALTH OR MULTIPLE DISEASES
Drugs for Neglected Diseases Initiative (2003):
    http://www.dndi.org/
Institute for One World Health (2000):
    http://www.oneworldhealth.org/
Foundation for Innovative New Diagnostics (2003):
    http://www.finddiagnostics.org/
International Partnership for Microbicides (2002):
    http://www.ipm-microbicides.org/

and **polio**. The United Nations and WHO consider good health to be a fundamental human right and a positive goal for their activities. The WHO is thus proactive and not merely reactive to dangerous outbreaks of disease. Though headquartered in Geneva, Switzerland, WHO has six regional offices through which many of its efforts are directed. In the Western Hemisphere it is the Pan American Health Organization (Washington, D.C.; formerly the PASB). WHO also maintains offices in countries that have needs being met by the organization. Collaboration with host countries is of utmost importance, as is collaboration with non-governmental organizations, especially those that can provide technical expertise or funding. The Bill and Melinda Gates Foundation is a good example of the latter. WHO also works with other international organizations—such as the Food and Agriculture Organization (FAO), UNICEF, and UNESCO—in areas such as nutrition, health and **personal hygiene** education, prenatal care, **children**'s diseases, and **vaccinations**.

In Volume 2 of his *National Health Systems of the World*, Milton Roemer lists eight general principles that currently guide international health care efforts: 1) Multinational organizations are established by autonomous national states and may only operate in a country with its permission. 2) All who work for an international agency must be dedicated to the agency and not to their home countries. 3) An organization must respond to the needs of any country that applies for help, no matter the nature of the government (though South Africa was made a pariah because of racial segregation [apartheid]). 4) A healthy population is a key to social and economic development. 5) Within a country many parts of government and society need to collaborate to maintain good general health. 6) In a given country highest priority should be given to the problems that affect the most people, with an emphasis on primary care facilities. 7) Both preventive care and treatment must be allocated equitably throughout the society. 8) Though international concerns originated in communicable disease control, efforts must address a much wider range of diseases and disabilities. *See also* Cholera: First through Third Pandemics, 1816–1861; Colonialism and Epidemic Disease; Demographic Data Collection and Analysis, History of; Epidemiology, History of; Geopolitics, International Relations, and Epidemic Disease; Leprosy, Societal Reactions to; Measles, Efforts to Eradicate; Non-Governmental Organizations (NGOs) and Epidemic Disease; Poverty, Wealth, and Epidemic Disease; Trade, Travel, and Epidemic Disease; Yellow Fever in Latin America and the Caribbean, 1830–1940.

Further Reading

Baldwin, Peter. *Contagion and the State in Europe, 1830–1930*. New York: Cambridge University Press, 1999.

Harvard University Library. *Contagion: Sanitary Conferences*. http://ocp.hul.harvard.edu/contagion/sanitaryconferences.html

Howard-Jones, Norman. *The Pan American Health Organization*. Geneva: World Health Organization, 1981.

Huber, Valeska. "The Unification of the Globe by Disease? The International Sanitary Conventions on Cholera, 1851–1894." *The Historical Journal* 49 (2006): 453–476.

Merson, Michael. *International Public Health: Diseases, Programs, Systems and Policies*. Boston: Jones & Bartlett, 2006.

Pan-American Health Organization. http://www.paho.org/

Siddiqi, Javed. *World Health and World Politics: The World Health Organization and the U.N. System*. Columbia: University of South Carolina Press, 1995.

Stern, Alexandra Minna, and Howard Merkel. "International Efforts to Control Infectious Diseases, 1851 to the Present." *Journal of the American Medical Association* 292 (2004): 1474–1479.

UNICEF. http://www.unicef.org/

Weindling, Paul, ed. *International Health Organizations and Movements, 1918–1939*. New York: Cambridge University Press, 1995.

World Health Organization. http://www.who.int/en/

Joseph P. Byrne

IRISH POTATO FAMINE AND EPIDEMIC DISEASE, 1845–1850. Between 1845 and 1850, the failure of the potato crop marked the worst famine in Irish history, with over 2 million dying from starvation and accompanying disease and an equal number emigrating. The Irish famine has continued to inspire narration, interpretation, and discussion by historians because of the scope of the human tragedy and the wealth of primary source material.

The famine in Ireland was both a warning of the dangers of monoculture—in this case, the potato—and a response to a colonial legacy that had created social, economic, and political dislocation on an unprecedented scale. The colonization of Ireland by England had been born out of a fear of invasion. Consequently, by the early nineteenth century, the bulk of the Irish people had lost political autonomy and religious freedom and had suffered severe limitations on land ownership, which created an underclass that faced a precarious existence as tenants with no security. The problems were further exacerbated by rapid population growth. By the 1840s this showed signs of slowing, but with a total population estimated at 8.5 million, issues such as housing, food, employment, and well being alone were a constant concern to the authorities in both Westminster and Dublin.

For many Irish, daily subsistence meant a life of **poverty**. The staple food was the potato, a crop with advantages including two harvests a year, plants that grew in most soil, and a relatively high nutritional value. It is believed that the average adult male had a **diet** of over 13 pounds of potatoes a week, supplemented with meat and dairy products when available. Despite the occasional poor harvest, wide scale potato crop failures were unknown, and the popular image of Ireland with its rich, fertile soil meant that many outsiders refused to accept the horrific accounts of starvation once the famine had taken a fatal grip on the country. The irony of the great hunger was that there was always sufficient food being produced in Ireland, but little of it ever reached the mouths of the indigenous population because of its value as an export commodity.

In 1843 reports of a blight affecting potatoes appeared in the United States. Rapid transmission to Europe occurred in contaminated seed crops. In 1845 the blight was recorded among potato crops in southeast Britain, where it thrived in the damp, temperate climate. Farmers recognized the ominous signs of black spots on one side of the leaf, while underneath lurked the telltale white mold. When the potatoes were lifted from the ground, they were already rotten and stinking. Years later the blight was identified as *Phytophhora infestans*, a fungus that still has the potential to devastate crops.

Conservative British Prime Minister Robert Peel (1788–1850) was sufficiently concerned to direct the government to consider the blight a priority and ordered further investigation. The accepted conclusion that this was a temporary failure, however, resulted in the decision not to establish long-term government relief programs.

In Ireland, the spring potato crop of 1845 was sound; only the autumn harvest showed signs of blight. The dire reports at this time were localized, and potatoes were stored for the oncoming winter. News soon spread, however, of stored potatoes becoming rotten. Those who attempted to eat the contaminated crop were the first medical victims, struck down by severe vomiting and bowel disorders. As winter set in, reports of starvation reached the authorities, followed by inevitable accounts of fevers. By early 1846 potato crops were earnestly planted, but unlike previous crops they showed few signs of being healthy. Peel, sensing the impending disaster in Ireland, surreptitiously purchased £100,000 of American corn (maize), to be shipped directly to Cork. The clandestine nature of this purchase reflected the full extent of anti-Irish feeling found throughout Britain and the continued reluctance to set aside prejudice and provide help for the millions of innocent victims struck down by disease and starvation.

On arrival in the Irish ports, the dried corn could not be distributed until it had been made fit for human consumption by a long and complicated process. Failure to prepare it properly resulted in severe gastric disorders, with the general agreement that the corn was not so much food but Peel's "brimstone." By 1846 there was widespread failure of the potato crop throughout the United Kingdom. However, Ireland stood alone in facing the dire consequence of starvation. The fall of Peel's government and the return of the liberal Whig party initially provided a sense of optimism in Ireland. However, Lord John Russell (1792–1878) led a minority government and was still very much at the mercy of public opinion. Relief now took the form of a variety of public works that provided food in return for honest toil. This did little to feed the most vulnerable and needy.

The high incidence of death from disease as opposed to actual starvation is one of the most harrowing features of famine in general, and Ireland was spared none of the horror. As evictions of penniless tenants became common, entire families could be found sleeping in the open and scavenging for food, thereby further weakening their resistance to illness. A formidable list of diseases was recorded, with many reaching epidemic proportions. The evidence for this can be found in the 1851 *Census for Ireland* (see sidebar). The final publication covered 10 volumes, with two being specifically allocated to "Status of Disease" and "Tables of Death." The compiler was Sir William Wilde (1815–1876), a skilled Irish medical practitioner. In 1841 Wilde had been appointed Medical Commissioner to the Irish Census, though unbeknown to him, much of his time in office would be spent recording the terrible famine years and their grim aftermath. Few were better trained to make sense of this grim legacy, but Wilde himself was also aware that for each of the thousands of deaths that were recorded, many more died without any official notification of cause or even identification.

OFFICIAL BRITISH GOVERNMENT REPORT ON DISEASE DURING THE GREAT FAMINE (1856)

Concurrent with the foregoing state of famine, and the disruption of the social condition of the people, pestilence came upon the nation in the following order: Fever, Scurvy, Diarrhea and Dysentery, Cholera, Influenza, and Ophthalmia . . .

On reviewing the history of epidemic pestilence in Ireland, we are struck by the frequency with which **dysentery** has been an element of destruction, in lessening its population . . . The Census Returns have afforded a total of 93,232 deaths from dysentery, in the proportion of 75.06 females to 100 males. Of these, more than one half occurred in workhouses . . . Of 283,765 persons who died in the workhouses between 1841 and 1851, as many as 70,526 were returned as having sunk under dysentery or diarrhea . . . When we remember the masses of debilitated people that were, of necessity, congregated in the parent and auxiliary workhouses during the years of famine, we cannot wonder at the great mortality from these diseases . . .

When the famine was most severely felt, and when fever and dysentery raged with the greatest violence, Asiatic **cholera** again invaded the continent of Europe . . . and reached our shores at the end of 1848. For some wide and inscrutable reason, upon which man can only speculate, it seemed good to the Great Disposer of events [God] to mitigate considerably its fatality, compared with that of its first invasion, sixteen years before, for the returns only give as many as 35, 989 deaths, in which the sexes were in the proportion of 95.57 males to 100 females.

Although **small-pox** has decreased in Ireland, both in virulence and extent, since the publication of the Census Report in 1841, there was some increase in that disease during the pestilential period of 1847, '48, and '49; yet the deaths returned to us (amounting to 35,275) in ten years) are not, considering the present state of **vaccination** in this country, of sufficient amount to warrant the assertion that small-pox influenced the great mortality of which this . . . is the analysis, although during a portion of the period it prevailed epidemically and was also very fatal in England.

An epidemic of **influenza** pervaded Great Britain in 1847 and 1848; where, although of brief duration it was of unusual fatality. The total deaths registered from influenza [in Ireland, 1841–1851] were 10,753, in the proportion of 85.5 females to 100 males.

The total deaths returned to us under the head of Starvation amounted to 21,770 . . . 70.6 females to 100 males . . . [Yet] many more must have perished from disease remotely induced by privation during the years of famine and pestilence.

From the British Government's *Census of Ireland for the Year 1851* (Dublin, 1856).

The first group to fall victim to disease was, not surprisingly, infants and children. Descriptions of marasmus, a form of severe protein deficiency affecting the very young, became common throughout Ireland. The victims are vividly portrayed in the sketches made at the time by illustrators working for the popular press. The same images also provided evidence of dropsy (currently known as edema). This was identifiable by the painfully bloated stomachs of young victims suffering from fluid retention in response to the lack of nutrition. Today over 50 million children still suffer from marasmus and other similar conditions caused by malnutrition.

Of all the diseases that affected the Irish population at this time, **cholera** and **typhus** were undoubtedly the most virulent. Cholera decimated the urban areas that previously had avoided the worst of the famine, whereas typhus was far more widespread as a result of it being highly infectious and thriving in poverty-stricken environments such as slums and workhouses. As the displaced population sought food and shelter, people unwittingly became carriers of typhus. Among the cruelest of outbreaks was that which occurred at sea. Refugee passengers who had survived the perils of starvation and disease in Ireland often found themselves succumbing to typhus fever when confined in overcrowded ships. Thousands died as they fled in search of a better existence in the aptly named "coffin ships," only to be cast overboard or hastily buried in the foreign soil they had believed would offer a new life.

As the famine showed no sign of abating, those with the opportunity increasingly took advantage of the chance to emigrate. The most popular options were North America and England although many countries recorded high Irish immigration at this time. The route to North America required money to purchase a single ticket, whereas the crossing to England was often free so long as passengers were prepared to act as ballast in ships returning to ports such as Liverpool. In 1847 alone, over 300,000 Irish were recorded as having entered Britain. However, they soon met with increasing hostility by both the public and the authorities. In their weakened and desperate state, they brought disease and a sense of unrest. City after city began to demand an end to the waves of immigrants, and many demanded that they be returned to Ireland. The Liverpool Poor Law Authority was the first to voice its concerns as over 90,000 homeless and often sick Irish flocked into the city, creating ghettoes in urban environments that were already rife with public health concerns.

The most tragic of all emigration tales was that of Grosse Île, Canada. During the cholera epidemic in 1832, a **quarantine** station had been established on Grosse Île, a small island in the St. Lawrence River. An increasing number of Irish found themselves heading for Canada rather than the United States as the passage was cheaper, and American ports on the eastern seaboard had begun imposing restrictions on immigrants in order to avoid additional strains on local providers of social welfare and medical care. Though all passengers were supposed to be inspected for disease prior to any sea passage, few British medical officers risked carrying out this duty in Irish ports. Consequently when *The Syria* headed out for Canada in March 1847, it had on board 241 passengers, some of whom were infected with typhus. When the passengers disembarked on the island, over 200 were so ill that they had to be admitted to the small hospital. Most never recovered. On Gross Île over 4,000 Irish immigrants died of disease within a two-month period in 1847, though many more were to perish throughout the remaining famine years. The tragedy symbolizes the dangers faced by many of the Irish diaspora who chose to flee the famine, only to face suffering and tragedy on foreign soil.

The medical officer of the station, Dr. George Douglas (director from 1836 to 1864), was utterly unprepared for the scenes he witnessed on *The Syria* and other ships that followed. Soon, any attempt to enforce disembarkation on the small island had to be abandoned. By the end of May 1847, 36 "coffin" ships lay at anchor off the island, with over 12,000 passengers waiting for permission to land. As typhus claimed its victims, bodies were brought onto the island for burial, although it soon became necessary to import soil from the mainland to ensure that rotting **corpses** were sufficiently covered. The Canadian Legislative Assembly eventually abandoned the practice of quarantine, and Irish immigrants were soon landing directly in Quebec and other cities. Little help was forthcoming, however, and destitution along with the ravages of the Canadian winters saw many of the Irish perish within the first few months of their new lives. *See also* Capitalism and Epidemic Disease; Cholera: First through Third Pandemics, 1816–1861; Colonialism and Epidemic Disease; Contagion and Transmission; Diet, Nutrition, and Epidemic Disease; Disease, Social Construction of; Environment, Ecology, and Epidemic Disease; Human Immunity and Resistance to Disease; Malthusianism; Public Health Agencies in Britain since 1800; Race, Ethnicity, and Epidemic Disease.

Further Reading

Gallman, J. Matthew. *Receiving Erin's Children: Philadelphia, Liverpool, and the Irish Famine Migration, 1845–1855.* Chapel Hill: University of North Carolina Press, 2003.

Gray, Peter. *The Irish Famine.* New York: Thames & Hudson, 1995.

Kennedy, L., P. S. Ell, E. M. Crawford, and L. A. Clarkson. *Mapping the Great Irish Famine: A Survey of the Famine Decades.* Bodmin: Four Courts Press, 1999.

Kinealy, Christine. *This Great Calamity: The Irish Famine 1845–52.* Boulder, CO: Roberts Rinehart, 1995.

Macarthur, William P. "Medical History of the Famine." In *The Great Famine: Studies in Irish History, 1845–1952,* edited by I. R. Dudley and T. Desmond Williams, pp. 263–315. New York: New York University Press, 1957.

Ó Gráda, Cormac. *Black '47 and Beyond: The Great Irish Famine in History, Economy and Memory.* Princeton: Princeton University Press, 1999.

HILARY S. MORRIS

ISLAMIC DISEASE THEORY AND MEDICINE. Islamic medicine has been historically shaped by a variety of medical traditions. Although it was solidly rooted in ancient **Greco-Roman medical theories and practices**, Islamic medicine was also influenced by pre-Islamic medical beliefs and practices, prophetic medicine, and medical practices from the Indian subcontinent. In turn, Islamic medicine had a profound impact on pre-modern European medical theory and practice.

Not much is known about Islamic medicine during the first centuries of Islamic history. A massive translation movement began under the patronage of the Abbasid caliphs in the ninth century. Ancient Greek medical texts were translated first into Syriac and then into Arabic, mostly by Nestorian scholars and court physicians. Hunayn b. Ishak (d. 873) was the most accomplished translator of this period. Works of adaptations from foreign medical texts soon followed translations, and before long, Baghdad became the center of medical learning. By the late ninth century, Hellenistic and Byzantine medical theories and practices were already integrated into Islamic medical learning. The most influential works were the *materia medica* of Dioscorides, c. 40–90), writings of Rufus of Ephesus (late first century CE), and above all those of **Galen** (even more so than those of **Hippocrates**). Overall, Islamic medical learning came to be dominated by Galenic teachings of **humoral theory**, according to which disease emerged in a human body because of an imbalance of bodily humors and could be cured by restoring the balance.

As an effort to counterbalance the dominance of secular and pagan Greco-Roman medical tradition on Islamic medicine, a new genre of medical writing called "prophetic medicine" emerged during the ninth century. These texts were mostly written by religious scholars of Islam, who gathered medical information from the Quran and *hadith* literature (which contained teachings of Muhammad). Although the authors of these texts were not opposed to medicine in principle, they wanted to give it an Islamic character. Although the genre became popular in the thirteenth and fourteenth centuries, it is hard to estimate to what extent Muslim **physicians** followed these texts.

During the tenth and eleventh centuries, there was a constant effort to organize the vast corpus of medical knowledge produced in the Islamic world. Several major medical compendia were written in this period—mainly in Arabic, but also in Persian. The works of al-Razi (**Rhazes**), al-Majusi (Haly Abbas, d. 994), and **Avicenna (Ibn Sina)** mark the apogee of Islamic medical compendia. Also, from the tenth century onwards, the Islamic world saw the emergence of **hospitals** known as **bimaristan**. The finest examples of medieval Islamic hospitals were established first in Baghdad, and then in Damascus and Cairo. The rise of hospitals prompted the development of institutional medical education, which had been informally practiced within family circles. The first medical school in the Islamic world opened in Damascus in the early thirteenth century.

Islamic medicine was exposed to influences from Indian and Chinese medical systems, mostly because of the geographic reach of Islamic Empires. As early as the ninth century, pharmaceutical substances brought to Muslim lands from India and China began to influence Islamic medicine. Muslim **pharmacists** contributed to pharmacological knowledge by integrating Indian and Chinese medicinal substances to the Hellenistic heritage of Dioscorides' *materia medica*. Especially, during the Ilkhanid period (1256–1353), Chinese medicine began to influence Islamic medicine via the translations of Chinese medical texts into Persian.

When the **Black Death (1347–1352)** struck the Islamic world, many plague treatises were written. Compiling current knowledge about the disease, these works typically discussed the notion of **contagion** and transmissibility of plague, as well as proper conduct in times of outbreaks, on the basis of *hadith* literature. Generally written by Muslim religious scholars, medieval plague treatises held that plague was a mercy or a blessing of God, and that those who died of it attained martyrdom. Therefore, Muslims were advised not to flee but to bear the plague with patience.

Plague epidemics also triggered the practice of alternative systems of healing. People resorted to **magic** and **astrology**, as well as to pre-Islamic folkloric elements, in the search for a cure. Charms, amulets, incantations, magical squares, magic-medicinal bowls with engravings of Quranic verses and magical symbols, and talismanic shirts were all used for protection against plague. Patience, prayer, fasting, and recitations of the Quran were commonly recommended during times of epidemics.

Islamic medical literature referred to several diseases including fevers, **malaria, leprosy**, melancholy, eye diseases, hemorrhoids, and dietetics. Leprosy, elephantiasis, scabs, consumption, **smallpox, measles**, and various forms of **plague** were classified as transmissible diseases, based on the long experience of the Islamic world with them. A variety of treatises were specifically devoted to diseases such as smallpox, measles, and plague. As new diseases such as **syphilis** emerged, the topics of treatises by Muslim authors also expanded to cover these new ailments.

In the seventeenth century, Islamic medicine began to be influenced by **Paracelsianism** advocated in Europe by the followers of **Paracelsus**. This movement came to be known in the Islamic world through the translation of these works and soon became very popular. The chemical medicine, as it was referred to, entailed the use of inorganic salts, mineral acids, and alchemical techniques for the production of its remedies. These translations also introduced to the Islamic medical literature a number of other new diseases seen in Europe, such as scurvy, chlorosis, anemia, and **sweating sickness**.

It is only in the nineteenth century that Islamic medicine underwent a substantial transformation of modernization and westernization. Many European medical texts were translated into Arabic and Persian in this period. European-style medical schools were established in Cairo and Tehran. Yet traditional elements of medicine still continued to survive and be widely practiced. In the Indian subcontinent, traditional Islamic medicine was referred to as Unani medicine and became very popular in the twentieth century, as an alternative to western medicine. *See also* Apothecary/Pharmacist; Leprosy, Societal Reactions to; Physician; Pilgrimage and Epidemic Disease; Plague in the Islamic World, 1360–1500; Plague in the Islamic World, 1500–1850; Public Health in the Islamic World, 1000–1600; Quacks, Charlatans, and Their Remedies.

Further Reading

Conrad, Lawrence I. "The Arab-Islamic Medical Tradition." In *The Western Medical Tradition: 800 BC to AD 1800*, edited by Lawrence et al., pp. 93–138. New York: Cambridge University Press, 1994.

———. "Epidemic Diseases in Formal and Popular Thought in Early Islamic Society." In *Epidemics and Ideas*, edited by Terence Ranger and Paul Slack, pp. 77–99. New York: Cambridge University Press, 1992.

———. "TĀ'ŪN and WABĀ': Conceptions of Plague and Pestilence in Early Islam." *Journal of the Economic and Social History of the Orient* 25 (1982): 268–307.

Dols, Michael W. *The Black Death in the Middle East*. Princeton: Princeton University Press, 1977.

———. trans. *Medieval Islamic Medicine: Ibn Ridwān's Treatise "On the Prevention of Ills in Egypt."* Berkeley: University of California Press, 1984.

Elgood, Cyril. *Safavid Medical Practice: The Practice of Medicine, Surgery and Gynecology in Persia Between 1500 AD and 1750 AD*. London: Luzac and Co., 1970.

Leiser, G. "Medical Education in Islamic Lands from the Seventh to the Fourteenth Century." *Journal of the History of Medicine and Allied Sciences* 38 (1983): 48–75.

Majeed, A. "How Islam Changed Medicine." *British Medical Journal* 351 (December 24–31, 2005): 1486–1487.

Murphey, R. "Ottoman Medicine and Transculturalism for the Sixteenth through the Eighteenth Century." *Bulletin of the History of Medicine* 66 (1992): 376–403.

Pormann, Peter E., and Emilie Savage-Smith. *Medieval Islamic Medicine*. Washington, DC: Georgetown University Press, 2007.

Rahman, Fazlur. *Health and Medicine in the Islamic Tradition: Change and Identity*. Chicago: Kazi, 1998.

Strohmeier, G. "Reception and Tradition: Medicine in the Byzantine and Islamic World." In *Western Medical Thought from Antiquity to the Middle Ages*, edited by M. D. Grmek, pp. 139–169. Cambridge, MA: Harvard University Press, 1998.

Ullmann, Manfred. *Islamic Medicine*. Edinburgh: University of Edinburgh, 1978.

NÜKHET VARLIK

J

JENNER, EDWARD (1749–1823). English physician Edward Jenner discovered the vaccine for **smallpox** in 1796. Discovering the vaccine to protect humans against smallpox has saved more human lives than perhaps anything else that any individual has ever done.

Edward Jenner was born May 17, 1749, in a small village, Berkley, in Gloucestershire, England. At age 14, he became an apprentice to a **surgeon**, and at age 21 he became the resident pupil of the famous surgeon John Hunter (1728–1793) in London. He returned to Berkley to practice medicine in 1773 and obtained a M.D. degree from the University of St. Andrews in 1792. He studied plants, birds, and animals, and collected fossils throughout much of his life. He also played the violin and flute, and wrote poetry.

In many rural areas of the world, it was well known that milkmaids were immune to smallpox after having cowpox. Edward Jenner heard of this at a young age, and it intrigued him for many years. After planning to use the scientific method to test his hypothesis, he waited for the right moment. On May 14, 1796, he saw a pustule on the hand of a milkmaid, Sarah Nelmes, and he took some material from this cowpox lesion and vaccinated an eight-year-old farm boy named James Phipps, after getting approval from the boy's father. Six weeks later he inoculated James with smallpox. James did not catch smallpox. Over the next several months, he carried out several more successful vaccine trials. Jenner published his findings in 1798. His success with cowpox elevated **vaccination** from **folk medicine** to scientific status and popularized it as a medical procedure. Parliament awarded Jenner £30,000 to develop and promote the vaccine. Cotton threads were dipped into vaccinial pus, or the pus was put on glass, allowed to dry, and then transported. By 1799 many people in England had been vaccinated, and the technique rapidly spread to several European countries.

**EDWARD JENNER'S EARLY EXPERIMENTS WITH INOCULATION, FROM HIS
"AN INQUIRY INTO THE CAUSES AND EFFECTS OF THE VARIOLAE VACCINAE,
OR COW-POX" (1798)**

A mare, the property of a person who keeps a dairy in the neighboring parish, began to have sore heels the latter end of the month of February, 1798, which were occasionally washed by the servant man of the farm, Thomas Virgoe . . . who in consequence became affected with sores in [his] hands, followed by inflamed lymphatic glands in the arms and axillae, shiverings succeeded by heat, lassitude, and general pains in the limbs . . .

Case XVIII.—John Baker, a child of five years old, was inoculated March 16, 1798, with matter taken from the pustule on the hand of Thomas Virgoe . . . He became ill on the sixth day with symptoms similar to those excited by cow-pox matter. On the eighth day he was free from indisposition.

Case XIX.—William Summers, a child of five years and a half old, was inoculated the same day with Baker, with matter taken from the nipples of one of the infected cows, at the farm alluded to.

Case XX.—From William Summers the disease was transferred to William Pead, a boy of eight years old, who was inoculated March 28th.

Case XXI.—April 5th: Several children and adults were inoculated from the arm of William Pead. The greater part of them sickened on the sixth day, and were well on the seventh, but in three of the number a secondary indisposition arose in consequence of an extensive erysipelatous inflammation which appeared on the inoculated arms. One of these patients was an infant of half a year old. Hannah Excell, a healthy girl of seven years old, and one of the patients above mentioned, received the infection from the insertion of the virus under the cuticle of the arm in three distinct points.

Case XXII.—From the arm of this girl matter was taken and inserted April 12th into the arms of John Macklove, one year and a half old, and Mary James, six years old.

From *The Harvard Classics: Scientific Papers*, edited by Charles W. Eliot (New York: P. F. Collier and Son, 1910).

In 1800 some vaccine material was sent to Benjamin Waterhouse (1754–1846) in the United States, and he was the first to test the smallpox vaccine in the United States. In 1967 the **World Health Organization** (WHO) started a worldwide smallpox vaccination program against the 15 million cases in 33 countries with endemic smallpox. The last case of smallpox was found in Somalia in 1977.

The University of Oxford awarded Jenner an honorary M.D. in 1813. Jenner practiced medicine in his hometown of Berkley from 1773 to his death at age 74. *See also* Scientific Revolution and Epidemic Disease; Smallpox Eradication; Smallpox in Premodern Europe.

Further Reading

Bazin, Hervé. *The Eradication of Small Pox: Edward Jenner and the First and Only Eradication of a Human Infectious Disease.* New York: Academic Press, 2000.

Jenner, Edward. *Vaccination against Smallpox.* Amherst, NY: Prometheus Books, 1996.

Rodriguez, Anna Maria. *Edward Jenner: Conqueror of Smallpox.* Berkeley Heights, NJ: Enslow Publishers, 2006.

Saunders, Paul. *Edward Jenner: The Cheltenham Years, 1795–1823: Being a Chronicle of the Vaccination Campaign.* Hanover, NH: University Press of New Hampshire, 1982.

MARK A. BEST

JEWS. *See* Biblical Plagues; Black Death, Flagellants, and Jews.

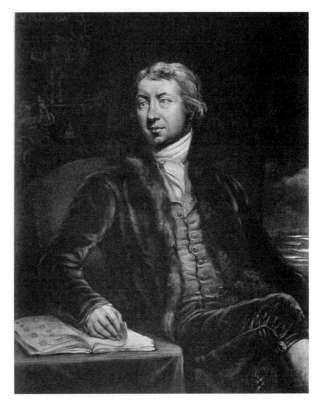

Edward Jenner, M.D. Original painting by J. Northcote. Courtesy of the National Library of Medicine.

K

KITASATO, SHIBASABURO (1852–1931). One of the first microbiologists in Japan, where he helped to open up the field of scientific medicine, Shibasaburo Kitasato's goal in life was the advancement of public health through scientific investigation. He contributed to the development of **immunology** through his early work with **diphtheria** and tetanus. He and French-Swiss bacteriologist **Alexandre Yersin** are both credited with the discovery of the microscopic bacterial organism that causes **bubonic plague**.

Kitasato was born in a village on the Japanese island of Kyushu and graduated from medical school in Tokyo. A German professor, from whom he learned that language, influenced his interest in medicine. The Japanese government sponsored his travel to Germany, which allowed him to realize his goal of working with bacteriologist **Robert Koch**. For six years, he studied **cholera**, anthrax, **typhoid fever, dysentery, tuberculosis**, and tetanus in Koch's laboratory, where he helped to establish the importance of pure cultures (a culture containing the growth or descendents of only one organism, and free of all other organisms). He and German bacteriologist **Emil von Behring** made a pioneering discovery in 1890, when they applied to diphtheria the knowledge they gained from their studies of tetanus antitoxin and showed how the blood can work to neutralize toxins.

The German government gave Kitasato the title of Professor, making him the first non-German ever to receive that honor, and when he returned home in 1892, he established his own laboratory. It was Japan's first scientific research institution, but because the Japanese government would not fund his work, he had to rely on a wealthy benefactor. When bubonic plague erupted in 1894 in Hong Kong, which was at that time a British colony, Kitasato was asked to find the cause.

Kitasato, who was assisted by a team, and Alexandre Yersin, who was working alone, were caught up in British-French political intrigue, and they met together only once. Kitasato's findings were translated into English and published in the esteemed British medical journal, *The Lancet*. Most scholars consider that he and Yersin, who had arrived in Hong Kong at the same time, separately discovered the causal bacterium (named *Yersinia pestis* for Yersin) at virtually the same time.

In 1898 Kitasato and Kiyoshi Shiga (1871–1957), Kitasato's Japanese student, were the first to isolate the **bacterium**, named for Shiga (*Shigellosis*), which causes **dysentery**. When **pneumonic plague** broke out in Manchuria in 1911, a region on the northeast coast of China, Kitasato was sent to find ways to prevent its spread. By 1914 Kitasato's laboratory had, to his dismay, been made a branch of the Ministry of Education. He founded a private laboratory, the Kitasato Institute, a nonprofit organization that has evolved into the Kitasato University. Like von Behring, Kitasato was raised by his government to nobility in recognition of his accomplishments. *See also* Plague in China; Plague in East Asia: Third Pandemic.

Further Reading

Bibel, D. J., and T. H. Chen. "Diagnosis of Plague: An Analysis of the Yersin-Kitasato Controversy." *Bacteriological Reviews* 40, 3 (September 1976): 633–651. http://pubmedcentral.gov/.

"The Late Baron Shibasaburo Kitasato." *Canadian Medical Association Journal* 25, 2 (August 1931): 206–206. http://pubmedcentral.gov/.

Marriott, Edward. *Plague: A Story of Science, Rivalry, and the Scourge that Won't Go Away.* New York: Metropolitan Books, 2002.

MARTHA STONE

KOCH, ROBERT (1843–1910).   Robert Koch discovered the causal agents of **tuberculosis** and **cholera** and made numerous technological advances in the study of microorganisms. Born in 1843 in Clausthal in northern Germany, Koch completed a medical degree at the University of Göttingen. After serving in several inconsequential medical posts and on a tour of duty in the military during the Franco-Prussian war of 1870–1871, Koch was appointed as a district **physician** in Wollstein, a small town in Polish-speaking Prussia. Once established in Wollstein, he set up his own laboratory and launched vigorously into a study of **bacteria**.

By the middle of the nineteenth century, no diseases had been conclusively traced to bacteria. However, there was growing evidence that anthrax was bacterial in origin. Anthrax was an ideal research target partly because it had enormous economic ramifications for the European livestock industry and partly because the anthrax bacillus was gigantic in comparison to other bacteria and relatively easy to identify. As throughout his career, Koch's work on anthrax exploited his own technical innovations such as the hanging-drop method for microscopic investigations and, later, the use of photography, new staining techniques, and solid-culture media. Koch was able to trace the life cycle of the anthrax bacillus and to answer numerous questions that had clouded earlier attempts to understand the disease. He presented his research in 1876, and its significance was immediately apparent. Soon thereafter Koch accepted an appointment at the Imperial *Gesundheitsamt* (Health Office) in Berlin.

Koch's anthrax research brought him into direct competition with French microbiologist **Louis Pasteur** who, in contrast to the young and aspiring Koch, was at the crest of a long and distinguished career. At first, Pasteur praised Koch's innovations, but later, largely because of Koch's harsh and often personal attacks, their relations became hostile. Ultimately, each claimed to have provided the final proof that the anthrax bacillus caused anthrax. Pasteur's argument rested on isolating the suspected causal organism and on inoculating pure strains into otherwise healthy animals—a procedure later codified under the name "Koch's Postulates" (which he probably adopted from his friend Edwin Klebs [1834–1913]). Once Koch adopted the Postulates, he repeatedly insisted that only by following those steps could causation be conclusively established. Ironically, although he also continued to claim that he had been the first to prove that the anthrax bacterium caused anthrax, at no point in his work on anthrax did Koch ever actually follow the Postulates. In fact, his failure to isolate and inoculate the organism was one basis for Pasteur's criticism of Koch's purported proof.

In the late nineteenth century, the disease now known as tuberculosis was the single most prominent disease in the western world. There had been repeated, but unsuccessful, attempts to show that it was bacterial in origin. Koch began studying the disease in August 1881. His work was kept absolutely secret and was conducted at a frantic pace. Relying, as usual, on technological innovations, Koch identified the causal organism and proved causation by meticulously following the Postulates. His first paper on tuberculosis, which was presented on March 24, 1882, in a meeting of the Berlin Physiological Society, was a stunning success. The younger biologist **Paul Ehrlich** described the meeting as his greatest experience in science. Within two years, Koch had also identified the causal organism for cholera. These achievements, together with Pasteur's successful anthrax and rabies inoculations, which came at about the same time, probably did more than anything else to persuade the world of the **germ theory** of disease in particular and of what has been called the etiological research program in general.

In 1891 the German government opened the Institute for Infectious Diseases and appointed Koch as the first director. Among Koch's students and colleagues at the Institute were **Emil Adolf von Behring**, who discovered **diphtheria** antitoxin; William Henry Welch (1850–1934), who was central to the rise of American bacteriology; **Shibasaburo Kitasato**, who helped develop tetanus antitoxin and identified the plague bacillus; **Gerhard Hansen**, who discovered the **leprosy**

ROBERT KOCH ON THE PREPARATION OF TUBERCULOSIS CULTURES (1882)

The simplest case in which the experiment is successful is presented, almost without exception, when an animal which has just died of tuberculosis, or a tuberculous animal which has just been killed for this purpose, is at one's disposal. First, the skin is deflected over the thorax and abdomen with instruments flamed just before use. With similarly prepared scissors and forceps, the ribs are cut in the middle, and the anterior chest wall is removed without opening the abdominal cavity, so that the lungs are to a large extent laid free. Then the instruments are again exchanged for freshly disinfected ones and single tubercules or particles of them, of the size of a millet seed, are quickly excised with scissors from the lung tissue, and immediately transferred to the surface of the solidified blood serum [coating the side of a test tube] with a platinum wire, which has been melted into a glass rod which must be flamed immediately before use. Of course, the cotton stopper [of the tube] may be removed for only a minimal time. In this manner a number of test tubes, about six to ten, are implanted with tuberculous material, because, with even the most cautious manipulation, not all test tubes remain free from accidental contamination.

Cultures that result from a growth of tubercule bacilli do not appear to the naked eye until the second week after the seeding, and ordinarily not until after the tenth day. They come into view as very small points and dry-looking scales.

From Koch's "The Etiology of Tuberculosis," translated by Berna and Max Pinner in *American Review of Tuberculosis* 25 (1932): 285–323.

bacillus; Christiaan Eijkman (1858–1930), whose work led to the discovery of vitamins; and August von Wasserman (1866–1925) and Paul Ehrlich, who made important contributions to **immunology**. All of this work brought world recognition to Koch, but there were clouds on the horizon. Probably hoping to emulate Pasteur's heralded and lucrative anthrax inoculations, in 1890 Koch had prematurely announced discovery of a substance, called tuberculin, which was expected to have prophylactic (preventive) or therapeutic significance for tuberculosis. As evidence accumulated that tuberculin was ineffective, Koch's professional credibility was tarnished. His reputation was also compromised by developments in his personal life. Around 1890 Koch fell in love with a 17-year-old actress named Hedwig Freiberg (1873–1945); he hastily divorced his wife and married Freiberg. Such behavior was incompatible with contemporary expectations, and society ostracized the couple.

Embarrassed by professional setbacks, rejected by Berlin society, and dogged by endless squabbles with competitors and former students, Koch spent more and more time away from Berlin. In 1896 he was invited to investigate *Rinderpest*, a disease that was ravaging cattle in the British colony of South Africa. He next traveled to Asia to study the **bubonic plague**. In 1898 and 1899, he visited Italy, Indonesia, and New Guinea. Between 1902 and 1907, he made several trips to Africa to investigate a range of human and animal diseases. In 1908 Koch visited America and Japan.

In 1910 Koch suffered a severe heart attack; he died a short time later. His body was cremated and the ashes deposited in a mausoleum in the Institute for Infectious Diseases in Berlin. *See also* Cholera: Fourth through Sixth Pandemics, 1862–1947; Contagion Theory of Disease, Premodern; Microscope.

Further Reading

Brock, Thomas D. *Koch: A Life in Medicine and Bacteriology*. Madison, WI: Science Tech Publishers, 1988.

Carter, K. Codell, trans. *Essays of Robert Koch*. Westport, CT: Greenwood Press, 1987.

———. *The Rise of Causal Concepts of Disease*. Burlington, VT: Ashgate, 2003.

K. CODELL CARTER

L

LASSA FEVER. *See* Hemorrhagic Fevers; Hemorrhagic Fevers in Africa.

LATIN AMERICA, COLONIAL: DEMOGRAPHIC EFFECTS OF IMPORTED DISEASES. Epidemics of imported diseases had a significant impact on demographic patterns throughout Latin America during the colonial period. Shortly after the arrival of Europeans in the Caribbean in 1492, the transfer of diseases from the Old World to the New began. During the next three centuries, epidemics of **smallpox, measles, bubonic plague, yellow fever**, and **malaria** appeared at regular intervals. Patterns of epidemic disease varied significantly by region, influenced by such factors as geography, climate, and population density. Some diseases such as smallpox, measles, yellow fever, and malaria eventually became endemic in specific areas. The first appearance of imported diseases resulted in virgin-soil epidemics (initial outbreaks of a disease previously unknown or absent from a particular area for many generations) that often produced morbidity rates over 50 percent and mortality rates of 25 to 50 percent. In general, throughout Latin America, indigenous populations declined 75 to 90 percent in the first century following contact with Old World diseases. Although the demographic impact of imported diseases on people of African or European origin was less severe, overall, epidemic disease had a devastating impact on human populations throughout Latin America between 1492 and 1800. The combination of epidemic disease and the violence and dislocation of European conquest ultimately produced significant social, demographic, economic, and political changes among indigenous populations, facilitating European conquest and colonization of the region.

The Historical Record. The historical record regarding the demographic impact of imported diseases varies significantly by region. Because Spanish **colonialism** in much of Latin America depended on a steady supply of indigenous labor, Spanish officials attempted to document the size of native populations in particular areas. Given that the largest indigenous populations resided in central Mexico and the Andean highlands, the most numerous and detailed records concerning epidemics of imported diseases and their demographic effects can be found in these areas. Although not as numerous, similar documents are also available for the Caribbean and Brazil, where Jesuit missionaries also recorded their observations of the demographic destruction visited upon native communities by diseases of Old World origin.

Spanish attempts to document the size of indigenous populations took a variety of forms during this early period. Some Spanish officials and settlers included estimates of the size of native populations in their written accounts. For example, Hernán Cortés (1485–1547), the conqueror of Mexico, offered estimates of the size of Aztec armies in his famous letters to the king of Spain. But the most detailed and numerous sources of demographic data during the sixteenth and seventeenth centuries derive from the efforts of royal officials to ascertain the size of indigenous populations for purposes of taxation and labor drafts. Following the military conquest of specific regions, Spanish conquerors and officials moved quickly to impose a system of tribute collection, and the first step in this process was to determine the number of Indians subject to this onerous tax. The censuses and tribute lists that resulted focused primarily on the number of adult males in a community, but in some cases they were organized by household and included the names and ages of everyone in the family. In some of the larger cities and towns of the Spanish empire, parish registers also recorded valuable information on demographic trends.

Just as the historical record varies by region, it also varies over time, with more detailed descriptions of epidemics and more complete census documents appearing during the second half of the eighteenth century. Historians and demographers have struggled with these problematic sources, especially those for the sixteenth and seventeenth centuries, for many years, and the controversy surrounding their reliability and usefulness is far from settled.

Nature of the Diseases.   Before the arrival of Europeans at the end of the fifteenth century, the disease environment of the Americas resembled that of other parts of the world in many significant respects. Acute respiratory and gastrointestinal diseases posed the greatest threats to human health, just as they did among Old World populations. Archaeological and documentary evidence also indicates that epidemics of **typhus** and **influenza** probably existed in the Americas before 1492. In addition, periodic famines, accompanied by high rates of secondary infections and mortality, also claimed the lives of significant numbers of native Americans. Finally, archaeological evidence suggests that high levels of violence, often as the result of **warfare**, played an important role in reducing indigenous populations before the end of the fifteenth century. But in spite of these similarities, the native peoples of the Americas were not immunologically prepared for the advent of a number of new, virulent infections that arrived along with European colonists and African slaves beginning in the early sixteenth century.

Smallpox, measles, bubonic and **pneumonic plague**, malaria, and yellow fever, all played a role in reducing the size of native populations throughout the New World. Smallpox and measles, both viral infections with attendant skin eruptions or rashes, were among the first of these diseases to make the trans-Atlantic journey. Both infections triggered virgin-soil epidemics, with accompanying mortality rates of 25 to 50 percent. Bubonic plague and its more virulent form, pneumonic plague, were often more difficult for observers to identify because their symptoms could be confused with other illnesses. Bubonic plague is caused by a bacillus that is transmitted to humans through the bites of infected fleas; whereas pneumonic plague, also caused by the plague bacillus, is spread directly through airborne droplets inhaled by those who come into contact with the sick. This more virulent form of the disease is characterized by high fever, headache, and sudden death, often claiming the lives of close to 100 percent of those infected.

Malaria was another imported disease that decimated American populations, both indigenous and European. Common in Europe, the disease, characterized by high fever and in some cases delirium, may have been introduced early in the sixteenth century and quickly became endemic in many areas. Although malaria is often a chronic disease, lying dormant in the human body for long periods, it can prove fatal to individuals already weakened by other infections or malnutrition.

Yellow fever was introduced from Africa as a result of the slave trade, probably during the 1640s. Symptoms of the disease, transmitted by the female *Aedes aegypti* mosquito, included sudden onset, fever, lethargy, jaundice, and sometimes the vomiting of blood. Although the disease proved especially lethal for Europeans and native Americans, Africans also succumbed, albeit in smaller numbers.

Origins and Spread.   Historians have identified numerous outbreaks of disease among both European and indigenous populations in the two decades following Christopher Columbus's (1451–1506) arrival in the Caribbean. But the first clearly documented epidemic of a disease imported from the Old World began in 1518 when smallpox appeared among the native population of Hispaniola. From this seat of Spanish colonial control, the disease spread quickly to other islands and finally to the Mexican mainland in 1520, arriving in time to play a major role in Cortés's siege of the Aztec capital, Tenochtitlán. From central Mexico, smallpox made its way south into Guatemala the following year. From there the disease probably continued into other areas of Central America and eventually into the Andean highlands. Although the arrival of smallpox is less clearly documented in South America, the disease may have arrived sometime between 1524 and 1530 when an epidemic swept through the Inca Empire, claiming the lives of several members of the Inca royal family and thousands of their subjects. The first recorded epidemic of smallpox in Brazil occurred in 1562, and thereafter, the disease reappeared at regular intervals for the remainder of the colonial period. Mortality rates associated with these first outbreaks of smallpox ranged between 25 and 50 percent for native Americans.

Initial epidemics of measles were more difficult to identify because the symptoms of the disease were often confused with those of smallpox. But given the long history of these diseases among European populations, the documentary evidence suggests that both viral infections had arrived in the Americas by the 1530s. Like smallpox, epidemics of measles often resulted in mortality rates of 25 to 50 percent. In some instances, both diseases appeared simultaneously, raising mortality rates even higher.

Given the challenges of distinguishing the symptoms of bubonic and pneumonic plague from other illnesses, the arrival of plague in the Americas is difficult to pinpoint. Epidemics of an illness that triggered severe hemorrhaging from mucous membranes occurred in Mexico and Peru in the 1540s and again in Mexico in the 1570s. Some scholars have also suggested that plague may have appeared in Brazil between 1559 and 1563, as the disease was epidemic in Portugal at the time and because observers described fever and hemorrhaging as symptoms of an illness then ravaging the indigenous population.

Although the documentary record is far from conclusive, malaria may have been the first of the imported diseases to appear in the New World, possibly arriving along with Columbus's fourth expedition in 1502. Columbus recorded that he, his son, and members of his crew became seriously ill, suffering from severe fevers. Because malaria was endemic throughout the Iberian Peninsula, many Europeans carried the plasmodium that caused the infection in their blood. Many explorers also recorded their encounters with swarms of mosquitoes, and research has revealed that the New World was home to species of the mosquito required to transmit the disease. Once introduced, malaria quickly became endemic and posed a severe threat to the health of both indigenous and European populations throughout the colonial period, especially in lowland tropical areas.

Yellow fever appears to have been the last of the Old World diseases imported to the Americas during the colonial period. Endemic to parts of Africa, the spread of this disease to other parts of the world followed the route of the African slave trade. The first documented outbreak of yellow fever occurred on the island of Barbados in 1647. From there the disease spread to other islands in the Caribbean and onto the mainland of Mexico and northern South America by the 1650s. Records indicate that epidemics of yellow fever did not reach Brazil or the Pacific coast of South America until the 1740s or even later. Both Europeans and natives proved highly susceptible to yellow fever, whereas long-term exposure to the disease among African populations conferred some measure of immunity.

The rapid and dramatic decline of native populations in response to the violence of European **colonialism** and the introduction of Old World diseases transformed the economic and political structures of indigenous societies. Migration, both forced and voluntary, altered settlement patterns and facilitated Spanish and Portuguese access to valuable natural resources. Warfare, famine, and epidemics led to declining birth rates, shrinking households, and rising rates of morbidity and mortality. Indigenous political structures changed as traditional native leaders collaborated with, or were replaced by, Spanish and Portuguese officials intent on implementing policies originating in European capitals. The responses of indigenous societies to epidemics of imported diseases and institutions of European colonialism also changed over time and included warfare and other forms of violence, messianic movements, **flight**, recourse to Spanish and Portuguese law courts, and the selective adoption and adaptation of various aspects of European culture, including Christianity.

It is interesting to note that although the history of European colonialism in Latin America has been rewritten by generations of scholars, few topics have generated the heated and often acrimonious rhetoric that surrounds the debate over the demographic history of the region on the eve of European contact. The controversy over estimating the size of New World populations began during the early sixteenth century, but the debate has been especially passionate since the 1960s. Many authors have published their calculations, some based on written records, others on mathematical formulas and computer simulations, and others on no apparent evidence at all. A review of some of the most widely cited figures reveals estimates that range from a low of 8.4 million to a high of 200 million.

Although the numbers themselves are significant, this emotional debate centers around three broad issues: First, what was the level of social, political, demographic, and economic development of New World societies before 1492? Second, to what extent did European colonialism and the introduction of Old World diseases devastate native American populations? And third, what is the nature of and appropriate use of the historical record? At the heart of this debate is a political schism between "high counters," those who view the aftermath of 1492 as the largest genocide in human history perpetrated by Europeans against the indigenous peoples of the Americas, and "low counters," those on the other side who argue that the native population of the New World was never large and that Europeans crossed the Atlantic to encounter a sparsely populated wilderness. The notion of the Americas as wilderness strengthens the argument that the political and economic benefits of Western civilization outweighed the destruction occasioned by the European conquest of the Americas.

The research of the later twentieth and early twenty-first centuries has revealed much about the social, political, and economic development of native American peoples before the arrival of Europeans; but the number of people who inhabited this hemisphere at the end of the fifteenth century will probably never be known for certain. What cannot be disputed, however, is that European colonialism and the introduction of diseases from the Old World reduced native American populations by 75 to 90 percent during the first century following contact. Furthermore, although the demographic impact of imported diseases on people of African or European origin was less severe, overall, epidemic disease had a devastating impact on human populations throughout Latin America between 1492 and 1800. *See also* Demographic Data Collection and Analysis, History of; Diagnosis of Historical Diseases; Disease in the Pre-Columbian Americas; Environment, Ecology, and Epidemic Disease; Historical Epidemiology; Human Immunity and Resistance to Disease; Insects, Other Arthropods, and Epidemic Disease; Malaria in the Americas; Measles in the Colonial Americas; Slavery and Epidemic Disease; Smallpox in Colonial Latin America; Yellow Fever in Colonial Latin America and the Caribbean.

Further Readings

Alchón, Suzanne Austin. *A Pest in the Land: New World Epidemics in a Global Perspective.* Albuquerque: University of New Mexico Press, 2003.

———. *Native Society and Disease in Colonial Ecuador.* Cambridge: Cambridge University Press, 1991.

Cook, Noble David. *Born to Die: Disease and New World Conquest, 1492–1650.* Cambridge: Cambridge University Press, 1998.

Cook, Noble David, and W. George Lovell, eds. *The Secret Judgments of God: Native Peoples and Old World Disease in Colonial Spanish America.* Norman: University of Oklahoma Press, 2001.

Henige, David. *Numbers from Nowhere: The American Indian Contact Population Debate.* Norman: University of Oklahoma Press, 1998.

Livi-Bacci, Massimo. "The Depopulation of Hispanic America after the Conquest." *Population and Development Review* 32, 2 (2006): 199–232.

McCaa, Robert. "Paleodemography of the Americas: From Ancient Times to Colonialism and Beyond." In *The Backbone of History: Health and Nutrition in the Western Hemisphere,* edited by Richard C. Steckel and Jerome C. Rose, pp. 94–124. New York: Cambridge University Press, 2002.

Verano, John W., and Douglas H. Ubelaker. *Disease and Demography in the Americas.* Washington, DC: Smithsonian Institution Press, 1992.

Suzanne Austin

LAVERAN, CHARLES LOUIS ALPHONSE (1845–1922). Alphonse Laveran was awarded the Nobel Prize for Physiology or Medicine in 1907 for his discovery of the **malaria** parasite that led to the identification of the mosquito's role in **transmission** of the disease. He was born in Paris, France, but when he was only five, his family moved to French Colonial Algeria, where his father had been transferred by the French army's medical service. Like his father and grandfather, Laveran elected to pursue a career in military medicine and completed his medical studies at the School of the Health Service of the Armies at Strasbourg in 1867. He served in the Franco-Prussian **War** (1870–1871) and was at the siege of Metz, where he helped care for the wounded.

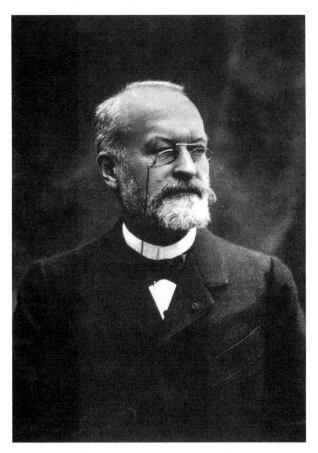

Alphonse Laveran. Courtesy of the National Library of Medicine.

When the city surrendered to the Prussians, Laveran was released and returned to France. He was then sent to the military hospital at Lille where he remained until the end of the war.

By age 29, Laveran was Professor of Diseases and Epidemics of Armies at the Val-de-Grâce Hospital in Paris, and when his appointment ended in 1878, he was reassigned to Algeria. He knew that about 30 percent of army personnel suffered from malaria. Deaths from malaria were higher than those from any other cause, so he began to autopsy malaria victims and examine the blood of individuals who suffered from the disease. Laveran began his study with the black malarial pigment, an iron-containing product from infected red blood cells, found in livers, spleens, and brains of malaria victims. It was during his studies, on November 6, 1880, that he made his first observations of the living malaria parasite. While examining freshly drawn blood from his patients, he clearly saw moving parasites that could not be seen in fixed and stained preparations. At the time, Laveran still accepted the long-standing theory that malaria was some sort of toxic vapor (mal'aria, "bad air") that arose in tropical swamps and was spread through the air. The connection between malarial fevers and marshes was very old, but, as Laveran realized, there were parts of the world where marshes existed without malaria, and conversely malaria could occur where there were no marshes. For a time, Laveran also considered the possibility that the malaria "germ" was in drinking **water** and that it would not occur if drinking water were first boiled. However, two years before Laveran's discovery of the malarial parasite, **Patrick Manson** had determined that the mosquito played a role in the development of another parasitic disease, and this ultimately led to the discovery of the role of the *Anopheles* mosquito in the transmission of malaria. Laveran spent his later years as a scientist studying **trypanosomiasis** and other tropical diseases caused by **protozoa**. *See also* Germ Theory of Disease; Insects, Other Arthropods, and Epidemic Disease; Ross, Ronald.

Further Reading

Bruce-Chuvatt, L. J. "Alphonse Laveran's Discovery 100 Years Ago and Today's Global Fight against Malaria." *Journal of the Royal Society of Medicine* 74 (1981): 531–536.

Jarcho, S. "Laveran's Discovery in the Retrospect of a Century." *Bulletin of the History of Medicine* 58 (1984): 215–224.

Nye, E. R. "Alphonse Laveran (1845–1922): Discoverer of the Malarial Parasite and Nobel Laureate, 1907." *Journal of Medical Biography* 10 (2002): 81–87.

RICHARD EIMAS

LAZARETTO. *See* Leprosarium; Pest Houses and Lazarettos.

LEEUWENHOEK, ANTONY VAN (1632–1723). Antony van Leeuwenhoek, a deeply curious man without a university education, is considered the father of bacteriology. In 1676, using a single lens **microscope** that he ground himself, he described the existence of what was later labeled by the German botanist Ferdinand Cohn (1828–1898) as **bacteria**. He believed that there was a similarity of form and function among all living things.

Leeuwenhoek was born in Delft, Holland, and prospered in the cloth trade, in which he had to use microscopes, available in Holland since the early seventeenth century, to look for flaws in material. It is possible that his interest in science was sparked by a visit to England, when he saw English scientist Robert Hooke's (1635–1703) book, *Micrographia* (1665), illustrating plants and animals seen with a compound (two lenses) microscope. Starting in 1671, Leeuwenhoek, who would not use a compound microscope, made the first of about 500 microscopes, most of them tiny, and many holding only one specimen permanently. As historian J. R. Porter puts it, his "special skill lay in polishing and mounting the lens between the metal plates, in obtaining the proper source of light, and in focusing on the object. Objects to be viewed were mounted on a small pin or specimen holder and brought into focus by adjusting two or three threaded screws, which moved the specimen in various ways in front of the lens."

Leeuwenhoek was friendly with some noted Dutch scientists, who encouraged him to share his finding with the world's oldest national scientific society, the Royal Society in England, and they translated hundreds of letters from one language to another. Leeuwenhoek used nonscientific terminology, illustrated all his letters, and described "animalcules" (the "little animals" or microorganisms) that he saw with his microscopes. He carried out experiments on bacteria, which he obtained from a variety of locations, including all his own bodily secretions. He discovered that both vinegar and hot coffee would kill bacteria and that heat would harm it. He examined bacteria that grew in sealed containers of pure rainwater infused with pepper and was the first person to see that bacteria would grow without exposure to air.

Though scientists throughout Europe were using compound microscopes to study organisms, Leeuwenhoek's work was not surpassed until the nineteenth century. Leeuwenhoek did not train any scientific apprentices, and his secrets died with him. *See also* Germ Theory of Disease; Scientific Revolution and Epidemic Disease.

Further Reading

Ford, Brian J. *The Revealing Lens: Mankind and the Microscope*. London: Harrap, 1973.

Porter, J. R. "Antony van Leeuwenhoek: Tercentenary of his Discovery of Bacteria." *Bacteriological Reviews* 40, 2 (June 1976): 260–226. http://pubmedcentral.gov/.

MARTHA STONE

LEGIONNAIRES' DISEASE.   Legionnaires' Disease is a potentially fatal pneumonia caused by infection with the Gram-negative **bacterium** *Legionella pneumophilia*. Mortality is highest among the elderly and individuals with compromised **immunity**. It is named for a famous outbreak among attendees at a national convention of the American Legion, an American military veterans organization, in Philadelphia during the summer of 1976. Prior to that outbreak, this organism and its association with human disease were unknown. In 1968 a similar flu-like illness with very rapid onset (2 to 48 hours after exposure) was detected among people in the Health Department Building in Pontiac, Michigan, which was later found to have been caused by *L. pneumophilia*. This illness has been called Pontiac Fever; it is self-limited, resolves without treatment, and does not result in pneumonia. It is considered a less severe form of infection with *Legionella*.

The **Centers for Disease Control and Prevention** (CDC) report that the disease affects 8,000 to 18,000 individuals per year (and probably more because of underreporting). Only about 10 to 20 percent of cases are identified with outbreaks, and about 20 percent are nosocomial (hospital-acquired). The majority of cases are sporadic, not associated with clustered outbreaks. Case fatality rates have been reported between 1 and 40 percent and appear to depend on the rapidity of **diagnosis**, institution of preventive measures, and appropriate **antibiotic** treatment. No person-to-person spread has ever been noted.

The organism of Legionnaires' Disease, *L. pneumophilia*, is a facultative intracellular pathogen, which means that it is able to grow within cells, but it does not have to do so. In the natural ecology of the organism, it appears that *L. pneumophilia* can infect free-living amoebae in warm freshwater, especially air-conditioning cooling **water**. Its ability to grow inside of other cells explains some of its pathogenicity in humans. The organism invades and multiplies inside macrophages, especially those in the lung, eventually killing these immune defense cells. The bacteria inhibit the normal mechanisms the macrophages use for attacking bacteria—that is, they prevent fusion of the phagosomes with the lysosomes within the macrophages. In this way, *L. pneumophilia* escapes the usual **immunity** provided by the macrophage system.

The nearest relative to the *Legionella* group of organisms is *Coxiella burnetii*, the pathogen responsible for Q-fever. Although *Coxiella* also invades macrophages, it appears to be able to survive within the acidic lysosomes, using a slightly different mechanism from *Legionella* for evasion of host cell destruction. Even so, the two groups of bacteria share many related genes.

Because of its intracellular location, the susceptibility of *L. pneumophilia* to antibiotics in laboratory cultures is not a good guide to clinical utility. Drugs must achieve high intracellular concentrations to be effective in the infected patients. Antibiotics with good intracellular penetration include the macrolides (e.g., erythromycin), quinolones (e.g., ciprofloxacin), tetracyclines (e.g., doxycycline), and rifampin.

The outbreak from which this disease gets it name started in Bloomsburg, Pennsylvania, on July 30, 1976, with the diagnosis of pneumonia of unknown origin in three men who had attended the national convention of the American Legion in Philadelphia a few days earlier. By August 2, 1976, the Pennsylvania State Health Department realized that a new disease was occurring among other attendees at the convention. Within the week, however, investigators had provisionally ruled out most known bacteria, fungi, and **viruses** as possible causes of these pneumonia cases. Causes discussed in the scientific and popular media at that time ranged from toxic chemicals to **bioterrorism** (domestic or foreign) aimed at the veterans. By September 1976, the focus had shifted from outside causes, such as a disease carrier, to the hotel environment itself, especially on toxins such as nickel carbonyl. For about six months, it appeared that little progress was being made, and public anxiety grew with alarmist newspaper accounts and congressional hearings. In January 1977, however, the CDC identified a previously unrecognized bacterium as being associated with the outbreak. This organism was subsequently classified as *Legionella pneumophilia.* With the realization that this organism was sensitive to several known antibiotics, public anxiety abated, but not before an estimated 180 cases resulting in 29 deaths had been studied. The convention hotel was closed as well (later to reopen).

Since this initial 1976 outbreak, other outbreaks have been identified around the world: United Kingdom, 1985 and 2002; Netherlands, 1999; Spain, 2001 and 2006; Norway, 2001 and 2005; France, 2004; New Zealand, 2005; Canada, 2005; Australia, 2007; and the United States (New York), 2007. *See also* Disease, Social Construction of; Environment, Ecology, and Epidemic Disease.

Further Reading

Bartram, Jamie, et al., eds. *Legionella and the Prevention of Legionellosis.* Geneva: World Health Organization, 2007.

Centers for Disease Control and Prevention. *Legionellosis.* http://www.cdc.gov/ncidod/dbmd/diseaseinfo/legionellosis_g.htm

Mayo Clinic. *Legionnaires' Disease.* http://www.mayoclinic.com/health/legionnaires-disease/DS00853

Stout, Janet E., and Victor L. Yu. "Legionellosis." *The New England Journal of Medicine* 337 (1997): 682–687.

Thomas, Gordon, and Max Morgan-Witts. *Anatomy of an Epidemic.* Garden City, NY: Doubleday, 1982.

World Health Organization. *Legionellosis.* http://www.who.int/mediacentre/factsheets/fs285/en/

WILLIAM C. SUMMERS

LEPROSARIUM.   Leprosaria have also been known as leper houses, leper colonies, and in the European Middle Ages lazar houses (also lazaretto, lazarette, or lazaret; after Lazarus, a biblical figure whom Christians believed was cured of his **leprosy** by Jesus). Modern leprosaria are hospitals and infirmaries that treat victims of leprosy, more properly known as Hansen's disease. Most leprosaria are residential hospitals, which is why they are also known as leper colonies. There are hundreds of leprosaria actively housing patients around the world, most notably in India, Africa, Brazil, and China. The last leprosarium in the continental United States was established in 1894 by the State of Louisiana in Carville, Louisiana. The site chosen was an abandoned plantation with a dilapidated mansion and seven old slave cabins. Known initially as the Louisiana Leper Home and staffed by Catholic nuns, the U.S. Public Health Service took over its management in 1921. Recently it was closed, but some of its research, education, and treatment functions were moved to Louisiana State University at Baton Rouge.

In the European Middle Ages leper houses were usually run by monastic houses and were thus organized in a similar fashion. The leper in effect took religious vows and removed him or herself from the community at large. Once diagnosed with leprosy (which in fact was often a misdiagnoses of other skin conditions), the medieval leper was pronounced dead and forced to enter a leprosarium. He or she was then enjoined to pray for absolution of whatever may have caused the leprosy, as all diseases in the Middle

Ages were viewed as punishments from God for sin. There were also strict laws limiting the leper's contact with the healthy; lepers were not allowed to enter most European towns during the day and usually had to ring a bell or a clapper to announce their presence, to limit physical contact with others. European experience with lepers set the pattern for isolating plague victims, and during plague outbreaks empty leprosaria often became **pest houses**.

Elsewhere in the world, and in time, other cultures also built leprosaria to isolate those afflicted with the disease. Because leprosy is a disfiguring disease, and the physically disfiguring symptoms have often been deemed too disturbing to look upon, and because the disease was generally feared as highly contagious, leper houses were created to remove the leper and protect the community. Many leprosaria were built far away from communities, to isolate the patients further. Others were built near major settlements, to ensure ease of collecting donations to support the leprosaria. Because medical science has now determined that Hansen's disease is not as contagious as once thought, and a there has been a general change in attitude toward people disfigured by disease, many leprosaria worldwide have closed, and patients have been integrated into other medical facilities or into society at large. *See also* Leprosy in the Premodern World; Leprosy in the United States; Leprosy, Societal Reactions to; Scapegoats and Epidemic Disease.

Further Reading

Edmond, Rod. *Leprosy and Empire: A Medical and Cultural History*. New York: Cambridge University Press, 2007.

Gaudet, Marcia. *Carville: Remembering Leprosy in America*. Jackson: University Press of Mississippi, 2004.

Gould, Tony. *A Disease Apart: Leprosy in the Modern World*. New York: St. Martin's Press, 2005.

Rawcliffe, Carole. *Leprosy in Medieval England*. Rochester, NY: Boydell, 2006.

Tayman, John. *The Colony: The Harrowing True Story of the Exiles of Molokai*. New York: Scribners, 2007.

CANDACE GREGORY-ABBOTT

LEPROSY.   Leprosy is a **bacterial** infection that causes damage to skin and nerves, with resulting disfigurement and deformity. Although leprosy is now curable, and the risk to exposed individuals is extremely low, the very word leprosy continues to evoke strong emotions. The disease remains endemic in some tropical countries.

Leprosy is caused by *Mycobacterium leprae* (M. *leprae*), a slow-growing, rod-shaped bacterium. Bacteriologists classify M. *leprae* as acid-fast bacteria (AFB) because it is resistant to decolorization by acids during conventional staining. With the commonly used Fite stain, M. *leprae* appears bright red under the microscope.

Norwegian researcher **Gerhard Hansen** first identified the leprosy bacillus microscopically in 1873. M. *leprae* lives within human cells, preferring the cooler temperatures in the nerves and skin of the extremities. Scientists have never succeeded in growing cultures of M. *leprae* in nutrient broths or on agar, hampering research into the disease. M. *leprae* can be grown in nine-banded armadillos (*Dasypus movemcinctus*), the only natural nonhuman reservoirs of the disease, and in laboratory mice. Recent sequencing of the M. *leprae* genome should lead to advances in treatment and prevention.

Most people who become infected with M. *leprae* mount an immunological defense that eliminates the infection. In progressive cases, symptoms are caused not only by invasion of bacteria, but also by immune responses triggered by the bacteria. M. *leprae* is transmitted through respiratory secretions. Transmission through skin patches or sores rarely, if ever, occurs. Close contact with an infected person increases the risk of transmission. Mothers do not infect their children in the uterus, but children in crowded households are susceptible to M. *leprae*. Most victims have no known contact with the disease. Even before the introduction of antimicrobial therapy, nurses and other caregivers were rarely infected. Some individuals appear to have increased genetic susceptibility to the disease.

> **NAMING THE UNSPEAKABLE**
>
> Near the end of the twentieth century, victims, caregivers, and the medical community at large decided that use of the term "leper," with its centuries-old stigmatizing power, should be abandoned in favor of "Hansen's Disease," a name recognizing the central role of Norwegian biologist Gerhard Hansen in leprosy research. Around the globe and across time, however, Hansen's Disease has had many different labels. The term in Old Norse, ancestor of Hansen's Norwegian, is directly related to the verb "to suffer." In Mali it is "the big disease," while Brazilians refer to it as "the spot disease." In the southern United States some folks refer to it as "this package," but among Cajuns in Louisiana it is "the disease you do not name." Arabic has long had two labels: one is *djudham*, which derives from the verb to cut off or mutilate, and the other is *al-baras*, a reference to the hypopigmented white blotches on the victim's skin.

The incubation period of leprosy averages four to ten years. The diagnosis is usually confirmed by identification of M. *leprae* in skin scrapings or tissue samples. In untreated patients, progressive nerve damage causes loss of sensation, especially in the hands and feet. Patients are unable to feel trauma such as burns, cuts, or painful pressure leading to chronic skin ulcerations with destruction of underlying bone. In time, the tissues become contracted or deformed, and fingers and toes may be destroyed (autoamputation). Further disability results from damage to motor nerves with subsequent muscle weakness in the hands and feet. Leprosy is usually not fatal, but many victims have died from neglect, uncontrolled infections, and behavior related to their despair.

There are two major forms of leprosy as well as several intermediate or borderline forms. Tuberculoid leprosy produces pale, dry, scaling skin patches with decreased or absent feeling as a result of nerve damage. Hypertrophied (enlarged) nerves may be felt through the skin. Tuberculoid leprosy is also called paucibacillary leprosy (*pauci-*, few) because there are very few M. *leprae* present in the skin and nerves.

The more severe form of leprosy is called lepromatous leprosy. These patients develop skin thickening and nodules as well as damage to the motor and sensory peripheral nerves. The number of M. *leprae* bacteria in the body of the patient is very high (multibacillary leprosy), thus rendering untreated patients more infectious. In addition to skin and nerves, M. *leprae* may attack the eyes, nasal cartilage, and larynx causing, respectively, blindness, collapse of the nasal bridge, and hoarseness. In some patients, skin nodules on the face produce a characteristic lion-like facial expression (leonine facies).

Historically, leprosy has tended to cluster in certain geographic areas. In North America the disease was once prevalent in Louisiana and New Brunswick, Canada. Although leprosy is generally endemic rather than **epidemic**, major population dislocations under conditions of **war** or natural disaster expose more people to the disease. For example,

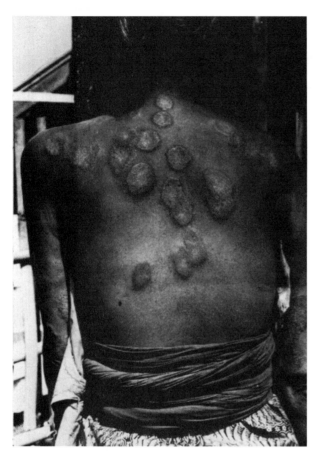

A woman, naked to the waist, shows the lesions resulting from leprosy on her back and arms, 1979. WHO photo. Courtesy of the National Library of Medicine.

dozens of American servicemen contracted leprosy in the Philippines during the Spanish-American War. Theories explaining the sharp decline in leprosy in Europe in the fourteenth century include improved standard of living, advances in hygiene, crossover immunity from **tuberculosis**, depopulation from **bubonic plague**, and the effectiveness of isolation measures. In retrospect, isolation was probably never very effective in preventing spread of the disease. The last endemic focus of leprosy in Western Europe was in Norway, where the disease lingered into the early twentieth century.

It is not surprising that scores of ineffective drugs and treatments have been tried over the centuries in an effort to control leprosy. Chaulmoogra oil, obtained from the seeds of several species of trees, was used for hundreds of years to treat leprosy in Asia and India. Western physicians introduced injectable forms of chaulmoogra oil in the first half of the twentieth century with unpleasant side effects and questionable benefits.

In 1940, Drs. Guy Faget (1891–1947) and Frederick Johansen at the U.S. Public Health Service Hospital in Carville, Louisiana (the national leprosy hospital), discovered that new injectable drugs Promin and DDS (dapsone) could help some patients, despite severe side effects.

Physicians in a number of countries soon devised effective, tolerable regimens of oral dapsone. In many patients, years of dapsone therapy eliminated M. *leprae* and reversed or improved symptoms. Outpatient treatments ended years of forced hospitalization and isolation. Within a few decades, single drug therapy with dapsone led to **drug resistance** and relapses. In some patients, therapy was complicated by severe inflammatory reactions.

Since the 1980s, the key to treatment and cure of leprosy has been multidrug therapy (MDT). Standard MDT includes dapsone, rifampin, and clofazimime, usually self-administered under medical supervision. Rifampin rapidly kills M. *leprae*. Clofazimime and dapsone slow the growth of the bacteria; clofazimime also helps prevent inflammatory reactions. **World Health Organization** regimens, designed for maximum ease of administration in medically underserved areas, range from 6 to 12 months, although treatment is usually given for longer periods in the United States. Isolation is unnecessary because patients are rendered noninfectious within a matter of weeks. Ideally, patients should be identified and treated before nerve damage leads to irreversible ulcers, deformities, or loss of digits. Bacille Calmette-Guerin (BCG) vaccine, widely used outside the United States to prevent tuberculosis, may protect some household contacts.

In medieval Europe, leprosy was variously seen as a loathsome disease, a biblical scourge, a venereal affliction, a divine punishment, or paradoxically a symbol of divine grace. Because disease clusters occurred in households, leprosy was also considered a hereditary disorder. Today, the term "leper," with its layers of historical meaning, is avoided because it is offensive to victims of leprosy. Some patients and advocates prefer the term Hansen's disease.

Leprosy may have originated in antiquity, but historians are cautious in making modern diagnoses based on ancient descriptions. Biblical use of the ancient Hebrew word for scaly skin disease (tsara-ath) was mistranslated as "leprosy." Prior to the introduction of effective antimicrobial therapy in the 1940s, the fundamental and almost universal response to leprosy was banishment of the victims from society to protect the community. In the prison-like setting of many government-mandated facilities for the forced isolation of leprosy victims, such as the colony established on Molokai in the Hawaiian Islands in 1865, complete neglect of hygiene and basic care resulted in foul-smelling ulcerations complicated by malnutrition and exposure. Members of religious orders and medical missionaries often assumed the onerous task of establishing and staffing hospitals or medical colonies. The best known of these was the Belgian priest Father Damien (1840–1889), who arrived at Molokai in 1873. Nineteenth-century imperialist governments frequently established isolation institutions and policies, as the Americans did in the Philippines. In every society, some victims lived secretly or remained hidden rather than face a grim future in **leprosaria**. Even the best leprosy hospitals were both haven and prison for their stigmatized residents.

Since 2000 the number of new cases has decreased by about 100,000 annually, with 300,000 new cases diagnosed in 2005. Most of these cases occur in places where the disease is endemic, led by India and Brazil. Political, social, logistical, and informational barriers continue to challenge international efforts to eradicate leprosy. Fewer than 200 cases of leprosy were detected in the United States in 2005, with most occurring in immigrants from endemic areas. *See also* Diet, Nutrition, and Epidemic Disease; Leprosy in the Premodern World; Leprosy in the United States; Leprosy, Societal Reactions to; Scapegoats and Epidemic Disease.

Further Reading

Boggild, A. K., J. S. Keystone, and K. C. Kain. "Leprosy: A Primer for Canadian Physicians." *Canadian Medical Association Journal* 170 (2004): 71–78.

Buckingham, Jane. *Leprosy in Colonial India: Medicine and Confinement.* New York: Palgrave Macmillan, 2002.

Centers for Disease Control and Prevention. *Hansen's Disease (Leprosy).* http://www.cdc.gov/ncidod/dbmd/diseaseinfo/hansens_t.htm

Demaitre, Luke. *Leprosy in Premodern Medicine: A Malady of the Whole Body.* Baltimore: Johns Hopkins University Press, 2007.

Edmond, Rod. *Leprosy and Empire: A Medical and Cultural History.* New York: Cambridge University Press, 2007.

Gaudet, Marcia. *Carville: Remembering Leprosy in America.* Jackson: University Press of Mississippi, 2004.

Gould, Tony. *A Disease Apart: Leprosy in the Modern World*. New York: St. Martin's Press, 2005.

Levis, W. R., and J. D. Erns "Mycobacterium leprae." In *Principles and Practices of Infectious Diseases*, 6th edition, edited by Gerald L. Mandell, John E. Bennett, and Raphael Dolin. London: Churchill Livingstone, 2004.

Rawcliffe, Carole. *Leprosy in Medieval England*. Rochester, NY: Boydell, 2006.

Sehgal, Alfica. *Leprosy*. Philadelphia: Chelsea House, 2005.

Tayman, John. *The Colony: The Harrowing True Story of the Exiles of Molokai*. New York: Scribners, 2007.

World Health Organization. *Leprosy*. http://www.who.int/mediacentre/factsheets/fs101/en/

SANDRA W. MOSS

LEPROSY IN THE PREMODERN WORLD. Research in molecular evolution suggests that *Mycobacterium leprae*, the pathogen responsible for **leprosy** or Hansen's disease, probably evolved in east Africa or the Near East as a single clone that was then spread by human migrations, acquiring a very small amount of genetic diversity along the way. It probably first moved eastward to India and China and the Pacific, and then northwestward to Europe. Leprosy strains in the Americas are closely related to strains from Europe and North Africa and from West Africa, not to strains from East Asia. This indicates that leprosy was introduced to the Western Hemisphere by European settlers (especially from the Scandinavian countries, the last stronghold of the disease in Europe) and by the slave trade from West Africa. In other words, leprosy reached the Americas after Christopher Columbus (1451–1506). However leprosy was known to all the great ancient civilizations in the Old World

China, India, and the Western Pacific. Leprosy was well known in China from the middle of the first millennium BCE onward. An anecdote dating to the "Warring States" period (475–221 BCE) shows that people were frightened to approach lepers. In 1975 archeologists working on the tomb of a local official who died in 217 BCE unearthed a text on a bamboo strip describing sanctions against lepers who committed crimes. This text shows that China had a complex body of legal regulations for dealing with lepers by that time. Lepers who committed capital crimes were to be executed by drowning, an otherwise unknown method of execution that was thought to wash away ritual impurity, whereas those who committed less serious offenses were to be sent to special penal colonies for lepers. From the time of the Han dynasty onwards (206 BCE–220 CE) there are references to individuals of high social status who were thought to be suffering from the disease. Leprosy was a problem for all social classes. The philosopher Confucius (551–479 BCE) attributed leprosy to the will of heaven, but doctors sought naturalistic explanations for the disease from an early stage. The *Neijing*, a classic early Chinese work of medicine dating to the Warring States period, attributed leprosy to a factor called "*feng*." By the time of the *Neijing* it had already been recognized in China that many people who come into contact with leprosy cases fail to develop the disease themselves; in other words they are resistant to leprosy. Human genetic factors appear to play a very important role in determining susceptibility to leprosy. In 610 CE the doctor Chao Yuanfang (550–630) tried to explain leprosy in terms of a living pathogen that was thought to attack people. During the Song dynasty (960–1279 CE) Chen Yan (fl. c. 1174) was the first Chinese doctor to describe leprosy as an infectious disease. From China movements of peoples speaking Austronesian languages carried leprosy eastward to the Pacific Islands. Skeletons of medieval date with bone deformations typical of leprosy were excavated on Guam in the Pacific. Leprosy ("kustha") is clearly described in the great early medical texts of India and Ceylon such as the *Susruta Samhita*. "Kustha" was an infectious disease thought to be transmitted by respiration or touch, through sexual intercourse, or through handling objects previously touched by a person with leprosy. In certain respects this analysis was extremely perceptive, because leprosy is now known to be acquired primarily by inhalation. Skeletons exhibiting symptoms of leprosy have been excavated at an Iron Age archeological site in Thailand (500 BCE–300 CE).

Ancient Near East and Egypt.   There has been a considerable amount of scholarly controversy regarding the presence of leprosy in the ancient Near East. Nevertheless, the balance of probability is that it was present. One cuneiform text from ancient Mesopotamia, which mentions the destruction of fingers and toes, sounds like a description of leprosy. There is also mention of white patches or nodules on the body, possibly a distinction between tuberculoid and lepromatous leprosy, the two principal forms of the disease. There has been plenty of discussion about how to interpret the term *tsara'ath* found in the Biblical book of Leviticus. Though generally translated into English as "leprosy," it seems preferable to interpret this word as a designation of ritual impurity in general, thought to require social exclusion, rather than as a description of a specific disease such as leprosy. However the term probably covered cases of leprosy in practice alongside sufferers from other skin diseases such as psoriasis. The Greek historian Herodotus (c. 484–425 BCE) states that social exclusion measures were taken against victims of a "white disease" in Persia in the fifth century BCE. The so-called "Phoenician disease" mentioned in a **Hippocratic** text of the fifth or fourth centuries BCE was leprosy, according to **Galen's** commentary from the second century CE, but no detailed information about it is available. There are no clear descriptions of leprosy in ancient Egyptian medical texts, such as the papyrus Ebers, dating to the time of the Pharaohs.

Ancient Greece and Rome.   The argument from the silence of the ancient Egyptian sources, which seldom describe any recognizable disease, is not conclusive. As soon as Greek migration to Egypt commenced in the late fourth century BCE, after the conquests of Alexander the Great (356–323 BCE), the Greeks started to notice the high prevalence in Egypt of leprosy, which to them was a new disease. Four skeletons, dating to the second century BCE and showing symptoms of leprosy, were excavated in the Dakhleh oasis in Egypt, possibly a colony for exiled lepers. There are no references to leprosy in the texts of the Hippocratic corpus, dating to the fourth and fifth centuries BCE, apart from the "Phoenician disease." The physician Straton (c. 340–268 BCE) was the first Greek author to describe leprosy. Because the new disease lacked a name in Greek, Straton called it "kakochymia," but this new term did not catch on. It was soon replaced by "elephantiasis," which became the standard ancient Greek word for leprosy. It was also sometimes called the "sacred disease," a euphemism also covering epilepsy. The Hippocratic word "lepra" originally had nothing to do with leprosy but was employed to translate the Hebrew *tsara'ath* into Greek and so eventually came to be associated with the new disease. The Roman encyclopedist Pliny the Elder (23–79) described leprosy as a new disease, which had only been known since the time of the doctor Asclepiades of Bithynia (late second century BCE). Similarly the medical writer Celsus (25 BCE–50 CE) regarded leprosy as a foreign disease in the first century CE. By that time the Greeks and Romans were becoming sufficiently familiar with the new disease to give good clinical descriptions of the lepromatous form, starting with Aretaeus in the first century CE, followed by Rufus of Ephesus (fl. late first c. CE) and Galen in the second century CE. Galen stated that leprosy was common in Alexandria in Egypt, an opinion repeated by **Avicenna** in the medieval period. In the fourth century CE, the sermons of the bishops of Cappadocia (in modern Turkey), such as St. Basil (c. 330–379), demonstrate a preoccupation with the social problems created by leprosy. The slow spread of leprosy is in fact the best-documented example of the spread of a new disease into the Greco-Roman world. Leprosy spreads slowly because *Mycobacterium leprae* is a very slow-growing species of bacterium.

Medieval Europe.   The spread of leprosy throughout Europe principally occurred in late antiquity and the medieval period. There were notable additions to Western knowledge about leprosy in the early medieval period. Arab physicians, such as Abul-Qasim (c. 936–1015) in Spain, and Byzantine doctors such as Paul of Aegina (c. 625–690) began to realize the importance of the neurological symptoms of tuberculoid leprosy, which is the least virulent form and had been overlooked by earlier writers. Archeological excavations of several cemeteries attached to leprosaria in Denmark and Britain have confirmed the reality of leprosy in northwestern Europe in the medieval period. The skeletal remains at Odense in Denmark show that lepers with facial symptoms were singled out for inclusion in the leprosarium, following the diagnostic criteria given by literary sources. Leprosy was not just a social construct, as has been suggested; it was a real disease in Europe at that time, although some accusations of being a leper were doubtless employed to exclude individuals from wider society. Research on ancient DNA from *Mycobacterium leprae* is also starting to make a contribution to knowledge of medieval leprosy. *See also* Ayurvedic Disease Theory and Medicine; Chinese Disease Theory and Medicine; Colonialism and Epidemic Disease; Contagion Theory of Disease, Premodern; Diagnosis of Historical Diseases; Greco-Roman Medical Theory and Practice; Hansen, Gerhard Armauer; Heredity and Epidemic Disease; Human Immunity and Resistance to Disease; Islamic Disease Theory and Medicine; Latin America, Colonial: Demographic Effects of Imported Diseases; Leprosy, Societal Reactions to; Paleopathology; Personal Liberties and Epidemic Disease; Religion and Epidemic Disease; Scapegoats and Epidemic Disease.

Further Reading

Bodde, Derk. "Forensic Medicine in Pre-imperial China." *Journal of the American Oriental Society* 102 (1982): 1–15.

Demaitre, Luke. *Leprosy in Premodern Medicine: A Malady of the Whole Body.* Baltimore: Johns Hopkins University Press, 2007.

Dols, Michael. "The Leper in Medieval Islamic Society." *Journal of the History of Medicine* 34 (1979): 314–333.

Grmek, Mirko. *Diseases in the Ancient Greek World.* Baltimore: Johns Hopkins University Press, 1989.

Rawcliffe, Carole. *Leprosy in Medieval England.* Woodbridge: Boydell & Brewer, 2006.

Roberts, Charlotte, Mary Lewis, and Keith Manchester, eds. *The Past and Present of Leprosy: Archaeological, Historical, Paleopathological and Clinical Approaches.* Oxford: Archaeopress, 2002.

ROBERT SALLARES

LEPROSY IN THE UNITED STATES.   Leprosy, now known as **Hansen's** disease, has had a low rate of incidence in the United States. Until the period following the Civil War, American leprosy sufferers were managed locally, within their immediate communities. As the disease's symptoms take years to manifest, if they become visible at all, some individuals were able to conceal the disease. Others lived under improvised **quarantine** in homes, hospitals, or **leprosaria**. In the late nineteenth and early twentieth centuries, however, individuals with leprosy were consolidated within a few institutions. Massachusetts briefly operated an institution for those with leprosy from 1905 until 1921, but the primary locales in which individuals were confined and treated were Carville, Louisiana, 85 miles north of New Orleans, and the Kalaupapa colony on the island of Molokai, Hawaii.

Of the 37 patients admitted to Massachusetts' Penikese Hospital over its 15-year tenure, most were immigrants and/or had no place of legal residence. Offering little in the way of therapeutic intervention, the Penikese authorities focused on regulating patients' **diets** and arranging regimens of outdoor activity thought to be beneficial. The Board of Charity of Massachusetts struggled with retaining trained staff, maintaining suitable quarters and laboratory space, and meeting the needs and desires of residents. Attuned to the facility's shortcomings, the Board repeatedly concluded that residents could not be well served. In 1913 the legislature allowed for the parole of patients not considered public health threats. After 1917, when Congress passed a law providing for the creation of a national leprosarium, Penikese had even greater difficulty obtaining appropriations, and four years later the hospital's 13 patients were transferred to Carville.

When the Louisiana Leper Home in Carville originally opened in 1894, it was the first state facility exclusively intended for the maintenance of leprosy sufferers. The state opened the home after press coverage highlighted the high incidence of leprosy in the state and exposed poor conditions within the New Orleans leprosarium. The Board of Control for the home engaged four nuns to care for the first seven patients, who moved into the slave quarters of a former plantation. When Carville was chosen to become the national leprosarium to provide "care, detention, and treatment" in 1921, the institution received a Medical Officer-in-Charge (MOC), **physicians**, and medical staff, as well as an infusion of funds for expanding and improving its facilities. Those diagnosed with leprosy in any state (except for New York, where isolation was not mandatory) could legally be apprehended and forced to reside at Carville, which was now administered by the U.S. Public Health Service (USPHS). Many who came to live in Carville, however, came of their own volition. Some came after having been reported to the health or police departments, whereas others came as a result of their own or their intimates' fears that they might spread infection. The patient census ranged between 200 and 400 individuals from the 1920s through the 1960s.

As in Massachusetts, Carville's medical staff could do little to alter the course of patients' illnesses before the development of sulfone drugs in the 1940s. The only treatment for leprosy thought to be of any value was Chaulmoogra oil, a nauseating and largely ineffective tree extract that patients could take orally or by injection. Given the lack of effective treatment, Carville's staff and administrators' primary objective was to control the movements of their charges. Beginning in 1921, patients had to adhere to rules that made their isolation more pronounced. There was no telephone designated for their use, the road to Carville was unpaved, and although small numbers of patients were permitted short vacations, they could only travel with the permission of their destinations' state health officers and had to avoid all public transportation. They also did not have the right to vote. Residents faced indefinite terms of confinement, as medical discharge was secured only by testing negative for the presence of Hansen's bacillus for 12 consecutive months.

Despite its penal features, Carville was not a sealed institution. Although the facility was surrounded by a high barbed-wire fence with a 24-hour guard, patients regularly slipped though the fence to hunt, visit Baton Rouge, or try to survive independently on the outside.

Patients cultivated a semblance of community, autonomy, and comfort that was permitted insofar as it did not interfere with Carville's priority of containing **contagion**. In the 1920s and 1930s, patients constructed cottages on the facility's grounds. A resident described Carville as "complete in its confines, with churches, shops, a theater, a morgue, the little cemetery, even a jail. Operating inside its fences are all the activities of a tiny city" (Martin, 1950, p. 75). The early Carville population was 40 percent foreign-born, two-thirds female, and less than 10 percent African American. Three quarters of patients were Catholic, a handful were Jewish, and most of the remainder were Protestant. Patient dormitories were racially segregated, but the facility's school was not.

The "tiny city" underwent a great deal of change in the 1940s, 1950s, and 1960s. During the Great Depression, patients at Carville generally did not challenge the medical-paternal order that provided for them, and they cooperated in enforcing their own seclusion. But during the Second World War and its aftermath, new therapeutics simultaneously increased patients' gratitude for the benefits they received as federal wards and, by instilling a new hope for recovery, fostered a vocal critique of the government's approach to fulfilling its mandate to care, detain, and treat.

In 1941 trials with **sulfa drugs** and sulfones were conducted at Carville, and the latter resulted in marked improvement in early cases within several months. Within two to three years, many patients were medically discharged. Equipped with these powerful new treatments, Carville's administrators continued to assert their authority over residents over the next several years, but the patient body began to organize, to resist breaches of **personal liberty**, and to demand changes. *The Star*, Carville's community newsletter, became a forum for articulating demands and a mode for circumventing the institutional hierarchy, allowing patients to communicate directly with decision-makers at the federal level and with a fascinated, and increasingly sympathetic, general public. The Surgeon-General appointed a National Advisory Committee on Leprosy to consider the recommendations made by Carville's United Patient's Committee. Ultimately, in 1947, a new MOC satisfied patients' key demands, increasing the length and frequency of holiday leave, establishing a post office branch at the complex, relaxing the terms of discharge, and hiring an occupational therapist.

In the early 1950s, patients continued to struggle to participate in setting the terms of their confinement and to assert their rights as community residents. By 1956, when residents had achieved their most complete recognition as partners in running the facility, Carville's census began to diminish, as treatment increasingly facilitated medical discharge. In the 1960s and 1970s, Carville remained an active and prolific research institute, producing pioneering investigations of techniques for rehabilitation and surgical reconstruction, as well as seminal trials of the drugs thalidomide and Rifampin. In 1981 the USPHS created a National Outreach Program for Hansen's disease, establishing 11 outpatient clinics to provide diagnosis, treatment, and ongoing care. Carville was decommissioned in the late 1990s, with some of its research programs being moved to Louisiana State University at Baton Rouge.

The other site to which the U.S. government historically confined patients with leprosy was Kalaupapa, on the Hawaiian island of Molokai. In 1909 the USPHS assumed

RULES FOR THE INMATES OF THE LOUISIANA LEPER HOME (CARVILLE, 1913)

1. PATIENTS must be in their respective rooms and places when the physician makes his visits.
2. PATIENTS must not laundry [sic], cook, bathe, nor store food and working tools in their rooms, or clothes rooms; the laundry, bathrooms, clinic and dining and ante-rooms being destined for such purposes. Living rooms and bedding must be aired daily, clothes rooms and individual clothes lockers must be aired weekly. Patients will deposit refuse bandages and dressing in receptacles designated for such, and same to be disposed of in incinerators.
3. PATIENTS will adhere to the regulations made prohibiting the men visiting the women in their enclosure and the women visiting the men in theirs. Inmates (relatives) will be allowed occasional visits in the place assigned for visitors; patients violating rules governing these visits will be denied further visits.
4. PATIENTS will be required to be in their respective rooms for the purpose of retiring at nine o'clock. Patients are prohibited the use of lamps or candles in their rooms. Lamps from halls will light rooms; book cases, desks and rolling chairs must be kept in halls. Patients are prohibited from throwing cigarette or cigar stubs upon the floor of the rooms, halls, or galleries, but same must be placed in receptacles for such or thrown upon the ground.
5. PATIENTS must assist according to their strength in the general care of the home and its inmates, and behave to one another with proper decorum. Inmates disturbing the peace by striking one another will be put in the GUARD HOUSE. Patients are prohibited the holding or keeping in their possession of FIRE ARMS. Packages intended for patients which have the appearance of containing articles prohibited to patients will be opened and inspected in the presence of one of the Sisters.
6. In order to avoid the spread of leprosy, patients are forbidden to go out of their enclosure or send out articles in their possession and prohibited trading directly with peddlers, employees, or any other persons outside the premises.
7. Guards are for the purpose of preventing patients leaving the premises without proper authority, and any guard who permits or allows a patient to violate this rule shall forfeit not less than two days' pay for same, subject to the approval of the Board.
8. A violation of any of the above rules by the patients will subject the violator to be detained in the Detention Room for a length of time commensurate with said violation, and any inmate communicating with a patient while in said Detention Room, without proper permission, will be deemed an offender and subject to be placed in said Detention Room. All reasonable complaints will be made to the Sister in charge, and same will be reported by her to the Board for its action.
9. No particular mode of religion or worship is required of any patient, but all patients are urged, for their own welfare, to attend religious services.
10. The Sisters are in charge of the Home as the representatives of this Board, and for the decorum and management of the Home they may adopt rules not herein enumerated, and not in conflict with these rules; and the rules and orders as adopted must be obeyed by the inmates and all employees.

By the order of the Board of Control Louisiana Leper Home.

J. J. Prowell, President
R. Stagg, Secretary

Courtesy of the National Hansen's Disease Museum, Carville, Louisiana control over Kalaupapa, which had begun as a leper settlement in 1866. The experiences of the residents of the Hawaiian facility paralleled Carville's inhabitants' in some respects. In others, however, it reflected the facility's radically different surroundings: a politically volatile, essentially colonial, environment in which first Britain and then the United States sought to tighten an imperial grip on the territory. The vast majority of Kalaupapa's residents—an average of 135 new cases were detained each year following the 1865 Act to Prevent the Spread of Leprosy—were native Hawaiians. Hawaiians were politically and economically disenfranchised by native- and foreign-born whites and suffered severe social marginalization.

Unlike the population of Carville, which was economically and ethnically mixed, the Kalaupapa settlement was made up largely of native Hawaiians, with only a small minority of Asian immigrants and a very few *haoles* (how-lees)—that is, white foreigners and native-born whites. Because whites with the disease were allowed to leave the island, and because of systemic discrimination by whites throughout Hawaiian society, Kalaupapa's patient population was largely homogenous socially and economically.

During the 1880s and 1890s, Hawaii underwent profound political and social change as *haoles* began to assert increasing control over the island—eventually overthrowing the Hawaiian monarchy, founding a short-lived independent republic, and finally paving the way for annexation by the United States. Native Hawaiians became ever more socially, politically, and economically marginalized. At the same time, public health authorities implemented more stringent quarantine measures that disrupted the community and family structures of patients at Kalaupapa. Physicians conducted experimental procedures, often in gross violation of even the lax ethical standards of the era. Although considerable medical experimentation took place at Carville as well, patients in Louisiana were generally the beneficiaries of that research and felt invested in the process. This was not so in Kalaupapa, where medical experimentation included efforts to infect the healthy with leprosy or the already infected with other diseases such as **syphilis**.

Ultimately, discontent fueled rebellion. Some patients engaged in relatively benign displays of civil disobedience such as vandalism, whereas others took a more aggressive stance, taking up arms and engaging in gun battles with police authorities sent to enforce public health quarantine. They assassinated physicians who championed rigid isolation policies, such as removing uninfected family members from the settlement, isolating individuals, often children, at Kalaupapa without their families. Violent protest culminated in the "Leper War" between the army of the Hawaiian Republic and armed leper "rebels" who had fled from the Hawaiian Board of Health—a conflict which ended in victory for the small but determined band of resistance fighters.

American annexation of the islands in 1898 and creation of a central government with strong law enforcement and public health capabilities neutralized rebellion during the first decade of the twentieth century, but the policy of strict isolation remained in place. Those with leprosy gained more freedoms within the settlement, particularly after Hawaiians were granted American citizenship, but stigmatization of the disease outside the facility deepened. As part of an effort to make Kalaupapa more of a medical institution on par with Carville, the United States Leprosy Investigation Station was built there in 1909. But whereas patients at the settlement had largely acquiesced to experimentation during the previous decades, the research station closed in 1913 after only 9 of 900 patients would consent to serve as research subjects. Kalaupapa residents resented USPHS experiments and intrusion into their lives and became an even more insular, self-sustaining community. Throughout the twentieth century, especially after the introduction of sulfone drugs in the 1940s, the population of Kalaupapa dwindled, but isolation laws were not abolished until 1969. During the twentieth century, the facility became, and for a small number of individuals remains, a refuge. *See also* Leprosy, Societal Reactions to; Medical Ethics and Epidemic Disease; Public Health Agencies, U.S. Federal.

Further Reading

Fairchild, Amy. "Community and Confinement: The Evolving Experience of Isolation for Leprosy in Carville, Louisiana." *Public Health Reports* 119 (2004): 362–370.

Furman, Bess. *A Profile of the United States Public Health Service, 1798–1945*. Washington, DC: U.S. Department of Health and Human Services, 1973.

Hasseltine, Herman E. "History of Leprosy in the New England States." *Public Health Reports* 12 (1944): 67–78.

Martin, Betty. *Miracle at Carville*. New York: Doubleday and Co., 1950.

Moran, Michelle T. *Colonizing Leprosy: Imperialism and the Politics of Public Health in the United States*. Chapel Hill: University of North Carolina Press, 2007.

Tayman, John. *The Colony*. New York: Scribner, 2006.

Turse, Nick. "Experimental Dreams, Ethical Nightmares: Leprosy, Isolation and Human Experimentation in Nineteenth Century Hawaii." In *Imagining Our Americas: Toward a Transnational Frame*, edited by Sandhya Shukla and Heidi Tinsman, pp. 138–167. Durham: Duke University Press, 2007.

AVA ALKON, NICK TURSE, AND AMY FAIRCHILD

LEPROSY, SOCIETAL REACTIONS TO. "Stigma" is Greek for a distinguishing mark, and few diseases present with the range of physical marks or symptoms that **leprosy**, or **Hansen's** disease, can. From its early stages with discolored skin patches to later development of open sores, terrible body odor, and disfigurement of face and extremities, the disease has long marked its sufferer as one to be shunned by the healthy. Death was rarely swift and cure or recovery unusual, so unlike the victim of plague, smallpox, or tuberculosis, one became a leper. Historically, societies have responded to leprosy, often a label for a broad category of skin diseases, by setting those afflicted with the disease apart from the healthy—and often even from other sufferers—in ways ranging from social ostracism to physical isolation on remote islands.

Cultural explanations of how and why one is afflicted with leprosy are key to understanding the levels of stigma attached to the disease. In many cultures, as diverse as ancient China and modern Mali, Thailand, and Paraguay, traditional explanations include heredity, sorcery, diet, and accidents. In such societies, the leper may be shunned for aesthetic reasons, for begging, or for supposedly breaking a food taboo, but the stigma tends to be light, and physical banishment is rare. As the disease progresses, however, the sufferer becomes less able to work, more physically abhorrent, and often is reduced to begging for sustenance. If married, divorce is often prescribed, lest spouse and children acquire the disease.

In ancient Israel early religious (Levitical) law prescribed that priests examine those with suspicious skin patches. If found to be ritually unclean—*tsara'ath* or *zara'ath*, a term used over 20 times in the Hebrew Scriptures that included but was not limited to people with skin ailments—they were to be placed outside the camp enclosure. When these Hebrew (Old Testament) texts were translated into Greek in the third century BCE, *tsara'ath* became *lepra*, the term for a recognized skin disease, and the leprous became a special class to be shunned, for religious no less than aesthetic reasons. When Jesus (c. 6 BCE–27 CE) healed ("cleansed") 10 lepers, he was displaying divine power to undo ritual impurity as well as healing illness. That he sent those he healed to the priests is further recognition of the religious nature of the condition and its place in Jewish society.

Medieval Christianity retained the notion of the ritually impure leper but blended it with the charity demanded by the Gospel and exemplified by Jesus. But God inflicted leprosy, as all diseases, perhaps because of terrible personal sins. Ritual impurity evolved into sinfulness and moral failure, and the leper's outer deformity became a sign of spiritual depravity. By contrast, early Islam, which could ignore the Old Testament in favor of the Quran and Muhammad's (570–632) doctrines, taught that Allah imposed leprosy freely as either a blessing or a curse, with no relation to the victim's moral status. Even so, the victim was stripped of many legal rights and reduced to the status of a minor or an insane person. Though Muhammad rejected the notion of contagion, he nevertheless urged his followers "to flee the leper as you would the lion." Supporting the leprous was an act of charity, and this ranged from handing out alms at the mosque to donating land to support a **leprosarium**. Muslim towns and cities often had leper quarters established outside their walls, which may have contradictorily served to increase victims' self esteem as members of a minority community while increasing stigma by isolation from the full community. In Fez, Morocco, all lepers had to reside in the quarter, though this sort of regulation seems to have been rare.

Chinese lepers were traditionally cast out of their towns and villages and collected in walled colonies whose conditions were so dreadful that many committed suicide. Indian lepers, believed to have been cursed by God, traditionally had no refuge, begging and dying in streets or alleyways, or being aided by the charitable to commit suicide by burial alive, incineration, or drowning. Believing the devil caused leprosy, premodern Russian Yakuts drove their lepers away from villages to live in solitary huts.

Though Christian saints like Francis of Assisi might embrace and even suck the pus from the wounds of lepers, high medieval Church authorities increasingly insisted on segregation and isolation of lepers from wider society. As in ancient Israel, determination of this status remained in the hands of the clergy, even after the emergence of professionalized medicine in the West. Charitable hospitals in major cities had long served as refuges for those disabled by the disease, especially in the Byzantine world. As with Jews, Muslims, and heretics, lepers fell into the category of those not well tolerated in open society, and from 1215 they had to wear distinctive clothing in the Catholic world. To the moral and aesthetic bases for segregation was added fear of physical contagion, especially with the descent of the **Black Death** from 1347. Coincidently, the incidence of leprosy in Europe declined with the new regime of plague (perhaps as a result of improving nutrition), and many leprosaria were soon filling with plague victims, becoming **pest houses**. Keener diagnoses, left to **physicians** from the early fourteenth century, also seem to have separated out victims of related diseases, reducing the number of lepers even further.

European colonization and the **slave** trade probably brought leprosy to the New World, and with it the Christian **social construction** of the disease. Catholic clergy and religious dominated the mission fields, and native lepers were treated as had been their European cousins. In Africa Christian missionaries often encountered societies whose attitudes to lepers had been shaped by Islamic ambivalence and native tolerance. Along with colonial

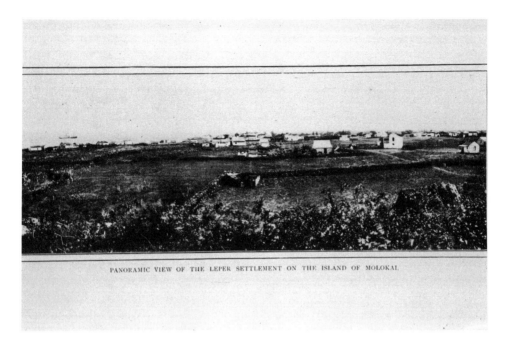

PANORAMIC VIEW OF THE LEPER SETTLEMENT ON THE ISLAND OF MOLOKAI.

Panoramic view of leper settlement on Molokai. *Harper's Weekly*, August 18, 1899. Courtesy of the National Library of Medicine.

governments and Christian missionaries came the stigmatization of the leper on religious grounds.

By the early nineteenth century, many experts believed leprosy to be hereditary and noncontagious, whereas others believed in its contagious nature. British debate revived interest in medieval lepers and leprosaria, generating many myths about both. After the discovery in 1873 of the *Mycobacterium leprae* by **Gerhard Hansen**, the debate over whether leprosy was contagious tipped to the "contagionists." Both the Royal Commission on Leprosy in India in 1891, and the First International Congress on Leprosy, held in Berlin in 1897 (presided over by **Rudolf Virchow**), adopted the contagionist position. Medical science therefore seemed to dictate segregation and isolation, and imperial governments, as well as those of free states, began imposing strict segregation measures. In 1877 Norway passed legislation restricting the movement of lepers and in 1885 required isolation in leprosaria or colonies. Sometimes brutal, sometimes welcoming, isolation prevented "contagion", controlled vagrancy, allowed forced medical treatment and experimentation, controlled reproduction of lepers, often provided care in a communal setting and an accepting atmosphere, allowed religious proselytizing to a captive audience, and provided an alternative to life among the judgmental.

Concern for the health of white colonists and native workers in Africa and Asia began to trump vaguer notions of the lepers' moral state, and it was voiced in popular books like H. P. Wright's 1889 *Leprosy: An Imperial Danger*. Imperialism, racism, social Darwinism, missionary Christianity, and the new **germ theory** interacted to provide potent support for segregation. If a germ caused leprosy, then the disease was spread by filth and sex in squalid native conditions, or so reasoned colonial physicians such as the French doctor Eduard Jeanselme (1858–1935). British Parliament considered Leprosy Acts for India in 1889 and 1896, and passed the Lepers Act in 1898. South Africa mandated isolation in 1891, and by the 1890s Kalaupapa leper colony on Hawaii's Molokai Island housed 700 residents. The Louisiana Leper Home in Carville opened in 1894 on a dilapidated plantation rented for $750 per year; run by Sisters of Charity nuns, it became the national leper hospital in 1921.

French Catholic Father Germain-Leger Testevuide (1849–1891) opened the first leprosarium in Japan on Mount Fuji in 1888 as a refuge. Two more followed in 1892, and the state established five more in 1907. Conditions were prison-like, and because the Japanese accepted hereditary theory rather than contagion they sterilized men and aborted fetuses of pregnant women. Forced isolation of lepers returned to Japan after World War II, and by 1956 some 11,000 were housed in numerous facilities that officially closed in 1996. In 2001 the practice was declared unconstitutional, and 127 plaintiffs were awarded the equivalent of $20 million in damages.

By the late 1980s the age of mandatory isolation was waning. Even after colonies or leprosaria are closed and patients healed, however, the problems of adjusting to the broader world lead many to remain in or near their former institutional homes. Many of China's estimated 60,000 leper colonists remain because of family abandonment and attendant shame. In a 2004 Japanese poll, only 2 percent of 4,300 current inmates desire to return home, and at Kalaupapa many remain as tour guides. At about the same time, a study of leprosy in Thai society showed that even after obvious lepers disappeared from view with effective medical treatment, the pejorative use of "leper" in daily language increased, which reinforced the psychological stigma of patients.

Since the early 1980s, a new outpatient multidrug therapy has provided a cure in two years or less with no physical deformities. In 1991 the **World Health Organization** set the goal of global elimination of Hansen's disease as a public health problem (cases reduced to 1 per 10,000 population) by 2000. Though efforts fell short, between 1985 and 2005 over 14 million cases were cured, largely thanks to donated drugs, and the number of current cases fell from 5,200,000 to 286,000 (95.5 percent). Yet stigmatization continues to keep victims from seeking effective treatment at early stages and minimizing the disease's effects. An anti-stigmatization media campaign drew 12,000 people to treatment centers in Nepal over a six-day period in 1999.

From the early 2000s, researchers have been working to develop means of quantifying leprosy-related stigma across cultures in order to understand and counteract this factor. In 2003 the generally biomedical *International Journal of Leprosy and Other Mycobacterial Diseases* committed itself to supporting social science research into the "social facets" of the disease. In a letter to the United Nations Commission on Human Rights dated January 29, 2006, Jimmy Carter (b. 1924), the Dalai Lama (b. 1935), Bishop Desmond Tutu (b. 1931), and other global activists urged "people all over the world to change their perception and foster an environment in which leprosy patients, cured persons, and their families can lead normal lives free from stigma and discrimination." *See also* Leprosy in the Premodern World; Leprosy in the United States; Medical Ethics and Epidemic Disease; Personal Liberties and Epidemic Disease; Religion and Epidemic Disease; Scapegoats and Epidemic Disease.

Further Reading

de Baroncelli, Jacques. *L'Homme du Niger* [film]. 1939.

Brody, Saul N. *Disease of the Soul: Leprosy in Medieval Literature*. Ithaca: Cornell University Press, 1974.

Bruno, Ellen. *Leper: Life beyond Stigma* [film]. 2000.

Cox, Paul. *Molokai—The Story of Father Damien* [film]. 1999.

Dols, Michael W. "The Leper in Medieval Islamic Society." *Speculum* 58 (1983): 891–916.

Edmond, Rod. *Leprosy and Empire: A Medical and Cultural History*. New York: Cambridge University Press, 2007.

Farrokhzad, Forough. *The House is Black* [film]. 1962.

Gethers, Steven. *Damien the Leper Priest* [film]. 1980.

Gould, Tony. *A Disease Apart: Leprosy in the Modern World*. New York: St. Martin's Press, 2005.

Grön, K. "Leprosy in Literature and Art." *International Journal of Leprosy* 41 (1973): 249–283.

Gussow, Zachary. *Leprosy, Racism and Public Health: Social Policy and Chronic Disease Control*. Boulder: University of Colorado Press, 1989.

Kagan, Daryn. *Breaking the Curse* [film]. 2007.

Lieber, Elinor. "Old Testament 'Leprosy,' Contagion and Sin." In *Contagion*, edited by Lawrence I. Conrad and Dominik Wujastyk, pp. 99–136. Burlington, VT: Ashgate, 2000.

Navon, Liora. "Beggars, Metaphors, and Stigma: A Missing Link in the Social History of Leprosy." *Social History of Medicine* 11 (1998): 89–105.

Rawcliffe, Carole. *Leprosy in Medieval England*. Rochester, NY: Boydell, 2006.

Richards, Peter. *The Medieval Leper and His Northern Heirs*. New York: Barnes and Noble, 1995.

Silla, Eric. *People Are Not the Same: Leprosy and Identity in Twentieth-Century Mali*. Portsmouth, NH: Heinemann, 1998.

Touati, François-Olivier. "Contagion and Leprosy: Myth, Ideas, and Evolution in Medieval Minds and Societies." In *Contagion*, edited by Lawrence I. Conrad and Dominik Wujastyk, pp. 179–202. Burlington, VT: Ashgate, 2000.

JOSEPH P. BYRNE

LITERATURE, DISEASE IN MODERN.   Literary works are rooted in the human endeavor and its challenges, so the prominence of disease among human populations ensured that **epidemics**, plagues, and other diseases would play a significant role in literature. Many of literary history's most memorable characters are those suffering from or dying with a catastrophic illness—Roderick and Madeline Usher in Edgar Allen Poe's (1809–1849) "The Fall of the House of Usher" (1839) or Benjy Compson in William Faulkner's (1897–1962) *The Sound and the Fury* (1929), for example. Additionally, some of history's greatest works of poetry are rooted in the struggle with disease or impending death, often the poet's own, as in John Milton's (1608–1674) "On His Blindness" (1652) or John Keats's (1795–1821) "La Belle Dame Sans Merci" (1819). In spite of the frequency with which plagues and illnesses appear in novels, plays, and poems, disease is significantly less common in literature than in the course of real human lives. For example, the common cold is extremely rare in literary contexts. The literary demand for conflict and economy of detail requires that diseases in literature be virulent enough to alter a character's life or the social dynamic of a story, or be worthy of the solemn reflection of a poem. As a result, disease has limited uses in literature, most often in a symbolic capacity.

The effect of disease on the social fabric of society, particularly during epidemics, has been a frequent theme of literary works. In one of the earliest such works, *The Decameron*

(1350–1353), by Giovanni Boccaccio (1313–1375), 10 young men and women are forced by the **Black Death** to leave Florence for a villa in the country, where they tell stories offering a window into Italy's changing social dynamics, such as a declining trust in the church brought on by the epidemic. Alessandro Manzoni's (1785–1873) 1825 novel *The Betrothed*, often considered one of Italy's greatest literary works, used the epidemic of **bubonic plague** that swept Milan in 1630 to convey the sort of social anarchy that an epidemic could bring to a culture during the early modern period. In Manzoni's work the plague becomes a major obstacle to his protagonists' marriage. Though outbreaks of epidemic disease declined dramatically in the Western world during the nineteenth and twentieth centuries, the complex social dynamics brought on by **industrialization** and **urbanization** made the prospect of an epidemic even more of a threat to society. Henrick Ibsen (1828–1906), in his play *An Enemy of the People* (1882), explored the potential for an epidemic to alter a society's economy and, as a result, its social relationships. In the controversial drama, a **physician** who seeks to close his town's public baths after discovering that they are the source of an epidemic among tourists is destroyed by a society determined to preserve its lucrative tourist trade. Albert Camus (1913–1960), a French writer deeply influenced by his nation's experience fighting the Nazis, examined the socially unifying power of an epidemic in his 1947 novel *The Plague*. Though true to Camus's existentialist beliefs, the novel ends with the population returning to their same selfish lifestyles once the threat has passed. By the end of the twentieth century, works of popular fiction, such as Robin Cook's (b. 1940) *Outbreak* (1987) and *Contagion* (1995), were exploring scenarios in which rapidly spreading and incurable diseases such as **Ebola** and **smallpox** become weapons of political intrigue, terrorism, or evil entrepreneurs.

Catastrophic diseases have occasionally stricken artistic and literary communities with such impact that the diseases become romanticized and mythologized in the literary works of that period, and consequently, in the public imagination. **Tuberculosis** during the Romantic Era and **Acquired Immune Deficiency Syndrome** (AIDS) near the end of the twentieth century are two of the most prominent examples. Because the diseases appeared to affect artists and writers at the peak of their careers, the mythology that developed around the diseases tended to associate them with greater creativity, a heightened emotional sensitivity, or a deeper understanding of the human condition. T. S. Eliot (1899–1965), whose 1922 poem *The Waste Land* is considered one of modernism's greatest works, was among those who believed that serious disease, in the right circumstances, could produce a flood of poetic creativity. Though humankind has been victimized throughout history by a variety of horrifying epidemics, including bubonic plague, smallpox, **cholera, influenza, polio,** and **malaria**, the frequency with which tuberculosis appears in nineteenth-century literature or AIDS appears in late-twentieth-century literature creates the impression that those diseases were far more prevalent than may actually have been the case; that they were a bigger threat to public health than were other epidemics; or, most problematic of all, that they were the price to be paid for creativity or empathy. By contrast, those epidemic and catastrophic diseases without such a mythology surrounding them, in spite of their prevalence or their threat to public health, have generally been considered in the public imagination to be merely cruel and unfortunate aspects of the human experience.

The early deaths from tuberculosis of Romantic artists as prominent as British poet John Keats and Polish composer Frédéric Chopin (1810–1849) played a major role in the mythology that grew up around "consumption," as tuberculosis was called at that time, and eventually led to the disease being associated with creativity throughout the nineteenth century. The effects of urbanization and the impoverishment brought on by the **Industrial Revolution** had, by the middle of the century, led to consumption becoming so common in the general population that the frequent tubercular characters in literary works, such as the kind-hearted Little Eva in Harriet Beecher Stowe's (1811–1896) *Uncle Tom's Cabin* (1952) or the young Paul Dombey in Charles Dickens's (1812–1870) *Dombey and Son* (1846–1848), did not even require having their disease identified. The symptoms alone were sufficient evidence for a reader to conclude that the characters were afflicted, though both the literary and social implications were, as Dickens notes in describing Dombey, that the sufferer possessed a moral weakness of some sort. Over time, the romanticized notion of tuberculosis became so ingrained in the public imagination that it continued far into the twentieth century. Writers as renowned as Franz Kafka (1883–1924) and D. H. Lawrence (1885–1930) continued to fall victim to the disease through the period between the world wars, and major literary works of the era, such as Thomas Mann's (1875–1955) *The Magic Mountain* and Lawrence's *Women in Love*, offered perhaps even more idealized portrayals of the disease than works of the nineteenth century.

AIDS became the focal point of a similar public fascination after its discovery in the early 1980s. Its prevalence among artistic communities was soon echoed in a number of prominent literary works in which characters struggle with the physical and social consequences of their condition. The first book to capture a broad audience, journalist Randy Shilts's (1951–1994) *And the Band Played On* (1987), was a chronicle of the emergence of the disease in and around San Francisco's gay community and the frantic search by medical research teams to identify the disease and locate its source. The candor with which Shilts examined the impact of AIDS on the gay community and the subsequent search for its origins dramatically altered the public and political conversation regarding the disease. By the 1990s, many of Broadway's most celebrated plays and musicals featured AIDS themes, including Tony Kushner's (b. 1956) two-part drama *Angels in America* (1990), which won both the Pulitzer Prize for Drama and the Antoinette Perry (Tony) Award for best play; William Finn (b. 1952) and James Lapine's (b. 1949) 1992 drama *Falsettos*, winner of a Tony Award for best book of a musical; Paul Rudnick's (b. 1957) critically praised 1993 Obie (Off-Broadway) Award-winning play *Jeffrey*; and Jonathan Larson's (1960–1996) nearly iconic musical *Rent* (1996), winner of four Tony Awards, including best musical.

Some diseases manifest symptoms that authors have found especially useful for allowing literary characters to engage in philosophical reflection, theological questioning, or heightened spiritual awareness. Ernest Hemingway's (1899–1961) 1936 short story "The Snows of Kilimanjaro" uses the bodily decay of gangrene to inspire a man dying in the African wilderness, identified only as "Harry," to reflect on the vast experiences of his unfulfilled and too-brief life. Similarly, in "The Death of Ivan Ilych" (1886), Leo Tolstoy (1828–1910) explored the experience of a slow and agonizing death from abdominal cancer and its power to inspire a profound self-examination on the part of its victim. Ilych, the title character, is shunned by his family and forced by the disgusting symptoms of his disease to confront the isolation and loneliness that the disease and his lifetime of selfishness have brought upon him. For both Hemingway and Tolstoy, the physical effects of their protagonists' diseases paralleled an unexamined moral decay brought to light only by the suffering of the disease. In Peter De Vries's (1910–1993) 1961 novel *Blood of the Lamb*, a brother's death from pneumonia and a young daughter's death from leukemia become the impetus for De Vries's protagonist, Don Wanderlust, to confront his rationalistic self-assurance and his doubts about faith. Like Hemingway and Tolstoy, De Vries uses the specific nature of the illnesses in *Blood of the Lamb* as symbols of his protagonist's emotional struggles—*pneumonia*, from the Greek word for "spirit," and *leukemia*, a disease that robs the blood of its life-sustaining quality. The unusual physical effects of epilepsy, with its uncontrollable seizures, suggest a heightened spiritual awareness that was utilized by Fyodor Dostoevsky (1821–1881) in his 1869 novel *The Idiot*. Dostoevsky, himself an epileptic, described the onset of the seizures experienced by his protagonist, Prince Myshkin, as a few moments of extraordinary insight into the nature of life, a doorway to spiritual apotheosis. That heightened appreciation of life (even as the protagonist may be taking his final breath) is the case with most works exploring a theological or philosophical introspection prompted by disease, though occasionally the experience of disease is portrayed as having an embittering effect on its victim, as in Joseph Conrad's (1857–1924) *Heart of Darkness* (1899) or Andre Gide's (1869–1951) *The Immoralist* (1902).

Among literary history's most memorable characters are those afflicted with mental illness. The appearance of psychological disorders—"madness"—in literature dates back to the ancient world, where in Euripides' (480 BC–406 BC) *The Bacchae* (405 BC), Dionysus, the god of wine and ecstasy, inspires a frenzied dancing, an implied temporary insanity, among the women of Thebes. In much of the literature involving a character's mental stability, the dramatic tension lies in whether the character is, in fact, mentally ill, or if instead he or she is feigning the illness, or is misdiagnosed, or is the victim of misguided social expectations. As early as William Shakespeare (1564–1616), the issue of feigned mental illness was a subject of literary intrigue. The question lies at the core of two of Shakespeare's best-known plays—Hamlet (1602) and King Lear (1606). In both cases, the illusion of insanity allows the "mad" characters—Hamlet and Edgar—to pursue surreptitious plots against the plays' powerful villains. By the nineteenth century, mentally ill characters were more often portrayed as disturbing antagonists or even villains. In Charlotte Bronte's (1816–1855) *Jane Eyre* (1847), the title character's love for Rochester is thwarted by his undisclosed marriage to a ghoulish woman he keeps locked in the attic to conceal her insanity. Yet another female character—women were portrayed as suffering from an ill-defined psychological illness much more often than were male characters—was kept locked away in an attic in Charlotte Perkins Gilman's (1860–1935) "The Yellow Wallpaper" (1892), eventually becoming delusional and experiencing hallucinations. Though only inferentially portrayed as mentally ill, Captain Ahab, the commander of the whaling ship *Pequod* in Herman Melville's (1819–1891) *Moby Dick* (1851), is afflicted by a frighteningly irrational obsession with killing one specific whale, destroying his ship and killing many of his crew in the process. Several works have utilized protagonists presumed by their society to be mentally ill to question whether such social judgments are reliable, including Fyodor Dostoevsky's *Notes from Underground* (1864) and Ken Kesey's (1935–2001) *One Flew over the Cuckoo's Nest* (1962). In both works, the protagonists manifest incidents of extraordinary mental clarity even though their insanity is largely assumed by those surrounding them.

Occasionally, authors have even invented diseases as a channel for exploring social themes. Nobel laureate José Saramago's (b. 1922) 1995 novel *Blindness* deals with the aftermath of a disease that causes instantaneous and complete blindness, leaving the victim with the sensation of seeing nothing but a milky white film. This "white darkness" quickly strikes the entire population, with one exception who is forced to conceal her continued ability to see, leading to a dramatic social upheaval as the society tries to cope with its pandemic sightlessness. In his famous short story "The Masque of the Red Death," Edgar Allen Poe utilizes an epidemic of "red death" to explore the depth of fear and societal indifference in the face of a plague. According to the narrator, Red Death is a hemorrhagic disease causing convulsions and severe pain and leading to death within a half-hour of the onset of profuse bleeding through the pores of the skin. In Poe's story, a large group of nobles attempts to escape the disease by quarantining themselves inside a castle, only to be infected and die when a mysterious guest at a masquerade ball turns out to be the disease itself in human form. *See also* AIDS, Literature, and the Arts in the United States; Biblical Plagues; Black Death: Literature and Art; Cinema and Epidemic Disease; Disease, Social Construction of ; Leprosy, Societal Reactions to; Plague Literature and Art, Early Modern European; Popular Media and Epidemic Disease: Recent Trends; Sexuality, Gender, and Epidemic Disease; Syphilis in Sixteenth-Century Europe; Tuberculosis and Romanticism.

Further Reading

Healy, Margaret. *Fictions of Disease in Early Modern England: Bodies, Plagues and Politics*. New York: Palgrave Macmillan, 2002.

Meyers, Jeffrey. *Disease and the Novel, 1880–1960*. New York: Palgrave Macmillan, 1985.

Pastore, Judith L., ed. *Confronting AIDS through Literature: The Responsibilities of Representation*. Urbana: University of Illinois Press, 1993.

Sontag, Susan. *AIDS and its Metaphors*. New York: Farrar, Straus, and Giroux, 1989.

———. *Illness as Metaphor*. New York: Farrar, Straus, and Giroux, 1978.

Torgerson, Beth. *Reading the Bronte Body: Disease, Desire, and the Constraints of Culture*. New York: Palgrave Macmillan, 2005.

DEVON BOAN

LONDON, GREAT PLAGUE OF (1665–1666). The **bubonic plague** outbreak that struck London, a city of 500,000 inhabitants, and other English urban centers in 1665 and 1666 was the last such **epidemic** in the British Isles. With a death toll of over 100,000, it was the deadliest since the **Black Death** of 1349, though in percentage terms it was less severe than earlier English plagues.

Though some scholars disagree, most accept that the plague deaths were the result of the *Yersinia pestis* **bacterium** spread among humans by rat-borne fleas that found new human hosts. The high mortality rates suggest that some cases may have become contagious **pneumonic plague**, by settling in victims' lungs, and lethal **septicemic plague**, by rapidly infecting the bloodstream of others. Bills of mortality, which were published weekly and listed all local deaths by parish and cause, also show dramatic increases in the incidence of other diseases that probably flourished among the physically weakened population.

In general, the catastrophe was well documented, and historians have recourse to official sources such as the bills, parish records, and a stream of governmental directives, as well as many personal sources. Diarists such as the Royal Navy bureaucrats Samuel Pepys (1633–1703) and John Evelyn (1620–1706) privately chronicled the event, and surviving correspondence from many other sources sheds light on personal tragedies. Plague tracts from previous outbreaks were circulated anew, while **surgeons, physicians**, and **apothecaries** published their own manuals of prevention and treatment, and preachers' sermons inveighed against sin and demanded the repentance that would placate the angry Deity whose responsibility for the disease was undoubted. Finally, many wrote in the wake of the plague, urging the adoption of policies and actions they believed would dampen the effects of the next epidemic. The best known of these was the novelist Daniel Defoe (1660–1731), author of *Journal of the Plague Year* (1720). Though largely fictionalized and written 55 years after the event by one who was only four years old at the time, it is the iconic description of the Great Plague.

Ironically, the English government had ample warning that plague was in the neighborhood. In the early 1660s it had swept among England's trading partners (and competitors) in the Baltic and North Sea regions and had struck Dutch cities hard in 1663 and 1664 killing 35,000 in Amsterdam. Early on, royal authorities established inspection and **quarantine** stations at the mouth of the Thames and in eastern port cities such as Great Yarmouth and restricted maritime trade with cities known to be stricken. **War** with the Dutch Republic—from March 1665—lessened the likelihood of contamination through **trade**, but victories brought Dutch prisoners to English towns, especially in East Anglia.

England suffered a few dozen scattered plague deaths in 1664, but an especially long and brutal winter raised hopes that plague would be kept at bay. Fears began to rise in London in May 1665, with 43 reported plague fatalities, but royal authorities dismissed their importance in order to prevent mass **flight** from the capital and reassure commercial and diplomatic partners. Nonetheless, theaters were closed on June 5, the Inns of Court shut their doors on June 15, and on June 21 a *cordon sanitaire* of warders appeared around the parish with the highest concentration of plague victims, St.-Giles-in-the-Fields. By mid-June, however, the bills of mortality were reporting over 100 plague deaths per week, and the flight of the frightened and wealthy began in earnest. The royal court began to abandon Westminster for Hampton Court as early as June 20, though King Charles II (1630–1685) remained until July 7.

Fear turned to horror as death counts mounted and incidences of the disease spread from poorer outlying parishes like St. Giles inward to the city itself. By late July, 86 of greater London's 130 parishes had reported a grand total of over 6,300 plague fatalities, 5,667 in July alone (of a reported total of 8,828 deaths in July). August numbers rose to 17,036 plague deaths in 113 parishes among a total of 22,413, and September fatalities spiked at a total of 30,899 with 26,230 attributed to plague, including the epidemic's worst week during which the bills reported 7,165 fatalities. They tapered off in October, and by late November fewer than 1,000 plague deaths appeared weekly. However accurate such numbers appear, both contemporaries and historians have treated them as low estimates, because parish-level reporting was inexpert, and non-Anglicans (Catholics, Quakers, Jews) were generally not counted.

Efforts to stem the deadly tide repeated past patterns: victims and family members were shut up in their houses; a few **pest houses** (with a total capacity of only 600) were opened; burials were conducted at night—at least for a time—to avoid funerary gatherings; dogs (around 40,000) and cats (perhaps 200,000) were killed as possible sources of the disease; 46 new medical publications on plague and its treatment appeared alongside dozens of reissued older works; and **quacks** confidently hawked their useless wares. Early September's terrifying numbers prompted the only attempt to cleanse the open, "miasmatic" **air** with bonfires, an effort dowsed by nature after a few days. Mass graves swallowed up victims by the hundreds, the poorer folk, servants, and laborers with nowhere else to go far outnumbering the more affluent.

River ports along the Thames suffered along with London, as did East Anglian towns such as Ipswich, with some 1,700 plague deaths, and Colchester, which lost over 4,800 to plague from a total population of around 11,000. Despite cordons and flight, Cambridge, Great Yarmouth, and Norwich each lost over 15 percent of their populations, and Dover about 30 percent. Famously, the North Derbyshire parish of Eyam contracted the plague, and in June 1666 Reverend William Mompesson (1639–1709) convinced all residents of the village to accept self-sacrificing voluntary isolation lest plague spread elsewhere. In the end the village suffered 259 deaths in 76 families, or about half its population, but its neighborhood was spared the ordeal.

London regained much of its population during the winter of 1665–1666, though the following year saw an additional 2,000 succumb to the disease. All told perhaps 2 percent of England's population died of plague. The economic costs of the plague were huge and included both expenses and lost revenues. England's governing bodies and philanthropists provided as needed during the epidemic, however, and Britain's economy rebounded rapidly afterward. Wealth was redistributed through inheritance, and baptisms of newborns soared in the years that followed. Despite occurring during the **Scientific Revolution**, few if any medical insights resulted from the disaster, but reformers resolved to enhance quarantine provisions, provide pest houses in place of household isolation, and better regulate slum housing in poorer neighborhoods where the plague seemed to fester first. *See also* Apothecary/Pharmacist; Astrology and Medicine; Black Death: Modern Medical Debate; Contagion Theory of Disease, Premodern; Corpses and Epidemic Disease; Diagnosis of Historical Diseases; Disinfection and Fumigation; Personal Liberties and Epidemic Disease; Plague: End of the Second Pandemic; Plague in Britain, 1500–1647; Plague in Europe, 1500–1770s; Plague Literature and Art, Early Modern European; Public Health Agencies in the West before 1900; Religion and Epidemic Disease; Sydenham, Thomas; Urbanization and Epidemic Disease.

Further Reading

Boghurst, William. *Loimographia: An Account of the Great Plague of London in the Year 1665* (1665). New York: AMS Press, 1976.

Champion, Justin A. I. *London's Dreaded Visitation: The Social Geography of the Great Plague in 1665*. London: Historical Geography Research Paper Series 31, 1995.

Defoe, Daniel. *A Journal of the Plague Year*. New York: Oxford University Press, 1999.

Harvard University Library. *Contagion*. http://ocp.hul.harvard.edu/contagion/plague.html

Hodges, Nathaniel. *Loimologia: Or, an Historical Account of the Plague in London in 1665* (1720). New York: AMS Press, 1994.

Latham, Robert, and William Matthews, trans. and ed. *The Diary of Samuel Pepys*. 11 vols. Berkeley: University of California Press, 2000.

Moote, A. Lloyd, and Dorothy C. Moote. *The Great Plague: The Story of London's Most Deadly Year*. Baltimore: Johns Hopkins University Press, 2004.

Porter, Stephen. *The Great Plague*. Stroud: Sutton, 1999.

Wear, Andrew. *Knowledge and Practice in English Medicine, 1550–1680*. New York: Cambridge University Press, 2000.

JOSEPH P. BYRNE

LYME DISEASE.   A spiral shaped **bacterium** related to that responsible for **syphilis** causes Lyme disease. Both of these related bacteria have many forms and shapes, but the corkscrew shape of the spirochete seems to predominate. Lyme is caused by the genus *Borrelia* and has many different species found around the world. It gains access to virtually the entire body in days to weeks, so fast treatment is critical. Lyme bacteria also have many ways to undermine treatment and harm humans by the use of a huge number of **antibiotic**-defeating plasmids, in addition to releasing biotoxins and slimy biofilms. Although it is found in many different ticks, the most common carrier appears to be various forms of the deer tick, a very tiny period-sized tick, which injects a painkiller, antihistamine, and anticoagulant when it bites. This is why patients often miss it. Although large mammals like deer are famous for dispersal of Lyme, it appears that smaller mammals such as chipmunks, specific mice, and other small mammals are also carriers.

Lyme disease is not a new infection; it has been found in preserved ticks from the nineteenth century. But infection rates have likely changed radically as a result of the increase of deer in some countries, together with the building of homes or other structures in areas with brush and wild fields. These factors have served only to increase the risk of infections.

Lyme is found in many countries and has been described in detail by dozens of medical papers in the last hundred years. Serious attention to Lyme disease began with Polly Murray, an artist and mother of four. Murray resides in Lyme, Connecticut, and noticed as early as the 1960s that she and her family and many local youth were sick with a special type of arthritis. In her book, *The Widening Circle*, she reports her tenacious struggle to convince **doctors** that she and her family were indeed sick, and not hypochondriacs, after having becoming infected with Lyme. In the 1960s, Lyme disease, and other tick infections like **Babesia** and **Bartonella**, were not part of routine clinical medicine. In 1971, Murray, criticized as a "doctor-chaser," began her own systematic research, seeking out investigative medical personnel and sharing stories with fellow sufferers. Finally, she received media attention and the attention of rheumatologist Allen Steere at nearby Yale, who discovered through preliminary studies that Lyme disease was indeed the cause of much illness in Lyme, Connecticut. This attracted the attention of the medical community to this unusual infection. Doctors began to appreciate that it was not simply a psychiatric problem.

Another major milestone in the treatment of Lyme disease was the discovery that it was not a **virus** or parasite, but a bacterium. Dr. Willy Burgdorfer, working at the Rocky Mountain Laboratories, discovered that it was a bacterial spirochete. This important discovery explained why some studies using antibiotics showed some improvement with Lyme disease, and why non-bacteria-targeted treatments would probably not be effective.

Diagnosis.   If a person has a bulls-eye rash, it is likely that he/she has Lyme or a related bacterial infection called "STARI." But the bulls-eye rash is not found in most patients with Lyme. Some Lyme rashes are diagnosed as "ring worm" or are ignored. Often, bulls-eye rashes simply do not appear. However, the appearance of a bulls-eye rash is a sign to start immediate treatment, because Lyme and other possible deer tick infections may have been inserted into the human body in recent days or weeks. Often, the Lyme bacteria are already disseminated throughout the body by the time a bulls-eye rash appears.

Debates on the reliability of testing are ongoing. The most common tests are the ELISA, the Western Blot, and DNA or PCR tests. Some countries use a two-step practice: if an ELISA screening test is positive, then they run a Western Blot to confirm the positive nature of the test. Although this is the generally accepted approach internationally, some physicians, scientists, and patients advocate that groups should report that the ELISA is unreliable and misses large numbers of obviously positive patients. Likewise, blind testing of laboratories is felt to show varying degrees of accuracy in diagnosing Lyme according to some skeptical scientists and physicians.

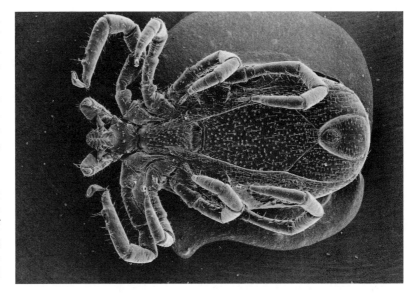

Scanning electron microscope ventral view of adult female castor bean tick, Ixodes ricinus, a vector of viruses and babesiosus. It is parasitic on sheep, cattle, and wild animals. Larvae are found on many wild birds and mammals. Carries many diseases and is thought to be the main vector for transmitting Lyme disease to humans. Courtesy of David Gregory and Debbie Marshall.

Traditional medical societies and agencies feel the Western Blot is a credible test, and yet a minority of scientists, tick infection specialty physicians, and vocal Lyme patient advocates feel most laboratories have adjusted some of the tests in a manner that yields fewer positives. Published studies seem to show a wide variety of accuracy of tests in picking up positive Lyme, with most being over 85 percent reliable. In the context of the debate over testing accuracy, both camps agree that because Lyme primarily lives in the tissues, DNA testing of body fluids such as blood, urine, saliva, and breast milk typically will be negative.

Another way to diagnose is by ruling out other causes and determining whether the patient has had exposure to tick bites. Some individuals think nothing of routine tick bites and do not realize that they are at risk for many tick borne infections. Others have minimal risk. Those who live near deer or similar large animals, or have hobbies that take them into wild fields and brush (such as campers or hunters) are at much higher risk for Lyme than are individuals who live in cities. Also, ticks are unable to infect when the temperature is under 4.4°C (40°F). However ticks can be on logs and other items brought into a home from a cold outdoor environment, and these ticks can be active (e.g., firewood can release tiny active deer ticks as the logs thaw).

An additional way to determine if someone has Lyme disease is to rule out all the other potential causes of a patient's complaints. Like syphilis a hundred years ago, however, Lyme is felt to be the "Great Imposter" and can cause virtually any problem with the body. Therefore, looking only for arthritis, or for a specific rash or new psychiatric symptoms, will cause many infected patients to be missed.

If a medical problem has virtually all of the other possible causes ruled out, and if Lyme disease seems to be the only likely cause left, some consider a treatment trial. However, many traditional physicians worry about the growth of resistant infections to unnecessary antibiotics (e.g., antibiotics used for viral sore throats) and would oppose the use of antibiotics in *possible* Lyme infection patients unless strong evidence exists.

Treatment.   Treatments suggested vary depending on ideology. Most infection societies and government agencies feel a three- to four-week course of doxycycline should kill most Lyme, whereas a minority group of clinical Lyme disease experts feels that, because Lyme replicates so much more slowly than other routine bacteria, treatment should be based on patient improvement on not on a set time. Both groups agree that after four weeks some patients report still not feeling well. Yet it is not clear why this residual illness occurs. Some feel it is the result of Lyme biotoxins causing inflammation like the patented BbTox1 (a problem first suggested to exist in the 1990s by Sam Donta, M.D.). Others feel incomplete cure is the result of biofilms or bacterial slimes covering the Lyme, such that antibiotics penetrate poorly (Eva Sapi, Ph.D., and Alan McDonald, M.D.). Some feel that advanced and disseminated Lyme found deep in body tissues simply cannot be cured in four weeks, whereas others believe there is a mysterious residual bacterial debris with inflammation that takes months to be cleared from the body.

Another issue that is critical to Lyme treatment is the emerging realization that deer ticks do not carry just one infection, but many, and that it is routine for a patient with Lyme to also be infected with *Babesia, Bartonella, Anaplasma*, or *Ehrlichia*. These infections clearly make treatment of Lyme disease more difficult and some, like *Babesia*, require entirely different treatments because they are not bacteria but tiny red blood cell parasites living inside red blood cells. It is well established that these coinfections, or parallel infections, slow the speed of Lyme elimination from the body.

Avoiding Lyme disease is relatively easy. Techniques include avoiding tick endemic areas from early spring until winter, covering one's skin fully with light-colored clothing to see ticks better, and tucking long pants into socks. One should consider using the insect repellent DEET, especially on feet, ankles, and legs, and applying Permethrin to cloths. *See also* Personal Hygiene and Epidemic Disease.

Further Reading

Centers for Disease Control and Prevention. http://www.cdc.gov/ncidod/dvbid/lyme/

Infectious Disease Society of America. http://www.idsociety.org

International Lyme and Associated Diseases Society. http://www.ilads.org

Murray, Polly. *The Widening Circle: A Lyme Disease Pioneer Tells Her Story*. New York: St. Martin's Press, 1996.

Schaller, James, P. J. Langhoff, and Randall Blackwell. *Chronic Treatment Resistant Tick and Flea-born Infections*. Tampa: Hope Academic Press, 2008.

Vanderhoof-Forschner, Karen. *Everything You Need to Know About Lyme Disease*. Hoboken, NJ: John Wiley and Sons, 2003

JAMES SCHALLER

M

MAGIC AND HEALING. All societies have some belief in magic, particularly in the service of healing. Magic is the use of ritual objects, actions, or words that are believed to influence the natural world. Most magical beliefs feature a body of secret knowledge known only to the practitioner. The earliest medical beliefs were spiritual/magical in nature. Practitioners had specialized metaphysical knowledge. There are surviving magical medical texts from the earliest civilizations in all ancient languages, and magical beliefs are still incorporated into many people's medical practices.

Magic and medicine worked in two ways, in combination. One way was through the use of herbs and physical substances, such as honey or various foods. The other was through the use of ritual. For instance, an herbal healing potion might be required for a particular medical need. The herbs for that potion would have to be gathered in a ritualistic manner during times of day or seasons that were deemed magically auspicious. The herbal healing potion would then be made while incantations were recited, and further incantations might be necessary while the potion was consumed or the poultice applied.

The choice of which herb to use for healing was determined by folk wisdom based on years of observation and magical beliefs about how the physical world worked. For instance, if a plant looked like a body part, imitative magic beliefs held that it would heal wounds or cure illnesses in that part of the body. Recent studies by pharmacologists have determined that many of the magical healing cures included elements that do have healing properties. For instance, honey was used in many potions and cures, usually to make them more palatable. It was also used in poultices, because it is viscous and sticky, and the poultice would adhere better to the wound. However, it turns out that honey has natural antibacterial and antifungal properties; using honey in these cures has a real pharmacological effect.

Another type of magical healing involves prayer. Although the faithful of any **religion** do not view their use of prayer as magic, for scholars of comparative religion and anthropology, prayer is a type of charm and ritualized behavior. Stories of miraculous cures exist in all major world religions. Sometimes the rituals become so ingrained in a culture that they persist even when the religion changes; long after England converted to Protestantism, Latin Catholic formulaic prayers were repeated over the sick and dying, in the belief that the language itself had magical healing properties. Rituals and prayer have been shown to have palliative psychological effects. Magic was used through ritual application of healing charms and medicines, and through **astrology**, which was used to predict and explain outbreaks of disease. People afraid of catching the **Black Death** sought out the protection of amulets, which they wore, and relics, which they touched as talismans in order to receive protection. A more modern example is found in Africa, where people infected with **AIDS** frequently turn to sorcerers and magicians for healing. *See also* Contagion Theory of Disease, Premodern; Folk Medicine; Pilgrimage and Epidemic Disease.

Further Reading

Baldwin, Martha. "Toads and Plague: Amulet Therapy in Seventeenth-century Medicine." *Bulletin of the History of Medicine* 67 (1993): 227–247.

Jolly, Karen Louise. *Popular Religion in Late Saxon England: Elf Charms in Context.* Chapel Hill: The University of North Carolina Press, 1996.

Thomas, Keith. *Religion & the Decline of Magic.* New York: Macmillan Publishing Company, 1971.

Vyse, Stuart. *Believing in Magic: The Psychology of Superstition.* New York: Oxford University Press, 1997.

CANDACE GREGORY-ABBOTT

MALARIA.   The word "malaria" is derived from the Italian phrase "mal'aria" (bad **air**), which was regarded as the cause of the excess mortality in many marshy areas of Italy before **Alphonse Laveran's** discovery of malarial parasites in 1880. The first attested use of the Italian phrase was by Marco Cornaro (1406–1479) in a book published in Venice in 1440. Horace Walpole (1717–1797) introduced the phrase into English literature in 1740. However, the disease is much older than that. Malaria was known to all the major ancient Old World civilizations under names like tertian fever or quartan fever, which refer to its most characteristic symptoms, namely intense fevers (alternating with chills) with a periodicity of 48 or 72 hours, a response to the synchronous reproduction of generations of parasites.

Biological Agent and Its Effects.   There are four species of human malaria: *Plasmodium falciparum*, *Plasmodium vivax*, *Plasmodium malariae*, and *Plasmodium ovale*. *P. falciparum* (malignant tertian fever) is the most dangerous species, occurring principally today in Africa, India, Southeast Asia, and some parts of Oceania and South America. Its temperature requirements for reproduction in vector mosquitoes largely confine it to tropical regions, although it was common in the past in southern Europe. *P. falciparum* produces a disease that can be rapidly fatal in nonimmune individuals and can cause chronic ill-health in individuals with some immunity (acquired or inherited). Its most dangerous clinical syndrome is cerebral malaria, whereas anemia is a common manifestation in less serious cases. *P. falciparum* has a periodicity of 48 hours. However, in practice there are frequently overlapping generations of parasites producing quotidian fevers (every 24 hours) that are often hard to distinguish, both in clinical practice today and in historical literature, from other acute infectious diseases such as typhoid fever.

Plasmodium vivax also has a 48-hour periodicity but lower temperature requirements than *P. falciparum*. Consequently it had a broader geographical distribution in the past, extending across large parts of Europe and Asia as far as the northern coast of Russia. After Columbus's arrival it became widely distributed in the Americas. Today it is most frequent in India. *P. vivax* is commonly regarded as a less serious disease (benign tertian fever) than *P. falciparum*, producing chronic ill-health but rarely causing death directly. This view presumably arose because most malaria research has concentrated on the effects of *P. falciparum* in Africa. However, there are increasing reports from India of cases manifesting the severe symptoms usually associated with *P. falciparum*, but in which only *P. vivax* parasites could be detected. The modern Indian evidence is congruent with historical evidence from Europe—for example, from the marshlands of Kent and Essex in early modern England—showing extremely high mortality rates in regions where *P. vivax* was present, but *P. falciparum* could not have been endemic for climatic reasons. In these areas *P. vivax* acted synergistically with other infectious diseases such as pneumonia and tuberculosis to produce its devastating effects.

Plasmodium malariae has a periodicity of 72 hours (quartan fever). Cases of quartan fever last for considerably longer than cases of the other types of human malaria; in fact the parasites of *P. malariae* can survive inside the human host for decades. Nevertheless, the resulting disease is overall less dangerous than *P. falciparum* or *P. vivax*, although *P. malariae* can cause severe kidney problems. *Plasmodium ovale*, the fourth species of human malaria, produces a benign tertian fever. This type of malaria is rare and has little significance.

Epidemiology and Transmission.   Malaria can be transmitted by any means in which contaminated blood is transferred from one person to another (blood transfusions, organ transplants, drug addicts sharing needles), but in practice it is generally transmitted by mosquitoes. Only a small proportion (certain members of the genus *Anopheles*) of all the known species of mosquito are capable of transmitting malaria efficiently. This often gave rise in the past to anophelism without malaria: localities in which there were large mosquito populations, but the wrong species of mosquito as far as the parasites are concerned. Consequently, there was no malaria. The phenomenon of anophelism without malaria helps to explain why people in the past often failed to associate malaria with mosquito bites and resorted instead to the explanation of "bad air." Malaria frequently has a very patchy distribution in ecological terms because mosquitoes rarely fly far, often no more than a few hundred yards from their breeding sites. Consequently, it is quite possible for one village to have intense malaria while another village a couple of miles away has no malaria at all. In most parts of the world where it occurs, malaria is predominantly a disease of the countryside because mosquito populations tend to be larger in rural areas than they are in the middle of large cities. In the wet tropics malaria occurs all the year round, whereas in the dry tropics infections occur mainly in the wet season. In temperate regions such as Europe, malaria had a distinctive seasonal pattern in the past because its temperature requirements confined new cases to the summer and autumn each year. The result was that agricultural laborers were often severely affected at the time of the harvest. The epidemiology of malaria varies because the mosquito species of different regions have different habits. In Europe, for example, malaria was strongly associated with marshy regions because European mosquito species like to breed in marshes. However, in tropical Africa today, *Anopheles gambiae*, the principal vector in Africa, breeds in small (often human-made) pools and avoids marshes. As a result, draining marshes to reduce mosquito populations played an important role in eliminating malaria from Europe, but unfortunately this technique does not work in Africa today. In Southeast Asia there are yet other mosquito species that flourish in forest environments.

Public Health Impact and Control of Malaria.   Malaria had an extraordinary impact on human populations all over the world in the past, wherever it occurred, and it still does today in many areas, especially in Africa south of the Sahara. Estimates of the direct mortality caused by malaria vary widely, but it seems that at least 1 million deaths a year can be attributed to it. In addition to direct deaths, malaria frequently acts by weakening the human body's immune response to other diseases; about two-thirds of all malaria-related mortality may be explained this way. Malaria's interactions with **tuberculosis** and pneumonia in historical populations and with **HIV** today in Africa are particularly important. The age distribution of mortality varies widely. In tropical Africa, where *Anopheles gambiae* is an extremely efficient vector, transmission rates are so high that malaria is a disease of childhood. It produces very high infant mortality rates, whereas those who survive childhood have developed or inherited immunity and so do not suffer from severe clinical symptoms in adulthood. However, in Europe in the past, transmission rates were much lower, and malaria transmission was highly seasonal in nature and frequently had an epidemic rather than an endemic character. Under these epidemiological conditions, it was possible for adults, too, to be severely affected.

Where malaria has been successfully eliminated, this was achieved above all by attacking the vector mosquitoes in the marshy environments where they breed. In Italy in the early twentieth century, for example, the widespread use of the drug quinine drastically reduced direct mortality from malaria, but it did not reduce morbidity very much, nor did it prevent disease transmission. Successful elimination was achieved principally in the 1920s and 1930s, when many marshes (for instance, the notorious Pontine Marshes south of Rome) were drained by Fascist dictator Benito Mussolini (1883–1945). The elimination of malaria in many parts of the world was achieved after the end of the Second World War by the use of the **pesticide** DDT to kill mosquitoes. For a time in the 1950s and 1960s, it seemed as if malaria could be completely eradicated. Then the use of DDT was stopped because of concerns about its impact on wildlife in general. Since then the mosquitoes have started to develop resistance to other insecticides, and malaria parasites have evolved widespread drug resistance. Consequently, malaria is once again an increasing problem, especially in many parts of Africa. Unfortunately, *Anopheles gambiae* in Africa has proven to be a more difficult target than mosquito species in other parts of the world. Attempts to produce a vaccine against malaria have so far not been successful, although this may still be achieved in the future. *See also* Malaria and Modern Military History; Malaria in Africa; Malaria in Medieval and Early Modern Europe; Malaria in the Americas; Malaria in the Ancient World.

Further Reading

Bruce-Chwatt, L., and J. Zulueta. *The Rise and Fall of Malaria in Europe.* Oxford: Oxford University Press, 1980.

Centers for Disease Control and Prevention. *Malaria.* http://www.cdc.gov/malaria/

Classic Malaria Films DVD: 1940s Malaria Disease Symptoms & Treatments History Films [film]. Quality Information Publishers, 2007.

Coluzzi, Mario, and David Bradley. *The Malaria Challenge after One Hundred Years of Malariology.* Rome: Lombardo Editore, 1999.

Cueto, Marcos. *Cold War, Deadly Fevers: Malaria Eradication in Mexico, 1955–1975*. Baltimore: Johns Hopkins University Press, 2007.

Honigsbaum, Mark. *The Fever Trail: In Search of the Cure for Malaria*. New York: Picador, 2003.

Humphreys, Margaret. *Malaria: Poverty, Race, and Public Health in the United States*. Baltimore: Johns Hopkins University Press, 2001.

Malaria: Fever Wars [film]. PBS Home Video, 2006.

Packard, Randall. *The Making of a Tropical Disease: A Short History of Malaria*. Baltimore: Johns Hopkins University Press, 2007.

Poser, C. M., and G. W. Bruyn. *An Illustrated History of Malaria*. New York: Informa Healthcare, 1999.

Sallares, Robert. *Malaria and Rome*. New York: Oxford University Press, 2002.

Smith, Alec. *Insect Man: The Fight against Malaria in Africa*. New York: Palgrave, 1993.

Snowden, Frank. *The Conquest of Malaria: Italy, 1900–1962*. New Haven: Yale University Press, 2006.

World Health Organization. *Malaria*. http://www.who.int/topics/malaria/en/

ROBERT SALLARES

MALARIA AND MODERN MILITARY HISTORY.   Throughout military history, battles have been won or lost because of the health or illness of the troops. **Malaria** is one of the diseases capable of decimating the ranks of a military force and continues to this day to be a severe and ongoing threat to military operations. Military campaigns can also have effects on local populations by forcing relocation to malarial areas and disrupting malaria prevention measures.

It is estimated that approximately half of the world's population lives in malaria-endemic areas. Many of these malarial areas are in militarily strategic locations or regions of unrest where the likelihood of military conflict is greatly increased. For every person who dies of malaria, there are 300 others infected with the disease. This large number of malaria carriers assures that there is a large reservoir of infection available to perpetuate the *Plasmodium* life cycle.

P. falciparum is the most widely spread and virulent form of malaria. This species predominates in the tropical areas of the world and is most capable of decimating a fighting force. Troops posted in a malarial region, after many years of exposure, will develop clinical **immunity** (premunition) to malaria through repeated exposure, but this premunition is rapidly lost once they leave the area where the disease is endemic. Armed forces and refugees from nonendemic areas are vulnerable in malarial areas because they have no acquired immunities to the disease.

Malaria in World War I (1914–1918).   The American military, having gained experience fighting mosquito-borne diseases (malaria and **yellow fever**) during earlier conflicts, entered the First World War better prepared to deal with malaria than most other combatants. Compared to the other allied and enemy forces, they did fare somewhat better. There were only 5,000 reported cases of malaria in the American overseas forces in 1917. In the spring of 1918, there were 420,000 American troops in Europe, with 10,000 troops arriving daily. By the end of the war, America had sent almost 1.2 million troops into the conflict. During the war there were 7.5 cases of malaria per 1,000 troops per year, as reported by U.S. authorities. By comparison, in the Macedonia campaign (1916–1918), malaria disabled the French, British, and German armies for a three-year period. Close to 80 percent of the 120,000 French troops were hospitalized with malaria, and the British army, with an average strength of 124,000 troops, had 162,512 hospital admissions for the treatment of malaria. In the same campaign, there were a total of only 23,762 British war casualties. Exact figures are not available for the German army, but it also suffered a high death (mortality) and illness (morbidity) rate from malaria during the same campaign.

The reason given for this disastrous epidemic in the Macedonia campaign was that the allied military planners had no way of knowing that the hundreds of thousands of Greek refugees, who had fled to Macedonia just prior to the landing of the British and French troops, were infected with *P. falciparum* malaria. The Allied armies, in a futile attempt to prevent or reduce a malaria outbreak, had timed their arrival in Macedonia for the end of the mosquito-breeding season, but the greatly increased availability of actively infected hosts (the refugees) provided the reservoir of infection needed for the *Anopheles* mosquitoes (the vectors) to spread malaria to the troops in epidemic proportions.

The American forces during World War I had the expertise of American military physicians such as Major **Ronald Ross** and Colonel **William Gorgas**, who had distinguished themselves in the fight against malaria during the U.S. military occupation of Cuba (1901) and the Panama Canal Action (1904–1914) and had brought their experience to the battlefields of "the War to end all Wars." Their method of controlling malaria was to impose sanitary drives so drastic that they were referred to as "sanitary Bolshevism." They established "mosquito brigades" to eliminate mosquito larvae from stagnant pools and marshes, and personal anti-mosquito defenses such as mosquito netting and repellants. These anti-malaria campaigns were carried out in high-risk areas in the theater of military operations and were the most effective methods available at the time. Quinine was the only effective medication during the First World War and was used in both the prevention and treatment of malaria by all of the warring armies.

Malaria in World War II (1939–1945).   By the time of the outbreak of World War II, many of the hard-learned lessons about the prevention and treatment of malaria had been forgotten. Malaria caused entire divisions of soldiers to become militarily ineffective on both sides. U.S. General Douglas MacArthur (1880–1964), commander of forces in the Pacific, said in 1943, "This will be a long war, if for every division I have facing the enemy, I must count on a second division in the hospital with malaria, and a third division convalescing from this debilitating disease."

At the outbreak of Word War II, quinine was still the only effective medication for the treatment and prevention of malaria. Realizing this, in 1942 the Japanese invaded Java and seized the Dutch plantations that produced 90 percent of the world's supply of cinchona bark from which quinine was extracted, and German forces seized the reserves of quinine stored in Amsterdam. This setback sent the Allied forces into a frenzy of activity to expand the remaining meager supply of cinchona trees, a process that could take years before the new trees matured or a viable substitute for quinine could be developed and produced.

By 1943 the United States military started using Atabrine, an unpleasant but adequate substitute for quinine that had been discovered by a German researcher prior to the war. The side effects of a bitter taste, nausea, vomiting, diarrhea, yellowing of the skin, and sometimes a temporary insanity (psychosis) were so bad that many soldiers discarded the pills and risked malaria, rather than take the medicine. In time, the side effects were overcome, and even better substitutes such as chloroquine were developed.

In the meantime, many tens of thousands of Allied troops suffered from the ravages of malaria. In some areas of the Pacific Theater, there was an American malaria rate of 4,000 cases per 1,000 troops—a figure made possible by counting each recurrence as a case.

Sixty thousand American soldiers died of malaria during the African and South Pacific campaigns. Even though the most disastrous effects of malaria occurred among the Allied forces in the South Pacific and African campaigns, the Allied campaign in Sicily, from July through September 1943, also suffered significant malarial casualties. There were 21,482 American hospital admissions for malaria compared with 17,375 admissions for war-related injuries. Most of the malaria infections were *P. vivax* and subsequently many infected allied soldiers suffered incapacitating relapses in the spring of 1944 just when they were needed most for the battles for Monte Cassino and Anzio.

For the Japanese military medical service, the greatest problem was the incidence of malaria in Burma. Even with the daily use of quinine and mosquito nets large enough to provide protection for a whole squad of soldiers, along with the use of anti-mosquito creams and sprays for those who had to leave the protection of the nets, malaria continued to be a problem in the Burma region. The overall incidence of malaria is not known, but one Japanese regiment had at least one incident of malaria for every member of the regiment.

The Italian army was taking Italchina pills for the prevention (prophylaxis) of malaria. When some Italian medical supplies, including Italchina pills, were captured in September of 1943, the pills were sent for analysis and were found to be identical to the American Atabrine. The German war machine encountered high rates of malaria in Greece and southern Ukraine and Russia after invading these areas in 1941. Medical officers distributed Atabrine and Plasmochine, but self-dosing proved impractical and ineffective. Both military and industrial labs experimented with effective insecticides and new drugs, whereas prisoner-of-war and concentration camp inmates and mental patients were subjected to often deadly experiments on proper Atabrine dosing.

Malaria in Biological Warfare. The only known attempt at biological warfare in Europe during the Second World War occurred in the autumn of 1943. The German army reversed the pumps draining the marshes just south of Anzio, and flooded the swamp area at the same time that they released millions of malaria carrying mosquitoes. The American and British forces attacked Anzio in January 1944 but avoided a massive outbreak of malaria by taking anti-malarial medication. The local Italian civilians, however, did not have access to the drugs and suffered from malaria on an epidemic scale.

Malaria in War Crimes. Following World War II, Dr. Klaus Schilling (1874–1946), a German physician and one of the world's leading experts on tropical diseases, was tried, convicted, and hanged for war crimes by the American Military Tribunal at Dachau, Germany, for conducting malaria experiments on inmates of the Dachau concentration camp. He would first infect the inmates using malaria-infected mosquitoes and then test a variety of drugs on the prisoners in an effort to find a cure for malaria. As a result of these experiments, 30 to 40 victims died from the direct result of the malaria itself and another 300 to 400 died later as a result of the debilitation brought on as a result of the malaria attacks. There were an additional unknown number of deaths as a result of overdosing with the drugs being tested.

Malaria in the Korean War (1950–1953). Malaria was endemic on the Korean peninsula prior to 1950. There are no specific figures of malaria morbidity and mortality available for the North Korean army, but it is known that the incidence of malaria increased during the conflict. In 1953, the last year of the war, South Korean Army medical records report 8,855 malaria cases, with a 35 percent decrease the following year. Foreign (United Nations) armies who participated in the war also had a significant malaria casualty rate. American troops, who received routine anti-malarial medication in the form of weekly chloroquine tablets, reported 1,513 cases of malaria between July 1951 and November 1952. Canadian soldiers had an 11 percent incidence rate (152 cases out of 1,350 soldiers) in 1952.

Malaria in the Vietnam War (1965–1975).   It was during the Vietnam War that the drug-resistant strains of malaria first emerged. In desperation American military physicians used combinations of anti-malarial medications that met with varying degrees of success. During the Vietnam War, malaria was responsible for more U.S. casualties than were combat injuries. The disease decreased the combat strength of some American units by as much as 50 percent. In 1965 the U.S. armed forces had a morbidity rate of 98 cases per 1,000 troops per year and a mortality rate of 1.7 per 1,000 troops per year.

Contemporary Conflicts.   During its nine-year military occupation of Afghanistan (1979–1988), the Soviet military suffered 469,685 casualties, and of this number, 415,932 were caused by infectious diseases, primarily malaria. No reliable figures exist for the Afghani fighters. Because malaria had been eradicated in northeastern Saudi Arabia and Kuwait, which was the primary theater of operations for 697,000 American forces during Operations Desert Shield (the build-up period) and Desert Storm (the six-week war to free Kuwait from Iraq), there were only seven American cases of malaria. These cases were only among troops who had crossed into southern Iraq.

Ongoing conflicts in or near African regions plagued by malaria result not only in victims among military personnel, but also in epidemic conditions among civilians whose environments are disrupted or who are forced to relocate. The year 2003 saw a major epidemic in the war-torn area of Ethiopia that killed perhaps 100,000 people. In the Darfur region of Sudan, among 2.5 million people dislocated by war and living in squalid camps, malaria, along with pneumonia and **enteric** diseases, killed an estimated 200,000 to 450,000 between 2003 and 2006 alone. Access to drugs is often made impossible by combatants' hijacking of medical transport and by the sheer isolation of refugee camps.

Anti-Malaria Vaccination Quest.   The ultimate defeat of malaria is expected to be the development of an effective vaccine. Unfortunately, development of a vaccine against the malaria **protozoon** with its myriad life stages is not a straightforward process. The U.S. military, as well as other modern military forces, has had very active vaccine development programs under way for many years. Several vaccines have been tested with mixed results, and several more advanced vaccines are in the developmental stages. *See also* Diet, Nutrition, and Epidemic Disease; Environment, Ecology, and Epidemic Disease; Human Immunity and Resistance to Disease; Insects, Other Arthropods, and Epidemic Disease; Malaria in Africa; Pesticides; Typhus and War; War, the Military, and Epidemic Disease.

Further Reading

B. S. Kakkilaya's Malaria Website. *History of Malaria Control.* http://www.malariasite.com/malaria/history_control.htm.

Bwire, Robert. *Bugs in Armor: A Tale of Malaria and Soldiering.* Lincoln: iUniverse, 2001.

Coates, John, and Paul Russell, Medical Department, United States Army. *Preventive Medicine in World War II*, Volume VI, Chapter 1, http://history.amedd.army.mil/booksdocs/wwii/malaria

Department of Health and Human Services, Center for Disease Control and Prevention. *History of Malaria, an Ancient Disease.* http://www.cdc.gov/malaria/history, accessed 5/15/2007

Graves, Patricia, and Myron Levine. *Battling Malaria.* Washington, DC: The National Academies Press, 2006.

Honigbaum, Mark. *The Fever Trail: In Search of the Cure for Malaria.* New York: Farrar, Straus, and Giroux, 2001.

THOMAS QUINN

MALARIA IN AFRICA.   A series of commercial interests followed by colonial motivations has attracted Europeans into Africa since the second half of the eighteenth century. While confronting an unfamiliar landscape in an alien land, European travelers frequently suffered from various forms of fever. However, it was not until the 1840s that the name **malaria** began to be used to refer to these fevers. In those days, malaria was not recognized as a specific disease. The word malaria derived from Italian words *mal'aria*, meaning "bad air." Malaria was believed to be a **miasma**, a poisonous form of putrid emanation that arose from decaying vegetable and animal matters. The presence of malaria was associated with marshlands and swamps. Malaria was then regarded more as a cause of diseases than as a disease itself.

"White Man's Grave".   Africa began to be acknowledged by Europeans as a land of malaria with the failure of the Niger expedition in 1841–1842. This was a British expedition commissioned to secure the abolition of **slavery** and establish networks of trade along the river Niger in West Africa. The mission failed because most of its personnel died of fever, attributed predominantly to malaria. Throughout most of the remaining nineteenth century, malaria figured consistently in the narratives of European traders, naval personnel, missionaries, colonial **surgeons**, and military men as a major deterrent to the healthy life of Europeans in Africa. In these narratives, Africa surfaced as a typically tropical mass of land that abounded in low-lying swampy areas. It was suggested that the banks of innumerable rivers in Africa were infested with excessive vegetation that produced unhealthy miasmic "exhalations." Together, these impressions converged to produce the image of Africa in the popular, and to some extent in the British official, mind as the "white man's grave" or the region of the "deadly climate." Malaria was believed to cause different forms of periodic fever (i.e., remittent and intermittent), in addition to subjecting the body to the risks of debilitating effects of black water fever. European medical officials serving in Africa pointed out that the ill effects of malaria manifested in European bodies in different ways. Anemia, formation of sallow yellowish tint on the skin, boils, absence of blood in the lips, occasional bleeding from the gums, dyspnea on slight exertion, cardiac weakness, enlarged spleen, edema in the ankles, some loss of memory, great debility along with giddiness and frequent insomnia, Carbuncles, dysentery, hematuria, renal complications, slight bronchitis, pulmonary congestion, Brow ague or neuralgia, chronic slight jaundice, and dyspepsia were seen as diverse expressions of malaria in the body. Malaria—along with acute yellow atrophy of the liver, insolation, and **yellow fever**—was believed to inflict the greatest mortalities among European colonials and soldiers in Africa.

Dealing with Malaria.   Despite the fear of malaria, Europeans continued to pursue their commercial and colonial interests in Africa. The explorations of David Livingstone (1813–1873), Richard F. Burton (1821–1890), and others opened up the vast interiors of the African continent. By the Ashanti War in 1874, different European powers had largely succeeded in dealing with the problem of malaria in Africa in different ways. The British palm oil trade in Africa, for instance, penetrated into the interior through specially devised river steamers and an ever-increasing consumption of quinine. Quinine, an extract from the bark of the cinchona plant, began to be appreciated as the best-known cure and preventive for malarial fevers. In British garrisons posted in Africa, daily consumption of smaller doses of quinine was made a key part of the mandatory **diet** for soldiers. In the nineteenth century there was an understanding that the natives in Africa were immune to the ill effects of malaria. It was argued that the natives in Africa were so frequently exposed to malaria in their daily lives that they had adapted themselves to its onerous effects. It was suggested that the delicate bodies of the Europeans in Africa were more vulnerable to the effects of malaria. Such a belief inspired the recruitment policies of the French army. In order to reduce figures of mortality from malarial diseases among the soldiers, the French devised a strategy of recruiting from within the indigenous African populations. In missionary publicity, such as that organized by the Universities' Mission to Central Africa, and in the speeches and writings of Livingstone and Burton, one finds European susceptibility to malaria in Africa explained as an indicator of lack in vigor caused by the delicacy of civilized living.

Malaria: A Protozoan Disease.   By the last decade of the nineteenth century, the meaning of the word malaria had undergone substantial transformation. The microbiological discoveries of **Louis Pasteur, Alphonse Laveran, Patrick Manson,** and Major **Ronald Ross** were received with respect among the dominant sections of the medical scientific community. Malaria began to be understood as a distinct form of fever-causing disease that was brought on by protozoan parasites in the blood. Henceforth, malaria came to be recognized as an infectious disease. Following Ronald Ross's researches, it has been proven that malarial parasites are transmitted from one body to another by female *Anopheles* mosquitoes. Therefore, with the advent of the twentieth century the history of malaria reached a new phase. Scientists and historians started to trace in historical records the presence of the fever-causing disease called malaria over the preceding centuries. In some of these writings, malaria had a very central place. It was suggested, for instance, that soldiers, merchants, or slaves coming from Africa introduced malaria into Greece in the fifth century BCE. Such writings acknowledged Africa as the ancient home of malaria. The image of Africa as a land of endemic malaria survived. Throughout the twentieth century, medical scientists and representatives of international health agencies conducting academic research on malaria frequently visited Africa. Africa was also seen as a geographical area that was perpetually in need of medical relief and philanthropy. Under the leadership of Ronald Ross, an expedition was dispatched to Sierra Leone in West Africa as early as 1899 to verify the results of his laboratory experiments pertaining to the mode of malaria **transmission**. The expedition was not merely inspired by an academic quest. In Freetown, Kissy, Wilberforce, and Lagos, Ross organized sustained assaults on the habitats of the mosquito vectors. This combination of research and relief has inspired an enduring presence of foreign medical professionals in the African continent to the present.

Malaria and the Colonial Political Economy.   Studies on African locales have indicated that malaria in Africa can be explained as an effect of drought, famine, and malnutrition. In Africa, malaria has been regarded as a companion of **poverty. Colonialism** has often been considered a crucial factor behind the patterns of malaria in Africa. A study of malarial epidemics in Swaziland, situated between Mozambique and South Africa, in 1923, 1932, 1939, 1942, and 1946, reveals one such pattern. The subordination of economic interests of the Swazi cultivators and herdsmen to those of the South African and local European settlers reduced the ability of many Swazi to feed themselves and made them vulnerable to climatic disasters. This often turned drought into famine. Excessive rainfall and vector (*Anopheles* mosquito) breeding often followed. Such convergences frequently resulted in massive upsurges in the incidence of malaria.

Black African society has been influenced by memories of racial discrimination and colonial oppression. Among natives, the association of the malarial elimination programs with white settlers has often bred suspicion and even contempt about the intent of such projects. In the 1930s, the South African Department of Public Health's (DPH) efforts to reduce mosquito larvae breeding areas in Zululand by pouring slicks of paraffin into streams and water supplies were interpreted as a white settler means of "poisoning" the Zulu in order to take their land and cattle. Rumors that malaria was caused by the whites, and that quinine caused sterility and abortions, spread rapidly through Zululand. Zulu people were highly suspicious of official motives for malaria control because of their previous experiences with conquest, land loss, and repression, which were rooted in the colonial context.

Malaria and Development.   Measures to eliminate malaria from Africa by promoting agricultural development often failed to achieve their intended purpose. A study of the impact of agricultural development on malaria in the *lowveld* region of the former Transvaal Province of South Africa reveals how the European settler commercial farmers benefited from projects of agricultural development. Such projects often failed to address the issues of poverty, malnutrition, and malaria successfully among the poorest of the Africans. Certain studies have attributed malaria in Africa to the development projects themselves. It is likely that a fisheries project undertaken in Kenya between 1957 and 1961 necessitated the digging of pits and ponds that eventually turned into breeding places for mosquitoes. Similarly, it has been alleged that the Kariba project in Zambia, the construction of the Kalimawe dam in Tanzania, and the Keno plain rice development scheme in Kenya were followed by long periods of malarial outbreaks triggered by the changes to the **environment**.

Malaria and WHO.   Although malaria continues to be a serious problem in eastern Africa, it is recognized as a hyperendemic disease throughout West Africa as well. Because biomedicine clearly understands the causes of malaria and is convinced about the proper ways to tackle it, the problem in responding to malaria is not so much medical as it is educational, bureaucratic, and financial. The **World Health Organization** (WHO) has declared malaria a target for global eradication since the 1950s. It has been reported that though malaria is a global issue, 90 percent of malaria-related deaths occur in Africa. The persistence of malaria in Africa has been explained in terms of limited resources, unfavorable ecological conditions, insufficient health coverage, extreme poverty, shortage of trained personnel, tragic misuse of resources, political instability, and disorganization of civil services. In 1998 the WHO started the "Roll Back Malaria" campaign. This campaign is not another attempt to eradicate Malaria but is a quest to halve malaria-related mortality by 2010 and again by 2015. Partners in this campaign include governments of malaria-endemic countries, donor governments, international organizations, the private sector, and several civil society bodies. In 1997 African scientists invited colleagues from other countries to a meeting in Dakar, and this led to the launch of a Multilateral Initiative on Malaria. Earlier, the regional office of WHO in Africa, the World Bank, and some nations providing development assistance led to the emergence of plans for a pan-African initiative for malaria control. This has evolved into the African Initiative on Malaria. Despite these efforts, *The Africa Malaria Report 2003* published by WHO maintained that malaria continues to be a major impediment to health in Africa south of the Sahara, where it is

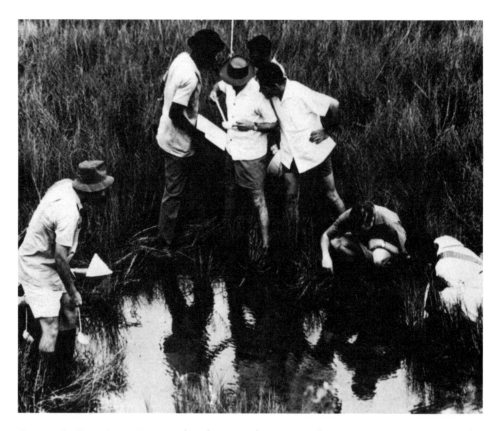

A team in Togo investigating the density of mosquito larvae in streams and marshy land. WHO photo. Courtesy of the National Library of Medicine.

believed to kill very young **children** and pregnant women; it has been shown to be the cause of at least one-fifth of all deaths of young children in Africa. Initiatives to tame malaria continue to emerge. Recently, the Global Fund to Fight **AIDS**, **Tuberculosis**, and Malaria (GFATM) has emerged as a major source of anti-malaria grant funds. Twenty-five countries are sharing a total of $256 million for an initial two years to invigorate malaria control activities. *See also* Colonialism and Epidemic Disease; Diagnosis of Historical Diseases; Disease in the Pre-Columbian Americas; Historical Epidemiology; Latin America, Colonial: Demographic Effects of Imported Diseases; Malaria and Modern Military History; Malaria in Africa; Malaria in Medieval and Early Modern Europe; Malaria in the Americas; Smallpox, Eradication of.

Further Reading

Abeku, Tarekegn A. "Response to Malaria Epidemics in Africa." *Emerging Infectious Diseases* 13 (2007): 681–687.

Carlson, Dennis G. *African Fever: A Study of British Science, Technology, and Politics in West Africa, 1787–1864.* Sagamore Beach, MA: Science History Publications, 1984.

Curtin, Phillip D. *The Image of Africa: British Ideas and Action, 1780–1850*. Madison: University of Wisconsin Press, 1964.

Packard, Randall M. *The Making of a Tropical Disease: A Short History of Malaria*. Baltimore: Johns Hopkins University Press, 2007.

Rocco, Fiammetta. *Quinine: Malaria and the Quest for a Cure That Changed the World*. New York: Harper, 2004.

Smith, Alec. *Insect Man: The Fight against Malaria in Africa*. New York: Palgrave, 1993.

ROHAN DEB-ROY

MALARIA IN MEDIEVAL AND EARLY MODERN EUROPE. Malaria posed a continuing health hazard in medieval and early modern Europe (c. 500 C.E.–1800). Although rarely a killer except among already vulnerable victims, medieval and early modern malaria caused reoccurring fevers that often weakened people, leaving them susceptible to other diseases. Some low-lying or swampy areas, such as the region around Rome and the Po valley in Italy, southeastern England, the Loire river valley and the Gironde in France, and the Don Delta in Ukraine, were particularly susceptible to malaria during this period, although the disease was found as far north as Scandinavia. European importation of slaves from Africa to its colonies in the New World opened the way for a more deadly strain of malaria to strike Europeans, one that reached epidemic proportions in the tropical Americas although not in Europe.

Where Was Malaria Found? Malaria, one of the oldest of human diseases, is caused by four species of fever-producing protozoan parasites of the genus *Plasmodium*. *Anopheles* mosquitoes transmit all four species. Two of the four species of malarial protozoa can be found in the temperate zone of Europe: *P. malariae* and *P. vivax*. Once Europeans began to import slaves from Africa to the West Indies, they exposed themselves to the much more virulent *P. falciparum* in tropical America but not in Europe.

Fevers were commonplace in medieval and early modern Europe and were caused by numerous diseases. In early modern Europe, the term ague came to stand for all of the summer fevers to which people were prone. In many low-lying, wet areas fevers were caused by *P. malariae* or *P. vivax*, and so malarial fever came to be almost synonymous with ague. Because fevers were commonplace and no germ theory of disease existed to explain the cause of disease, malarial fevers were often lumped in with other fevers and accepted as a matter of course for people living in some areas. Nonetheless, some observers did make the connection between the incidence of fever and swampy areas. However, the connection was not between mosquitoes and fever, but between the odors generated by swampy areas and the disease—hence the term bad **air** (*mal'aria* in Italian) used to describe the cause of fever. The eighteenth-century Scots physician William Cullen (1710–1790), for example, thought that fevers were generally caused by exposure to putrid air or bad weather; hence, the cause for fevers was viewed as being located in the atmosphere. At least governmental responses that were directed to removing the "bad air" problem associated with swamps also helped to remove the breeding ground for the mosquitoes that carried malaria.

Plasmodium vivax causes benign tertian fevers in humans. The blood cycle in this case is of 48 hours' duration, so fevers occur every two days, peaking on the third (hence "tertian"). *P. vivax* is generally not a killer, but it produces a recurring fever that saps the strength of its victims. This malaria species may appear to cure itself, only to reappear again over two or three years. *P. vivax* settles in the liver tissue and remains there to cause its victims periodic relapses. Although the parasite dies out in its victims, exposure conveys no immunity, so later mosquito bites cause a repeat of the cycle. A disease of the subtropics and temperate regions, it was found throughout southern Europe and as far north as southern England well into the early modern period. Many summer fevers were the product of *P. vivax*.

Plasmodium malariae was also commonplace in medieval and early modern Europe and was found throughout Europe except in the coldest climates. It produced a quartan fever that peaked every fourth day (counting the first day as day one, as did the Romans who coined the term). In this case the parasites had a 72-hour growth cycle, producing daughter parasites every third day and a high fever that followed. *P. malariae* has the ability to continue to reappear for as long as 10 years after an initial infection. This form of malaria was relatively mild and was often accepted as a normal part of life in some regions.

The Impact of Malaria.   Both *P. vivax* and *P. malariae* were endemic to several regions in medieval and early modern Europe. Swampy areas provided a breeding ground for mosquitoes, and people living near low-lying areas came to expect summer fevers as a matter of course. Because humans provided a host for the malaria parasite, the disease was continually replenished ensuring a reoccurring cycle of disease. In some areas summer fevers were so common, and generally mild, that many people considered them a normal occurrence rather than a sign of illness. Some places became well known for their summer fevers, such as the region around Rome. The Pontine Marshes near Rome provided an ideal environment for malaria until they were drained in the sixteenth century. Marshy areas along the Dutch coast and in Kent and East Anglia in southern England were also noted for their summer fevers throughout the period, as were the lower reaches of the Loire valley in France. In some areas of Kent, burials often exceeded baptisms throughout the period. Malaria was endemic in some parts of England, and some of the early English colonists in the New World transmitted malaria across the Atlantic in their bloodstream so that an early outbreak in Jamestown was caused by the English colonists.

Areas infected by malaria were, nonetheless, generally less healthy than other regions because of a variety of environmental factors. Infant mortality rates were especially high in many low-lying areas, often approaching 300 per 1,000 in southeastern England, for example (the usual infant mortality rate ranged from 150 to 300 per 1,000), although not all of these deaths were directly caused by malaria. Continued malaria infections served to debilitate a population leading to other health problems. Even when death did not result from malaria attacks, the productive capacity of the population was often low because of continued weakness generated by the summer fevers.

The clearing of land for agriculture that began to expand across Europe from the central Middle Ages onward helped to expand the environment for malaria. Small pools of stagnant **water** were an ideal breeding ground for mosquitoes, and land clearing often produced small puddles. As Europeans expanded their agricultural reach, they occupied newly cleared land that might become the breeding ground for malaria-carrying mosquitoes. The medieval warm epoch expanded the temperate zone farther north and higher into the mountains, increasing the potential reach of malaria. The gradual cooling cycle, which reached its high point in the seventeenth century, did help to reduce the environment for malaria in northern Europe from the late seventeenth century onward.

Although European colonization of the Americas exposed them to *P. falciparum*, it also enabled them to find a remedy for the fevers caused by malaria infections. The Spanish discovered the effectiveness of the bark from the cinchona bush, a remedy that Native

Americans may have used for treating fever (this point is debated among scholars, some crediting the Jesuits in Peru with discovering the medicinal use of cinchona). The Jesuits brought cinchona to Europe from Peru in the 1630s as a specific treatment for malaria, and it was often referred to as Jesuit bark or Jesuit powder. The religious connection was so strong that some Protestants with ague (such as Oliver Cromwell [1599–1658] in England) refused to be treated with "Jesuit bark" fearing that they would be poisoned. In the nineteenth century chemists were able to isolate a gummy product from yellow cinchona bark that was effective against malaria, a substance they labeled quinine from an old Peruvian name for the bark. *See also* Colonialism and Epidemic Disease; Insects, Other Arthropods, and Epidemic Disease; Malaria in Africa; Malaria in the Americas; Protozoon, –zoa; Slavery and Disease.

Further Reading

Bollet, Alfred J. *Plagues and Poxes*. New York: Demos Medical Publishing, Inc., 2004.

Bruce-Chwatt, Leonard J., and Julian de Zulueta. *The Rise and Fall of Malaria in Europe*. New York: Oxford University Press, 1980.

Dobson, Mary J. *Contours of Death and Disease in Early Modern England*. New York: Cambridge University Press, 1997.

Hays, J. N. *The Burdens of Disease*. New Brunswick: Rutgers University Press, 1998.

Packard, Randall M. *The Making of a Tropical Disease: A Short History of Malaria*. Baltimore: Johns Hopkins University Press, 2007.

JOHN M. THEILMANN

MALARIA IN THE AMERICAS.   Locating **malaria** in the colonial history of the Americas (from 1492) can be a difficult task. The word *malaria* hardly makes an appearance in the contemporary historical records. The fever-producing disease we now understand as malaria—caused by Plasmodium **viruses** spread by the *Anopheles* mosquito—seems to have been referred to in a variety of ways in the past. Historians have carefully searched for features of malarial fever in the records pertaining to the colonial Americas. In doing so, they have worked closely with demographers, archeologists, geologists, linguists, and medical researchers. They believe that they have been able to infer retrospectively the presence of malaria in the colonial history of the Western Hemisphere.

The Debate.   There has been a long debate involving the introduction of malaria in the Americas. Some scholars have argued that malaria was present prior to the invasion by the Spanish beginning in 1492. Some have interpreted linguistic evidence to suggest that fevers rampant in the armies of Pahacutec around 1378 CE were malarial. The presence of malaria in the pre-Columbian era in the Americas has been suggested from the discovery of pictures of mosquitoes on prehistoric pottery from New Mexico. Several ancient Mayan words have been translated to mean chills, fevers, and other symptoms associated with malaria.

Caribbean Islands.   The predominant view among historians, however, is that malaria was completely unknown in the Americas before the Spanish invasion. They suggest that malaria was imported first into the Caribbean islands and later into the American mainland by Spanish invaders and their African slaves after 1492. The massive movement of population, armies, explorers, slaves, cattle, and insects following the discovery of the sea route to the Americas from Europe resulted in the introduction and spread of malaria in the New World. But malaria was only one among many diseases introduced into the Americas in the sixteenth century. Viral diseases including **influenza**, **measles**, mumps, rubella, **smallpox**, and **yellow fever**, and bacterial diseases including pneumonia, scarlet fever, pertussis, anthrax, **bubonic plague**, and **typhus** are supposed to have been imported at the same time.

Colonial North America.   Spanish populations carried malaria with them as they moved beyond the Caribbean islands and across the American mainland. English colonists probably introduced the disease into the Chesapeake region at Jamestown in 1607, and French-Canadian records mention it in the later seventeenth century. A visitor to La Famine Jesuit mission in 1684 reported 150 cases. Along with smallpox, malaria was the biggest killer of northern Native Americans in the sixteenth century. Falciparum malaria and yellow fever played a major role in depopulating the warmer parts of the Americas once the European settlements began spreading. It has been estimated that mortality from malaria among the Amerindians may have been as high as 75 percent. The Indians were not the only ones to suffer the effects of malaria in the sixteenth and seventeenth centuries. Nonimmune European soldiers and sailors sent to fight colonial battles died more often from yellow fever and malaria than from battle wounds. Malaria was not always a fatal disease, of course. In some parts of northern America, as in the Mississippi Basin, it was more of an endemic debilitating condition. Some pockets in North America remained relatively free from malaria until the early eighteenth century. The first explorers and pioneers who entered the Mississippi Valley, for instance, found no malaria. In Illinois, there was almost no malaria through the whole period of French settlement up to the 1760s. Thereafter, the situation changed drastically.

Along the East Coast malaria spread with infected settlers, becoming more or less endemic from Massachusetts to Georgia. Though thriving in low-lying and warmer areas, the disease was no stranger to northern entry ports such as Philadelphia and New York City, especially in the warm, humid summer months. More than other southern regions, South Carolina proved a "graveyard" for colonists, thanks to endemic malaria. The low-lying, marshy ground and long summers that encouraged the cultivation of rice and indigo proved perfect for mosquito breeding. Malarial deaths and debilitation among the colonists and natives prompted the widespread use of immune African slave labor.

South America.   As in the North, there is considerable debate involving whether malaria was native to South America or imported. Some historians have argued that malaria may have been indigenous to South America. That ancient Peruvians built their houses far from the rivers has been attributed to the probable presence of malaria. Malaria might have been one of the fevers that attacked the invading pre-Columbian Inca armies in the Upper Amazon. However, such impressions are challenged by demographic figures for this region preceding the conquest: such densities of population in that region would have been impossible under the threat of malarial fevers. Alternatively, many historians have argued that malaria was imported into South America during and after the Spanish conquest.

Many places that have since then been repeatedly devastated by malarial fevers seem to have been free from malaria at the time of conquest. Historical records suggest that the invading troops under Hernán Cortés (1485–1547) and Francisco Pizarro (1471–1541) did not complain about malaria. Guyaquil, today still heavily infested, was a health resort during the sixteenth century. As late as the seventeenth century, Spanish expeditions in the Amazon valley did not suffer from malaria. This explains why the therapeutic powers of cinchona bark (a base for quinine) were unknown to the natives. Thus, the predominant opinion among historians is that malaria was an imported disease, and one or more strains of malarial parasites were undoubtedly imported into the Americas in the sixteenth century from endemic areas in Europe and Africa. The tropical lowlands of northern South America, the Amazon basin, and coastal Brazil are believed to have been particularly conducive to the development and propagation of mosquito-borne diseases. Studies have indicated that milder varieties of malarial parasites—for example, *Plasmodium vivax* and *Plasmodium malariae* mosquitoes—existed in several areas of Central and South America before the discovery of the New World, whereas the Spaniards and their slaves brought the fatal *Plasmodium falciparum*.

Malaria came to be referred to in South America by different names, such as *sezoes* in the eighteenth-century Brazilian interior. By the nineteenth century, malaria began to be referred to as intermittent or pernicious fever. Malarial epidemics felled huge portions of the native populations following the Spanish intrusion into Hispaniola, central Mexico, northwestern Mexico, Guatemala south of the Peten rainforest, and the central Andes. Sixteenth-century Jesuits recorded attacks of fever throughout the tropical regions. When, in the sixteenth century, Spaniards discovered that extractions from the bark of the cinchona plants provided a cure for malarial fevers, they exported it and popularized it as an anti-periodic in other parts of the world.

Malaria in the Colonial Americas and the African Slave Trade. The Indian population in the Americas died of European and African diseases, whereas the Europeans died of African diseases. The African slaves were perceived as being able to survive both. This resulted in the impression that the African slaves were immune to malaria. They were said to have survived malaria throughout their lives in their homelands. Europe was home to the milder variety of malarial parasite *Plasmodium vivax*. Thus, the malarial agents that had been transmitted by the European sailors and soldiers were seen as causing a general debilitating effect on the native Americans. In contrast, Africa has been home to the more deadly variety of malarial parasite, the *Plasmodium falciparum*. Historians have considered falciparum malaria to have been equally deadly to the Europeans and the Indians in the Americas, wherever it had been introduced to the local mosquitoes by the African slaves along the marshlands of the Atlantic and Gulf Coasts.

Malaria in the United States. By the late colonial period, malaria had receded from New England, and its incidence was falling in the Mid-Atlantic states. Westward emigration and pioneer agriculture, however, brought malaria to the Ohio and Mississippi River Valleys and beyond. Initial settlement along watercourses and the clearing of heavily forested land encouraged the *Anopheles*, and malaria soon became the dominant disease of the American Midwest. Thirty years before **Alphonse Laveran** discovered the role of Plasmodium, American pioneer naturalist and medical educator Daniel Drake (1785–1852) of Ohio concluded from his travel and study of regional wildlife that malaria ("autumn fever") was a result of "animalcules" rather than miasma. He published his findings and conclusion in *A Systematic Treatise, Historical, Etiological, and Practical, on the Principal Diseases of the Interior Valley of North America* (1850–1854). Malaria's slow decline in the Midwest from the 1860s resulted from such trends as urbanization, expansion of railroad service (which moved people away from waterways), local drainage efforts, better nutrition, and the spread of cattle raising, which provided the mosquitoes' preferred hosts.

Malaria remained a problem in the American South, however, especially in marshy areas dedicated to labor-intensive agriculture. Civil War soldiers, whose campaigns were generally in southern climes, suffered from malaria more often than from any other disease. In the 12 southern U.S. states between 1912 and 1915 there were still 1 million cases of malaria in a total population of 25 million people. Even so, the mechanization of agriculture and the draw of rural southerners to northern cities during World War I (1914–1918) reduced population densities, producing a dramatic reduction of 90 percent in deaths from the disease between 1910 and 1920. The application of mosquito control techniques developed during the Second World War (1939–1945) eliminated malaria from the American landscape by 1949. The **Centers for Disease Control and Prevention** (CDC) still report many annual cases in the United States (1,349 in 2005), but virtually all of them are attributed to immigration or travel by U.S. residents.

Modern Latin America.   Malaria continued to plague postcolonial Latin American societies well into the twentieth century. Nineteenth-century European and Creole elites across the continent demanded and attained improvements in water supply and drainage in their enclaves, but little was done for the rural masses. At the end of World War I, the young Rockefeller Foundation took on the elimination of malaria from Caribbean and Latin American sources, in part to prevent its reintroduction into the United States via migration (a fear that remains today). Others reinforced Rockefeller's efforts during the 1930s, and after 1945 anti-malarial spraying with DDT and provision of improved drug therapy for the sick became a major task of the Pan American Sanitation Bureau (PASB; later the Pan American Health Organization). In the 1950s the **World Health Organization** (WHO), UNICEF, and the U.S. State Department aided PASB. When WHO announced its initiative for the Global Eradication of Malaria in 1956, Mexico was among the first to sign on. Others followed, but by 1967 progress was disappointing, and the scope was reduced to providing for local control measures. By 1972 the initiative was declared moribund, despite nearly $1 billion in U.S. funding.

Malaria is still considered endemic in certain parts of Latin America. In the 1980s, a chloroquinine-resistant strain of parasite, along with massive deforestations in Rondonia and other parts of the Amazon, led to significant outbreaks of malaria among miners, Indians, and settlers in the region. In the early 2000s, regional governments and other agencies increased anti-malarial budgets in a concentrated effort to reduce the incidence of the disease dramatically by 2015. Between 2002 and 2006, the region's annual budgets rose from about $80 million to nearly $171 million. Reported malaria deaths dropped from 348 in 2000 to 101 in 2006, though reported cases only fell from 1,146,042 to 916,467, a reduction of 20 percent. Brazil accounted for 53.5 percent of the cases in 2000 and 60 percent in 2006. But progress has not been steady, and rising global temperatures might expand the geographical range of vector mosquitoes, increasing their rate of development and reducing the extrinsic incubation time of their pathogens. *See also* Colonialism and Epidemic Disease; Diagnosis of Historical Diseases; Disease in the Pre-Columbian Americas; Historical Epidemiology; Latin America, Colonial: Demographic Effects of Imported Diseases; Malaria and Modern Military History; Malaria in Africa; Malaria in Medieval and Early Modern Europe.

Further Reading

Cook, Noble David, and W. George Lovell. *"Secret Judgments of God": Old World Disease in Colonial Spanish America.* Norman: University of Oklahoma Press, 1992.

Cueto, Marcos. *Cold War, Deadly Fevers: Malaria Eradication in Mexico, 1955–1975.* Baltimore: Johns Hopkins University Press, 2007.

Dunn, Frederick L. "On the Antiquity of Malaria in the Western Hemisphere." *Human Biology* 57 (1965): 385–393.

Gehlbach, Stephen H. "Scourge of the Middle West: Autumnal Fever and Daniel Drake." In *American Plagues: Lessons from Our Battles with Disease*, edited by Stephen H. Gehlbach, pp. 93–122. New York: McGraw Hill, 2005.

Grob, Gerald N. *The Deadly Truth: A History of Disease in America.* Cambridge, MA: Harvard University Press, 2002.

Humphreys, Margaret. *Malaria: Poverty, Race, and Public Health in the United States.* Baltimore: Johns Hopkins University Press, 2000.

Packard, Randall M. *The Making of a Tropical Disease: A Short History of Malaria.* Baltimore: Johns Hopkins University Press, 2007.

Prothero, R. Mansell. "Malaria in Latin America: Human and Environmental Factors." *Bulletin for Latin American Research* 14 (1995): 357–365.

Rocco, Fiammetta. *Quinine: Malaria and the Quest for a Cure That Changed the World.* New York: Harper, 2004.

Rutman, Darrett B., and Anita H. Rutman. "Of Agues and Fevers: Malaria in the Early Chesapeake." *William and Mary Quarterly* 33 (1976): 31–60.

Stepan, Nancy Leys. "'The Only Serious Terror in These Regions': Malaria Control in the Brazilian Amazon." In *Disease in the History of Modern Latin America: From Malaria to AIDS*, edited by Diego Armus, pp. 25–50. Durham, NC: Duke University Press, 2003.

Rohan Deb-Roy

MALARIA IN THE ANCIENT WORLD.

China.   **Malaria** was already one of the most widespread diseases in the Old World by the time of the earliest historical records from all the major ancient civilizations. In China a fifth-century document written by Zuo Qiuming (Spring and Autumn period, 770–476 BCE) describes how a minister developed malaria following an **insect** bite. Other sources dating to the Warring States period (476–221 BCE) describe the typical seasonal pattern of the disease in temperate to subtropical climates, its 48- (tertian) or 72-hour (quartan) periodicity in humans, and its transmission. It was already known in ancient China that malaria was transmitted by mosquito bites, long before this was discovered in Europe. Fifth-century BCE Chinese author Zhan Guo, however, attributed the disease to the entry into the human body of an evil element called "*shui qi.*"

The Pacific and the Indian Oceans.   From China malaria was carried eastward by human migrations. Unlike the Chinese civilization, many of these cultures lack written records, so historians have to rely on research into the genetic makeup of many of these societies. The strong linkage of ovalocytosis (a human genetic mutation giving resistance to cerebral malaria) to populations of speakers of Austronesian (South Pacific Islander) languages has been used as evidence for the spread of malaria by the ancestors of these populations in prehistory. They probably moved from Taiwan throughout the western Pacific to Melanesia, where the disease reaches its greatest intensity today outside Africa. Malaria, however, was unable to establish itself on some of the more remote Pacific islands because of the absence of its vectors, *Anopheles* mosquitoes. Moving in the opposite direction as well, speakers of Austronesian languages spread eastward across the Indian Ocean from Indonesia, bringing ovalocytosis to Madagascar. Malaria was also well known in India in antiquity. It is described in the great ancient **Ayurvedic** medical text *Susruta Samhita*, which dates from before 500 CE. One passage in this Sanskrit text may attribute malaria to mosquito bites, although the text is difficult to interpret.

Egypt and Mesopotamia.   Egyptian papyri dating to the period of the Pharaohs do not mention the characteristic periodicity of malarial fevers. Nevertheless, the argument from silence is not decisive because hardly any diseases are clearly described in these documents. The presence of the disease from the dawn of Egyptian civilization has been confirmed by antibody tests to detect malaria antigens in tissues from desiccated bodies dating to the Predynastic Period about 3200 BCE and in later mummies as well. Greek papyri from Egypt dating to the Hellenistic and Roman periods (300 BCE–400 CE) do use the characteristic Greek terminology for malaria and describe **magic** spells that were used to try to ward off the disease. Malaria was also well known in ancient Mesopotamia. Both the symptoms of the benign tertian fevers caused by the microorganism *Plasmodium vivax* and the neurological symptoms of cerebral malaria caused by *Plasmodium falciparum* have been identified in ancient cuneiform texts from Mesopotamia.

Greece and Italy.   The greatest volume of surviving evidence for malaria in antiquity relates to the world of classical Greece and Rome around the Mediterranean (800 BCE– 500 CE), particularly to Rome. It is here that it is possible to appreciate most clearly the effects of the disease, its **epidemiology**, and human reactions and responses to the problems it created. The writings attributed to **Hippocrates**, those of **Galen** and other ancient medical writers, as well as those of nonmedical authors, provide abundant literary evidence. In the first century CE, the Roman author Celsus (c. 25 BCE–50 CE) clearly described and differentiated the symptoms of malignant tertian fevers, caused by *Plasmodium falciparum*; of benign tertian fevers, caused by *P. vivax*; and of quartan fevers caused by *P. malariae*. In addition, it is possible to examine human skeletal remains excavated from archaeological sites for malformations caused by inherited human genetic conditions associated with resistance to malaria, such as the anemia-causing, inherited blood disorder thalassemia, which is common in Mediterranean populations, and the sickle cell trait. Although the sickle cell trait undoubtedly first evolved in tropical Africa, the earliest direct evidence for it comes from Hellenistic burials dating to the third century BCE on the island of Failaka in the Persian Gulf, where fossilized sickle-shaped red blood cells have been directly observed under the electron microscope. This was probably the mild form of sickle cell disease found today from Arabia to India, rather than the more severe form of the disease that occurs in people from tropical Africa and in African Americans. A third avenue of research is provided by biomolecular archaeology (the study of ancient DNA and other ancient biomolecules, already alluded to above in relation to Egypt). Ancient DNA has been used to confirm an archaeologist's hypothesis that malaria was the cause of an epidemic that produced an infant cemetery in the ruins of an abandoned Roman villa at Lugnano in Umbria in central Italy in the fifth century CE.

For over 2,000 years, malaria was endemic in the countryside of central Italy around Rome. In the first century BCE, the Roman orator Cicero (106–43 BCE) records that Romulus, the legendary eighth-century founder of Rome, chose a healthy location in a pestilential region for his new city (traditional foundation date 753 BCE). The famous Seven Hills of Rome were healthy for those people, particularly the aristocracy, who lived on top of them. Though they did not make the connection, this was because mosquitoes, the vectors of malaria, only flew at the lower altitudes and around badly drained soils. In the lowlands surrounding the city of Rome in antiquity, however, malaria had as great an impact on the economy and the population as it does today in tropical Africa. Cato the Elder (234–149 BCE), one of the earliest Roman historians, indicated that building a villa in an unhealthy location in summer, the malaria season, would increase the cost of the construction work by a quarter. The chronic ill health produced by malaria led many of the Romans to want to migrate away from their own homes. The first-century Roman historian Livy (c. 59 BCE–17 CE) stated that when the Romans invaded Campania, the region around Naples, in the fourth century BCE, in their first major excursion outside their homeland of Latium, the Roman soldiers did not want to return home after the end of the war because their farms in Latium were unhealthy, whereas Campania was healthy. This was the result of differences in the distribution of various species of mosquito, not all of which are capable of transmitting malaria. As the Romans vacated their own farms around Rome to acquire an empire, a labor shortage developed on fertile agricultural lands around the city. Malaria was most intense in low-lying areas with the best land for agriculture. The Romans solved the labor problem by importing large numbers of non-Roman slaves, who were forced to work in the fields in chain gangs, under the whip. A whole economy based on mass chattel **slavery** developed in the countryside around ancient Rome, as a response to malaria. After the collapse of the Roman Empire, malaria continued to flourish around the city of Rome until Italian dictator Benito Mussolini (1883–1945) eliminated it in the 1920s and 1930s.

Africa South of the Sahara.   The historical record for Europe demonstrates what we can only assume in the case of Sub-Saharan Africa, given the scarcity of documentary evidence relating to tropical Africa before European colonization commenced. *Plasmodium falciparum*, the most dangerous of the four species of human malaria, had an extraordinary impact over a very long period of time on the development of civilization even in areas on the fringe of its geographical distribution, in southern Europe. In central Africa, where it evolved, it probably had an even greater impact in the past. Indeed, it is very likely that the presence of endemic malaria is a major reason why civilization failed to develop in antiquity in tropical Africa, where *Homo sapiens* first evolved.

Pre-Columbian New World.   Whether malaria was present in the Americas before Christopher Columbus (1451–1506) is a matter of controversy, as is the presence of numerous other diseases. However, the most significant argument that is currently available is that no native American population manifests any of the human genetic mutations conferring a degree of resistance to malaria (e.g., sickle trait, thalassemia, ovalocytosis) that are so common in the Old World wherever malaria occurs today or is known to have occurred in the past. Consequently, it seems that the exposure of Amerindian populations to malaria, which occurs today in parts of Central and South America, is very recent, indicating that the disease was either not present at all or at least was not very important in the New World before Columbus. Presumably, the necessary mosquito vectors of malaria, which is a temperature-dependent disease, could not survive the passage of the ancestors of the Amerindians from Asia to North America across the Bering Strait. *See also* Chinese Disease Theory and Medicine; Diagnosis of Historical Diseases; Environment, Ecology, and Epidemic Disease; Greco-Roman Medical Theory and Practice; Human Immunity and Resistance to Disease; Malaria in Africa; Malaria in Medieval and Early Modern Europe; Malaria in the Americas; Neolithic Revolution and Epidemic Disease; Paleopathology; War, the Military, and Epidemic Disease; Water and Epidemic Diseases.

Further Reading

Caldas de Castro, Marcia, and Burton Singer. "Was Malaria Present in the Amazon before the European Conquest?" *Journal of Archaeological Science* 32 (2005): 337–340.

Clark, Jeffrey, and Kevin Kelly. "Human Genetics, Paleoenvironments, and Malaria: Relationships and Implications for the Settlement of Oceania." *American Anthropologist* 95 (1993): 612–630.

Grmek, Mirko. *Diseases in the Ancient Greek World.* Baltimore: Johns Hopkins University Press, 1989.

Packard, Randall M. *The Making of a Tropical Disease: A Short History of Malaria.* Baltimore: Johns Hopkins University Press, 2007.

Sallares, Robert. *Malaria and Rome.* New York: Oxford University Press, 2002.

Webb Jr., James. "Malaria and the Peopling of Early Tropical Africa." *Journal of World History* 16 (2005): 269–291.

ROBERT SALLARES

MALLON, MARY (1869–1938).   Known as "Typhoid Mary," Mary Mallon is a significant figure in the history of epidemic disease because she was the first individual in the United States to be identified as a healthy carrier (a person who is contagious but has no symptoms) of **typhoid fever**. Mallon, whom the popular media of the day dubbed "The Most Dangerous Woman in America," rose to notoriety during the first decade of the twentieth century because her asymptomatic-carrier status allowed her to move freely throughout New York City and its suburbs, directly infecting 47 people (3 of whom died).

Mallon was born in 1869, in County Tyrone, Ireland. She immigrated to New York City in 1883 and worked her way through a series of menial jobs, until she eventually earned a reputation as a trustworthy and competent cook. Between 1900 and 1907, Mallon served as a cook for a number of wealthy New York–area families, infecting her employers with the typhoid bacillus (*Salmonella typhi*) through the meals she prepared.

Public health officials eventually caught up with Mallon in 1906, when an outbreak of typhoid occurred in Oyster Bay, Long Island, an affluent suburb of New York City. The outbreak attracted the attention of George Soper (1870–1948), a 37-year-old civil engineer turned public health specialist, who deduced that a local cook, Mallon, had caused the outbreak. In 1907 Soper tracked down Mallon, who was working for a family on Park Avenue (their only child eventually died of typhoid fever). Violently opposed to the idea that she could be a silent carrier, Mallon refused to cooperate with Soper. He enlisted the help of NYC Health Commissioner, Herman Biggs (1859–1923), and Dr. Sara Josephine Baker (1873–1945), an inspector from the Department of Health. Using their authority, Soper was able to take blood, urine, and stool samples, all of which tested positive for the typhoid bacillus. The emerging science of bacteriology thus proved that Mallon was in fact a healthy carrier.

Even though other healthy carriers of typhoid fever existed in New York City, Mallon was a foreign-born, Irish-Catholic, working-class woman at the peak of anti-immigrant nativism. She was automatically deemed a "threat to society" by the Department of Health. Denied her civil liberties, Mallon was forcibly isolated on North Brother Island in the East River near the Bronx. She remained a prisoner of the state until 1910.

In 1915, another typhoid outbreak occurred, this time at New York's prestigious Sloane Maternity Hospital. Twenty-five staff members contracted the disease, two of whom died. Soper determined that the cause of the outbreak was Mallon. Though she had been barred by the city authorities from ever working as a cook again, she was employed in the hospital kitchen. Once again she was isolated on North Brother Island. She remained there until her death in 1938 of pneumonia, at the age of 69. *See also* Medical Ethics and

Epidemic Disease; Public Health Agencies, U.S. Federal; Scapegoats and Epidemic Disease; Typhoid Fever in the West since 1800.

Further Reading

Bourdain, Anthony. *Typhoid Mary: An Urban Historical*. Collingdale, PA: Diane Publishing Company, 2004.

Leavitt, Judith Walzer. *Typhoid Mary: Captive to the Public's Health*. Boston: Beacon Press, 1997.

Kraut, Alan M. *Silent Travelers: Germs, Genes, and the Immigrant Menace*. Baltimore: Johns Hopkins University Press, 1995.

Typhoid Mary: The Most Dangerous Woman in America [film]. Nova, 2004.

TANFER EMIN TUNC

MALTHUSIANISM.   In nature it is common for populations of **animals** and **insects** to undergo "boom and bust" cycles, in response to fluctuations in food availability. It is inherent in the process of biological evolution and natural selection that individuals, families, or groups of organisms compete with one another, up to the limits of available food and other key resources.

The word "Malthusian" refers to the view that humans, too, are subject to food supply limits acting as a final, and "bust"-generating, constraint on population growth. Malthusianism envisages that, when such food limits are reached, starvation, social disorder, and heightened mortality are the inevitable natural checks on continuing population growth. Some scholars have interpreted the written accounts of past famines and social breakdowns as illustrations of Malthusian depopulating crises. However, others have argued that the form of a crisis is shaped more by social and economic forces than by laws of biological demography.

This perennially controversial idea came from the Reverend Thomas Robert Malthus (1766–1834), an English cleric, demographer, and political economist. Malthus developed his pessimistic but highly influential views on population growth largely as a reaction to what he regarded as the undue optimism of the French political scientist and philosopher Marquis de Condorcet (1743–1794) and of his own father and associates, who included the *philosophe* Jean-Jacques Rousseau (1712–1778). Those optimistic ideas reflected the enthusiastic populist ideals behind the French Revolution. In 1798 Malthus published his famous *An Essay on the Principle of Population*, predicting that the multiplicative growth of population would outrun the usually linear increase in food supply. His "Principle of Population" stated that population, if unchecked, increases at a geometric rate (i.e., 1, 2, 4, 8, etc.), whereas the food supply grows at a much slower arithmetic rate (i.e., 1, 2, 3, 4, etc.).

This disparity, Malthus argued, must lead to a decrease in available food per person, with consequent starvation, **epidemic** disease, and worse. His phraseology was dire:

> The power of population is so superior to the power of the earth to produce subsistence for man, that premature death must in some shape or other visit the human race. The vices of mankind are active and able ministers of depopulation. They are the precursors in the great army of destruction, and often finish the dreadful work themselves. But should they fail in this war of extermination, sickly seasons, epidemics, pestilence, and plague advance in terrific array, and sweep off their thousands and tens of thousands. Should success be still incomplete,

gigantic inevitable famine stalks in the rear, and with one mighty blow levels the population with the food of the world.

Writing at a time when periodic famine persisted in Europe, Malthus anticipated a food-shortage disaster during the nineteenth century. However, largely because of the gains of the second agricultural revolution in Europe and the higher food yields from cultivars brought back from Europe's adventures overseas (e.g., the potato from the Andes), this prediction did not eventuate. Further, his classically static analyses, with simple forward extrapolations of recent trends, were unsuited to the nonlinear behavior of complex social, economic, and agricultural systems.

Malthus favored moral restraint as a preemptive check on population growth. This restraint included late marriage and sexual abstinence—which he advocated particularly for the poor and working classes. The young Charles Darwin (1809–1882) was influenced by his reading about the dynamics of the Malthusian process, wherein, with limited food supplies, those who were the most politically powerful and privileged were most likely to survive. Here lay the seeds of an idea: the natural selection processes of biological evolution. *See also* Diet, Nutrition, and Epidemic Disease; Environment, Ecology, and Epidemic Disease; Human Immunity and Resistance to Disease; Irish Potato Famine and Epidemic Disease, 1845–50; Poverty, Wealth, and Epidemic Disease; Water and Epidemic Diseases.

Further Reading

Malthus, Thomas Robert. *An Essay on the Principle of Population.* New York: Oxford, 1999. See also http://www.faculty.rsu.edu/~felwell/Theorists/Malthus/essay2.htm

Peterson, William. *Malthus, Founder of Modern Demography*, 2nd edition. Edison, NJ: Transaction, 1999.

Ross, Eric B. *The Malthus Factor: Population, Poverty, and Politics in Capitalist Development.* London: Zed Books, 1998.

ANTHONY MCMICHAEL

MANSON, PATRICK (1844–1922). A **physician** and expert on tropical medicine, Patrick Manson was born in Aberdeenshire, Scotland. He graduated in 1865 from Aberdeen University and in 1866 was awarded his M.D. degree. Manson spent 23 years in China and Hong Kong, where at various points he was a government health officer, had a private practice, and founded the Hong Kong School of Medicine. He eventually returned to London where he helped establish the discipline of tropical medicine.

Appointed in 1866 to the Chinese Imperial Maritime Customs as medical officer for Formosa (Taiwan), he resigned in 1871and moved to Amoy, where he joined a missionary hospital. In this period he began to conduct research on the *filaria* worm and diseases affecting the lymphatic system. He concluded that the mosquito was an intermediary host necessary for the development of *filaria* worms, organisms responsible for causing elephantiasis. He retired to Scotland in 1889 but in 1892 moved London where he was appointed **physician** to the Albert Docks of the Royal Naval Hospital. There he took the opportunity to continue his research on tropical medicine. He thought that there might be a similar mosquito-parasite relationship for **malaria** and in 1894 published a hypothesis about the role of the mosquito in the transmission of malaria. **Alphonse Laveran** had also speculated about the role of the mosquito in the transmission of malaria, but it was **Ronald Ross** who built on the work of Manson and others to demonstrate it.

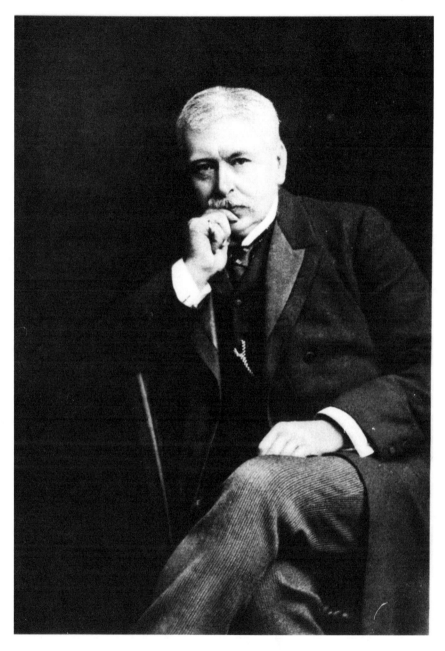

Dr. Patrick Manson. Courtesy of the National Library of Medicine.

While he was in London, Manson developed programs to control **epidemic** diseases in the British Empire. In 1894 he was appointed medical advisor to the Colonial Office, providing memoranda on public health and epidemic disease control as well as names of experts to make trips to the Empire to dispense advice to local governments. He also elicited the support of Joseph Chamberlain (1836–1914), the Colonial Secretary, for a scheme to improve research opportunities in tropical medicine and education in the discipline for physicians and public health officers. In 1898 Manson published his seminal *Tropical Diseases: A Manual of the Diseases of Warm Climates*. With support from the Colonial Office and the help of **William Simpson** and James Cantlie (1851–1946), in 1899 Manson founded the London School of Tropical Medicine, which became an important reference for the study of the control, prevention, and cure of epidemic diseases in the tropics.

Further Reading

Haynes, Douglas. *Imperial Medicine: Patrick Manson and the Conquest of Tropical Disease*. Philadelphia: University of Pennsylvania Press, 2001.

Hewa, Soma. *Colonialism, Tropical Disease and Imperial Medicine*. New York: University Press of America, 1995.

MARY P. SUTPHEN

MARBURG VIRUS.   *See* Hemorrhagic Fevers; Hemorrhagic Fevers in Modern Africa.

MATHER, INCREASE (1639–1723) AND COTTON (1663–1728).   The New England "Mather Dynasty" dominated Massachusetts religious and political life during most the seventeenth century and into the first quarter of the eighteenth. The son of Richard Mather (1596–1669), who had emigrated from England because of religious persecution for his Puritan views, Increase Mather was raised and educated in Massachusetts, preached in Congregationalist churches in England during the Puritan Commonwealth (1649–1660), and returned to New England after the restoration of the monarchy in 1660. Although his hesitation to intervene against the Salem witch trials caused some to blame him for persecution, Increase Mather held to the view that it was better for those guilty of witchcraft to go free rather than to punish the innocent, and he was skeptical of so-called "spectre (spirit) evidence." This rather rational ethos was also evident in his promotion of a society to advance scientific knowledge and, upon his appointment as rector of Harvard College from 1686 to 1701, his encouragement of scientific study at the college. He, along with his son Cotton, also pioneered in advocacy of inoculation during a **smallpox** epidemic, an unpopular and controversial position at the time.

Like his father, Cotton Mather is chiefly known as a Congregationalist religious leader, although a speech impediment nearly discouraged him from a career as a preacher and inclined him toward the profession of medicine, a field in which he maintained an active interest. When he inoculated his own son against smallpox, nearly causing the young man to die, Cotton Mather drew the ire of his fellow citizens, including Dr. William Douglass (1691–1752), the only **physician** in Boston with a medical degree. His account of these events was published in the transactions of the Royal Society of London, which had admitted him into its membership upon the publication of his study of American natural phenomena, *Curiosa Americana* (1712–1724). As evidence of his wide-ranging interests,

Cotton Mather possessed the largest private library in colonial America. He was the author of numerous works on a variety of topics, including *Sentiments on the Small Pox Inoculated* (1721) and *An Account . . . of Inoculating the Small-Pox* (1722).

Unpublished in his lifetime was the medical manual *The Angel of Bethesda* (c. 1724). This manual discusses the general causes of illness and prescribes regimens for wellness, and it proposes an early form of **germ theory**, noting the ubiquity of microscopic organisms. It discusses specific diseases and speculates upon their causes while proposing treatments. Concerning smallpox, he attributes the cause to an "Animalculated Business" (what we would call microorganisms) and suggests a variety of treatments once the disease is contracted. As a clergyman, Cotton Mather took pains to associate disease and **epidemics** with moral and spiritual concerns, both attributing a link between sick souls and sick bodies and admonishing readers to employ the trial and suffering of illness as an occasion for repentance. *See also* Jenner, Edward; Religion and Epidemic Disease; Smallpox in Colonial North America; Vaccination and Inoculation.

Further Reading

Hall, Michael G. *The Last American Puritan: The Life of Increase Mather, 1639–1723.* Middletown, CT: Wesleyan University Press, 1988.

Levin, David. *Cotton Mather: The Young Life of the Lord's Remembrancer, 1663–1703.* Cambridge, MA: Harvard University Press, 1978.

Silverman, Kenneth. *The Life and Times of Cotton Mather.* New York: Welcome Rain, 1984.

THOMAS LAWRENCE LONG

MEASLES.   Measles is the English-language term for a systemic fever-producing exanthematous disease and for the **virus** that causes it. Measles is known as *la rougeole* in French, *Masern* in German, and *sarampión* in Spanish. Over the past four centuries, measles terminology has been complicated by the fact that the three major exanthematous diseases of childhood (measles, scarlet fever, and rubella) had not always been distinguished from each other. Certain terms for measles "wandered" among what we now know to be different diseases, a situation that did not resolve until the three were formally distinguished from each other in 1881. In examining the historical literature on measles published before 1900, it is advisable to review historical terminology first.

Measles Virus.   Measles virus is a member of the paramyxovirus family, which includes a number of other viruses that infect a diversity of animals, with the expectation that many other related viruses remain to be identified. Within the Paramyxoviridae are the viruses that cause mumps, parainfluenza virus infection, respiratory syncytial virus infection, and metapneumovirus infection (all human diseases), as well as zoonotic henipaviruses such as Hendra virus, which has caused occasional human **epidemics**. It is believed that thousands of years ago, an ancestral virus evolved in different directions, leading to the now-diverse morbillivirus group of which measles is a member, within the larger paramyxovirus group. The morbilliviruses also include viruses of carnivores (e.g., canine distemper virus), ruminants (e.g., rinderpest virus), and cetaceans (e.g., dolphin morbillivirus). Measles disease was first purposely transmitted to humans by the virus-infected blood of ill persons in 1905; six years later, the virus was serially passaged in monkeys given respiratory secretions that contained the infectious agent. The virus was finally cultivated in tissue culture in 1954 by **John Franklin Enders** and a colleague.

A close relative of rinderpest morbillivirus, which causes a serious epizootic disease of cattle, measles virus probably arose from a common viral ancestor several thousand years ago, at some time after early human civilizations began to settle into fixed communities and to domesticate animals (c. 10,000–8,000 BCE). Thus, measles virus is undoubtedly a descendant of an animal virus that evolved to switch to a human host. It is now a uniquely human virus, although some other primate species develop disease upon experimental infection.

Measles Disease.   In the absence of **vaccination**, almost all persons infected with measles virus will develop a "full blown" disease. Measles has long been regarded as a so-called "textbook disease" not only because of its unvarying clinical picture but also because of its clear epidemiologic features of extreme respiratory transmissibility, relatively fixed period of incubation time to prodromal illness (10 days) and to appearance of rash (14 days), and, in the pre-vaccine era, its propensity to infect urban infants and small children in 2- to 3-year cyclic waves.

Clinically, measles begins with nonspecific prodromal signs and symptoms: fever, malaise, and the classic "three C's" of cough, coryza (upper respiratory inflammation and mucous development), and **conjunctivitis**. Measles also features a classical "pathognomonic sign" (a clinical finding that points to only one disease) in the appearance of Koplik spots, first described by Russian pediatrician Nil Filatov (1847–1902) but known in English by the surname of the American pediatrician who popularized the spots as a diagnostic feature (Henry Koplik, 1858–1927). Koplik spots are small bluish-white dots on a red background in the cheek mucosa, appearing about two days before the rash, and lasting a day or two after the rash appears. The rash itself is characteristically red, spotted, and raised, starting at the hairline and moving down the body over the first day or so, tending to recede in old areas of skin as it appears and develops in new areas.

Although measles has been considered a benign disease of childhood, it has long been associated with a number of severe complications whose incidences may vary widely with host and environmental factors, including severe and fatal pneumonia, corneal ulceration and blindness, acute disseminated encephalomyelitis, and subacute sclerosing panencephalitis (SSPE).

Measles History.   The Persian-born **physician Rhazes** first distinguished measles from smallpox, and claimed that the same disease had been prevalent several hundred years before his time. In the early Middle Ages, reports of possible measles were further recorded, with mention of it being a childhood disease in 1224.

During the Age of Exploration, measles was one of the principal diseases, along with smallpox, to devastate New World and Pacific populations, including the loss of tens of millions of Central and South Americans in the sixteenth century, following the conquests of Hernán Cortés (1485–1547) and Francisco Pizarro (1475–1541), and of many Native Americans in what are now the United States and Canada. Medical history books contain a bewildering catalog of fatal measles epidemics that have devastated populations small and large over the past five centuries. Among these was the "virgin-soil" **measles epidemic in Fiji** of 1875. Japan apparently suffered a number of major imported measles epidemics over the past millennium, culminating in one of the most highly fatal in recorded history, appearing in 1862. Measles was so deadly in Japan that it gave rise to the folk saying: "Hōsō (smallpox) determines one's looks, but *hasika* (measles) determines one's life." Also worthy of mention are the fatal epidemics that occurred in 1917 in the U.S. military training camps across the country, concentrated in the southern United

AN ACCOUNT OF THE MEASLES AS THEY APPEARED IN PHILADELPHIA IN THE SPRING OF 1789

This disease, like many others, had its precursor. It was either a gum-boil, or a sore on the tongue. They were very common but not universal. They occurred in some instances, several days before the fever, but in general, they made their appearance during the eruptive fever, and were a sure mark of the approaching eruption of the measles. I was first led to observe this fact, from having read Dr. Quin's accurate account of the measles in Jamaica. I shall now proceed to mention the symptoms of the measles as they appeared in the different parts of the body.

1. In the head, they produced great pain, swelling of the eye-lids, so as to obstruct the eye-sight, tooth-ache, bleeding at the nose, tinnitus aurium, and deafness; also coma for two days, and convulsions. I saw the last symptom only in one instance. It was brought on by the stoppage of a running from the ear.
2. In the throat and lungs, they produced a soreness and hoarseness, acute or dull pains in the breast and sides, and a painful or distressing cough. In one case, this cough continued for two hours without any intermission, attended by copious expectoration. In two cases I saw a constant involuntary discharge of phlegm and mucus from the mouth without any cough. One of them terminated fatally. Spitting of blood occurred in several instances. The symptoms of pneumonia vera notha [bronchial] and typhoid were very common. I saw two fatal cases from pneumonia notha, in both of which, the patients died with the trunk of the body in an erect posture. I met with two cases in which there was no cough at all till the eruption made its appearance on the fourth day, and one which was accompanied by all the usual symptoms of the cynanche trachealis humoralism [swollen upper airway].
3. In the stomach the measles produced, in many instances, sickness and vomiting. And,
4. In the bowels, griping, diarrhea, and in some instances, bloody stools. The diarrhea occurred in every stage of the disorder, but it was bloody and most painful in its decline. I attended a black girl who discharged a great many worms, but without the least relief of any of her symptoms.

There was a great variety in this disease.

From *Medical Inquires and Observations* by Dr. Benjamin Rush of Philadelphia (Philadelphia, 1796; see Google Books).

States, where recruits were more likely to have escaped childhood measles by virtue of growing up on isolated farms and in very small towns. That the rate of complication and death was so high in this healthiest segment of the population (young men prescreened for underlying physical and infectious diseases) attests to the pathogenic vigor of measles.

Measles has also figured in important advances in medicine. In 1758, three decades after smallpox inoculation had been introduced into Europe, Scots physician Francis Home (1719–1813) began inoculating subjects to prevent measles (apparently without much success). In 1846 Danish medical student (and later renowned physiologist) Peter Panum (1820–1885) conducted a measles outbreak investigation in the Faroe Islands that not only established the epidemiology and duration of protective immunity of measles, but also became a classic example of epidemiologic methods, still read by epidemiologists

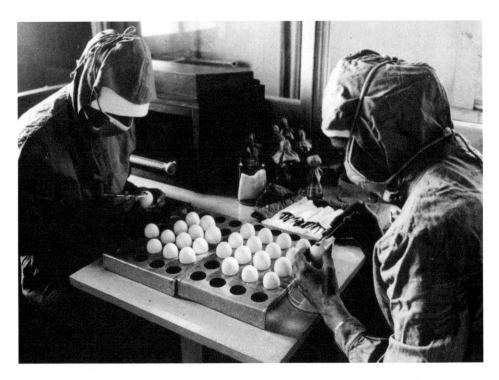

Lab technicians at the Tirana Institute of Hygiene and Epidemiology in Albania inject chicken eggs with the measles virus to produce the vaccine. Courtesy of the National Library of Medicine.

more than 150 years later. Finally, it should be noted that it was chiefly the experience with severe and fatal measles pneumonia in the 1917 Army camp epidemics that led to the remarkable bacterial and pathological studies of the 1918 "Spanish influenza" by U.S. military physicians a year later, in both instances establishing as the cause of most fatalities a "one-two punch" by a respiratory virus (measles or influenza) and one or more resident pathogenic bacteria.

Measles Vaccines.   Although measles immune globulin was administered early in the twentieth century, it was not until the early 1960s that measles vaccines were licensed and became widely available in the developed world. First-generation vaccines were inactivated; over several years' time, their protective ability declined to the point where breakthrough infections occurred and resulted in an altered disease often featuring severe pneumonitis ("atypical measles"). Second-generation vaccines containing live attenuated measles viruses are now used worldwide and have been gradually reducing the burden of measles mortality in the developing world. Recent figures of the **World Health Organization** estimate 454,000 measles deaths in 2004, down 48 percent from the 871,000 annual deaths estimated five years earlier. These figures nevertheless put measles in the same category of high childhood fatality as **malaria**, general respiratory diseases, and diarrheal diseases. Given the extreme transmissibility of measles, vigorous vaccination campaigns must be ongoing in order to prevent disease in individuals and to achieve disease elimination, a goal which appears feasible though not likely to be met by 2010. A disturbing trend in recent years has been for parents to refuse measles vaccination for their children in favor of natural exposure, sometimes at staged "measles parties" where healthy children are deliberately exposed to children with measles. This is a dangerous practice because the negligible risk of vaccination is grossly outweighed by the well-known risk of death, neurologic disease, and other morbidity caused by natural measles infection.

The Interaction of Agent, Host, and Environment. The 454,000 estimated annual measles deaths reflect the high rate with which measles complications may occur under conditions of deprivation and coinfection. It was recognized 130 years ago that acute measles fatalities were typically associated with either severe pulmonary or gastrointestinal complications. During World War I, investigators of a measles epidemic at Camp Zachary Taylor, in Louisville, Kentucky, showed that virtually 100 percent of severe and fatal measles cases were associated with streptococcal coinfection, and that bacterial pneumonia was the proximate cause of death in most of those who died. More than 75 years ago, it was recognized that measles severity was associated with vitamin A deficiency, and in more recent times it has become apparent that even low levels of vitamin A, not yet reaching clinical deficiency status, predispose individuals to more severe measles disease. Observations in Africa and elsewhere have shown that severe measles, including "hemorrhagic measles" and "black measles," may be associated with marasmus, kwashiorkor, and underlying infections. Measles in persons with deficiencies of cell-mediated immunity can result in either severe giant cell pneumonia, often in association with multi-organ involvement, or measles inclusion body **encephalitis** (MIBE), associated with chronic replication of a defective virus. A clinically similar condition, SSPE, is now uncommon in the developing world because widespread measles vaccination has prevented early childhood infection with wild virus. SSPE is a progressive fatal neurologic disease in children with normally functioning immune systems who are infected at an early age with measles virus and like MIBE is associated with persistence of a defective virus. *See also* Children and Childhood Epidemic Diseases; Measles, Efforts to Eradicate; Measles in the Colonial Americas.

Further Reading

Caulfield, E. A. "Early Measles Epidemics in America." *Yale Journal of Biology and Medicine* 15 (1942–1943): 531–536.

Griffin, D. E. "Measles Virus." In *Fields Virology*, 5th edition, edited by D. M. Knipe et al., pp. 1551–1585. Philadelphia: Lippincott, Williams, and Wilkins, 2007.

Morens, David. M. "Measles in Fiji, 1875: Thoughts on the History of Emerging Infectious Diseases." *Pacific Health Dialog* 5 (1998): 119–128.

DAVID M. MORENS

MEASLES, EFFORTS TO ERADICATE. Given the success with eradicating **smallpox**, the huge strides in eliminating **polio**, and certain epidemiological elements of **measles**, there has been a series of regional and global campaigns to eliminate and eventually eradicate measles from the world by mass immunization and close surveillance.

Measles is an acute disease that is caused by a **virus** and is highly contagious. The patient is infectious for about a week, and the disease or **vaccinations** will confer immunity on recipients. Most common among children, it can wreak havoc among nonimmune adults, as happened to indigenous peoples during periods of European colonization. Deaths are usually the result of complications from the disease. In 1954, **John Enders** and a colleague isolated the measles virus, and a safe vaccine was ready for use in humans by the early 1960s. In the United States, the vaccination program began in earnest in 1963.

In the midst of early success, the director of the U.S. **Centers for Disease Control** (CDC) announced in 1966 its first goal of eliminating measles from the United States during the following year. Four factors made elimination of the disease seem possible: very widespread incidence of measles meant widespread immunity among older children and adults who had contracted it; measles only affects humans (though some primates can carry it), so no animal reservoir has to be considered; no one carries the disease long term, or chronically; and the herd immunity threshold, or the rate of immunity in the population below which a disease would continue to spread, was believed to be around 55 percent.

The campaign consisted of four tactics: routine infant immunization; upon entry into school, vaccination of those who had not been immunized; close surveillance of cases; and vigorous reaction to major outbreaks. In 1967 one of the two types of vaccines being used was withdrawn for having proven to provide only short periods of immunity and a tendency to predispose the recipient to atypical measles. Even so, between 1963 and 1968 reported cases in the United States fell by over 90 percent. An initiative against rubella with a new vaccine interrupted the measles program in 1969, and cases spiked from 22,000 in 1968 to over 70,000 in 1971. In the same year, the MMR (Measles, Mumps, Rubella) vaccine began to replace the more limited one for measles alone.

The campaign revealed that measles was more contagious than previously believed, and thus the herd immunity threshold was closer to 90 percent than 55; the current level of coverage was estimated to be only around 78 percent, with lowest levels in poorer inner city neighborhoods. In addition, though the surveillance system was adequate, schools were in no position to verify and immunize as required. In 1978 the CDC's goal of elimination was repeated, this time with a four-year window (by 1982). Reduction was again dramatic, with the 1978 figure of 27,000 cases falling to 1,497 in 1983, though elimination remained evasive. This time success was soured with the realization that a single dose of vaccine was insufficient, and that booster shots would be needed. All shots had to be administered after the infant was nine months old, because up to that point, the child of an immune mother retained its mother's antigens, which negated the effect of the vaccination.

In 1977 the **World Health Organization**–affiliated Pan American Health Organization (PAHO) began the Expanded Program on Immunization (EPI), which included measles coverage. With the early successes of the anti-polio campaign in the Western Hemisphere as a model, in 1987 PAHO began "catch-up" programs to immunize children between nine months and 14 years of age against measles. In 1994 PAHO set a target date of 2000 for elimination of measles from the Western Hemisphere. Between 1990 and 1995, confirmed cases of measles in Latin America and the Caribbean fell from 218,000 to 3,382. In 1995, however, Canada alone reported 2,362 cases, which prompted public health authorities there to initiate "catch-up" activities that reduced the number to 324, an 86 percent drop in one year. Meanwhile, the CDC reported a total of 55,622 U.S. cases in 1989–1991, so in 1994 the Childhood Immunization Initiative—part of the PAHO six-year initiative—established targets of 90 percent coverage and elimination of indigenous (exclusive of imported) cases by 1996. 1995 saw 309 reported cases.

The advances against measles in the Americas prompted the consideration of a global program for eradication, along the lines of the ongoing effort against polio. In July 1996 representatives of PAHO, WHO, and CDC met in Atlanta, Georgia, and decided to recommend a goal of worldwide eradication of measles within a 10- to 15-year framework.

A Measles quarantine warning. Courtesy of the National Library of Medicine.

At that time, an estimated 800,000 died of the disease annually, 500,000 in Africa, where immunization coverage was generally less than 50 percent. Globally, measles accounted for about 10 percent of mortality for children less than five years old and remained a major cause of blindness. Some efforts yielded spectacular results: in Malawi reported cases dropped from 7,000 to 2 between 1997 and 1999. But progress was never consistent: after steady reductions, in 1997 Brazil relapsed and produced some 50,000 cases, mostly around São Paolo.

As the millennium turned, and the global target date was moved back five years (to 2005), critics expressed their doubts that measles could be eradicated, but 2001 saw the launch of the Measles Initiative, signed by the WHO, UNICEF, the United Nations Foundation, the American Red Cross, and the CDC. Among the shared goals is a drop in global measles deaths of 90 percent by 2010 (from a base of 2000). Global deaths caused by measles fell by 59 percent, from about 871,000 in 1999 to about 354,000 in 2005. Africa showed the most progress, with reductions in cases and deaths estimated to be 75 percent. *See also* Children and Childhood Epidemic Diseases; Measles in the Colonial Americas; Poliomyelitis, Campaign Against; Smallpox Eradication.

Further Reading

Carabin, H., and W. J. Edmunds. "Future Savings from Measles Eradication in Industrialized Countries." *Journal of Infectious Diseases* 187 (2003): 29–35.

Gay, N. J. "The Theory of Measles Elimination: Implications for the Design of Elimination Strategies." *Journal of Infectious Diseases* 189 (Suppl 1) (2004): 27–35.

Hinman, Alan R., Walter A. Orenstein, and Mark J. Papania. "Evolution of Measles Elimination Strategies in the United States." *Journal of Infectious Diseases* 189 (2004): 17–22.

Measles Eradication Field Guide. Washington, DC: Pan American Health Organization, 1999.

Measles Mortality Reduction and Regional Elimination Strategic Plan 2001–2005. Geneva: World Health Organization and United Nations Children's Fund, 2001.

Orenstein, Walter A. "The Role of Measles Elimination in Development of a National Immunization Program." *Pediatric Infectious Disease Journal* 25 (2006): 1093–1101.

Strebel, P. M., et al. "Global Measles Elimination Efforts: The Significance of United States Measles Elimination. *Journal of Infectious Diseases* 189 (Suppl 1) (2004): 251–257.

JOSEPH P. BYRNE

MEASLES EPIDEMIC IN FIJI (1875) AND EUGENICS.   The 1875 Fiji **measles epidemic** represents a tragic landmark in epidemic history. Beyond the large number of deaths of native peoples who had never before encountered measles, the epidemic has served as a multipurpose metaphor for the terrible human and cultural losses to imported diseases during the Age of Discovery, for the still-confused epidemiological concept of "virgin-soil epidemics," and for the extent to which science could be coopted by eugenics theory during a time of great scientific change and discovery.

In the fall of 1874, its native ruler ceded the South Pacific island of Fiji to Britain as a Crown Colony, and the British government began the slow process (nine months, as it turned out) of sending out a new government from London to Fiji via Australia. In the interim, Queen Victoria (1819–1901) wished to send the ceding "Cannibal King" Cakobau ("Destroyer of Bau"; d. 1883), along with his family and a party of about 100 Fijians, to Sydney, Australia, the nearest seat of government, on a State Visit and sightseeing vacation. The voyage between Fiji and Sydney, on the *HMS Dido*, took 19 days each way. On the 13th day of the return trip back to Fiji, Cakobau's 25-year-old son developed a rash and fever. The ship surgeon diagnosed measles, then prevalent in Sydney but unknown in Fiji, and placed the son in isolation in a hastily built shack on the deck.

Against international regulations, the ship's yellow **quarantine** flag was not flying when the *Dido* sailed into port. British functionaries arriving in a small boat worsened the mistake by focusing on a seemingly more pressing problem: while in Sydney the just-married son had acquired not only measles, from which he was by then recovering, but also "a drip" (**gonorrhea**). This discovery had to be kept from newspaper reporters: Cakobau had forsaken cannibalism and converted to Christianity, and his sons had been baptized. The possibility that Queen Victoria's first gift to Fiji might be a venereal disease in the royal household was unthinkable. During the ensuing confusion on board, no one noticed that boats were bringing impatient passengers to shore, or that most of Fiji's police force had sailed out to celebrate with the doubly infected son. And despite common knowledge about the **epidemiology** of measles in 1875, no one seems to have considered the problem of 100 Fijians potentially incubating the disease.

The problems were soon to be greatly magnified. While the king was away, the mountain cannibal chiefs had threatened to revolt against cession. The king's brother had been asked to arrange an unprecedented national meeting at which the chiefs might be persuaded to join the government. It was to be the largest gathering in Fiji's history. On January 25, 1875, 13 days (about one measles incubation period) after the *Dido*'s return, the meeting was attended by 69 chiefs, 800 others, and the same 143-man police force that had greeted the royal party's return two weeks earlier, many of them already developing fevers and rashes.

Those who attended the meeting returned to their homes throughout Fiji, seeding a deadly measles epidemic that spread like wildfire throughout the country and to all of the outlying islands, and indeed widely throughout the Pacific. In an effort to reduce fever, terrified Fijians lay down in the ocean and in streams and wrapped small children in wet grass. To stop epidemic spread, those few who remained healthy burned the homes and villages of the ill, who lay trapped inside. **Corpses** lay everywhere in the open, scavenged by dogs and wild pigs. The stench of destroyed villages was notable at a mile's distance. The king survived but his brother, the elder statesman who had arranged the fateful meeting, succumbed, and his body was thrown into a communal pit. An estimated 40,000 people, one-third of Fiji's population, died within a few weeks' time. In response, the mountain chiefs revolted, killing (and sometimes eating) British subjects, provoking an all-out war. A British military force defeated the rebels and hung their leaders.

An inquiry initiated by the angry British queen was derailed by that war, and there was never any accounting for the deadly mistakes. The term "virgin-soil epidemic" seems to have taken hold following an 1875 British parliamentary speech in which Colonial Secretary Henry Herbert Lord Carnarvon (1831–1890), seeking to understand what had happened, used the term to describe the epidemic. Twenty years later, when Queen Victoria commissioned a study of Fiji's population decrease, the measles epidemic was barely mentioned, but the cautionary tale of the quintessential "virgin-soil epidemic" remained in textbooks for another century.

"Virgin-soil epidemic" now refers simply to the reemergent introduction of an infectious disease into a completely susceptible population. However, the term came to take on a more complicated meaning during the "eugenics era," which lasted from roughly 1879 to 1933. The 1875 Fiji epidemic occurred at a time when Darwinian evolutionary theory was being imperfectly digested by scientists and the public alike. It was common supposed knowledge at the time, even among some physicians and scientists, that traits like musicality, susceptibility to **tuberculosis**, criminality, and even **poverty** were a matter of **heredity**. Eugenics theory, based on incomplete and sometimes erroneous interpretations of human genetics knowledge, sought to promote civic actions and public policies aimed at improving the human "race" by supporting procreation of the most fit and discouraging or preventing it in the least fit. In its most extreme and odious form, eugenics led to sterilization of persons with mental illnesses in the United States and to the Nazi euthanasia program, the "legal" basis of murders in the extermination camps in German-occupied territories during the years of World War II. In the United States, Great Britain, and elsewhere in Europe, eugenics theory became a refuge for "respectable" racism, and the 1875 epidemic was often cited as an argument in favor of eugenics activism.

Despite much evidence to the contrary, which continued to mount in the succeeding decades, eugenics theories led to the notion that the much higher mortality in native Fijians in 1875 was the result of "racial degeneracy," a conclusion that led directly to schemes to import Caribbean "racial groups" and force them to interbreed with Fijians. The scientific study of the current notion that populations long in isolation from infectious diseases fail to develop natural resistance to them is incomplete, and some of the evidence in favor of it is clearly erroneous or overstated. Presumably, this 130-year-old question will become better understood as genomics studies of human susceptibility and microbial evolution advance further. Other evidence suggests that incipient vitamin A deficiency, starvation, exposure to cold and wetness, lack of nursing care, and secondary bacterial pneumonias probably caused most of the 40,000 Fijian deaths. That Fijian mortality in later measles epidemics was low suggests that "virgin-soil" theories of immune susceptibility to this infectious disease are difficult to support.

The Fijian epidemic was taught to medical students well into the 1970s (a century after it occurred), but is now gradually becoming an historical footnote of confused and uncertain meaning. Even in Fiji itself, the epidemic is only vaguely remembered. If we view it in modern terms, however, it is easy to see a different metaphor, that of the many complexities and uncertainties underlying epidemic disease emergence, which incorporates complex interactions between the microbial agent, the human host, and the **environment**. *See also* Colonialism and Epidemic Disease; Disease, Social Construction of; Historical Epidemiology; Measles, Efforts to Eradicate; Race, Ethnicity, and Epidemic Disease.

Further Reading

Cliff, Andrew D., and Peter Haggett. *The Spread of Measles in Fiji and the Pacific: Spatial Components in the Transmission of Epidemic Waves through Island Communities*. Canberra: Australian National University, 1985.

Morens, David M. "Measles in Fiji, 1875: Thoughts on the History of Emerging Infectious Diseases." *Pacific Health Dialog* 5 (1998): 119–128.

DAVID M. MORENS

MEASLES IN THE COLONIAL AMERICAS.   The effect on the Amerindian populations of the introduction of Old World diseases to the Western Hemisphere in the late fifteenth and sixteenth centuries was far more devastating than that of the **Black Death** on the Old World. **Epidemic measles** ran second only to **smallpox** as a biological agent of death, especially among the virgin native populations when first contact was made. It sporadically ravaged the Amerindians and American-born European colonists, however, long after it had become endemic.

Measles is caused by a **virus** that is easily acquired through respiration and has an incubation period of 10 to 14 days. Symptoms include coughing, a red rash, and high fever. The acute phase usually lasts about a week, though full recuperation may take months, especially if followed by a secondary disease. In societies in which it is common, measles generally becomes a childhood disease with mild effects and very low mortality for those over three years of age who receive appropriate care; lifetime **immunity** or high resistance is generally conferred. In a virgin population, however, it can spread very rapidly and kill adults, children, and even fetuses readily, especially when proper treatment is not provided, and a population is weakened by malnutrition.

Native Americans had never experienced measles before the arrival of Europeans. They did not domesticate the sheep, goats, and cattle from whose rinderpest disease measles seems to have developed, nor did the earliest migrants carry it with them through Alaska. In the early sixteenth century, measles was endemic in many Spanish cities, including Seville, from which city most voyages to the Spanish Americas originated. Measles was also widespread and endemic in other colonizing countries such as England, France, and Portugal. This meant that most colonists were immune.

Spanish America.   A deadly epidemic in Hispaniola in 1518 of what many think was measles, however, spread to the Mayans of Guatemala as early as 1519 (see sidebar). A participant in Hernán Cortés's (1485–1547) attack on Tenochtitlán (Mexico City) in 1520 wrote of the devastating impact of "the pestilence of measles and smallpox" that struck down their foes. Pandemic measles had arrived in New Spain with colonists' **children** from the Caribbean islands by 1530. Subsequent outbreaks and its appearance in other parts of the Spanish American Empire are attributable to the continuous trans-Atlantic traffic from Spain and Africa; to the expeditions of conquistadors; to slaving expeditions and the forced movements of populations in response to local labor shortages; and to travel by native carriers, a factor that probably explains its first appearance in the Andes in the 1520s. Contemporary Spanish authors ultimately attributed the disease to God but also recognized its "stickiness," or ability to pass from one person to another.

Named by the Nahuatl-speaking Indians in Mexico *zahuatltepiton* (awkwardly translated "little leprosy (*lepra*)" by the Spanish; smallpox was the "great *lepra*"), measles is often difficult to tease out of contemporary reports on diseases and epidemics. Descriptions are usually from untrained observers who provide minimal or even contradictory accounts, and vocabulary is fluid, often forcing the historian to conjecture about the disease described. Typically the Spanish word *serampión* indicates measles, but at times the attendant description of symptoms suggests another disease. In addition, during epidemics, measles

---

EFFECTS OF EARLY MEASLES EPIDEMICS IN THE NEW WORLD (1519 AND 1532)

Mayan description of measles (?) in Guatemala, 1519:

In the course of the fifth year the pestilence began, O my children. First there was a cough, then the blood was corrupted, and the urine became yellow. The number of deaths at this time was truly terrible. The Chief Vakaki Ahmak died, and we ourselves were plunged in great darkness and deep grief, our fathers and ancestors having contracted the plague [measles], O my children.

Truly the number of deaths among the people was terrible, nor did the people escape from the pestilence.

The ancients and the fathers died alike, and the stench was such that men died of it alone. Then perished our fathers and ancestors. Half the people threw themselves into the ravines, and the dogs and foxes lived off the bodies of the men. The fear of death destroyed the old people, and the oldest son of the king at the same time as his young brother. Thus did we become poor, O my children, and thus did we survive, being but a little child—and we were all that remained.

From *Annals of the Cakchiquels,* trans by Daniel Brinton (Philadelphia: Library of Aboriginal American Literature, 1885) p. 171.

Measles in Central America, 1532:

Throughout New Spain there passed a sickness that they say is measles, which struck the Indians and swept the land, leaving it totally empty. It arrived in this province some three months ago.

From letter of *Conquistador* Pedro de Alvarado from Santiago de Guatemala; in Cook, *Born to Die,* p. 88.

---

seems often to have accompanied smallpox, **typhus**, exanthemous typhus, **diphtheria**, and mumps; and measles itself was not clearly identified clinically in Europe until the eighteenth century. Weakened by measles, the recovering victim might well fall prey to other opportunistic secondary diseases, including **encephalitis**, **influenza**, and **enteric fevers**. Colonial fatality figures are notoriously unreliable, for numerous reasons, especially when reporting mortality among Amerindian populations.

Measles may have been the disease that struck down two-thirds of the remaining Indians on Cuba in 1529. The earliest pandemic of measles occurred in New Spain between 1530 and 1534, and returned in 30-year cycles. Initially it seems that children suffered most, but in 1532 the disease was indiscriminate. By 1534 measles, dysentery, and typhoid reportedly had killed 130,000 of 150,000 natives in Culiacán alone. Further south in

Central America, measles followed influenza and smallpox from 1532 to 1534, and in Nicaragua measles followed 1531 outbreaks of bubonic and possibly pneumonic plague. As always, Indians bore the brunt, and Honduran reports lament death tolls of 50 percent and the loss of thousands of mine workers and household servants. In Guatemala a royal treasurer reported smallpox and measles in 1533, and local authorities were soon urging those using Indian labor to reduce their demands so the natives could rest and recover. Between 1558 and 1562, measles and influenza swept across Guatemala, spreading in 1563 and 1564 to central Mexico with death tolls of 50 percent in Chalco but much lower elsewhere. Guatemala suffered again in 1576–1577 from measles plus smallpox and typhus, with children most commonly struck down. From 1592 to 1597, measles, accompanied variously by smallpox, mumps and typhus, hit Mexico as far north as the Pueblo people. These victims blamed their Jesuit guests, burning down the mission and murdering a missionary in 1594.

Measles reached South America as early as the mid-1520s, probably from Guatemala. Disease fatally disrupted Incan society by killing the Inca ruler Huayna Capac around 1525 and sparking dynastic wars that weakened the Empire. A wider and deadlier pandemic spread south between 1531 and 1533 across the Andes killing perhaps a quarter of the native population. African slaves who arrived from Hispaniola may have sparked a large-scale epidemic of measles, influenza, and smallpox in Peru and Ecuador in 1558. New Granada claimed death tolls of 40,000, and with secondary influenza, Peru lost 15 to 20 percent of its native population. Such losses led to mass relocations of natives in 1570 and to the importation of ever more black slaves. This led to widespread exposure and immunization, so measles may have become endemic in parts of the north by the 1580s. Other areas were struck hard, however, between 1585 and 1592. Lima and Cuzco suffered high mortalities from measles, smallpox, and mumps. Ecuador was hit in 1586–1591, but the source is thought to have been African slaves or Francis Drake's (1540–1596) raiders in Cartagena. Moving inland, the epidemic killed 30,000 of Quito's population of 80,000 between 1587 and 1591, with 4,000 dead in three months. Children suffered most, but literally countless Indian laborers died in rural areas, and along the coast villages were extinguished or abandoned. All told, perhaps half the native population died. Because so many victims were children and young people, birth rates declined precipitously, and the population could never replace itself.

The seventeenth century opened with an epidemic outbreak of measles in New Spain accompanied by mumps and typhus in 1604. A wider pandemic with typhus, diphtheria, and scarlet fever began in the Andes in 1611. This may have spread to Guatemala in 1613, central Mexico (with smallpox) in 1615, and Nicaragua (with typhus and smallpox) in 1617. Colombia, Bolivia, Peru, and Chile suffered again in 1617–1619, with disease compounded by locust infestations and famine. High death rates resulted in entire mining operations being shut down for lack of labor. In Paraguay, Indians were collected into the Jesuit "reductions" in which diseases could spread wildly. In the 1630s, 1,000 of 7,000 died in Candelaria alone. Lima was hit by measles again in 1628 and 1634–1635, and Peru more widely in 1645 and 1648 by measles and diphtheria. A pandemic that included measles, diphtheria, typhus, and smallpox swept Colombia, Ecuador, Peru, and Bolivia between 1691 and 1695. Records suggest that between 25 and 50 percent of the Indian population died, especially children and young adults.

By the eighteenth century, pandemics should have immunized much of Spanish America's population, though the worst measles epidemic in a century occurred in

Ecuador and Colombia from 1785 to 1788. Poor crops and little labor for the harvest led to famines that weakened people's resistance. The eighteenth century also saw Spanish colonial authorities organize efforts to deal with diseases. Urban public hygiene and sanitation became priorities, at least in theory. **Physicians** were consulted and employed to treat cases and to try to determine the causes and reasons for dissemination of the diseases. In 1764 Ecuador received a medical examiner (*protomédico*), and during the virulent outbreak of 1785, he saw that **apothecaries** and physicians provided for the poor as well as the wealthy. But Quito itself had only one **hospital** for patients (another was for lepers), and this was chronically underfunded.

The English and French Colonies in North America.   European contact with North America before the formal settlement of Virginia (1607) and Plymouth (1620) colonies planted infectious diseases among Amerindian populations. Florida suffered from the early 1530s, and the disease may have traveled northward through many of the Eastern Woodland tribes. Between 1592 and 1596, the Seneca Indians of Cameron Village in western New York experienced at least hundreds of casualties from measles originating in the Spanish-held American Southwest. From 1616 to 1619, an epidemic of diseases (the "great dying"), possibly including measles, destroyed perhaps 90 percent of the native population in the coastal Massachusetts region. Pilgrims discovered abandoned villages and crops before they met the local natives. English colonists in both New England and Virginia brought with them the full panoply of European diseases, and after 1619 enslaved Africans unwittingly contributed their share in the Chesapeake.

The specific impact of measles on the native population is far more difficult to ascertain for the English colonies than for the Spanish and Portuguese. The English had neither the missionaries nor government agents to keep records, nor were English-Indian relations nearly as close as were those in Latin America. Unlike the far-ranging conquistadors, English adventurers tended to remain relatively close to home. On the other hand, French fur trappers and missionaries penetrated deep inland and may have spread the disease widely.

In the seventeenth century, reports of measles outbreaks among colonists are sporadic and rare. French Jesuit missionaries north and west of the English reported "a sort of measles" and other diseases among both French and Huron Indians as early as 1634. The Hurons suffered gravely and repeatedly until 1640, losing perhaps 80 percent of their population according to the French. In the 1640s the diseases spread south and westward, leaving vast areas depopulated by death and migration. The Huron Confederation lay in ruins and the Iroquois extended their hegemony. Boston was struck first in 1657 and Connecticut during the following year, having allowed a generation of young people to be born and mature away from the measles reservoirs of Europe. Despite many cases, fatalities were few. Measles broke out widely among Canadians in 1687, reportedly after a French royal ship with at least one carrier docked on the St. Lawrence. This probably spread to the English, who suffered later the same year and in 1688. Measles struck Williamsburg, Virginia, in 1693, with an English ship being the probable source of the infection. This prompted a day of "humiliation and prayer" among the Anglican populace, a religious response usually reserved for times of plague or war.

As a result of increasingly higher levels of immigration, Boston saw the intervals between major outbreaks fall from three decades after 1657 to 11 years by the 1730s. New Englanders suffered from 1713 to 1715, with at least 150 measles-related deaths reported in Boston's bills of mortality. Though Boston seems to have been struck hardest, adults as well as children contracted the disease in Connecticut, New York, New Jersey, and Pennsylvania. Letters from Virginia record the disease striking mostly adults in 1716 and 1717. 1729 saw another light outbreak in Boston (15 reported fatalities), and in New York City most patients were children. A decade later, Boston hosted a much more severe outbreak that may have been spread by those fleeing the city. Puritan preacher **Cotton Mather**, who lost his maid and four children, took the occasion to pen his humane and useful "A Letter about a Good Management under the Distemper of the Measles" (1739). Over the following two years, colonists in New England, New York, and New Jersey were infected as well.

In 1747 and 1748, New England, New York, Pennsylvania, and South Carolina were revisited. Patients in Charleston tended to suffer further from enteric problems, whereas those in Boston reported secondary throat "distemper." Children in Philadelphia suffered additionally from "the flux," whereas adults caught secondary **yellow fever**. Between 1750 and 1775, one-third of those buried in Christ Church cemetery were victims of measles. 1759 saw a mild outbreak among children in South Carolina, New York City, and Philadelphia, though Fairfield, New Jersey, experienced a severe outbreak with several attendant diseases including smallpox. Dedham, Massachusetts, on the other hand, reported 260 cases with but a single fatality. A general outbreak in the colonies occurred in 1772 and 1773, with insignificant fatalities outside the south; the *South Carolina Gazette*, however, reported "8[00] to 900" young fatalities from a population of 14,000. Among other remedies and treatments, **doctors** recommended opiates, asses' milk, and bloodletting. The final outbreak in colonial U.S. history occurred in 1775 with broad morbidity but mild mortality, at least among whites. A study of Philadelphia's Anglican bills of mortality (1722–1775) revealed that slaves in Philadelphia were roughly twice as likely to die of measles during epidemics as whites (crude death rates of 106 and 56 respectively), though immunity did raise a slave's price in the market, an incentive to provide adequate care. Around 1800, measles became endemic in the United States. *See also* Animal Diseases (Zoonoses) and Epidemic Disease; Children and Childhood Epidemic Diseases; Colonialism and Epidemic Disease; Contagion and Transmission; Demographic Data Collection and Analysis, History of; Diagnosis of Historic Diseases; Disease in the Pre-Columbian Americas; Historical Epidemiology; Latin America, Colonial: Demographic Effects of Imported Diseases; Measles Epidemic in Fiji (1875) and Eugenics; Race, Ethnicity, and Epidemic Disease; Slavery and Disease; Smallpox in Colonial Latin America; Smallpox in Colonial North America; Trade, Travel, and Epidemic Disease; War, the Military, and Epidemic Disease.

Further Reading

Alchón, Suzanne Austin. *A Pest in the Land: New World Epidemics in a Global Perspective.* Albuquerque: University of New Mexico Press, 2003.

Black, Francis L., et al. "Epidemiology of Infectious Disease: The Example of Measles." In *Health and Disease in Tribal Societies.* (Amsterdam: Elsevier, 1977), pp. 115–35.

Caulfield, Ernest. "Early Measles Epidemics in America." *Yale Journal of Biology and Medicine* 15 (1943): 531–538.

Cook, David Noble. *Born to Die: Disease and New World Conquest, 1492–1650.* New York: Cambridge University Press, 1998.

Cook, David Noble, and W. George Lovell. *"Secret Judgments of God": Old World Disease in Colonial Spanish America.* Norman: University of Oklahoma Press, 1992.

Duffy, John. *Epidemics in Colonial America.* Baton Rouge: Louisiana State University, 1971.

Grob, Gerald N. *The Deadly Truth: A History of Disease in America.* Cambridge, MA: Harvard University Press, 2002.

Livi Bacci, Massimo. "Return to Hispaniola: Reassessing a Demographic Catastrophe." *Hispanic American Historical Review* 83 (2003): 3–51.

JOSEPH P. BYRNE

MEDIA.   *See* News Media and Epidemic Disease; Popular Media and Epidemic Disease: Recent Trends.

MEDICAL EDUCATION IN THE WEST, 1100–1500.   In early medieval Europe, few healers had access to learned medical writings from Greek and Roman antiquity. Medical practitioners were trained in practical healing through apprenticeship and did not rely upon broad theoretical systems to explain the functioning of the body, the processes of disease, or the rationalization for therapeutic practices. Only a small number of monks, trained in a few prominent monastic centers, had access to the limited number of Greek medical texts available in Latin, the language of scholarship. Beginning in the eleventh century, however, western Europe received a flood of translations of previously unknown texts from Greek and Arabic into Latin. These translations provided a more intellectually sophisticated theoretical foundation for the basic **Greco-Roman** medical learning already familiar in the Latin West. Spurred in part by the influx of this new knowledge, Europe witnessed the development of universities in the thirteenth century that provided new opportunities for medical education and ultimately for the professionalization of medicine.

The school in the southern Italian town of Salerno was the earliest center of medical education to incorporate the newly translated materials in its teaching. Salerno, a crossroads of Christian, Jewish, and Arabic cultures, had gained a reputation as a place for acquiring practical medical skills and successful cures as early as the tenth century. During the twelfth century, the school began to shift from practical to theoretical medical instruction based upon a select group of the newly available medical and philosophical texts. Salernitan doctors assembled a collection of treatises known as the *Articella*, which introduced basic elements of the medical theories ascribed to **Hippocrates** and **Galen** and formed the core texts for advanced medical knowledge in the Middle Ages. Salerno's emphasis on teaching medicine through books elevated the importance of theoretical medical knowledge in relation to empirical medical knowledge gained through practical experience.

By the thirteenth century, Salerno had been eclipsed as a center for medical learning as medicine became one of the subjects available for study at the newly founded universities in Italy, France, England, and Spain. During this period, the universities most renowned as centers for medical education were those in Bologna, Montpellier, and Paris. Students at these and other universities would pursue a preliminary education in the seven liberal arts (grammar, logic, rhetoric, arithmetic, geometry, astronomy, and music), after which they could pursue a bachelor's degree in medicine. They could also continue toward a medical doctorate which would require at least 10 years of study, and which conferred the right to teach medicine anywhere in Europe.

The instruction provided at the universities was primarily based upon the study of authoritative texts. Students attended lectures where teachers would read and provide commentaries on specific passages from the books of the *Articella*, supplemented with material from **Avicenna's** *Canon of Medicine* and increasingly with some longer works by Galen. In addition to reading and hearing lectures on these medical authorities, students would also be expected to engage in disputations, or formal debates, concerning textual interpretations or aimed at reconciling conflicting opinions among the authoritative texts. This style of teaching through the use of commentaries and disputations around a set of authoritative texts is often referred to as the "scholastic" method. Even in the teaching of human anatomy, in which students had the opportunity to observe public anatomical demonstrations, greater emphasis was placed on learning by reading the authoritative texts than on the careful examination of human cadavers. The importance of learning from texts did not mean that students failed to receive any practical training, however; indeed, they were often required to spend some time in medical practice or in attendance with a practicing physician before earning their degrees.

The subjects of the university medical curriculum were divided into courses in *theorica* and those in *practica*. Under *theorica*, or theoretical medicine, students learned about the philosophical basis of medicine, contemporary concepts of physiology, general pathology, and **humoral theory**. Courses in *practica* also dealt with what one might otherwise consider "theoretical" knowledge, but they emphasized material that had direct practical applications for the **diagnosis** and treatment of specific diseases. A number of *practica* manuals provided lists of diseases in order from head-to-foot, with detailed discussions as to their causes, and advice on how to diagnose and treat them. From the mid-fourteenth century, tracts (*consilia*) were also written specifically to address the disease known as the plague or pest. Together, these medical texts provided young physicians with guidance on how to recognize diseases based on a variety of signs, including the careful study of the pulse and urine, and how to prepare the appropriate medicines or dietary menus to treat them. In addition to these subjects, medical students were expected to gain some competence in astronomy, including what today is termed **astrology**, in order to understand the cosmological influences on individual health. **Epidemic** diseases were often thought to result from astrological influences, and so a proper knowledge of astronomy was deemed necessary for those seeking to recognize and treat them.

Despite the development of university medical education, the number of **physicians** trained at universities remained small throughout this period. Most medical practitioners continued to be trained through apprenticeship and received little or no theoretical education from books. The range of non–university trained healers who learned through experience included **surgeons, apothecaries,** midwives, and a variety of other kinds of **empirics** including those who specialized in treating eye diseases, pulling teeth, setting bones, or selling religious and magical cures. Thus, although university trained physicians became the new elites among medical practitioners in the later Middle Ages, they were only a small minority in the overall medical community. *See also* Air and Epidemic Diseases; Black Death (1347–1352); Corpses and Epidemic Disease; Diet, Nutrition, and Epidemic Disease; Folk Medicine; Hospitals in the West to 1900; Islamic Disease Theory and Medicine; Medical Education in the West, 1500–1900; Plague and Developments in Public Health, 1348–1600; Plague in Medieval Europe, 1360–1500; Quacks, Charlatans, and Their Remedies.

Further Reading

Bullough, Vern L. *Universities, Medicine, and Science in the Medieval West.* Burlington, VT: Ashgate, 2004.
Conrad, Lawrence I., Michael Neve, Vivian Nutton, Roy Porter, and Andrew Wear. *The Western Medical Tradition 800 BC to AD 1800.* New York: Cambridge University Press, 1995.

Jacquart, Danielle. "Medical Scholasticism." In *Western Medical Thought from Antiquity to the Middle Ages*, edited by Mirko D. Grmek and translated by Antony Shugaar, pp. 197–240. Cambridge, MA: Harvard University Press, 1998.

Leiser, G. "Medical Education in Islamic Lands from the Seventh to the Fourteenth Century." *Journal of the History of Medicine and Allied Sciences* 38 (1983): 48–75.

Siraisi, Nancy G. *Medicine at the Italian Universities, 1250–1600*. Leiden: Brill, 2001.

WILLIAM H. YORK

MEDICAL EDUCATION IN THE WEST, 1500–1900.   The ideal form of medical education has always been a mixture of theory, practice, and hands-on experience. Between 1500 and 1700, there were two formal and many informal methods of medical education. Those aiming to become **physicians**, the elite of the medical practitioners, attended university lectures—almost exclusively on Greco-Roman and Islamic medical texts—for several years in order to acquire the prestigious M.D., Doctorate of Medicine. From the sixteenth century, the scope of these lectures expanded to include hands-on training in anatomical dissection. Andreas Vesalius's (1514–1564) *De humani corporis fabrica* (On the Structure of the Human Body, 1543) was both a representation of and an advertisement for the value of dissection, and by the end of the seventeenth century, every prominent medical school and many hospitals provided lectures on anatomy illustrated by cadavers. Physicians' erudition, as well as the social and economic status conveyed by the M.D., led them to claim authority over all other medical practitioners, as the head had authority over all other parts of the body.

The second type of formal education was apprenticeship to a **surgeon**, a legally-contracted relationship in which the master surgeon agreed to teach the young man his craft over a period of years, in exchange for a specified fee. If physicians were the "head" of the medical profession, then surgeons were its skillful hands. Though elite surgeons in Italy might attend anatomy classes at the universities of Padua or Bologna, few surgeons elsewhere took courses or studied the scholarly literature. Instead, they honed their manual skills by serving first as their masters' servants, and gradually taking on more and more complex tasks.

There were also many informal methods of medical education, for outside of urban jurisdictions there was little government regulation of medical treatment. Medical students might travel from university to university, attending lectures by the most famous professors. Or they might learn their "business," as it was often referred to, from fathers or uncles. Women, excluded from both university and guild, learned to be midwives through formal or informal apprenticeship with an experienced midwife, often treating a range of women's and children's ailments as **empirics**.

Yet when an epidemic arose, formal education mattered less than administrative ability, presence of mind, and courage in the face of certain danger. In 1630 Diacinto Gramigna was apprenticed to his father, a municipal surgeon in Prato, Italy, when the **plague** arrived. When the town's physicians left with their elite patients, Gramigna's father died, and no other surgeon would agree to work in the town's **pest house**, Prato's Town Council appointed Gramigna as surgeon. He served faithfully for the eight months that the hospital was open, even catching and recovering from the plague himself. His reward was enough money so that he could have a new suit of clothes made and burn those he had been wearing as Public Health surgeon.

By the 1700s, a new pedagogical innovation had taken hold, the introduction of clinical lectures—based upon human bodies instead of classical texts—into university medical curricula. This was a modification of traditional medical apprenticeship, and one that caught on quickly for medical students: instead of being formally bound to a master for a number of years, they could attend university lectures in which the professor used hospital patients as living case histories of specific diseases. Hermann Boerhaave (1668–1738) at the University of Leyden, Holland, gave clinical lectures using the local charity hospital, and from there the innovation was picked up by every major medical school. Other innovations followed by the early 1800s. Surgeon's apprentices increasingly attended medical lectures, and medical schools in major cities offered courses in clinical surgery. Distinctions between medical students and surgical apprentices blurred as both groups "walked the wards" for clinical experience, attended postmortem dissection in the hospital morgue, and debated James Lind's (1716–1794) use of lime juice for scurvy (1762) and **Edward Jenner's** vaccination for smallpox (1798).

By the mid-nineteenth century, the best medical education lasted between three and four years and included classes in basic science—anatomy, organic and inorganic chemistry, physiology—as well as in medical practice—pathology, pharmacology, obstetrics. Clinical and surgical courses might require another year or two. New instruments, like the stethoscope, were introduced to the medical school curriculum, as was the **microscope** for examining minute structures of the **human body**. No wonder one nineteenth-century medical student wrote that "time was all too short and often we wished the twenty-four-hour day might be stretched to thirty-six" (Rosner, 1997, p. 154).

Some of the innovations brought their own risks, however. In 1861, **Ignaz Semmelweis**, working at the teaching facility of the Vienna General Hospital, attributed the high incidence of puerperal fever to the practice of medical students moving from anatomical theater to morgue to obstetrics ward without properly washing their hands. His research was later vindicated by the antiseptic principles of Joseph Lister (1827–1912), working at teaching hospitals first in Glasgow and then in Edinburgh. Modern **germ theory**, developed by **Louis Pasteur** and **Robert Koch** in the 1870s, provided for the first time a consistent, biologically based answer to the basic question of medical theory and practice: "What is the cause of disease?" It was rapidly adopted by medical schools, requiring sweeping revision of the curricula in pathology and clinical subjects. By the time of Abraham Flexner's (1866–1959) influential report, *Medical Education in the United States and Canada* (1911), the laboratory had taken its place beside the lecture hall, anatomical theater, and hospital as an essential component of medical education.

By 1900 the medical school curriculum encompassed more subjects than ever before. Medical education was also becoming more socially diverse. Middle-class women had been calling for access to the same medical education as their brothers since the mid-nineteenth century. The world-renowned Swiss universities began admitting women on an equal footing with men from the 1860s. The Écoles de Médécine in Paris followed suit in the 1870s, as did many of the German universities by 1910. In Great Britain and the United States, where universities were generally treated as private institutions, women had a harder time gaining admittance. In both countries, they founded their own institutions, such as the Women's Medical College of Philadelphia (1850) and the New Hospital for Women in London (1874). African American students in the United States faced similar obstacles and also founded their own institutions, such as Howard University in Washington, D.C., (1868). Full acceptance of diverse social groups into medical schools

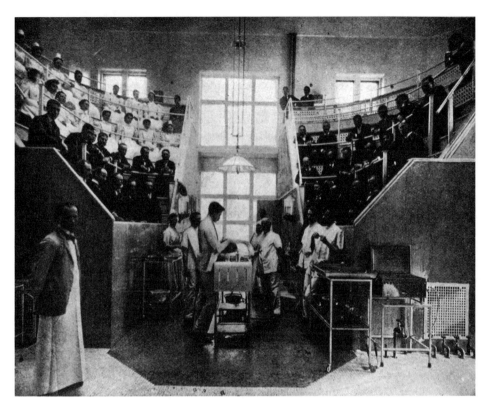

Operating theater at New York's Presbyterian Hospital, 1898. Interior view of an amphitheater with an operation in progress; medical students and/or physicians and nurses are observing the surgical procedure. Courtesy of the National Library of Medicine.

remained a contentious issue throughout the twentieth century. *See also* Astrology and Medicine; Contagion Theory of Disease, Premodern; Corpses and Epidemic Disease; Hospitals and Medical Education in Britain and the United States; Hospitals in the West to 1900; Humoral Theory; Medical Education in the West, 1100–1500; Plague and Developments in Public Health, 1348–1600.

Further Reading

Bonner, Thomas Neville. *Becoming a Physician: Medical Education in Britain, France, Germany, and the United States, 1750–1945*. Baltimore: Johns Hopkins University Press, 2000.

Ludmerer, Kenneth. *Learning to Heal: The Development of American Medical Education*. Baltimore: Johns Hopkins University Press, 1996.

Rosner, Lisa. "The Growth of Medical Education and the Medical Profession." In *Western Medicine: An Illustrated History*, edited by Irvine Loudon, pp. 147–159. New York: Oxford University Press, 1997.

LISA ROSNER

MEDICAL EDUCATION IN THE WEST, 1900–PRESENT.   *See* Hospitals and Medical Education in Britain and the United States.

MEDICAL ETHICS AND EPIDEMIC DISEASE.   Medical ethics consists of the ethical standards that medical professionals—doctors, nurses, public health professionals, and professionals in allied health-related fields—set for themselves to govern their conduct in their relations with each other, with patients, and with the public. These standards are usually stated in professional codes of medical ethics (see sidebar). They stipulate the professional's obligations to the public and patients with respect to care, confidentiality, dignity, protecting health, and preventing harm. They can also stipulate the extent to which health providers have a professional obligation to risk their lives or their health to treat patients afflicted by infectious disease.

Contagion Theory and Medical Ethics during Epidemics.   Discussions of the medical ethics in the context of pestilence were largely absent from the medical literature until the eighteenth century. They begin to surface in conjunction with the development of medical **contagion theory**, an idea attributed to the Veronese **physician Girolamo Fracastoro**, who published a book on the subject, *On Contagion and Contagious Diseases*, in 1546. Fracastoro explained the spread of pestilence in terms of "contagion," by which he meant transmission of diseases by minute particles in the atmosphere, on objects, and from person to person.

The introduction of contagion theory into the comparatively isolated environment of the British Isles in the early eighteenth century sheds light on why Fracastoro's theory generated medical ethical debate. Before this period, many considered doctors useless during outbreaks of **plague in Britain**. Thomas Dekker (c. 1570–1632), a well known seventeenth-century English pamphleteer, observed that during an outbreak of **bubonic plague** in London, in 1603, "our Phisitions [physicians] . . . hid their Synodicall heads . . . and I can not blame them, for their . . . drugs turned to dirt: . . . not one of them durst peepe abroad; and if anyone take upon him to play the venturous Knight, the Plague put him to his Nonplus [confounded him]." In his *Journal of the Plague Year* (1722) English novelist Daniel Defoe (1660–1731) offered a similarly bleak assessment of the efficacy of medicine during the **Great Plague of London** in 1665: "The plague defied all medicines; the very physicians were seized with it, with their preservatives in their mouths; and men went about prescribing to others and telling them what to do, 'till . . . they dropped down dead, destroyed by that very enemy they directed others to oppose."

Attitudes changed after 1720, when the English government commissioned Richard Mead (1673–1754), a fellow of the College of Physicians, to recommend a policy for preventing an outbreak of bubonic plague, then raging in and around Marseilles, France, from reaching British shores. Mead's report, *A Short Discourse Concerning Pestilential Contagion, and the Methods to Be Used to Prevent It* (1720), the first book of epidemiological advice produced by a medical practitioner at the request of a state, analyzed the risk of pestilence in terms of a medical theory of contagion. Heeding Mead's advice, Parliament passed several acts in 1720 and 1721, requiring the **quarantine** of ships and the **isolation** of towns suspected of infection by means of a *cordon sanitaire*. These acts were too great an imposition on the British sense of **personal liberties** and were quickly repealed.

This vignette illustrates how the medical theory of contagion changed the relationship between physicians and pestilence. The most important change was the higher regard in which doctors were held. Unlike the seventeenth-century physicians dismissed by Dekker and Defoe, contagion theory gave the eighteenth-century physician a role—prevention.

Meade became, in effect, England's first public health commissioner, advising the government regarding how best to protect the public from contagious disease. The change also meant that Meade and other physicians were in a position to dismiss as medically irrelevant some public reactions to pestilence—penance, flagellation, scapegoating, massacres—even as they validated other traditional practices, like isolation and quarantine, as properly scientific.

Public Health Ethics.   The new public health medicine embraced an ethical perspective that focused on the relationship between governmental institutions and the public. Conventional medical ethics, in contrast, had always focused on the relationship between the individual physician and the individual patient. One consequence of this difference is that, whereas conventional medical ethics can ignore politics, political considerations have infused public health medicine and ethics from their inception. Mead's recommendation of a *cordon sanitaire*, for example, whatever effects it may or may not have had in controlling a rat-borne disease transmitted by fleas, failed because the measure was unacceptable to the public. In another example of the fusion of politics with public health, Philadelphia physician, **Benjamin Rush**, a signatory to the American Declaration of Independence, preferred **environmental** (miasmatic) explanations of **yellow fever** to contagion theory in large measure because he believed that contagion theory would give governments too much power to control the lives of the governed. As the famous historian of medicine, Erwin Ackerknecht (1906–1988), observed, public health medicine has been politicized from the moment of its conception. It remains so today.

The Physician's Duty to Treat the Epidemic-Stricken.   Public health medicine shares common goals with conventional medicine: preventing disease, promoting health, and healing the sick. It also shares a common moral commitment of caring for the ill. Physicians in eighteenth-century England accepted an ethical "[d]uty to come when . . . call'd whether to Rich or Poor . . . to Distant Places as well as Near, to Prisons as well as Palaces . . . in a word, to all Mankind without Exception." The same author, however, wrote in 1715 that "'tis [physicians'] Duty to consult their own Safety first . . . to visit [only] where they have Reason to believe that their Presence may be of the utmost Consequence to the Recovery of others, and not extreamly or immediately Dangerous to themselves." Thus by offering a medical model for the spread of epidemics, contagion theory created an ethical expectation that physicians would provide medical care for the pestilence stricken, if they could do so at minimal risk to themselves.

Not surprisingly, since anti-contagionists (like Rush) believed that they faced minimal risk in providing medical care for the epidemic-stricken, they tended to provide a great deal of the medical care offered during epidemics. Rush, for example, became an exemplar of medical heroism because, while many other physicians fled, he remained in Philadelphia to tend yellow fever victims during the great epidemic of **yellow fever in North America** in 1793, which killed approximately 10 percent of the city's population. As the type of pestilence common in the nineteenth century shifted from bubonic plague to **cholera** and **typhoid**, there was a correlative decline in the risks to physicians and other caregivers. As the risks to caregivers declined, it became less acceptable for physicians to practice **flight** from epidemics, and staying to care for the epidemic stricken came to be viewed as almost obligatory. At mid-century the formal statement of medical ethics of the American Medical Association (AMA; 1847), stated that "When pestilence prevails, it is [members] duty to face the danger, and to continue their labors for the alleviation of the suffering, even at the jeopardy of their own lives."

A commitment to caring for the epidemic stricken remained integral to medical ethics through the mid-twentieth century, even during outbreaks of highly contagious diseases, like the **influenza pandemic of 1918–1919**. When it struck the United States, William Henry Welch (1850–1934), President of the AMA (1910–1911) and founding director of the Johns Hopkins School of Hygiene and Public Health, set the standard for the nation's doctors by personally taking the lead in providing day-to-day care for influenza patients. Through 1976 the AMA's code of ethics stipulated some version of the duty to tend to the epidemic stricken, even at risk of the physician's life.

When it revised its code of ethics in 1977, however, the AMA deleted the statement that physicians were obligated to risk their lives to treat the epidemic stricken. Thus, when the **AIDS** epidemic struck the United States in the 1980s, there was no authoritative professional ethical guidance on physicians' obligation to put themselves at risk to treat AIDS patients, and some physicians refused to provide care for HIV-positive patients. Responding to this situation, the AMA issued a point of clarification: "A physician may not ethically refuse to treat a patient whose condition is within the physician's realm of competence solely because the patient is seropositive."

The AMA's statement, however, only addressed care for HIV-positive patients. It left open the question of whether physicians were obligated to treat other epidemic-stricken patients. The American College of Physicians, however, stated a broader commitment of caring for the epidemic stricken—irrespective of risk to the caregiver: "It is unethical for a physician to refuse to see a patient solely because of medical risk, or perceived risk, to the physician."

Public Health Ethics, Conventional Medical Ethics, and Confidentiality. On certain issues, public health ethics and conventional medical ethics have differed. Confidentiality, the physician's duty to protect the secrecy of a patient's medical information, is the most prominent of these. For conventional physicians to practice medicine effectively, patients need to entrust them with sensitive personal information about their lifestyles and their symptoms. This trust is facilitated because physicians promise to maintain the confidentiality of the information that patients impart to them. Through 1903 the AMA "Principles of Medical Ethics" conventional practitioners promised patients, "secrecy [is] to be Inviolate," and "no infirmity . . . observed during medical attendance, should ever be divulged by physicians." In the case of infectious diseases, however, individual patients often seek to assert confidentiality where communal protection demands publicity. Thus, public health ethics stressed the need to make information about infectious diseases public in order to prevent the spread of contagious diseases, whereas conventional medical ethics tended to stress physicians' obligations to protect patient confidentiality.

Public health ethics and conventional medical ethics remained at odds on the need to protect patient confidentiality through most of the twentieth century. When the AIDS epidemic was recognized in the 1980s, however, their positions reversed. Seeking to maximize treatment of a heavily stigmatized disease, public health medicine tended to promise HIV-positive patients complete confidentiality. In contrast, the AMA, seeking to protect physicians' health, proclaimed in its "Principles of Medical Ethics" that, "exceptions to confidentiality are appropriate when necessary to protect the public health or . . . to protect . . . health-care workers, who are endangered by persons with HIV." The AMA also holds that "when a health care provider is at risk for HIV infection because of . . . contact with potentially infected bodily fluids, it is acceptable to test the patient for HIV infection even if the patient refuses consent" (1999).

The Ethics of Vaccination.   In 1721, when Richard Mead played the role of England's first public health commissioner, he not only dealt with the pestilential threat of the Plague of Marseilles but also with another pestilence: **smallpox**. Seeking to verify anecdotal evidence that **inoculation** with pus from smallpox pustules would confer **immunity**, Mead recruited Newgate prisoners to serve as research subjects. To reward their "voluntary" service, he arranged for the commutation of their sentences. When Mead had established that inoculation typically resulted in a mild immunity-conferring case of smallpox, he recommended the practice to Parliament and to the Royal Family (which dutifully followed his advice). This episode touches on two of the most ethically charged aspects of public health medicine: experimentation and **vaccination**. Vaccination requires intentionally subjecting someone to the risks associated with a vaccine in order to confer some level of immunity against a disease to which that person may, or may not, be exposed. Smallpox inoculation, for example, can result in a virulent or even fatal case of the disease itself. The point to appreciate is that, although not all vaccines are as risky as smallpox inoculations, they all entail some level of associated risk. Assessing the safety of vaccination (i.e., the levels of risk appropriate to the potential benefits of vaccination) has been controversial from Mead's day to the present.

Some individuals and families seek to minimize these risks by declining vaccination. This is a relatively safe option if 75 percent to 95 percent of the rest of the population has been vaccinated. Under these circumstances, the entire population is usually protected because of a phenomenon known as herd or community immunity. Those who decline vaccination thus have a "free ride," benefiting from the immunity conferred by the communal acceptance of the risks of vaccination without themselves undertaking any of those risks. However, free riders are at risk of contracting the disease if they become a sizeable percentage of the community. Should a large segment of the community join the "no vaccine bandwagon" and attempt to minimize their own risks by declining vaccination for themselves or their **children**, community immunity will weaken, and the unvaccinated portion of the community would be exposed to the disease. This happened in Ireland and the Netherlands in 1999–2000 when the level of communal immunity declined to well below the 95 percent internationally accepted level for controlling measles—falling to 72 percent in Ireland and to 63 percent in parts of Dublin. Reported cases of measles increased from a few hundred to 1,603 cases in Ireland and 3,292 cases in the Netherlands.

To insure that all members share the risks and benefits of vaccination fairly, some communities make vaccination mandatory for the entire population (e.g., as a condition of entering school). Mandating vaccination, however, raises issues about individuals' rights to refuse medical treatment and about the civil liberties of religious dissenters, such as Christian Scientists. Moreover, because most vaccines are administered to minor children, mandatory vaccination also raises questions about parental prerogatives to act on behalf of their minor children. Communities balance these interests in different ways. Some communities merely recommend vaccination. Some communities mandate vaccination but offer formal mechanisms for parents to decline vaccination for their minor children. Other communities consider parental refusals of vaccination for certain life-threatening diseases a form of child abuse.

The Ethics of Experimentation.   As the Mead smallpox vignette illustrates, medical innovations, including the development of new vaccines, require experimentation on **human subjects**. Many subjects have been willing volunteers. As early as 1900, for example, the

American military physician **Walter Reed** used consenting volunteers to conduct experiments to confirm Carlos Finlay's (1833–1915) hypothesis that mosquitoes transmitted yellow fever. Most people, however, are reluctant to serve as human subjects for vaccines against pestilential diseases. To deal with the anticipated difficulties of recruiting volunteers for experiments on these diseases, some researchers have experimented on people without their knowledge or their consent—at times claiming that the public's good outweighed the individual's rights. Ironically, these experiments have often served the public good, not as the researcher intended, but by provoking scandals that led to major reforms in research ethics.

Scandals associated with research on pestilential diseases have led to some of the most significant reforms in modern research ethics. In the early twentieth century, for example, Germany led the world in medical research on epidemic disease. In 1898 a scandal over the surreptitious inoculation of patients with an experimental vaccine against **syphilis** led to the world's first governmental prohibition of unconsented experiments on patients. In 1911 a scandal erupted over the involuntary internment of thousands of "natives" in German East Africa. Nobel Laureate **Robert Koch** and other physicians had imprisoned unconsenting natives in a camp to test an arsenic compound's efficacy in preventing **sleeping sickness**. The compound proved dangerous and ineffective. The researchers' internment of natives provoked a scandal, which, in turn, led to the first regulation protecting the rights and freedoms of colonial natives against scientific researchers.

Yet another scandal, the death of 72 children in the German city of Lübeck from **tuberculosis** as result of receiving an experimental BCG vaccine, led to the 1932 German Research Regulations. These regulations—at the time the most advanced in the world—required scientific validity, the informed voluntary consent of research subjects, prior animal experimentation, and a host of other protections for human subjects. A form of these regulations eventually found its way into international law because it became the basis of the Nuremberg Code of Research, which was formulated because of another scandal—the Nazi medical experiments that led to the 1947 Nuremberg War Crime Trials of German physicians and medical researchers. One of the accusations leveled at one trial involved research on an anti-**typhus** vaccine. Between 1942 and 1944, a German **pharmaceutical** company, *Behringwerke* AG, and the Robert Koch Institute in Berlin infected a population of 450 previously healthy concentration camp inmates with typhus to test the efficacy of experimental anti-typhus vaccines—leading to the deaths of one-third of them. The Nuremberg tribunal condemned the researchers who conducted these and other experiments, sentencing some to death and others to prison. In justifying their condemnation, the tribunal reformulated the 1932 German research ethics regulations as the Nuremberg Code of Research Ethics—making them part of international law. This code reiterated that the primary obligation of researchers was to obtain the informed voluntary consent of their subjects.

After the Second World War, the United States became the world leader in medical research. New scandals involving research on epidemic disease again generated new reforms. U.S. researchers had rejected the Nuremberg Code as "a good code of Nazis" but unnecessary for American researchers—until a headline scandal led to congressional hearings. The scandal was as follows: from 1932 to 1972, the U.S. Public Health Service had conducted a study of the natural evolution of syphilis in 399 African American men, the Tuskegee Syphilis Study, misinforming the subjects of their diagnosis, conducting

CODES OF MEDICAL ETHICS

Professions are self-regulating fields whose members are committed to using their specialized expertise in the service of some common good, such as providing health care. Until the nineteenth century, professions regulated themselves through oaths of induction like the ancient Greek Hippocratic Oath—the very word "profession" derives from the Latin term for having sworn (professed) an oath. In the nineteenth century, however, professional oaths were relegated to a ceremonial role, and the real standards governing professional conduct began to be set forth in professional codes of ethics. These codes were public statements of the specific obligations binding on everyone in a profession. Violations of professional codes of ethics can lead to censure or expulsion from professional bodies, termination of employment, and loss of licensure. Because courts typically recognize the authority of professional codes, the standards of professional conduct set out in these codes often have the force of law, and code violations can create legal liabilities, such as malpractice lawsuits.

Although professional standards for physicians get the most public attention, almost all the professionals involved in preparing for and responding to epidemics—from researchers and public health professionals, to paramedics and emergency medical technicians (EMTs), to physicians, nurses, and various allied health professionals—subscribe to formal codes of professional ethics. The National Association of Emergency Medical Technicians (NAEMT; founded in 1975), for example, has a code of ethics that commits EMTs to conserving life, alleviating suffering, promoting health, doing no harm, and encouraging the quality and equal availability of emergency medical care based on human need, with respect for human dignity, unrestricted by consideration of nationality, race, creed, color, or status. There is also an international code of nursing ethics, as well as codes from various national nursing associations. The American Public Health Association (APHA; 1872) has an elaborate code of ethics, as does the American Medical Association (AMA; 1847).

Professional standards for research on human subjects provide a good example of internationally recognized codes of professional ethics. The major research ethics codes were developed by two international professional organizations: the Council of International Organizations of Medical Science (CIOMS; founded in 1949 but issuing research ethics guidelines since 1982) of the **World Health Organization** (WHO), and the World Medical Association (WMA; founded in 1947 but issuing research ethics guidelines since 1964). Governmental and quasi-non-governmental agencies ("quangos," such as the Medical Research Council of Britain and the U.S. National Institutes of Health) and professional societies (such as the APHA) typically align their policies and regulations with these international standards. This creates, in effect, a worldwide set of professional standards for research involving human and animal subjects, recognized and enforced by the professions and their journals and by private, governmental, and quango funding agencies.

Robert Baker

lumbar punctures (spinal taps) without informed consent, and, in some cases, denying subjects access to potentially curative antibiotics. After these hearings, the U.S. government developed a common rule for ethical research on human subjects.

The U.S. government research regulations were justified initially, and are still justified today, by a set of three basic principles. These principles were articulated in the

1979 Belmont Report. The principle of respect for persons justifies regulations mandating the informed consent of the research subject (because failure to ask people to volunteer knowingly to become research subjects shows a fundamental disrespect for them as persons). The principle of beneficence requires that experiments produce more good than harm. The principle of justice requires a fair distribution between the benefits and burdens of research, so that the affluent and well-placed do not benefit inequitably from research burdens born disproportionately by the poor and disenfranchised. The World Medical Association (WMA) adopted similar standards with the Declaration of Helsinki (1975–2002) as did the Council of International Organizations of Medical Science (CIOMS) of the World Health Organization (WHO), which has also offered guidelines for ethical research since 1982. These three codes set national and international standards for ethical research on vaccines for AIDS, **Bird flu**, **Ebola**, **SARS**, and other modern pestilences. *See also* AIDS in Africa; AIDS in America; Animal Research; Capitalism and Epidemic Disease; Disease, Social Construction of; Geopolitics, International Relations, and Epidemic Disease; International Health Agencies and Conventions; Leprosy, Societal Reactions to; Mallon, Mary; Pest Houses and Lazarettos; Popular Media and Epidemic Disease: Recent Trends; Tuberculosis in the Contemporary World; War, the Military, and Epidemic Disease.

Further Reading

Baker, Robert. "Codes of Ethics: Some History." *Perspectives on the Professions* 19 (1999), http://ethics.iit.edu/perspective/pers19_1fall99_2.html

———. "Medical Ethics and Epidemics: A Historical Perspective." In *Ethics and Epidemics*, edited by John Balint, Sean Philpott, Robert Baker, and Martin Strosberg, pp. 93–134. Amsterdam: Elsevier, 2006.

Baker, Robert, Arthur Caplan, Linda Emanuel, and Stephen Latham, eds. *The American Medical Ethics Revolution: How the AMA's Code of Ethics Has Transformed Physicians' Relationships to Patients, Professionals, and Society.* Baltimore: Johns Hopkins University Press, 1999.

Bayer, Ronald, et al., eds. *Public Health Ethics: Theory, Policy, and Practice.* New York: Oxford University Press, 2006.

Beauchamp, Dan, and Bonnie Steinbock, eds. *New Ethics for the Public's Health.* New York: Oxford University Press, 1999.

Emanuel, Ezekiel, et al., eds. *Ethical and Regulatory Aspects of Clinical Research: Readings and Commentary.* Baltimore: Johns Hopkins University Press, 2003.

Grady, Christine. "Ethics of Vaccine Research." *Nature Immunology* 5 (2004): 465–468.

Grell, Ole Peter. "Conflicting Duties: Plague and the Obligations of Early Modern Physicians towards Patients and Commonwealth in England and The Netherlands." *Clio Medica* 24 (1993): 131–152.

Hazelgrove, Jenny. "The Old Faith and the New Science: The Nuremberg Code and Human Experimentation Ethics in Britain, 1946–73." *Social History of Medicine* 15 (2002): 109–136.

Roelcke, Volker, and Giovanni Maio, eds. *Twentieth-Century Ethics of Human Subjects Research: Historical Perspectives on Values, Practices, and Regulations.* Stuttgart: Franz Steiner Verlag, 2004.

Schneider, Winfried. *Medical Ethics in the Renaissance.* Washington, DC: Georgetown University Press, 1995.

Weindling, Paul. *Nazi Medicine and the Nuremberg Trials: From Medical War Crimes to Informed Consent.* New York: Palgrave Macmillan, 2004.

ROBERT BAKER

MENINGITIS.   Meningitis is an inflammation of the meninges, the membranes covering the brain and spinal cord, and may have first been described by medieval **physicians**. Symptoms can be **influenza**-like, with fever, headache, and nausea common, but, depending on the cause, they can be more severe and even fatal. Meningitis can be caused by a diverse range of agents including certain drugs and cancer, but it is most commonly caused by microorganisms. Most meningitis is caused by a group of **viruses** known as enteroviruses and is often mild, not requiring treatment. Fungi also commonly cause meningitis in immunocompromised individuals, for example **HIV/AIDS** patients. Bacterial meningitis, which is endemic in most countries, is much more severe, however. It can be a rapidly progressing, life-threatening infection that primarily affects the young and has been the focus of major public health control efforts and vaccine development programs.

Biological Agents.   **Bacteria** are the most clinically important and severe cause of meningitis, with just four species causing the majority of cases. *Neisseria meningitidis* (the meningococcus) causes large **epidemics** and even intercontinental pandemics; *Streptococcus pneumoniae* (the pneumococcus) is also a major cause of pneumonia; *Haemophilus influenzae*, of which serotype B causes almost all disease; and *Streptococcus agalactiae* (Group B Streptococcus or GBS) is the leading cause of meningitis in newborns.

Humans are the only known reservoir for these bacteria, which all commonly colonize the nose and throat without symptoms. GBS, which also colonizes the lower gastrointestinal tract and vagina, is transmitted from person to person by skin contact, whereas the other three species are transmitted in aerosolized respiratory droplets. **Transmission** is most efficient in closed or semi-closed communities, such as university campuses or military recruit camps, and is facilitated by factors that promote damage to the cellular lining of the nose and throat (including smoking), close contact among individuals (including overcrowded living conditions), and sharing of respiratory secretions (including coughing, sneezing, and kissing).

Importantly, disease is not part of the life cycles of these bacteria, but for largely unknown reasons, they occasionally cause systemic disease. This occurs when the bacteria invade the epithelial cells in the nose and throat and enter the bloodstream, before eventually entering the cerebrospinal fluid (the fluid between the meninges) *via* the meninges. A number of virulence factors, including polysaccharide capsules and outer membrane proteins, have been identified in each species. These also have normal roles in asymptomatic colonization including adhesion to host cells, modulation or diversion of the host immune response, and scavenging of host nutrients.

Symptoms, Morbidity, and Mortality.   Different bacterial causes of meningitis cannot be easily differentiated from one another based on symptoms alone. Early in infection symptoms can resemble influenza, making **diagnosis** difficult without further testing of blood or cerebrospinal fluid. Fever, nausea, headache, and dislike of strong lights and sounds are also common symptoms. All four species commonly cause other diseases as well as meningitis, including septicemia (blood poisoning) and ear infections. Without effective clinical management and **antibiotic** treatment, bacterial meningitis can be swift, resulting in toxic shock, major organ failure, and death. Mortality rates vary from approximately 2 to 6 percent with Hib, through 10 percent for meningococci and GBS, to 25 percent in pneumococci. Neurological side effects, including brain damage, hearing damage, and learning difficulties, are common because of the infection's location, in the central nervous system. Amputations are also often necessary because of the tissue-toxicity of bacterial surface molecules. Serious side effects in survivors are seen in approximately 20 percent of meningococcal cases, 30 percent of Hib cases, and up to 50 percent of pneumococcal and GBS cases.

Susceptibility to bacterial meningitis is strongly influenced by antibody levels, especially against the polysaccharide capsules as demonstrated by **epidemiology** studies, and a higher risk of disease exists in people with genetic antibody deficiencies. Protective antibody levels arise from passage of maternal antibody across the placenta, asymptomatic carriage of the bacteria, or antigenically cross-reactive species and **vaccination**. Genetic mutations in the host are important in determining susceptibility to all species and are thought to contribute a third of the risk of meningococcal disease.

There is very little social stigma attached to meningitis sufferers because asymptomatic bacterial carriage is common, transmission easy, and disease rare. Nevertheless, meningitis is often seen in the headlines of the regional or national press and has a huge impact on public consciousness, affecting the young, appearing at random, killing rapidly, and leaving survivors with terrible side effects.

Epidemiology.   The global disease rate of bacterial meningitis was approximately 171,000 deaths per year at the turn of the twenty-first century, with the meningococcus, the pneumococcus, and Hib accounting for over 90 percent of childhood bacterial meningitis. Although carriage of all four species occurs throughout the year, disease (apart from GBS) is seasonal, with the majority of cases occurring in winter and spring in temperate regions when the rate of respiratory infections is higher.

Meningococci are carried in around 10 percent of the general population and in up to 40 percent of 15–24 year olds. They can be classified into 13 "serogroups" based on antigenic differences in their capsular polysaccharide, with 5 serogroups being responsible for more than 90 percent of disease. There are also many genetic groups of meningococci which exchange capsular types easily, but around 10 "hyperinvasive lineages" cause the majority of disease. Two disease peaks exist, the first in infants and the second in young adults, the latter thought to be caused predominantly by the increased carriage rate in this age group. Developed countries have an endemic meningococcal disease rate of 1 to 5 per 100,000 population but this is much higher in the developing world. The "Meningitis Belt" of Sub-Saharan Africa is a region with hyper-endemic levels of meningococcal disease and where large-scale epidemics occur approximately every 10 to 14 years. The worst epidemic of the twentieth century occurred in 1996, with a quarter of a million cases and 25,000 deaths. Here, the disease also displays an altered seasonality, peaking in the dry season when the dusty conditions and crowding during the cold nights exacerbate damage to the cellular lining of the nose and throat and increase transmission. The immune status of the host population is a highly important determining factor in the development of epidemics. For example, population genetic data following a 1993 epidemic in the Czech Republic showed that antigenically related meningococci had not been seen there in the three previous decades.

Pneumococci are more likely to cause pneumonia and inner ear infections than meningitis. Carriage rates vary by age, and the duration of carriage is longer in children. Virulent strains belong to 90 serotypes, based on antigenic differences in the polysaccharide capsule, and approximately 60 percent of disease is caused by just 10 serotypes. In the United States before 2000, there were approximately 60,000 annual cases of invasive pneumococcal disease and 3,300 of pneumococcal meningitis. These numbers have since fallen with the introduction of new vaccines.

Hib disease occurs worldwide, but has highest incidence in the developing world. Before Hib vaccines became available in the 1980s and 1990s, it was the leading cause of invasive bacterial disease and meningitis in children under five years of age, with 40 to 100 annual cases per 100,000 population in the United States. Carriage of Hib is low, at 0.5 to 3 percent of healthy infants and children.

GBS is carried in approximately 40 percent of pregnant women and, since the 1970s, has replaced *Escherichia coli* as the leading cause of meningitis in newborns. The disease incidence is approximately 3 in 1,000 live births, striking before or just after birth (early onset disease) or, twice as frequently, in the first few months of life (late onset disease). There is a higher risk of disease in premature babies, in prolonged labor, or when the mother is infected. There are six immunologically distinct serotypes based on the capsular polysaccharide and surface proteins, and 60 percent of infants born to colonized mothers will be colonized with the mother's serotype.

History of Research on and Control of Meningitis.   Along with the descriptions by medieval Arab physicians, including Avenzoar of al-Andalus (Spain; 1091–1161) in the twelfth century, reports of "spotted fevers" go back to antiquity. It was not until the nineteenth century, though, that medical science started to understand and treat bacterial meningitis.

Meningococcal disease was first described by the Swiss physician Gaspard Vieusseux (1746–1814) in 1805 during an outbreak in Geneva, and the bacterium was first isolated by the Austrian pathologist Anton Weichselbaum (1845–1920) in 1887 in Vienna, who named it Diplococcus intracellularis meningitidis. *S. pneumoniae* was originally isolated by **Louis Pasteur** and pioneer American bacteriologist George Sternberg (1838–1915) independently in 1881, and the importance of the capsular polysaccharides for virulence was described in the early twentieth century. Richard Pfeiffer (1858–1945), German physician, first identified *H. influenzae* in 1892 during the **influenza pandemic** of that year. This led to *H. influenzae* being mistakenly proposed as the cause of influenza, and it was not until the 1930s, when the influenza virus was first isolated, that the bacterium was found to be a major cause of secondary infection. In the same decade the different capsular serotypes were identified, and it was found that the majority of disease was caused by serotype B (Hib).

GBS was originally known as *Streptococcus mastitidis* after it was identified as a cause of bovine mastitis (swelling of the mammary glands in cows) and was first isolated in 1887 by French veterinarian Edmond Nocard (1850–1903) (with a Charenton veterinarian named Mollereau). It was first identified in vaginal cultures by Rebecca Craighill Lancefield (1895–1981) and colleagues, who also classified the Streptococcus genus into groups, though it was only reported as a human pathogen by R. M. Fry in 1938. Antibiotics now play a major role in the control of this pathogen, but vaccines are being developed.

The first bacterial meningitis vaccines based on the polysaccharide capsules of meningococci, pneumococci, and Hib were introduced in the 1970s and 1980s. These were not effective in protecting infants and, since the 1990s, have been surpassed by a new generation of vaccines in which the capsular polysaccharides are conjugated (chemically linked) to immunity-boosting proteins. These have often been administered in population-scale vaccination campaigns and in infant immunization schedules, with significant impacts on disease, notably the 99 percent reduction in Hib disease to now negligible levels in the developed world. Pneumococcal vaccines are also effective and continue to change to keep pace with the disease prevalence of different serotypes. Conjugate meningococcal vaccines against serogroups A, C, Y, and W-135 are in development, but serogroup B vaccines have so far eluded science as a result of the similarity of the serogroup B polysaccharide to molecules on human cells. To combat this, as in other diseases, a number of vaccines are being developed based on outer membrane proteins on the bacterial surface. Furthermore, as for many other infectious diseases, reverse vaccinology (genome-based vaccine design) is also yielding new vaccine candidates against bacterial meningitis.

As we enter the twenty-first century, effective antibiotics and/or vaccines are available against all four of the major bacterial causes of meningitis. However, antibiotic resistance is known in all four species, and the often high cost of vaccines has prevented their use in the developing world, where much of the disease burden lies. New genomic data and knowledge of the bacterial population structures is providing novel vaccine development strategies, which are complemented by growing global experience of how to deploy them most effectively. The effectiveness of diagnosis and early detection of symptoms continues to benefit from increased awareness campaigns, improved clinical management programs, and the use of modern molecular diagnostic tests. In the developing world, global coordination of public health and economic efforts aim to provide more funds for meningitis vaccines, though there is significant competition for funding from other serious diseases including HIV/AIDS. For now, however, bacterial meningitis is very much still with us. *See also* Children and Childhood Diseases.

Further Reading

Centers for Disease Control and Prevention. *Meningococcal Disease*. http://www.cdc.gov/ncidod/dbmd/diseaseinfo/meningococcal_g.htm

Goldsmith, Connie. *Meningitis*. Brookfield, CT: Twenty-First Century Books, 2007.

ICON Health Publications. *Bacterial Meningitis: A Medical Dictionary, Bibliography, and Annotated Research Guide to Internet References*. San Diego: ICON Group International, Inc., 2004.

Mayo Clinic. *Meningitis*. http://www.mayoclinic.com/health/meningitis/DS00118

Meningitis Foundation of America. http://www.meningitisfoundationofamerica.org

Rappuoli R. "Bridging the Knowledge Gaps in Vaccine Design." *Nature Biotechnology* 25 (2007): 361–66.

Segal, Shelley, and Pollard Andrew. "Vaccines against Bacterial Meningitis." *British Medical Bulletin* 31 (2005): 65–81.

World Health Organization. *Meningitis*. http://www.who.int/topics/meningitis/en/

MARTIN CALLAGHAN

MIASMA THEORY.   *See* Air and Epidemic Diseases.

MICROSCOPE.   Archeologists have discovered magnifying lenses dating back thousands of years, but they were used for decorative, not scientific, purposes. In the early 1600s, the microscope's design evolved from the telescope, with lenses contained in a vertically mounted tube and an adjustable mirror to reflect light. The rays of light and magnifying lenses enable the observation of small objects, and thus these microscopes are called light microscopes. The microscope made its first appearance in compound form (two lenses), used most often today, near the end of the sixteenth century.

By the 1620s, microscopes began appearing in European cities, and in 1665, English scientist Robert Hooke (1635–1703) published his pioneering book *Micrographia*. It contained extremely detailed illustrations of a huge variety of microorganisms, seen through a compound microscope that magnified about 30 to 50 times. After wondering how cork, which looked solid, could be so soft, he observed it under his microscope, and was the first to use the word "cell" to describe the small air-filled chambers he consequently saw.

Hooke was a likely influence on Dutch microscopist **Antony van Leeuwenhoek**. Using a single-lens microscope that he ground himself and which magnified up to 275 times, Leeuwenhoek made the first discovery of what are now known to be **bacteria**, along with other single-celled organisms including **protozoa**. Protozoan diseases include **sleeping sickness** and **malaria**. With the aid of the more complex microscopes that became available in the 1840s, bacteriologists **Louis Pasteur**, in France, and **Robert Koch**, in Germany, discovered the role that bacteria played in disease. Koch was one of several scientists who discovered the importance of dying techniques, which made viewing of the organisms easier.

The invention of the oil immersion lens allowed for even higher magnifications, as it allowed for oil to be placed between the organism and lens, so as to reduce the bending of light. With this high magnification, individual bacteria were able to be seen. Bacteria can be seen to have different shapes, including spherical, rod-like, or spiral, and their shape is an important way to identify them. Examples of bacterial diseases include **bubonic plague, cholera, diphtheria, leprosy, typhoid fever**, and **whooping cough**.

In the 1930s, the electron microscope was developed. The electron microscope uses a stream of electrons to coat the object, and a "picture" of the outside of the organism is then made. One disadvantage to using an electron microscope is that it kills the organism being viewed. With an electron microscope, **viruses**, submicroscopic in size, were able to be seen for the first time. Viral diseases include **measles**, rubeola, rubella, **smallpox, poliomyelitis, influenza**, and **AIDS**. The electron microscope has also provided images of all other microorganisms of unprecedented clarity and detail, revolutionizing the understanding of cellular biology. *See also* Diagnosis and Diagnostic Tools.

Further Reading

Fournier, Marian. *The Fabric of Life: Microscopy in the Seventeenth Century*. Baltimore: Johns Hopkins University Press, 1996.

Rasmussen, Nicolas. *Picture Control: The Electron Microscope and the Transformation of Biology in America, 1940–1960*, new first edition. Stanford: Stanford University Press, 1999.

Ruestow, Edward G. *The Microscope in the Dutch Republic: The Shaping of Discovery*. New York: Cambridge University Press, 1996.

Wilson, Catherine. *The Invisible World: Early Modern Philosophy and the Invention of the Microscope*. Princeton, NJ: Princeton University Press, 1995.

MARTHA STONE

MILITARY.   *See* War, the Military, and Epidemic Disease.